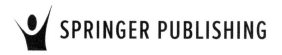 **SPRINGER PUBLISHING**

MW01200979

GET THE MOST FROM YOUR BOOK

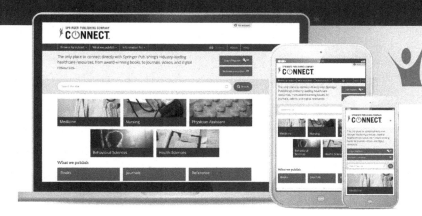

SPRINGER PUBLISHING
CONNECT™

VOUCHER CODE:

S07R85YD

Online Access

Your print purchase of *The Psychological and Social Impact of Chronic Illness and Disability, Eighth Edition*, includes **online access via Springer Publishing Connect™** to increase accessibility, portability, and searchability.

Insert the code at http://connect.springerpub.com/content/book/978-0-8261-5111-7 or scan the QR code and insert the voucher code today!

Having trouble? Contact our customer service department at cs@springerpub.com

Instructor Resource Access for Adopters

Let us do some of the heavy lifting to create an engaging classroom experience with a variety of instructor resources included in most textbooks SUCH AS:

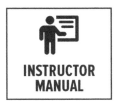

INSTRUCTOR MANUAL

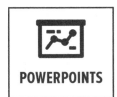

POWERPOINTS

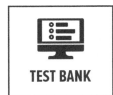

TEST BANK

Visit **https://connect.springerpub.com/** and look for the **"Show Supplementary"** button on your **book homepage** to see what is available to instructors! First time using Springer Publishing Connect?

Email **textbook@springerpub.com** to create an account and start unlocking valuable resources.

THE PSYCHOLOGICAL AND SOCIAL IMPACT OF CHRONIC ILLNESS AND DISABILITY

Irmo Marini, PhD, DSc, CRC, CLCP, is professor in the School of Rehabilitation at the University of Texas–Rio Grande Valley in Edinburg, Texas. He obtained his PhD in rehabilitation from Auburn University and a master's degree in clinical psychology from Lakehead University in Thunder Bay, Ontario, Canada. He is a 2009 recipient of the National Council on Rehabilitation Education's Distinguished Career Award in rehabilitation education and 2010 recipient of the American Rehabilitation Counseling Association's James F. Garrett Distinguished Career Award in rehabilitation research. In 2012, Dr. Marini was bestowed an honorary Doctor of Science (honoris causa) from his alma mater Lakehead University and was the recipient of the 2013 National Council on Rehabilitation Education's Educator of the Year award. In 2015, he was the recipient of the Patricia McCollom Distinguished Career Award in life care planning research, and in 2022 the Outstanding Educator of the Year Award with the International Academy of Life Care Planners. He is the coauthor and coeditor of seven books, 62 book chapters, and 97 refereed journal publications. He is the former chair of the Commission on Rehabilitation Counselor Certification and former president of the American Rehabilitation Counseling Association.

Allison R. Fleming, PhD, CRC, is associate professor in the Counseling, Educational Psychology, and Special Education Department at The Pennsylvania State University. She obtained her PhD in rehabilitation counselor education from Michigan State University and her master's degree in rehabilitation counseling from Springfield College in Western Massachusetts. She worked as a vocational rehabilitation (VR) counselor for the Massachusetts Rehabilitation Commission and for the Institute for Community Inclusion, providing continuing education for community rehabilitation providers and VR counselors prior to studying at Michigan State. Dr. Fleming conducts research in the areas of employment, quality of life, transition, and rehabilitation outcomes. She directs an inclusive postsecondary transition program for students with intellectual and developmental disabilities at Penn State. Dr. Fleming has authored 42 peer-reviewed publications, 10 book chapters, and co-edited two books. She has served on the CRCC Standards and Exam Committee and is past president of the National Council for Rehabilitation Education.

Malachy Bishop, PhD, CRC, is the Norman L. and Barbara M. Berven Professor of Rehabilitation Psychology in the Rehabilitation Psychology and Special Education Department at the University of Wisconsin–Madison. Previously, he served as professor and doctoral program coordinator in the rehabilitation counseling program at the University of Kentucky and as director of research for the University of Kentucky's University Center for Excellence in Developmental Disabilities, the Interdisciplinary Human Development Institute. He obtained his PhD in rehabilitation psychology from the University of Wisconsin–Madison and his master's degree in rehabilitation counseling from Portland State University. Dr. Bishop conducts research in employment and psychosocial aspects of chronic neurological conditions and the application of quality-of-life research to adaptation to chronic illness and disability. He was an appointed member of the Institute of Medicine Committee on Public Health Dimensions of the Epilepsies. Dr. Bishop has authored over 125 articles in professional journals, 30 book chapters in rehabilitation and healthcare, and co-edited six books. He was the 2020 recipient of the American Rehabilitation Counseling Association James F. Garrett Distinguished Career in Rehabilitation Research Award and the 2015 recipient of the George N. Wright Varsity Award.

THE PSYCHOLOGICAL AND SOCIAL IMPACT OF CHRONIC ILLNESS AND DISABILITY

EIGHTH EDITION

Irmo Marini, PhD, DSc, CRC, CLCP

Allison R. Fleming, PhD, CRC

Malachy Bishop, PhD, CRC

EDITORS

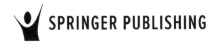 SPRINGER PUBLISHING

Springer Publishing Company, LLC
www.springerpub.com
connect.springerpub.com

Acquisitions Editor: Mindy Okura-Marszycki
Production Editor: Dennis Troutman
Compositor: Pajeflow

ISBN: 978-0-8261-5112-4
ebook ISBN: 978-0-8261-5111-7
DOI: 10.1891/9780826151117

SUPPLEMENTS:

 A robust set of instructor resources designed to supplement this text is located at **http://connect.springerpub.com/content/book/978-0-8261-5111-7**. Qualifying instructors may request access by emailing **textbook@springerpub.com**.

Instructor Materials:
LMS Common Cartridge: 978-0-8261-5112-5
Instructor Manual: 978-0-8261-5114-8
Test Banks: 978-0-8261-5115-5
Instructor Chapter PowerPoints: 978-0-8261-5116-2

23 24 25 26 / 5 4 3 2 1

The author and the publisher of this Work have made every effort to use sources believed to be reliable to provide information that is accurate and compatible with the standards generally accepted at the time of publication. Because medical science is continually advancing, our knowledge base continues to expand. Therefore, as new information becomes available, changes in procedures become necessary. We recommend that the reader always consult current research and specific institutional policies before performing any clinical procedure or delivering any medication. The author and publisher shall not be liable for any special, consequential, or exemplary damages resulting, in whole or in part, from the readers' use of, or reliance on, the information contained in this book. The publisher has no responsibility for the persistence or accuracy of URLs for external or third-party Internet websites referred to in this publication and does not guarantee that any content on such websites is, or will remain, accurate or appropriate.

Library of Congress Cataloging-in-Publication Data

Names: Marini, Irmo, author. | Fleming, Allison R., author. | Bishop,
    Malachy, author.
Title: The psychological and social impact of chronic illness and
    disability / Irmo Marini, PhD, DSc, CRC, CLCP, Allison R. Fleming, PhD,
    CRC, Malachy Bishop, PhD, CRC.
Description: Eighth edition. | New York, NY : Springer Publishing Company,
    LLC, [2024] | Includes bibliographical references and index.
Identifiers: LCCN 2023026648 (print) | LCCN 2023026649 (ebook) | ISBN
    9780826151124 (paperback) | ISBN 9780826151117 (ebook)
Subjects: LCSH: People with disabilities—United States—Psychology. |
    People with disabilities--Rehabilitation—United States. | People with
    disabilities—Family relationships—United States. | People with
    disabilities—Sexual behavior—United States. | People with
    disabilities—United States—Public opinion. | Public opinion—United States.
Classification: LCC HV1553 .P75 2024 (print) | LCC HV1553 (ebook) | DDC
    362.4—dc23/eng/20230703
LC record available at https://lccn.loc.gov/2023026648
LC ebook record available at https://lccn.loc.gov/2023026649

Contact sales@springerpub.com to receive discount rates on bulk purchases.

Publisher's Note: **New and used products purchased from third-party sellers are not guaranteed for quality, authenticity, or access to any included digital components.**

Printed in the United States of America by Hatteras, Inc.

This is my last book that I am dedicating solely to my wife Darlene, who I dated prior to my accident, married, and just celebrated our 40th anniversary with. You have saved me in more ways than you will ever know with your unconditional love, compassion, patience, and selflessness. I would not have ever accomplished nearly this much if you were not by my side the entire journey. You allowed me to lock myself up in my office bubble while you ran the entire household, leaving me to pursue my passions. There are no words that can accurately convey my love and gratitude I have for sharing the best part of my life with you. Thank you for loving me and not ever giving up on your optimism in knowing that we could survive that terrible day in 1981 that changed our lives. Everyone we've ever known can clearly see that we thrived and did not succumb.

—Irmo

I dedicate this book to my family, "the J's"—I love and appreciate our life together. Also, in memory of my dad, who always told me I could do anything I wanted. I wish you could have been here to see where I ended up.

—Allison

I dedicate this book to the rehabilitation educators and students with whom it has been my privilege and honor to work and to Art Dell Orto and Robert Marinelli. Thank you to my extraordinary wife, Lisa, for our extraordinary life.

—Malachy

CONTENTS

Contributors   xi
Foreword   xv
Preface   xvii
Acknowledgments   xix
Springer Publishing Connect™ Resources   xxi

PART I: HISTORICAL AND CULTURAL PERSPECTIVES ON ILLNESS AND DISABILITY

1. History of Treatment Toward Persons With Disabilities in America and Abroad   5
   Danielle D. Fox and Irmo Marini

2. Societal Attitudes and Myths About Disability: Improving the Social Consciousness   17
   Irmo Marini

3. History of Treatment Toward Persons With Psychiatric Disabilities   37
   Kim L. Nguyen-Finn

4. Disability Identity and Disability Culture   55
   Carlyn Mueller, Erin E. Andrews, and Bradley J. Minotti

5. Recognizing, Understanding, and Constructively Responding to Ableism   69
   Dana S. Dunn

6. The Evolution of Laws and Policies in the United States and Their Impact on Disabled People   85
   Allison R. Fleming, Sarah M. Roundtree, and K. Lynn Pierce

PART II: THE PERSONAL IMPACT OF DISABILITY

7. Psychosocial Adaptation to Chronic Illness and Disability: A Primer for Counselors   105
   Malachy Bishop, Sara Park, Hanoch Livneh, and Phillip Rumrill

8. Theories of Adjustment and Adaptation to Disability   123
   Irmo Marini and Laura A. Villarreal

9. Vulnerabilities, Abuse, and Psychosocial Disparities of Women With Disabilities   147
    Debra A. Harley and Carol E. Jordan

10. Sexuality and Disability   169
    Noreen M. Graf and Rory L. Glover

11. Ableist Microaggressions   197
    Deniz Aydemir-Döke

12. Quality of Life and Psychosocial Adaptation to Chronic Illness and Disability   215
    Malachy Bishop, Yunzhen (Judy) Huang, Kaiqi Zhou, and Megan Baumunk

PART III: FAMILY ISSUES IN ILLNESS AND DISABILITY

13. Family Adaptation Across Cultures Toward Loved Ones With Disability   235
    Noreen M. Graf and Jacqueline Mercado Lopez

14. Giving Parents a Voice: Challenges Experienced by Parents
    of Children With Disabilities   257
    Kathy Sheppard-Jones, Stephanie Meredith, and Constance Richard

15. Psychosocial Counseling Aspects of Grief, Dying, and Death   275
    Mark A. Stebnicki

16. Psychosocial Issues for Family Caregivers   291
    Gloria K. Lee, Eun-Jeong Lee, Kristin M. Rispoli, and Trisha L. Easley

PART IV: SPECIFIC TRAUMA AND STIGMATIZED POPULATIONS

17. Living With Substance Use Disorder: From Stigma to Recovery   311
    Mykal Leslie and Stuart Rumrill

18. Culturally Competent Service Provision: Considerations for Supporting
    Veterans and Family Reintegration   339
    Kellie Forziat-Pytel and Christina Dillahunt-Aspillaga

19. Responding Well to Individuals Experiencing Abuse and Relationship Violence   351
    J. Ruth Nelson

20. Immigrants, Refugees, and Asylum Seekers:
    The Psychosocial Cost of War on Civilians   365
    Mark A. Stebnicki

21. Key Concepts and Techniques for an Aging Population of Persons With Disabilities   *381*
Eva Miller and Susanne M. Bruyère

PART V: NEW DIRECTIONS, ISSUES, AND PERSPECTIVES

22. Interventions to Improve the Well-Being of People With Disabilities and Chronic Illness   *401*
Allison R. Fleming, Emre Umucu, and Brian N. Phillips

23. Users of Assistive Technology: The Human Component   *417*
Hung Jen Kou, Annemarie Connor, and Michael Yeomans

24. Religion and Disability   *435*
Bryan O. Gere, Nahal Salimi, Roy K. Chen, and Uzoamaka Okori

25. Social Justice, Oppression, and Disability Counseling   *451*
Irmo Marini, Kerra LaJoy Daniel, Uzoamaka Okori, and Tori Livingston

26. The Impact of Social Media Influence on Mental Health   *471*
Rigel Macarena Piñón and Kerra LaJoy Daniel

27. Reflections and Considerations   *483*
Irmo Marini, Allison R. Fleming, and Malachy Bishop

PART VI: PERSONAL PERSPECTIVES

My Experience as a Deaf Woman   *493*
Cassandra Cantu

Fires Are Not Drills   *494*
Donelle Henderlong

My Story of Becoming Blind   *497*
Macarena Pena

Multiple Sclerosis: Not Just Surviving but Thriving   *501*
Jessica Henry

Chris and His Mother: Hope and Home   *503*
Chris Moy

Karen—My Daughter Forever   *508*
Linda Stacey

Living in Spite of Multiple Sclerosis   *510*
Tosca Appel

Surviving Amyotrophic Lateral Sclerosis: A Daughter's Perspective   *513*
Judy Teplow

My Life With a Disability: Continued Opportunities   *517*
Paul Egan

Experiencing Sexuality as an Adolescent With Rheumatoid Arthritis   *519*
Robert J. Neumann

My Life With Muscular Dystrophy: Lessons and Opportunities   *524*
Robert P. Winske

Life Lessons Taught to Me by My Disability   *529*
Alfred H. DeGraff

Index   *535*

CONTRIBUTORS

Erin E. Andrews, PsyD, ABPP, Rehabilitation Psychologist, VA Texas Valley Coastal Bend Health Care System, University of Texas at Austin Dell Medical School, Harlingen, Texas

Tosca Appel, MS, Newton, Massachusetts

Deniz Aydemir-Döke, PhD, Assistant Professor, The Pennsylvania State University, State College, Pennsylvania

Megan Baumunk, MS, CRC, LPC-IT, PhD Student, University of Wisconsin–Madison, Madison, Wisconsin

Malachy Bishop, PhD, CRC, Professor of Rehabilitation Psychology, Rehabilitation Psychology and Special Education Department, University of Wisconsin–Madison, Madison, Wisconsin

Susanne M. Bruyère, PhD, CRC, Academic Director and Professor Disability Studies, Yang-Tan Institute on Employment and Disability, ILR School, Cornell University, Ithaca, New York

Cassandra Cantu, Student, University of Texas–Rio Grande Valley, Edinburg, Texas

Roy K. Chen, PhD, Professor, University of Texas–Rio Grande Valley, Edinburg, Texas

Annemarie Connor, PhD, Professor, Department of Rehabilitation Sciences, Florida Gulf Coast University, Fort Myers, Florida

Kerra LaJoy Daniel, CRC, PhD, Compliance Officer, Department of Labor, Kansas City, Missouri

Alfred H. DeGraff, EdD, Fort Collins, Colorado

Christina Dillahunt-Aspillaga, PhD, CRC, CVE, CLCP, IPEC, ICVE(D), CBIST, FACRM, Professor, University of South Florida, Tampa, Florida

Dana S. Dunn, PhD, Professor and Chair of Psychology, Moravian University, Bethlehem, Pennsylvania

Trisha L. Easley, MA, CRC, LLPC, Doctoral Candidate, Michigan State University, East Lansing, Michigan

Paul Egan, MS, Dracut, Massachusetts

Allison Fleming, PhD, CRC, Associate Professor, Counseling, Educational Psychology and Special Education Department, The Pennsylvania State University, State College, Pennsylvania

Kellie Forziat-Pytel, PhD, LPC-PA, NCC, ACS, Assistant Professor, Commonwealth University of Pennsylvania, Lock Haven, Lock Haven, Pennsylvania

Danielle D. Fox, PhD, CRC, NCC, NBC-HWC, Integrative Wellness Specialist, University of Texas–Rio Grande Valley, Edinburg, Texas

Bryan O. Gere, PhD, CRC, Associate Professor and Graduate Program Director, University of Maryland Eastern Shore, Princess Anne, Maryland

Rory L. Glover, MSW, Doctoral Student, Tulane University, New Orleans, Louisiana

Noreen M. Graf, PhD, CRC, Professor, School of Rehabilitation, University of Texas–Rio Grande Valley, Edinburg, Texas

Debra A. Harley, PhD, Professor, University of Kentucky, Lexington, Kentucky

Donelle Henderlong, MA, Disability Consultant, The Gregory S. Fehribach Center at Eskenazi Health, Indianapolis, Indiana

Jessica Henry, PhD, CRC, LPC, Associate Teaching Professor, The Pennsylvania State University, State College, Pennsylvania

Yunzhen (Judy) Huang, PhD, CRC, Assistant Professor, California State University–Los Angeles, Los Angeles, California

Carol E. Jordan, MS, Executive Director, Office for Policy Studies on Violence Against Women, University of Kentucky, Lexington, Kentucky

Hung Jen Kou, PhD, CRC, LPC, Assistant Professor, Michigan State University, East Lansing, Michigan

Eun-Jeong Lee, PhD, CRC, LCPC, Professor, Illinois Institute of Technology, Chicago, Illinois

Gloria K. Lee, PhD, CRC, Professor, Department of Counseling, Educational Psychology, and Special Education, Michigan State University, East Lansing, Michigan

Mykal Leslie, PhD, CRC, LPCC-S, Assistant Professor, Kent State University, Kent, Ohio

Tori Livingston, PhD candidate, LPC-A, LCDC-I, Research/Teacher Assistant, University of Texas—Rio Grande Valley, Edinburg, Texas

Hanoch Livneh, PhD, CRC, Professor Emeritus, Portland State University, Portland, Oregon

Jacqueline Mercado Lopez, MS, Research Assistant, School Of Rehabilitation Services and Counseling, University of Texas—Rio Grande Valley, Edinburg, Texas

Irmo Marini, PhD, DSc, CRC, CLCP, Professor, School of Rehabilitation, University of Texas—Rio Grande Valley, Edinburgh, Texas

Stephanie Meredith, MA, Director, National Center for Prenatal and Postnatal Resource and LEND Family Faculty, Human Development Institute, University of Kentucky, Lexington, Kentucky

Eva Miller, PhD, CRC, Professor and Licensed Psychologist, University of Texas—Rio Grande Valley, Edinburg, Texas

Bradley J. Minotti, MEd, PhD Student, School Psychology, University of Florida, Gainesville, Florida

Chris Moy, MS, Scranton, Pennsylvania

Carlyn Mueller, PhD, Assistant Professor of Special Education, University of Wisconsin–Madison, Madison, Wisconsin

J. Ruth Nelson, PhD, NCSP, LSP, Professor, Bethel University, St. Paul, Minnesota

Robert J. Neumann, Chicago, Illinois

Kim L. Nguyen-Finn, PhD, LPC-S, Lecturer II, Coordinator Expressive Arts Program, School of Rehabilitation, University of Texas—Rio Grande Valley, Edinburg, Texas

Uzoamaka Okori, MA, Research Assistant, University of Texas—Rio Grande Valley, Edinburg, Texas

Sara Park, MS, CRC, LPC-IT, Doctoral Student, University of Wisconsin–Madison, Madison, Wisconsin

Brian N. Phillips, PhD, CRC, Associate Professor, Utah State University, Logan, Utah

K. Lynn Pierce, PhD, CRC, LPC, Assistant Professor Counselor Education and Supervision PhD Program Coordinator, Mercer University, Macon, Georgia

Macarena Pena, Caseworker, Texas Workforce Solutions Vocational Rehabilitation Services, North Richland Hills, Texas

Rigel Macarena Piñón, PhD, CRC, Forensic Vocational Consultant, Marini and Associates, McAllen, Texas

Constance Richard, MS, CRC, Instructor, Rehabilitation Psychology and Special Education, University of Wisconsin–Madison, Madison, Wisconsin

Kristin M. Rispoli, PhD, NCSP, Associate Professor, Michigan State University, East Lansing, Michigan

Sarah M. Roundtree, MS, CRC, Doctoral Student, The Pennsylvania State University, State College, Pennsylvania

Phillip Rumrill, PhD, CRC, Professor and Director of Research, Human Development Institute, University of Kentucky, Lexington, Kentucky

Stuart Rumrill, PhD, CRC, Postdoctoral Research Associate, University of Illinois at Urbana-Champaign, Champaign, Illinois

Nahal Salimi, PhD, Assistant Professor, Northern Illinois University, DeKalb, Illinois

Kathy Sheppard-Jones, PhD, CRC, Executive Director, Human Development Institute, University of Kentucky, Lexington, Kentucky

Linda Stacey, Framingham, Massachusetts

Mark A. Stebnicki, PhD, LCMHC, DCMHS, CRC, CMCC, Professor Emeritus, Department of Addictions and Rehabilitation, East Carolina University, Greenville, North Carolina

Judy Teplow, MSW, Canton, Massachusetts

Emre Umucu, PhD, Associate Dean for Research at College of Health Sciences, Associate Professor of Public Health Sciences, University of Texas at El Paso, El Paso Texas

Laura A. Villarreal, MS, CRC, Workforce Absence Team Leader, University of Texas—Rio Grande Valley, Edinburg, Texas

Robert P. Winske, MS, Boston, Massachusetts

Michael Yeomans, MA, CRC, Doctoral Student, Michigan State University, East Lansing, Michigan

Kaiqi Zhou, PhD, CRC, LPC-IT, Assistant Professor, Department of Rehabilitation and Health Services, University of North Texas, Denton Texas

FOREWORD

Rehabilitation counseling is a systematic process that assists people with chronic health conditions and disabilities to achieve their personal, employment, and independent living goals through the application of the counseling process. The counseling process involves communication, goal setting, and beneficial growth or change through self-advocacy, psychological, vocational, social, and behavioral interventions (Certified Rehabilitation Counselor Commission [CRCC], 2021). Psychosocial aspects of disability and cultural diversity is a major knowledge domain in the curriculum of the Council for Accreditation of Counseling & Related Educational Programs (CACREP) accredited graduate programs in clinical rehabilitation counseling (CACREP, 2016). Psychosocial aspects of disability is a required course in graduate rehabilitation counseling programs and a major knowledge domain in the Certified Rehabilitation Counselor examination.

The ongoing coronavirus disease 2019 (COVID-19) pandemic has disproportionately affected the disability community, leading to exclusive sources of trauma, stressors, and challenges unique to people with chronic health conditions and disabilities. The American Psychological Association (2020) identified specific concerns of people with chronic health conditions and disabilities during the ongoing pandemic, including distress about unemployment, financial difficulties, and health care access as well as prolonged grieving, fear of death, social isolation, loneliness, and sadness that significantly affect their physical health, mental health, and well-being. The pandemic and the Black Lives Matter movement have unveiled unconscious bias (individual level) and systemic discrimination (organizational level) against Black/African Americans and other minority groups including people with disabilities (the largest minority group in the United States). The negative impact of the pandemic on physical health, mental health, and well-being is even more profound for individuals with multiple stigmatizing identities. Evidently, discrimination against people with disabilities, or ableism, is present across sectors of the society. There is an urgent need to refine and revise contents of the psychosocial aspects of disability course to include ableism and how to combat discrimination and negative reaction to people with chronic health conditions and disabilities, health promotion that can improve physical and mental health of people with disabilities, stress management interventions that can help people with disabilities cope with high levels of stressors and challenge during the ongoing COVID-19, and positive psychology interventions that can increase the character strengths, positive foundational human traits, PERMA (**P**ositive Emotion, **E**ngagement, **R**elationships, **M**eaning, and **A**ccomplishment), and well-being of people with disabilities. This popular textbook, now in its eighth edition, is widely adopted for the psychosocial aspects of disability course. This comprehensive and contemporary text continues to provide readers with a treatment of dominant theories, models, and techniques related to the psychosocial adjustment process of persons with chronic health conditions and disabilities. Importantly, it also includes new chapters to address the emerging issues related to psychosocial adjustment and disability. This textbook will enable instructors to help counselors-in-training develop state-of-the-science knowledge in their professional practice of clinical rehabilitation counseling. There are no more appropriate scholars than Irmo Marini, Allison Fleming, and Malachy Bishop to edit this comprehensive and contemporary textbook. They made this book a significant contribution to the rehabilitation counseling profession.

Fong Chan
Professor Emeritus, University of Wisconsin–Madison

REFERENCES

American Psychological Association. (2020, May 6). *How COVID-19 impacts people with disabilities.* https://www.apa.org/topics/covid-19/research-disabilities

CACREP. (2016). 2016 CACREP Standards. https://www.cacrep.org/for-programs/2016-cacrep-standards/

CRCC (2021). Scope of practice. https://crccertification.com/scope-of-practice/

PREFACE

The eighth edition of this classic text has been developed in and for a time that is seeing some of the most significant and fundamental shifts in the psychological and social experience of disability in human history. While prevailing ideas about the meaning of disability are being challenged and reconsidered and the personal, societal, and professional understanding of the experience of disability and chronic illness reexamined, many of the historical barriers and injustices faced by people with disabilities endure. At this critical period, and in the tradition of this series, the present edition comprehensively explores these issues, with new perspectives contributed by voices in disability and rehabilitation policy, research, and lived experience. Whether a student, educator, professional, or person living with a disability or chronic illness, this revised edition offers an informed, critical, and engaging exploration that will be relevant for those in the wide scope of professions concerned with the psychological and social experience of illness and disability. Readers of previous editions will appreciate the continued commitment to a diverse range of topics, from the historical and cultural perspectives on illness and disability, to the personal, familial, and social impacts of disability and from the most current rehabilitation and counseling approaches for working with specific populations to the broader social perspectives on disability issues.

OVERALL GOAL OF THE BOOK

The overall goal of this text is to provide the reader with a broad history of how people with chronic illness and disability (CID) have been viewed and treated throughout history and to examine and explore changes and developments over the last decade. Our goal is to provide students, educators, and professionals in rehabilitation counseling, disability studies, psychology, social work, sociology, and related disciplines a comprehensive and current understanding of CID topics ranging from the impact of laws and policies, social justice issues for persons with CID and minority populations, climate and immigration, to more specific personal and professional issues of rehabilitation and the psychosocial experiences of CID, including disability identity, microaggressions, ableism, and the mental health impact of the increased use of social media platforms.

CONTENTS

As with prior editions, this book is organized into five parts. Part I: Historical and Cultural Perspectives on Illness and Disability examines disability from a sociological and social psychological perspective, with chapters exploring the historical treatment of persons with disabilities, models of disability, disability identity, and ableism and discriminatory behavior toward people with disabilities. Part II: The Personal Impact of Disability includes chapters that explore theories and models of psychosocial adaptation and adjustment to disability; abuse, interpersonal violence, and psychosocial disparities among women with disabilities; sexuality and disability; and ableist microaggressions. Part

III: addresses Family Issues in Illness and Disability contains chapters that explore family adaptation across cultures; advocacy and challenges experienced by parents of children with disabilities; counseling aspects of grief, dying, and death; and psychosocial issues for family caregivers. In Part IV: Specific Trauma and Stigmatized Populations are examined, including the experience of living with substance use disorder and recovery; culturally competent service provision for veterans and family reintegration; responding to individuals experiencing abuse and relationship violence; the psychosocial cost of war and the experiences of immigrants, refugees, and asylum seekers; and working with the aging population of persons with disabilities. Finally, Part V: New Directions, Issues, and Perspectives contains six chapters that explore interventions to improve the well-being of people with CID, assistive technology, religion and disability, social justice and disability counseling, and the influence of social media on mental health and concludes with the editors' reflections and considerations on the topics in this text. Finally, a psychosocial text concerning illness and disability would not be complete without the stories and perspectives of persons with disabilities. As always, this text includes personal perspectives, and we have retained all of these timeless poignant personal accounts written by persons with disabilities and/or their loved ones. For this edition we have added several new perspectives from individuals reflecting on their lived experience.

DISTINGUISHING FEATURES AND LEARNING TOOLS

The distinguishing features of this text relative to the prior editions are that the content and coverage are all new and deal with contemporary situations involving persons with CID. We have carefully balanced retaining the features that have made this classic series so popular with students, educators, and professionals, including the comprehensive scope and inclusion of the leading thinkers, practitioners, and researchers on their chapter topics, with new and updated content and topics, including many topics are not addressed in other textbooks on the psychosocial aspects of disability. Each chapter provides class thinking and learning activities to promote student engagement, pre-reading and discussion questions, and PowerPoint presentations to summarize content and enhance instruction. We also provide an Instructor Manual and a Test Bank for each chapter.

The insights shared in the eighth edition continue to give students, rehabilitation educators, and practitioners a different perspective of life with a chronic illness and disability in the United States and internationally. It is our hope that this knowledge will be helpful for students, educators, and practitioners to continue to gain insights and strategies to assist persons with disabilities to live a satisfying and full life.

Irmo Marini, PhD, DSc, CRC, CLCP
Allison R. Fleming, PhD, CRC
Malachy Bishop, PhD, CRC

ACKNOWLEDGMENTS

We would like to most humbly thank several key people who made this book possible. Senior editor for the Behavioral Sciences program, Mindy Okura-Marszycki, who recently joined us in this venture and has been most supportive of this project. She replaced her predecessor, Rhonda Dearborn, who was with us and equally supportive, partway through this process. We also want to thank the lady who has continued to get deep into the weeds with the three of us, Kirsten Elmer, who is the assistant editor of the Behavioral Sciences program. Kirsten has provided us with so much assistance regarding content arrangement, contributors, and overall has kept us on track for our submission date. We also would like to thank all the unnamed Springer copyeditors and other employees who strive to make the contents of this book flawless. We also want to thank each of our chapter contributors for their time and expertise since for all of us, this is largely a labor of love and our passion. It is a privilege to be able to share our expertise with students, educators, and practitioners. From my personal perspective, I would also like to thank my two PhD assistants for assisting me in scouring the literature for information to update my chapters in this book, Tori Livingston and Laura Villarreal. I also must acknowledge my wife Darlene who always double-checks my citations and builds my reference list. This is tedious work, but she has assisted me with this part for 27+ years for which I am very grateful. And finally, to those new contributors who live with a disability and bring the empirical based literature to life in telling their stories, ultimately leading the reader to the conclusion that people with disabilities have lives like those without disabilities but largely have adapted to their disability and live otherwise normal lives if supported and not hampered by physical or societal barriers.

—*IM*

I would like to acknowledge and thank Drs. Irmo Marini and Malachy Bishop for inviting me to join this editorial team and for their kind and gracious mentorship as we completed this project. This has always been my favorite rehabilitation text and one that I have grown to appreciate more and more over the years—being asked to join this project is a true and humbling honor. I would also like to acknowledge our authors and contributors for their hard work and generosity of their time and ideas that brought so much life to this new edition.

—*AF*

I would like to acknowledge the PhD students whose hard work on this project made it happen, including Sara Park, Megan Baumunk, Connie Richard, Kaiqi Zhou, Yunzhen (Judy) Huang, and Stuart Rumrill Sr. Thank you, Hanoch Livneh and Phil Rumrill, for your gracious help and generosity. Thank you, Boo, for your support.

—*MB*

SPRINGER PUBLISHING CONNECT™ RESOURCES

 A robust set of instructor resources designed to supplement this text is located at http://connect.springerpub.com/content/book/978-0-8261-5111-7. Qualifying instructors may request access by emailing textbook@springerpub.com.

- **LMS Common Cartridge With All Instructor Resources**
- **Instructors Manual** containing learning objectives, chapter overview, and discussion questions.
- **Test Bank** with more than 250 multiple-choice questions of various types (including full rationales).
- **Instructor Chapter PowerPoints**

HISTORICAL AND CULTURAL PERSPECTIVES ON ILLNESS AND DISABILITY

The first part of this book addresses disability from a sociological or social-psychological perspective, focusing on exploring disability from the outside looking inward. A major premise for contemporary scholars in the field has been to examine the impact of the environment on the individual with a disability and his or her family. Somatopsychology and ecological and minority models of disability emphasize the positive and all-too-often negative psychosocial implications that societal attitudes, physical barriers, and social inequities can have on persons with disabilities. For this reason, we first explore past treatment of persons with disabilities and examine models of disability, disability identity, and understanding ableism as a construct

MAJOR HIGHLIGHTS IN PART I

- In Chapter 1, we explore how persons with disabilities have been treated throughout history up to present day both abroad and here in the United States. The chapter specifically addresses Darwinism and the concept of eugenics, particularly around the mass immigration to the United States in the early 20th century. At these ports of entry such as Ellis Island in New York, legislation was enforced to withhold or garnish payments to ship captains who were told not to bring immigrants to the United States who appeared to have any type of mobility impairments, visual impairments, and anyone else who might become a ward of the state. It also covers the political and establishment perceptions of disability and how those perceptions impacted legislation that followed. American legislation beginning in the 1920s, including and recently the Americans with Disabilities Act, is discussed. Still debated and considerations presently are what is considered the new eugenics movement regarding genetic testing and aborting a fetus with a disability, genetically engineered fetuses, and the current landscape regarding disability in the United States.

- Negative societal attitudes toward persons with disabilities are evident and have been reflected in disability policy and legislation. Chapter 2 discusses why some people in society as a whole are often anxious, reluctant, resistant, and in some cases afraid of people with disabilities and those who are different. Understanding the misperceptions that surround people with disabilities and how these attitudes originated is critical to understanding how we can move forward. The author of this chapter explores aspects of the conscious and subconscious human psyche at the root of the most common societal perceptions of disability.

■ The historical treatment of persons with psychiatric disabilities in the United States is particularly noteworthy, given the harsh treatment, discrimination, and institutional repression that have ensued. Psychiatric disability or mental illness has arguably been perceived and treated more harshly than any other diagnosed disability. Chapter 3 describes early beliefs of severe mental illness as demonic possession, the involuntary confinement of the mentally ill in subhumane "institutions," use of prefrontal lobotomies, and debate about the legal definition of *torture*. In the United States today, persons with a history of mental illness are often homeless or incarcerated. Indeed, psychiatric disability is a category unto itself. In this chapter, the author chronicles the often brutal and inhumane history of treatment toward those with psychiatric disabilities and what happens to individuals when they are perceived as less than human.

■ As is evident in the first three chapters in Part 1 of this text, in the broader culture, individuals with disabilities have historically been depicted and viewed from an inherently devaluing, medical model–based perspective, with policies, systems, and clinical perspectives reflecting an understanding of disability as negative, stigmatized, and isolating and of disabled people as passive recipients of care. Over the past three decades, a very different perspective has been emerging, and a growing body of scholarship has focused on exploring the processes of disability identity and disability culture development, reflecting an understanding of people with disabilities as active agents in creating and defining disability as a powerful positive identity and cultural category. In Chapter 4, disability identity is defined and explored as an individual, social, and cultural process involving a positive sense of self and feelings of connection with the broader disability community. The authors explore definitions of disability identity from several perspectives, including in the context of various extent models of disability; describe the history of disability identity and disability culture; and comprehensively review disability identity scholarship from the 1990s through the present. Models of disability identity are reviewed, and the authors describe relevant disability identity measures. Important counseling perspectives, approaches, and research are discussed, including the role of self-concept and disability identity in adaptation to congenital or acquired disability, and critically important content for counselors on supporting identity development in counseling. The chapter concludes with a consideration of future directions and means by which to support disability identity and culture through advocacy.

■ Chapter 5 is a thorough exploration of *ableism*, a term defined by stereotypes and prejudicial attitudes, oppression, and discriminatory behavior toward people with disabilities. In this chapter, the author explains the origins of ableism as a predictable response to disability, as well as the consequences of ableism for disabled people in their everyday lives. The author draws distinctions between intentional and unintentional ableism, providing examples of ways that individuals and even professionals promulgate ableism in how we react to and treat disabled people. He also outlines strategies to counter ableism by centering disability culture and identity, becoming effective disability allies, and pursuing advocacy in ways that have the potential to meaningfully alter long-held attitudes about the capabilities and value of disabled people.

■ Disability history in the United States is sometimes referred to as "hidden" and includes institutionalized segregation, exclusion, erasure, and abuse. However, people with disabilities have been at the center of many movements, including social welfare policy development, occupational health and safety, and civil rights. Victories won by the disability rights movement have resulted in legislative changes and advances in civil rights mandating greater access to public spaces and services and prohibiting discrimination in employment and educational opportunities. However, discrimination, exclusion, and reduced opportunity continue to hinder individuals with disabilities in the United States. Chapter 6 begins with a synthesis of historical gains in rights and access for disabled Americans and addresses areas of policy that continue to hinder equity in medical care, community life, and civil rights. The authors present approaches for continued advocacy and policy change to remove barriers for individuals with disabilities.

CHAPTER 1

HISTORY OF TREATMENT TOWARD PERSONS WITH DISABILITIES IN AMERICA AND ABROAD

DANIELLE D. FOX AND IRMO MARINI

LEARNING OBJECTIVES

After reading this chapter, you will be able to:

- Examine the history of treatment toward PWDs in the United States and abroad.
- Differentiate between and among the various types of discrimination toward PWDs.
- Compare the history of treatment toward PWDs to the treatment of PWDs today.
- Identify current forms of discrimination toward PWDs in the United States and abroad.

PRE-READING QUESTIONS

1. What is eugenics and how has the beliefs, laws, and practice of it impacted persons with various disabilities over the past 150 years?

2. How were PWDs treated differently than their nondisabled counterparts in previous centuries compared to today?

3. When was the first major disability civil rights legislation passed in the United States and what does it entail?

Despite the common ideal that the United States is a land of opportunity, the early history of America was not necessarily a welcoming one for everyone. The fear of diluting American bloodlines with potential hereditary diseases or illnesses had a huge impact on public and governmental beliefs and attitudes. This fear, combined with the eugenics movement of the early 19th century, led American lawmakers to pass laws that specifically restricted certain people or groups from entering the United States and, within some city ordinances, even kept them out of public view. Early American lawmakers believed that by doing this, they were protecting the welfare of the country and Americans as a whole. The purpose of this chapter is to review the history of treatment toward people with disabilities (PWDs) in the United States.

Give me your tired, your poor, your huddled masses yearning to breathe free, the wretched refuse of your teeming shore. Send these, the homeless, tempest-tosst to me. (Lazarus, 1883)

This is a section of the 14-line sonnet that is engraved on the Statue of Liberty in New York City. The statue was completed in 1886, and the verse was inscribed on her in 1945. These words symbolized an American ideal against oppression to all immigrants who entered the United States during the early 20th century. However, American immigration legislation and practice during that time were in direct opposition to the intended message engraved on the Statue of Liberty.

EARLY IMMIGRATION LEGISLATION

"It is often said, and with truth, that each of the different alien peoples coming to America has something to contribute to American civilization. But what America needs is desirable additions to, and not inferior substitutions for, what it already possesses" (Ward, 1924, p. 103). Early immigration literature and the apparent attitudes and treatment toward PWDs, as well as certain other immigrant populations, were blatantly prejudiced and discriminatory. Antidisability sentiment became more evident with immigration restriction, which began as early as the development of the first North American settlements. It was after 1838, when a large influx of immigrants came to the United States, that the issue of disability became more pressing to the early American settlers (Treadway, 1925).

Antidisability legislation began in 1882 and continued through 1924, with some of the original laws in effect until the 1980s. The concept behind early immigration legislation was to prevent the immigration of people who were considered undesirable. Early Americans believed that preventing people considered undesirable from entering the United States was a means of protecting not only the people but also the welfare of the country (Ward, 1907). Baynton (2005) states, "disability was a crucial factor in deciding whether or not an immigrant would be allowed to enter the United States" (p. 34). The term *"undesirable"* was used to describe people from any race, ethnicity, or religion and/ or with a disability, who were believed to be more likely to pass on less-than-desirable traits to their offspring. The purpose of early immigration legislation was to protect the American bloodlines, and, according to early lawmakers, this meant excluding people based on any trait that could be considered undesirable. Baynton (2005) states,

> One of the driving forces behind early federal immigration law, beginning with the first major Immigration Act in 1882, was the exclusion of people with mental and physical defects (as well as those considered criminal or immoral, problems seen at the time as closely related to mental defect). (p. 32)

This marked the beginning of the exclusion of PWDs in America.

In the years following 1882, early American lawmakers became more and more concerned about the bloodlines of immigrants seeking entrance into the United States and their possible effect on the bloodlines that were already present. With the 1891 revised Immigration Act, a key wording change made restrictions even more discretionary regarding excluding PWDs. Baynton (2005, p. 33) notes that the original 1882 law wording was "any lunatic, idiot, or any person *unable* to take care of himself or herself without becoming a public charge"; the phrase changed in the 1891 law from *unable* to "*likely* to become a public charge." In 1894, the Immigration Restriction League (IRL) was established in Boston. The primary focus of the IRL was to "carry on a general educational campaign for more effective restriction and selection" (Ward, 1924, p. 102). According to Ward, the league's fears were that the United States was becoming an "asylum for the poor and the oppressed of every land" (p. 100). Ward went on to explain:

Americans began to realize that the ideal of furnishing an asylum for all the world's oppressed was coming into conflict with changed economic and social conditions. The cold facts were that the supply of public land was practically exhausted; that acute labor problems, aggravated by the influx of ignorant and unskilled aliens, had arisen; that the large cities were becoming congested with foreigners; that large numbers of mentally and physically unfit, and of the economically undesirable, had come to the United States. (p. 102)

As such, by 1896, literacy requirements were imposed on all immigrants entering the United States, and then from 1903 through 1907, immigration laws were broadened and became more restrictive in scope. However, it was only after the 1917 revisions to the 1907 Immigration Act had occurred that more specific and harsher discriminatory language appeared in legislation. Before this, in 1903, persons with epilepsy were added to the list, as well as individuals who met the 1903 wording: "persons who have been insane within 5 years previous [or] who have had two or more attacks of insanity at any time previously" (Baynton, 2005, p. 33). Treadway (1925) cites the exclusionary language of the law in the 1907 Act:

The insane; idiots; imbeciles; feebleminded; chronic alcoholics; constitutional psychopathic inferiors; the mentally defective whose defect would modify their ability to earn a living; those with loathsome or dangerous contagious diseases, and those over sixteen years of age who were without a reading knowledge of some language. (p. 351)

The 1907 Act was also the first in which the law required a medical certificate for persons judged to be "mentally or physically defective, such mental or physical defect being of a nature which *may affect* the ability of such alien to earn a living" (Baynton, 2005, p. 33).

The subsequent years saw increasing restrictions, including financial penalties on transport companies and ship captains for the transportation of immigrants considered "unfit" for entry into the United States (Barkan, 1991; Baynton, 2005; Treadway, 1925). To gain better control of the immigration situation, ship captains at ports of entry were to examine prospective immigrants for "defects." Although they were neither physicians nor did they have any medical experience, the purpose of their inspections was to medically examine the immigrants. If a disability, either mental or physical, was observed or perceived, the ship captain at transit or the inspector at entry ports was authorized to either deny departure from the immigrant's country of origin or deny entry into the United States. If an immigrant was granted departure from his or her country of origin and, on arrival, entry into the United States was denied, the immigrant was to be deported back to his or her country of origin at the expense of the transport company that brought the individual (Baynton, 2005). For this reason, many ship captains likely denied numerous individuals for various vague reasons in order to not be fined or potentially lose their jobs. Baynton (2005) notes:

Inspectors prided themselves on their ability to make a "snapshot diagnosis" as immigrants streamed past them single file. For most immigrants, a normal appearance usually meant an uneventful passage through the immigration station. An abnormal appearance, however, meant a chalked letter on the back. Once chalked, a closer inspection was required for lameness, K for suspected hernia, G for goiter, X for suspected mental illness, and so on. (p. 37)

This process allowed for the discrimination and/or refusal of immigrants based on whether or not impairment was present. The commissioner general of immigration in his 1907 report regarding the governing immigration laws essentially laid out that the primary reason for the laws was to exclude anyone with a disability or anyone perceived as having a disability. The commissioner wrote, "The exclusion from this country of the morally, mentally, and physically deficient is the principal object to be accomplished by the immigration laws" (Baynton, 2005, p. 34). To exclude those with physical disabilities, the regulations stated that inspectors were to observe individuals at rest and then in motion to detect any irregularities or abnormalities in gait. Again, the wording for excluding individuals was vague and granted the inspectors full discretion in excluding anyone they wished. Baynton wrote about an Ellis Island medical inspector whose job was to "detect poorly built, defective or broken-down human beings" (2005, p. 34). A few examples of the physical impairments listed included spinal curvature, varicose veins, poor eyesight, hernia, flat feet, bunions, deafness, arthritis, hysteria, and, simply, poor physical development. Once again, as with all age-old debates on eugenics, ethnocentricity, and exactly who was considered the weaker species, there was no consistent consensus.

During this period, individuals were often excluded based on size or physical stature, or lack thereof, and abnormal sexual development. In addition, the commissioner and IRL, among others, were concerned about the public charge of becoming an economic drain because of perceived discrimination from employers in hiring. The surgeon general, in a letter to the commissioner, noted that such persons were:

> A bad economic risk . . . known to their associates who make them the butt of coarse jokes to their own despair, and to the impairment of the work in hand. Among employers, it is difficult for these unfortunates to get or retain jobs, their facial and bodily appearance at least in adult life, furnishing a patent advertisement of their condition. (Baynton, 2005, p. 38)

In all, it is difficult to determine exactly how many immigrants were excluded either before or on entering the United States. Baynton (2005) cites statistics that increased over the years and notes that the actual numbers were likely much higher. The number of individuals excluded because they were likely to become a public charge or were mentally or physically defective in 1895 was 1,720; in 1905 the number was greater than 8,000, and by 1910 it rose to more than 16,000. Individuals from certain countries were denied more often than the others. Individuals from Slovakia were viewed as slow witted; Jews were seen as having poor physique and being neurotic; and those of Portuguese, Greek, or Syrian ethnicity were described as undersized (Baynton, 2005).

For those individuals who were somehow allowed entry into the United States or were born in the United States with any type of perceived or real impairment, life was not generally favorable regarding societal attitudes. Specifically, Longmore and Goldberger (2000) noted court rulings in which railroads and public transit systems were essentially granted permission to deny access to transportation for these impaired people. School laws were upheld segregating PWDs by not allowing them to attend school or requiring that they be taught in a segregated room. Employers were also permitted to discriminate in hiring those with disabilities, and all public venues such as restaurants, theaters, and so on, could deny access and frequently did so. For all intents and purposes, many of those with disabilities during the early 20th century were relegated to being shut-ins in their own homes, and when venturing out were subject to ridicule and indignant comments.

Many PWDs were outraged by these political and societal attitudes and the blatant efforts to prejudice and discriminate against them. For many, it was not only the negative attitudes of being devalued and dehumanized but also the discrimination of being excluded from the workforce. Longmore and Goldberger (2000) cite the historic accounts during the spring of 1935 after 5 years of the Great Depression, in which a number of persons with physical and other disabilities demanded their voices be heard and protested against New York City's Emergency Relief Bureau, demanding jobs. Forming the League of the Physically Handicapped (LPH), this group focused on discrimination issues as opposed to their medical impairments. Media coverage back then was also largely discriminatory and prejudiced. Longmore and Goldberger cite how media and popular culture portrayals during the 1920s and 1930s perceived PWDs as villains, victims, sinners, charity cases, unsightly objects, dangerous denizens of society, and unworthy citizens (2000, p. 896).

Franklin D. Roosevelt was a member of the LPH, and although he largely hid his own paralysis from polio at age 39 years, he strived for the rehabilitation of those with disabilities. He epitomized what persons with a disability "can" do and is arguably one of America's greatest presidents, having presided for 12 years over troubling times, including the Great Depression, the signing of the 1935 Social Security Act, and World War II (in Gallagher, 1994). In his book, *FDR's Splendid Deception,* Gallagher cites how Roosevelt was intuitively aware of the negative societal attitudes toward disability and aware that if the public knew of both the extent of his disability and chronic pain, he would be perceived as a weak, ineffective leader. As such, Roosevelt had agreements with the media not to photograph or film him in his wheelchair or while ambulating with his leg braces. Ironically, he did not really have a disability agenda and in fact tried to reduce vocational rehabilitation funding by 25%, which was ultimately not supported by Congress (Gallagher, 1994).

THE EUGENICS MOVEMENT IN AMERICA

Driving the ideology of the early immigration acts was Charles Darwin's highly influential 1859 book, *On the Origin of Species by Means of Natural Selection, or the Preservation of Favored Races in the Struggle of Life,* which initially set out to explain the concept of heredity in plants and animals. Darwin refrained from applying his beliefs to humans out of fear of the reaction from the ruling religions. Sir Francis Galton, a cousin of Darwin's, whose own studies primarily focused on mathematics and meteorology, was inspired by Darwin's work and the implications of it. Galton applied mathematics to the study of heredity, and through this application he established not only some of the techniques of modern statistics but also the basis for what he later called *eugenics* (Pearson, 1995). Galton, who coined the term *eugenics* in 1883, believed that natural selection could rid mankind of problems such as disease, criminality, alcoholism, and poverty (Farrell, 1979). Farrell states that when Galton introduced the word *eugenics* in 1883, he did so with the following explanation:

> We greatly want a brief word to express the science of improving stock, which is by no means confined to questions of judicious mating, but which, especially in the case of man, takes cognizance of all influences that tend in however remote a degree to give to the more suitable races or strains of blood a better chance of prevailing speedily over the less suitable than they otherwise would have had. The word eugenics sufficiently expresses the idea; it is at least a neater word and a more generalized one than viriculture which I once ventured to use. (p. 112)

The concept of eugenics reached America around 1900, and many prominent politicians, physicians, and academics agreed with Galton's premise of essentially restricting the promulgation of those considered the weaker species. The notion of protecting and preserving healthy American bloodlines for the betterment of future generations was idealistic in theory and would later prove extremely difficult to implement. The central question contemplated for these powerful and predominantly Caucasian White males was to decide who exactly the weaker species was and how exactly could these undesirables be restricted from bearing children (Marini, 2011a). President Theodore Roosevelt also embraced eugenics in the United States along with other highly influential people such as Alexander Graham Bell, John Harvey Kellogg, and J. C. Penney, to name a few (Pearson, 1995).

STERILIZATION IN THE UNITED STATES AND BARBARISM ABROAD

Evidence of eugenic ideals became more obvious with the passage of sterilization laws in the early 20th century, the primary goal of which was to "improve the quality of the nation's citizenry by reducing the birth rate of individuals they considered to be 'feebleminded'" (Largent, 2002, p. 190). The term *feebleminded* was used at this time to describe anyone with any type of observed or perceived mental or physical disability. Eugenics continued to gain strength and support through the first quarter of the 20th century, with 27 of the 48 states adopting sterilization laws (Farrell, 1979). The state of Indiana was at the forefront of the sterilization movement, being the first to implement eugenic sterilization laws in 1907.

Although the first sterilization law was passed in 1907, Osgood (2001) noted that unauthorized sterilization of the so-called defectives had already occurred in institutions in several states as early as the 1890s (p. 257). In 1909, the state of Oregon also implemented eugenic sterilization laws, 5 years after Dr. Bethenia Owens-Adair had proposed sterilization in Oregon as a means of dealing with persons considered to be criminals and/or insane (Largent, 2002). Noll (2005) reports that the use of intelligence testing in the 1920s allowed medical and mental health doctors to identify "feeblemindedness" more accurately. As the years progressed, more states adopted eugenic sterilization laws, and, as the United States entered World War II, the nation's state mental health and prison authorities reported more than 38,000 sterilizations (Largent, 2002, p. 192). In the 1920s, the most notable Supreme Court sterilization case was *Buck v. Bell*. In 1927, Carrie Buck, a 17-year-old Virginia girl, became pregnant and was institutionalized by her foster parents in the Virginia State Colony for Epileptics and Feeble-Minded. Carrie's mother had already been committed and was deemed feebleminded and subsequently sterilized. Because Carrie's mother was deemed feebleminded, Carrie was also deemed feebleminded and was sterilized as well. Carrie had a younger sister who, under the pretense that she was undergoing an appendectomy, was also sterilized as a result of her mother's perceived mental capacity. Although there was no evidence to the accusations that Carrie Buck was promiscuous, the case went to the U.S. Supreme Court, where Judge Oliver Wendell Holmes, Jr., reported in an 8 to 1 decision that the state of Virginia was supported by its sterilization law and further stated, "three generations of imbeciles are enough" (Carlson, 2009, p. 178). The case of Carrie Buck was not an isolated incident at the time, and although other cases similar in nature were found in other states to be unconstitutional, *Buck v. Bell* was never overturned. Despite the injustice associated with forced sterilization of people considered to be developmentally disabled, mentally ill, or simply criminals, sterilization laws lasted well into the 1980s in some states (Largent, 2002). Although there was a focus on eugenic sterilization laws, other laws that specifically targeted persons with mental and physical disabilities were being passed.

Finally, Germany began its sterilization program of Germans with disabilities in 1933 as Hitler became chancellor and rose to power. The German elite also believed in Darwinism and the superior race philosophy following eugenics; however, these elites took sterilization one step further with top politicians, philosophers, physicians, and others who agreed to begin a secret program to exterminate German citizens with disabilities who they termed "useless eaters." It is estimated that approximately 300,000 German citizens were murdered between 1939 and 1941, when Hitler's "final medical assistance" program ended, with rising outcries from German citizens who learned their loved ones with disabilities were exterminated (Gallagher, 1995). The eugenics movement decreased and largely went underground after the dismal failure of eugenics and a superior race was taken to an extreme.

THE UGLY LAWS

Any person who is diseased, maimed, mutilated or in any way deformed so as to be an unsightly or disgusting object, or an improper person to be allowed in or on the streets, highways, thoroughfares or public places in this city shall not therein or thereon expose himself or herself to public view under penalty of one dollar for each offense. On the conviction of any person for a violation of this section, if it shall seem proper and just, the fine provided for may be suspended, and such person detained at the police station, where he shall be well cared for, until he can be committed to the county poor house. (Coco, 2010, p. 23)

This was a city of Chicago ordinance, originally passed in 1881. Unsightly beggar ordinances passed between the years 1867 and 1913 were otherwise known as *Ugly Laws*. The first unsightly beggar ordinance was passed in San Francisco in 1867. Although these ordinances had been in place for 14 years before the passage of the Chicago ordinance, it is the most well-known and considered "the most egregious example of discrimination against people with physical disabilities in the United States" (Coco, 2010, p. 23). The passing of these ordinances and laws allowed some insight into how disability was perceived. PWDs were generally thought of as a burden to society, as they lacked the ability to care for themselves or contribute in any way to society. This perception, however, was largely contingent on one's social standing and social contribution (Schweik, 2009). Although unsightly beggar ordinances were commonplace in cities throughout the country, Chicago's unsightly beggar ordinance remained on the law books until 1973 (Coco, 2010).

However, the soldiers returning from World War II with various disabilities provide a good example of how some PWDs were perceived. For example, soldiers were often viewed with sympathy but were nevertheless respected because of their contribution, whereas a civilian born with a disability would often not be perceived in the same way. The Industrial Revolution in the United States further increased the number of Americans with disabilities, as factory workers began to sustain injuries leading to chronic conditions. Without effective workers compensation laws early on, injured workers had to sue their employers, with the vast majority often losing their suits for contributory negligence and for knowingly accepting the hazards of the job, otherwise known as "assumption of risk" (Marini, 2011b).

For some PWDs with facial or physical deformities, performing in circus freak shows became the only employment they could obtain. These PWDs appeared to be more highly regarded and were often considered to be prominent citizens even though in certain parts of the country, where Ugly Laws were adopted, they were unable to show themselves in public.

THE NEW EUGENICS

While support of the eugenics movement appeared to decrease in the aftermath of the horrors of World War II Nazi Germany, the ideals of genetic enhancement have maintained a place in medicine, science, bioethics, and research (Carlson, 2019; Sparrow, 2011). What has emerged in the 70 years post WWII is the "new eugenics" school of thought. This is rooted in the idea that living with severe disability not only greatly diminishes the individual's overall quality of life but also brings great burden to the individual and their family (Brown et al., 2019). New eugenics places emphasis on genetic enhancement and is considered mainstream medical practice today (Brown, 2019). Supporters of new eugenics argue these "new" ideals differentiate from the "old" eugenics ideals in the sense that new eugenics takes into consideration individual well-being, versus the collective well-being promoted by the eugenics movement of the early 1900s (Brown et al., 2019; Carlson, 2019; Sparrow, 2011).

The practice of new eugenics can be seen today in the abortion of fetuses with genetic disorders that would otherwise result in a life of severe disability, the denial of lifesaving care to newborns and/or individuals with severe and profound disability, and the choice to end life-sustaining care for individuals during end-of-life processes based on the perceived lacking long-term benefit (Brown, 2019). Examples of new eugenics include genetic testing prior to term with the option to abort the fetus if deemed medically beneficial to do so by the individuals having the child and/or medical professionals, embryo splitting to maximize the most desirable traits of the embryo prior to implantation, and predetermining desired traits prior to fertilization of the egg. It further includes physicians withholding life-sustaining care as well as end-of-life decision-making based on disability severity and perceived quality-of-life outcomes (Brown, 2019; Brown at al., 2019; Carlson, 2019; Sparrow, 2011). Carlson (2019) argues that there are unchallenged assumptions surrounding the idea of diminished quality of life among PWDs, despite empirical-based research showing PWDs reporting perceived quality-of-life levels just as high as their nondisabled counterparts. Despite the strides made through the passing of the Americans with Disabilities Act (ADA) in 1990, the ideology of minimizing and/or eliminating disability remains and is evident in new eugenics ideology.

More recent examples of the practice of new eugenics can be seen in the 2019 to 2020 COVID-19 pandemic triage protocols. Triage is the allocation of resources and treatment based on the determination, by medical professionals, of who will best benefit from provided resources and/or treatments (Merriam-Webster, 2022).

Orfali (2021) states, "While triage protocols share a common goal, maximizing life by selecting patients who would most benefit from critical care, there are many variations in the selection criterion to respond to situations of scarcity of resources" (p. 77). Triage protocols inadvertently discriminate against individuals with advanced age and underlying chronic conditions. One of the most commonly used predictors for the determination of triage care is the Clinical Frailty Scale (CFS; Wilkinson, 2021). The CFS scale assesses an individual's level of frailty based on their level of physical independence, activity levels, ambulatory independence, and more. Higher CFS scores equate to less independent mobility and activity and correlate to a higher rate of mortality and lower perceived clinical outcomes, while lower CFS scores correlate to lower rates of mortality and higher perceived clinical outcomes (Wilkinson, 2021). Therefore, individuals with lower CFS scores are given preference with regard to medical resources and treatments, while individuals with higher CFS scores are deemed less likely to benefit from medical resources and treatments available.

The use of CFS scores as primary determiners of triage care has been criticized for not taking younger individuals with physical disabilities into account, thus carrying the potential of misdirecting care (Wilkinson, 2021). Another clinical instrument used to assess clinical outcomes is the Sequential Organ Failure Assessment (SOFA). The SOFA assesses a series of organ system metrics, including arterial pressure, oxygen saturation, the Glasgow Coma Scale, and various blood serum levels (Zhu et.al., 2022). Individuals with underlying disability typically score much higher on this scale, resulting in higher predicted mortality rates (Zhu et al., 2022). SOFA scores combined with CFS scores present an unfavorable picture of medical outcomes for individuals with underlying chronic conditions and/or physical disability (Zhu et al., 2022). This was evident at the start of the COVID-19 pandemic, where the elderly and disabled were left without lifesaving resources that were being rationed for more able-bodied individuals, particularly when it came to who would or would not benefit from a ventilator (Orfali, 2021; Wilkinson, 2021; Zhu et.al., 2022).

MOVEMENT TOWARD EQUALITY

As disability discrimination and sterilization laws were being passed concerning PWDs, helpful legislation was also being passed. The 1920s brought about the Smith–Fess Act (P.L. 66–236), allowing services to PWDs such as vocational guidance, occupational adjustment, and placement services. In 1935 the Social Security Act (P.L. 74–271) was passed and the state/federal Vocational Rehabilitation Program was established as a permanent program (Parker et al., 2005). Despite this early legislation and numerous additional laws over time designed to protect and employ PWDs in the workforce, the unemployment rate for PWDs has been dismally holding at around 70%. Yelin (1991) noted that the lowest unemployment rate for PWDs was during World War II because many able-bodied Americans were involved in the war, and manufacturing jobs for the war effort increased dramatically. Once the war was over, however, tens of thousands of able-bodied men and women in the armed services returned home looking for work, and thousands of workers with disabilities were subsequently replaced and suddenly unemployed. There was a shift in who was entering the workforce in the United States (Longmore & Goldberger, 2000).

The year 1943 marked the passage of landmark legislation with the Vocational Rehabilitation Act Amendments (P.L. 113), essentially increasing the amount of state vocational services available to PWDs (Parker et al., 2005). The Vocational Rehabilitation Act Amendments also broadened the definition of disability, allowing persons with mental illness or psychiatric disabilities to be eligible for services. Disability rights continued to make progress for the next 30 years without much fanfare, but unemployment rates remained relatively the same as they are today.

The 1973 Rehabilitation Act was also considered to be landmark legislation for PWDs, especially since President Nixon was considering abolishing the state/federal Vocational Rehabilitation Program altogether. After much debate and considerable outcry from disability groups, President Nixon signed into law what is believed to be the first civil rights laws for PWDs, from which the 1990 ADA was designed. Again, there was increased funding for public vocational rehabilitation programs and affirmative action in the hiring of federal employees (Parker et al., 2005). Although this landmark employment legislation was unprecedented, it was extremely difficult for employees to sue and win their claims against discriminatory employers. Colker (1999) noted that 94% of all court trials were decided in the employer's favor. The statistic remains high even today, as much of the burden of proof lies with the suing employee. Separately, Sections 501 to 504 of the Act also addressed access to transportation, removal of architectural barriers, and physical access to all newly constructed federal buildings. Perhaps one of the most criticized aspects of the 1973 Act was the fact that there was no enforcement entity designed to check whether policies were being followed or implemented.

In 1975, the Rehabilitation Act was combined with the Education for All Handicapped Children Act (P.L. 94–142), now known as the Individuals with Disabilities Education Act (IDEA). IDEA allowed for opportunities such as equal access to public education for all children with disabilities in the least restrictive environment. IDEA also allowed for children with disabilities to be tested through multiple means, such as being tested in their native language. The law also gave parents the right to view their children's school records (Olkin, 1999). The 1986 revision of IDEA extended services to provide early intervention for children from birth to preschool, help with equipment purchases, and provide legal assistance to families with children with disabilities (Olkin, 1999).

Perhaps the single most important legislation to date concerning the civil rights of PWDs was the 1990 passage of the ADA by President George H. W. Bush. The Act contains five titles: employment, extended access to state and federal government services including public or paratransit transportation access, public accommodations for physical access to all public venues (e.g., restaurants, theaters, sporting events), access to telecommunications (e.g., closed captioning, theater audio loops), and a miscellaneous title. The ADA has arguably been deemed a success as far as making communities more accessible; however, t complaints and lawsuits continue to be filed daily owing to employers and businesses that continue to discriminate knowingly or unknowingly (Blackwell et al., 2001). Some PWDs continue to see the glass as half-empty regarding physical access and societal attitudes; others see it as half-full (Marini, 2001). The United States Equal Employment Opportunity Commission's charge statistics website (n.d.) indicates that since 2009, there have been over 20,000 to 25,000 filed disability employment discrimination claims annually.

CURRENT PULSE ON AMERICA REGARDING DISABILITY

Attitudes, physical access, and the laws regarding PWDs have unquestionably improved in the last century. The eugenics movement essentially died down after World War II, primarily because of Social Darwinism and the Nazi extermination of an estimated 250,000 German citizens and war veterans with disabilities (Marini, 2011a). In America, many eugenicists realized that this extremist version was essentially a slippery slope and that continued forced sterilization, as well as forbidding those with epilepsy, mental illness, or mental retardation from marrying, could potentially lead them down a similar path.

Current attitudes of Americans without disabilities toward those with disabilities suggest contradictory sentiments of both admiration and pity (Harris, 1991). Similar sentiments about disability continue today since media coverage and depictions have not changed. Most likely influenced by media portrayals, the sentiment of admiration can be easily explained when we watch a documentary on FDR, Wilma Rudolph, Christopher Reeve, or Stephen Hawking. Conversely, the pity sentiment occurs when one watches any televised charitable event, particularly *Jerry's Kids Muscular Dystrophy* Labor Day telethon. Although Americans generally believe that it is right to hire a qualified individual with a disability, many nondisabled persons still believe that PWDs are fundamentally "different" from those without disabilities (Harris, 1991).

As previously noted, how much better conditions and attitudes toward those with disabilities have become is still open to debate. Although many outside observers anecdotally argue that PWDs get free benefits and healthcare without making a contribution to society, others are quick to point out a different reality. Specifically, with an approximately 65% unemployment rate and two-thirds of those with disabilities indicating they would work if they could, this population still has one of the highest poverty rates in America (Rubin & Roessler, 2008). Single minority females with children with a disability have the highest rate of poverty, along with single minority female parents with a disability (Brault, 2012). More than 25% of African Americans and Hispanics live under the federal poverty rate, and approximately 30% of caregivers who have a child with a disability live in poverty as well (Annual Disability Statistics Compendium, 2014; United States Department of Health and Human Services, 2014). This is compared to approximately 13% of those Caucasian families without a disabled loved one.

Although physical barriers and community access have improved exponentially since the 1990 ADA, several studies of persons with physical disabilities suggest that the United States still has a long way to go to become barrier free. Specifically, two recent studies have found that even 22 years after the ADA was signed into law, persons with physical disabilities still cite physical access barriers as the number-one frustration (Graf et al., 2009; Marini et al., 2009). Negative and ambivalent societal attitudes were not far behind in the rankings as perceived by those with disabilities. Although many outsiders or those without disabilities and no experience with disability view the proverbial glass as half-full, many persons with disabilities (insiders who live the experience) continue to see the glass as half-empty (Marini, 2011a). Many experience daily frustrations with healthcare, education, public accommodations, transportation, and employment. These are among the ongoing daily hassles many Americans with disabilities face (O'Day & Goldstein, 2005).

Eugenics has taken a different form in the 21st century. Today, scientists are improving medical technology to remove the so-called defective genes responsible for various neuromuscular diseases while an unborn fetus is still in the embryo stage (Marini, 2011a). Likewise, parents are now able to abort a fetus that may result in a child having a developmental disability and essentially start over. Roberts et al. (2002) found that when referred by their physician for genetic testing in relation to potential fetus birth defects, 65% of mothers elected to abort such a child. However, when mothers were provided with information and educational counseling about the disease or disability, many changed their minds. The authors found little effort to educate and counsel expectant mothers takes place in genetic testing clinics. Designer babies are also medically possible now, meaning parents can select gender, eye, and hair color. In one extreme example of the quest for the perfect human, a *Playboy* photographer auctioned off a supermodel's egg and 5 million people visited the website in one morning, offering $42,000 for the egg (Smart, 2009). For those who can afford to pay for a designer baby, the option has arrived.

The survival-of-the-fittest concept and natural selection in the 21st century appear to have morphed into a survival of the financially fittest ideology. The ramifications of the 2008 Great Recession, continual middle-class decline into poverty, and historical government actions to cut social programs like Social Security, Medicare, and Medicaid during financial downturns ultimately leave those who need the most assistance to fend for themselves (Huffington, 2010; Reich, 2010). Today the many persons with disabilities continue to face poor healthcare access and treatment, poor transportation options, unemployment or underemployment, and food insufficiency (Kellett et al., 2021). Indeed, the most disenfranchised of us, largely including those minorities with disabilities, may see their life expectancy shortened by 20+ years depending on one's ZIP Code (Hoffman et al., 2012). Those who live in poorly planned or discriminating ZIP Codes typically are grocery store food deserts; have few, if any, hospitals within the area; have few, if any, playgrounds or parks for children and adults to exercise; and have an abundance of fast-food restaurants and convenience stores. The Centers for Disease Control and Prevention, epidemiologists, and community planners have begun to deal with these blatant, discriminatory inequities of the past, including redlining. With the aging of America and millions of baby boomers moving into their golden years, the financial portfolios of these individuals dictate what the quality of their lives will be like at no time before in American history. Although many well-off Americans are living longer and healthier lives, those with disabilities and little income are facing precarious times ahead without better government assistance and community planning.

Relatedly, the COVID pandemic, with overwhelmed intensive care units (ICUs), forced emergency room (ER) physicians to make emergency triage decisions regarding who would and would not qualify for a ventilator since there was a mass shortage. Similar to wartime, physicians had to decide who was most likely going to benefit from lifesaving measures versus who would not. Although Americans will never know the numbers of persons with severe disabilities who may have been saved but were not selected for a ventilator and lifesaving measures, odds are that many were not. The Canadian government and Canadian hospitals formulated an order of selection regarding measures of frailty and disability versus just providing comfort measures only (Iezzoni et al., 2021; Ontario Health Ministry, 2020).

Although unquestionably attitudes and treatment toward persons with disabilities have improved over the last several decades, there arestill many in society who view people with disabilities as second-class citizens from their attitudes, legislative policies, and ongoing physical barriers barring full participation and social injustice. In order for this to change, there has to be a quantum shift in how PWDs are portrayed in the media, considered in policy making for full inclusion, and treated equitably across sectors of society. The rehabilitation counselor can advocate with and on behalf of their clients, educate the public and employers about the assets PWDs bring to the table, and be a rallying cry, fighting oppression by filing complaints with agencies blatantly denying a client's rights.

CONCLUSION

The history of treatment toward PWDs since the Greek and Roman era has often been brutal globally, from sterilization due to eugenic beliefs up until extermination by the Nazis in World War II. Despite more humane treatment of PWDs over the past half-century, many still feel like second-class citizens, and social inequities in terms of societal attitudes and government legislation continue to exist in many industrialized countries such as the United States. PWDs continue to be the most disenfranchised minority across the globe, often receiving inequitable healthcare, physical barriers to full access, and, most recently witnessed, being at the bottom of the list for lifesaving crises triage in overcrowded hospitals during COVID-19. The new eugenics has taken the form of genetic testing and termination of pregnancies when a disability is detected and where parents are now able to choose designer babies with the admired traits they desire their child to have. Although PWDs are no brutally exterminated, it leaves us to wonder whether the new eugenics era is just another way for us to contemplate our own selective master race.

CLASS ACTIVITIES

1. Have the class role-play that they are Caucasian American influential men of the 1890 to 1930s that includes politicians, psychiatrists, physicians, and academics. Your job on this policy-making committee is to decide who should be included as the weaker species and thus be sterilized and prevented from procreating or marrying. Use for fictitious examples (a) a single welfare mother of five; (b) a professor who acquires a spinal cord injury and teaches but requires a home health aide to complete activities of daily living; (c) a physically and mentally able-bodied homeless man; and (d) a physician who has epilepsy but works. Which among them would be considered the weaker species and why?

2. Have the class list how many politicians they can think of in the past 10 years who have campaigned on maintaining the Americans with Disabilities Act and advocating for people with disabilities.

3. Ask the class about the 2020 COVID pandemic, and if they were ER physicians and they had to deal with a lack of ICU beds and one remaining ventilator, which of the following two individuals would more likely receive a ventilator and give their reasons why: a 25-year-old nonvaccine believer and non-mask-wearing, otherwise healthy individual who is now in need of a ventilator or a 60-year-old professor with a spinal cord injury who has worn her mask and is a vaccine believer.

KEY REFERENCES

Only key references appear in the print edition. The full references appear in the digital product on Springer Publishing Connect™: https://connect.springerpub.com/content/book/978-0-8261-5111-7/part/partI/chapter/ch01

Baynton, D. (2005). Defectives in the land: Disability and American immigration policy, 1882–1924. *Journal of American Ethnic History, 24*(30), 31–44. https://www.jstor.org/stable/27501596

Brown, I. (2019). The new eugenics in human progress. *Journal of Policy and Practice in Intellectual Disabilities, 16*(2), 137–140. https://doi.org/10.1111/jppi.12304

Darwin, C. (1859). *On the origin of species by means of natural selection, or the preservation of favoured races in the struggle for life* (American ed.). D. Appleton & Co.

Kellett, K., Ligus, K., & Robison, J. (2021). "So glad to be home": Money follows the person participants' experiences after transitioning out of an institution. *Journal of Disability Policy Studies*, 1–11. https://doi.org/10.1177/10442073211043519

Longmore, P. K., & Goldberger, D. (2000). The League of the Physically Handicapped and the Great Depression: A case study in the new disability history. *Journal of American History, 87*(3), 888–921. https://doi.org/10.2307/2675276

Wilkinson, D.J.C. (2021). Frailty triage: Is rationing intensive medical treatment on the grounds of frailty ethical? *The American Journal of Bioethics, 21*(11), 48–63. https://doi.org/10.1080/15265161.2020.1851809

CHAPTER 2

SOCIETAL ATTITUDES AND MYTHS ABOUT DISABILITY: IMPROVING THE SOCIAL CONSCIOUSNESS

IRMO MARINI

LEARNING OBJECTIVES

After reading this chapter, you will be able to:

- Understand what the definition of attitudes entails.
- Identify the major research problems in being able to accurately measure attitudes.
- Differentiate the numerous theories of why persons without disabilities may have negative attitudes toward those who do.
- Implement various ways to enhance attitudes toward disability.

PRE-READING QUESTIONS

1. How does one measure a person's attitudes, and how is attitude defined?
2. What common personal attributes or traits do individuals typically have where others view them as physically and personally attractive or appealing?
3. What are the typical attitudes toward persons with disabilities?
4. How can an individual's attitudes toward disability be enhanced or made more positive?

ATTITUDES DEFINED: COMPONENTS AND CONCEPTS

It is first important to understand that some researchers argue that the concept of "attitude" is too abstract to accurately measure. It is further compounded by the fact that unless respondents' answers to attitude surveys are anonymous, many people respond in a way they believe to be *socially desirable* (Antonak & Livneh, 1988). In other words, people will claim they have positive attitudes toward persons with disabilities (even if they do not), because to state otherwise is not socially acceptable and considered to be prejudice. Attitude survey studies have further been criticized due to poorly validated measures being used, violations of internal validity, poor theoretical referents (not supported by theory), and making causal relationships from correlational studies (Antonak & Livneh, 1988, 2000; Chubon, 1994; Yuker, 1988). Regardless of such complaints, there have been hundreds of empirical studies devoted to studying attitudes toward disability (see Yuker, 1988).

Although there is no single definition pertaining to the concept of attitudes, there are certain commonalities that exist among these definitions (Ostrom et al., 1994). Plotnik defines attitude as "any belief or opinion that includes a positive or negative evaluation of some target (object, person, or event) and that predisposes us to act in a certain way toward the target" (Plotnik, 1996, p. 540). Ostrom et al. (1994) state that any definition of attitude shares three features: an *evaluative* feature that involves whether we like or dislike an object, person, or event; a *target* at which the attitude is aimed; and a *predisposition* to behaving or acting in a certain way toward the target. For example, if an individual likes or admires (evaluation feature) persons with spinal cord injuries (target feature), he or she is more apt to approach and talk to such an individual as opposed to avoiding him or her (predisposed feature).

Eagly et al. (1994) also differentiate the fact that attitudes have three components to their makeup. As with other aspects of human behavior, attitudes involve a cognitive, affective, and behavioral component. The *cognitive* component includes our beliefs and thoughts. The *affective* component pertains to the feelings or emotions that are conjured up when we think about a target (object, person, or event). The *behavioral* component again predisposes us to act in a certain way. So, in the case of persons with antisocial personality disorder, some people "believe" that those with antisocial personality disorders are rude and uncaring toward others. This may cause some people to "feel" anger toward persons with personality disorders and, in turn, also "behave" rudely or totally avoid contact with this population.

Ostrom et al. (1994) further distinguish between three ways in which attitudes influence or function for us in our daily lives. A previously formed attitude *predisposes* us to behaving in a certain way when encountering or anticipating an encounter with a target. We *interpret* new events or situations we encounter, which assists us in categorizing the target and deciding how to behave next time (i.e., "I don't like scary movies; therefore, I will avoid going to them"). We then *evaluate* or assess the new encounter, which, in turn, helps us form our opinions or beliefs about the target.

As such, attitudes function to minimize our discomfort in negotiating our environment from day to day because we continuously interpret and evaluate it, generally acting in ways that minimize our discomfort unless we have little choice, such as in a job interview or taking an examination. For example, some people feel uncomfortable or anxious about passing homeless persons without giving them money. This may lead them to avoid making eye contact or to ignore a homeless person as they walk by. Still others may believe that homeless persons are lazy (predisposition/interpretation/cognition), causing them to defiantly walk past a homeless person and give them a dirty look (behavior).

Finally, it is important to note that people are not always consistent in the three components that form attitudes. An individual's beliefs and affect toward another person or group of people may be very different from how he or she outwardly behaves. In situations where people perceive they have little control, they may behave in a way that is socially desirable and appear to like the person. For instance, an employee who despises his or her boss may nevertheless be outwardly very friendly to him or her for some perceived ulterior reason (e.g., being promoted or avoiding being fired). Having laid the foundation for how attitudes are defined and developed, we now turn our attention to attitude formation regarding persons with disabilities.

ATTITUDES TOWARD DISABILITY: POSITIVE, NEGATIVE, OR AMBIVALENT?

Inherent Problems in Attitude Measurement

There has been a great deal of debate among researchers as to not only whether we can accurately measure attitudes toward disability but also whether peoples' attitudes are positive, negative, or ambivalent (Antonak & Livneh, 2000; Makas, 1988). The answer to this question is too complex to ever be able to generalize about society as a whole. Chubon (1982), in a critical review of the literature on attitude measurement during the 1970s, found numerous problems with the findings researchers were making. First, only 60 of the 102 articles he reviewed were empirical studies; the remaining were editorials or conceptual papers having no empirical basis. Second, in the empirical studies, there appeared to be differing attitudes based on the type of disability being studied. For example, Sowa and Cutter (1974) found that persons with alcohol or substance abuse problems were viewed more negatively by some professionals. Tringo (1970) also found that respondents ranked physical disability more positively than sensory impairments or brain injury. As such, attitude surveys, many of which often essentially cluster all disabilities into one homogeneous group, contained little meaningful value. Chubon (1982) also noted that many attitude instruments were poorly validated and had poor internal validity, a sentiment also echoed by Antonak and Livneh (1988). Finally, a number of studies used college students as participants, which again had limited generalizability to the attitudes of the general public (Comer & Piliavin, 1975; Fichten & Bourdon, 1986; Makas, 1988).

Wright (1988) further argued that scientists have a predisposed "fundamental negative bias" (p. 3) when conducting attitude studies about disability. She indicated that some measurement instruments themselves are laden with negatively biased labels (e.g., former developmentally disabled patient, amputee). Researchers also tend to make the disability the most salient aspect of the survey without accounting for other factors that help form our attitudes toward others, such as age, education, physical appearance, socioeconomic status, and so on (Antonak & Livneh, 2000). Many of the attitude survey instruments focus solely on the disability. Wright (1988) further noted how people tend to rate relationships with a stranger more negatively than with someone they know. In other words, it is inaccurate to conclude that participants necessarily have a negative attitude toward persons with disabilities solely based on administering a survey where the disability is the most salient feature and where the person with the disability is a stranger.

We must take into account the effect of the stranger relationship. Indeed, this argument was confirmed in the 1991 Lou Harris poll, which showed that able-bodied persons had more favorable attitudes toward persons with disabilities when they knew someone with a disability (Harris, 1991). A third criticism Wright (1988) asserted pertains to negatively loaded statements about disability in surveys that connote something negative about disability (e.g., persons with disabilities should pay more for auto insurance). This example alludes to the myth that persons with disabilities are unsafe drivers, and Wright argues that such negatively laden statements perpetuate stereotypes. A fourth fundamental negative bias committed by researchers deals with ignoring findings that do not meet statistical significance. Researchers become so motivated to obtain statistically significant findings (which show differences and increase chances of publication) that they ignore the meaningfulness of obtaining no differences. Findings showing how persons with disabilities are similar to able-bodied persons have typically been ignored. As Goffman (1963) observed, persons with disabilities are stigmatized as being "different" and are therefore reduced or discounted as a people. This was further confirmed in the 1992 Harris survey where a majority of respondents reported that persons with disabilities were viewed as fundamentally different from those without disabilities.

Harold Yuker, in his 1988 book *Attitudes Toward Persons with Disabilities*, supported Wright's (1988) argument that researchers have a knowing or unknowing negative bias in developing and interpreting attitude survey findings by making the disability the most salient aspect of the survey, while ignoring other factors that social psychologists have long since shown affect people's attitudes. Yuker and others describe what some of these other important factors are.

PHYSICAL ATTRACTIVENESS

Research suggests that people rated as more physically attractive create more favorable impressions than those rated less attractive (Longo & Ashmore, 1995). Physically attractive people are also generally perceived to be more kind, intelligent, interesting, responsive, likable, competent, sociable, outgoing, and poised and more likely to be promoted in their jobs (Eagly et al., 1991; Longo & Ashmore, 1995; Yuker, 1988). American and other industrialized countries' societal values and corporate advertisers bombard the media with magazines, commercials, movies, and so on around the youthful perfect male and female body type as well as its perceived relationship to wealth, fame, and idolization. Conversely, older persons are perceived as having poor health and being wrinkled and ugly (Haboush et al., 2012; Halliwell & Dittmar, 2003).

COMPETENCE

Persons viewed as being competent are perceived as being more attractive and credible (Yuker, 1988). Like physical attractiveness, there is no empirical evidence to support the assumption that attractive persons are indeed any more competent or intelligent than persons perceived to be unattractive. Nonetheless, many in society continue to perceive persons with disabilities as incompetent. Wright (1983) described the concept of "spread" pertaining to how some persons without disabilities assume that someone with a physical disability may also be mentally developmentally delayed. This belief often plays out, for example, when a nondisabled person goes to a restaurant with someone who uses a wheelchair, and the waiter asks the nondisabled partner what the wheelchair user would like to order, thus erroneously perceiving the wheelchair user as mentally unable to order for himself or herself.

SOCIAL SKILLS

Social poise, including nonverbal behavior and the ability to interact with others, is also perceived as more attractive and likable (Gresham, 1982). Good social skills have been demonstrated to be important in mainstreaming children, as well as in employment and promotion (Collmann & Newlyn, 1957; Oberle, 1975). Conversely, poor social skills have been shown to lead to rejection or negative attitudes toward persons with developmental disabilities (MacMillan & Morrison, 1980).

Other important factors that influence attitudes that are not considered in attitude measurements are the relationship of age, education, socioeconomic status, and personality variables (Antonak & Livneh, 2000; Yuker, 1988). We tend to like and feel more comfortable with others who are similar to us. Therefore, being of the same ethnic background, age, education, and socioeconomic status all have an influence on our attitudes and lowers interaction anxiety because such individuals are much like us and we perceive to have more in common with them (Gosse & Sheppard, 1979; McGuire, 1969; Rabkin, 1972; Sue & Sue, 1999).

ATTITUDES TOWARD DISABILITY

There exists a plethora of empirical and anecdotal studies and books documenting that, for the most part, attitudes toward people with disabilities most often tend to be stereotypically negative in nature (Chan et al., 2009; Chubon, 1994; Donaldson, 1980; Livneh, 1988; Olkin, 1999; Wright, 1988). The next section addresses 16 commonly perceived origins or causes of negative attitudes, also identifying studies related to positive attitudes and those that indicate attitudes toward disability in general as neither positive nor negative, but rather ambivalent.

Mackelprang and Salsgiver (2009), for example, discuss common stereotypical attitudes toward persons with disabilities covering a variety of themes. First is the notion that persons with disabilities are perpetual children, citing the annual March of Dimes telethons and "Jerry's kids" years ago, referring to how Jerry Lewis used to portray people with muscular dystrophy, regardless of their age. This sentiment is also evident in the medical model paradigm today, in which some physicians treat their patients with disabilities as children. Second is the stereotype that people with disabilities are objects of pity, as evidenced again in telethons but also in news and media coverage where common descriptors such as "tragedy" and "victim" are overused. Third is the notion that people with severe mental illness are a menace or threat to society. This is portrayed in numerous movies and television characters, including psychotic serial killers in television police dramas concerning those with schizophrenia or described as psychopaths (Byrd et al., 1977). Group homes for those with developmental and intellectual disabilities are often vehemently protested by concerned parents who fear for their children's lives because they believe these populations will sexually assault or attack their children. Fourth is the perception by some that persons with disabilities are sick, asexual, helpless, and incompetent and therefore need to be cared for. They are also relieved of any responsibility to contribute to society because they are incapable of doing so. A fifth stereotype centers around disability as a psychological and economic burden to society, consuming resources without providing anything in return. This sentiment is similar to the ones held by the Nazis and eugenicists, which ultimately led to confinement, sterilization, and extermination.

Origins of Negative Attitudes

Livneh (1991) and others have postulated a number of reasons regarding the origins of negative attitudes toward persons with disabilities. These are discussed or combined with other plausible reasons as to why persons with and without disabilities may possess less favorable attitudes toward those with disabilities. In all, 16 different hypotheses are proposed and are adapted from Livneh's original work.

1. *Attributional origins*: Plotnik defines attributions as "the things we point to as the causes of events, other people's behaviors, and our own behaviors" (Plotnik, 1996, p. 537). Studies have shown that European Americans tend to attribute blame to internal reasons (i.e., Jack did not get the job because he lacked the qualifications), whereas persons of minority tend to attribute blame to external or environmental factors (i.e., Jack did not get the job because the employer discriminated against him; Sue & Sue, 1999). Similarly, individuals who are perceived as having caused their own disability receive more negative appraisals than those perceived as not having contributed to their situation (Bordieri, 1993; Marantz, 1990; Murphy, 1998; Obermann, 1965; Zola, 1983). In general, military veterans are viewed more positively, whereas persons with alcohol and substance abuse disorders, HIV/AIDS, and mental illness are viewed more negatively because of a common belief that their disability was self-inflicted or results from a weak personality (Bickenbach, 1993; Hayes et al., 1999; Safilios-Rothschild, 1982).

2. *Blaming the victim*: Wright (1983) defines the concept of blaming the victim, which, although sounding similar to attributional origins in definition, is distinctively different. Blaming the victim for his or her circumstances is not just limited to disabilities considered to be self-imposed (i.e., substance abuse). It is a psychological safety mechanism designed to minimize our fears and anxiety as to why something bad cannot happen to us. If I can justify to myself that I am a better driver than my reckless neighbor who was recently in an accident and fractured his neck, it serves to minimize my fears that such events can randomly occur anytime and happen to anyone.

3. *Disability as a punishment for sin*: Despite its early origins in beliefs, some people continue to believe that disability is a punishment from God for having sinned (Byrd, 1990). This may be especially true for those who follow the teachings of the Bible closely. As noted in Chapter 1, there are passages in the Bible that allude to persons being healed of their disability by repenting their sins (Gallagher, 1995). Meng (1938, as cited by Livneh, 1991) cited three

unconscious mechanisms of punishment for sin attributions. These relate to the belief that the individual has sinned; he or she is disabled unjustly and therefore is now motivated to sin; or, projecting one's own sinful impulses onto the person with a disability, he or she is evil.

4. *Anxiety-provoking situations*: Several research studies have explored the reported anxiety persons with and without disabilities express in unstructured (or even structured) interactions (Albrecht et al., 1982; Kleck, 1968; Marinelli, 1974; Marini, 1992). Anxiety or discomfort is typically experienced when people are in ambiguous social situations where they do not know what to say or how to behave (Albrecht et al., 1982). Nondisabled persons often have an irrational fear of unintentionally offending someone with a disability that might upset them (i.e., telling a person who is blind that you went to "see" a movie last night). In Leary's (1990) literature review regarding social anxiety, he indicated that people initially assess a social situation in terms of its costs and rewards. If the perceived costs of an anticipated interaction outweigh the rewards, individuals will most likely avoid the interaction altogether. As such, if persons with or without disabilities perceive that an interaction with the other has little value or reward attached to it and the anticipated interaction provokes discomfort or anxiety, social avoidance will likely occur (Piliavin & Piliavin, 1972). Kleck (1968) demonstrated how persons without disabilities held less eye contact and ended interactions sooner with persons with disabilities than they did with those without disabilities.

5. *Childhood influences*: Livneh (1991) and others also believe that young children are influenced as they grow up in forming attitudes toward others (Vash & Crewe, 2004). Sometimes when children hurt themselves for doing something they should not be doing, parents scold them by saying "God punishes you when you are bad," which can later be misconstrued when encountering someone with a disability. The authors state how young children are sometimes scurried away from interacting with someone with a disability in public; however, this action thwarts the child's natural curiosity and leaves him or her with a sense that "these people" (with disabilities) are somehow different and need to be avoided. Thus, if children grow up having had little opportunity to interact and learn about people with disabilities, they tend to fear what they do not understand and tend to derive their attitudes from prevailing myths or misconceptions (Begab, 1970).

6. *Sociocultural conditioning*: Livneh (1991) discussed several societal and cultural norms that have had a negative impact on attitudes toward disability. Western society is almost obsessed with physical appearance and the "body beautiful" concept (Buss, 1999). Seligman (1993) described how Americans spend billions of dollars each year on self-improvement programs and products, such as dieting, exercise devices, workout videos, cosmetic facial creams or surgery, hair coloring, liposuction, gastric bypass surgery, plastic surgery, and so on. Social media platforms and influencers have amplified this barrage of marketing. Television commercials and magazine ads depict young, athletic, healthy, medically inadvisably thin, physically attractive people promoting consumer products; however, none of the actors or, recently, influencers are persons with disabilities (Halliwell & Dittmar, 2003; Smart, 2009). As noted in Chapter 1, some people will pay thousands of dollars for a supermodel's ovarian egg. Western society also admires persons who are successful and wealthy (Haboush et al., 2012). Many celebrities, athletes, and musicians are highly admired and publicized in our culture (Safilios-Rothschild, 1968). Few people with disabilities seemingly fall into this esteemed category, and instead are perceived as objects of charity, many of whom are perceived as poor, helpless, sick, and incapable of making decisions (Biklen, 1986; Olkin & Howson, 1994).

7. *Psychodynamic factors*: These pertain to views held by nondisabled persons toward those with disabilities in relation to unconscious psychological processes developed during childhood. Wright (1960, 1983) first described a *requirement of mourning*, where an individual with a disability is expected to grieve the loss of body function and preinjury way of life. Nondisabled persons may inherently expect persons with disabilities to experience ongoing sadness, and, if they do not, they are accused of being in denial and may draw criticism from others (Dembo et al., 1956). Another psychodynamic variable relates to living in a *just world*: the perception that people generally get what they deserve (Walster, 1966; Yamamoto, 1971). We rationalize or justify why someone becomes disabled as either punishment for some misdeed (much like childhood influences) or because he or she was inept (attributional blame), which safely justifies why such an injury will not happen to us. This serves to reduce existential anxiety over the randomness of events and the fear that bad things can indeed happen to good people. This is similar to Wright's *blaming the victim* concept. The concept of *spread* is another unconscious origin of negative attitudes, whereby it is assumed that a disability envelops or spreads to define all aspects of the individual (Wright, 1960, 1983). Someone with a physical disability is believed to be mentally impaired as well; thus, the disability becomes the single most salient defining feature of the individual.

8. *Existential angst*: Smart (2009) describes the fear nondisabled persons experience in becoming disabled themselves. Being in the presence of someone with a disability reminds us of our vulnerability to also acquire a disability. Schilder (1935) viewed this unconscious fear as a threat to one's body image. This is similar to why many people do not like going to hospitals, nursing homes, or funerals or making their will. In all instances, we may experience discomfort in contemplating our own deterioration and eventual death. For some nondisabled persons, disability brings these unpleasant thoughts into consciousness, and such thoughts can be disturbing. Therefore, as a defense mechanism, some persons without disabilities may prefer to avoid those with disabilities to repress these fears (out of sight, out of mind; Siller et al., 1967). Siller et al. (1967) further discuss the concept of *fear of contamination*, whereby nondisabled persons fear that by interacting with someone with a disability, they too might become disabled, or by marrying someone with a disability, their offspring will be disabled. There is also a perceived related stigma that there must be something wrong with a nondisabled person if he or she has to associate with someone with a disability.

9. *Aesthetic aversion*: Livneh (1991) describes aesthetic-sexual aversion in relation to what society finds visually pleasing or repulsing to the eye. Certain disabilities, such as amputation, facial disfigurement, and deformity, are perceived as repulsive to look at, despite the fact that we have a morbid curiosity to stare. Fox and Marini (2018) cite the 1887–1913 "ugly laws" passed by various U.S. cities, including Chicago, where the law deemed that:

    Any person who is diseased, maimed, mutilated or in any way deformed so as to be unsightly or disgusting object, or an improper person to be allowed in or on the streets, highways, and thoroughfares or public places in this city shall not there in or thereof expose himself or herself in public view under penalty of one dollar for each offense. On the conviction of any person for violation of this section, if it shall seem proper and just, the fine provided may be suspended, and such person detained at the police station, where he shall be well cared for, until he can be committed to the County poorhouse (Coco, 2010, p. 25). The conflicting cognition of wanting to stare and concomitantly look away generates discomfort. Aesthetics relates to the concept of beauty as in the eye of the beholder, and as discussed earlier, Western society dictates that beautiful people are those who are deemed physically attractive, thin, wealthy, and successful.

10. *Minority status*: Despite an estimated 73 million persons reporting a disability (2020 U.S. Census) in the United States, persons with disabilities are marginalized and disenfranchised more than any other group in North America. As a member of a minority group, societal perceptions of people with disabilities are that they are poor, helpless, sick, and incapable (Biklen, 1986; Mackelprang & Salsgiver, 2009). Being an ethnic minority, having a disability, and being female triples misperceived stereotypes and is statistically evidenced by disparities in employment rates, education levels, and poverty levels (Szymanski et al., 1996; Wright, 1988).

11. *Prejudice-inviting behavior*: Wright (1960) described how some persons with disabilities behave in a way that strengthens negative stereotypes toward them. This includes acting fearful, helpless, passive, and dependent; not standing up for oneself; and seeking secondary gains, such as acting helpless to receive attention (Livneh, 1991). Such behaviors confirm society's views that persons with disabilities need to be cared for and are inferior.

12. *Disability-related factors*: Livneh (1991) and others described several disability-specific factors that suggest some disabilities or dynamics are viewed more negatively than others (Safilios-Rothschild, 1970). There are inconclusive results as to whether nondisabled persons have more negative attitudes toward certain disabilities as opposed to others (Goodyear, 1983; Schmelkin, 1984; Stovall & Sedlacek, 1983). Schmelkin (1984) concluded that preferences toward disability could not be hierarchically ranked due to the multidimensionality factors related to it (e.g., severity, cause, gender, age, type of disability). Smart (2009) asserts, however, that a hierarchy of stigma does exist toward disability, backed by several studies indicating that of four disability categories, persons with physical disabilities are least stigmatized, followed by those with cognitive disabilities, those with intellectual disabilities, and those with mental illness (Antonak, 1980; Charlton, 1998; Tringo, 1970). It further appears that individuals believed to have caused or contributed to their own misfortune are rated more negatively. Weiner et al. (1988) found that persons with physical disabilities were not viewed as having caused their disabilities, but those with emotional and behavioral disabilities were to blame due to perceptions of being weak-willed. Yamamoto (1971) found that curable and predictable disabilities were viewed less negatively than those that were chronic or unpredictable. There is also some support that the more severe, visible, and aesthetically aversive a disability is, the less favorable the attitudes may be (Shontz, 1964; Siller, 1963). Olkin (1999) noted that in initial contacts with someone with a disability, appearance and severity of the disability do influence attitudes. However, initial negative attitudes can be diminished once the individual with a disability becomes better known and is able to demonstrate the disability is just one trait. If the person with a disability is perceived as being attractive and competent and possesses good social poise, these factors create more positive attitudes.

    More recently, graduate social workers proffered similar disability-specific attitude preferences over working with certain disabilities. Jensen et al. (2017) found social workers had a more positive attitude working toward those with depression as opposed to those with schizophrenia, who they rated more negatively due to the perception of the unpredictability of dangerous behavior. Similarly, Werner and Araten-Bergman (2017) found their sample of social worker attitudes toward persons with mental illness received as being more responsible for their condition as well as dangerous compared to those with intellectual disabilities.

1. *Media portrayals of disability*: Perhaps the most influential factor in facilitating and perpetuating negative attitudes toward disability is the effect of the media (Anderson, 1988; Black & Pretes, 2007; Byrd et al., 1977; Hadley & Brodwin, 1988; Marini, 1992). Couldry and Hepp (2017) note that the media not only reflects the world we live in but

also contributes to the construction of social realities. There is no coincidence in the correlation between societal attitudes of those with disabilities being asexual, helpless, unemployed, or villains based on movies such as *Forrest Gump, Me before You, Phantom of the Opera, Hunchback of Notre Dame,* and *The Sessions,* to name a few. Television, newspapers, and magazines often reinforce negative stereotypes about disability. Byrd et al. (1977) found that of the 64 shows depicting disability, 51 were police dramas, movies, and comedies that made scant effort to educate viewers, and in a majority of the police dramas, the character with the disability often was a psychopathic killer. In a later study, Byrd (1989) found that 49 of 67 characters portrayed in 302 films had abnormal personalities. Other characteristics of portrayals indicated that in more than 50% of the films, the person with a disability was portrayed as being a victim, more than 50% of the characters with disabilities were not given an occupation, and the fate of the character with a disability was given a negative or neutral ending in 67% of the films. The absence of persons with disabilities in media also conveys a different message. Persons with disabilities are rarely seen in television commercials or magazine advertisements (Smart, 2009). The absence of persons with disabilities enjoying themselves, purchasing and consuming goods, and socializing in restaurants or other public venues indirectly conveys the message that people with disabilities do not get out much and are sick and helpless. Similarly, the typical language reporters use in newspapers and magazines pertaining to persons with disabilities also facilitates negative attitudes, while sensationalized news headlines often perpetuate society's fears about persons with mental illness. Whenever someone with schizophrenia injures or murders someone, and despite the fact that persons with mental illness are statistically less violent than the general population (Gostin, 2008), the lay public generalizes and fears all persons with schizophrenia. In addition, journalists and reporters often cover disability stories by making the disability the salient focus of the story to titillate the reader's emotions with the use of common descriptive words such as *victim, tragedy,* or *courage,* depending on the story angle (Margolis et al., 1990). In addition, because telethons receive more donations when viewers are made to feel for the recipients (e.g., muscular dystrophy telethon), it comes as no surprise when nondisabled Americans indicate the most common sentiments they feel toward persons with disabilities are pity and/or admiration (Harris, 1991).

2. *Demographic variables related to nondisabled persons*: A number of researchers have explored factors related to nondisabled persons and their attitudes toward disability. Findings reveal the following: (a) Females tend to have more positive attitudes toward persons with disabilities than do males (Antonak & Livneh, 2000; Chesler, 1965; English, 1971a; Keesler, 2021). (b) Young children (age 6 years) show a preference for playing with nondisabled children (Weinberg, 1978), whereas persons in late childhood and adulthood appear to have more positive attitudes than older persons (Ryan, 1981). (c) Persons with higher levels of education generally have more positive attitudes (Tunick et al., 1979). (d) Overlapping with education is socioeconomic status, where several studies have shown that those with higher incomes typically manifest more favorable attitudes (English, 1971b; Whiteman & Lukoff, 1965), although Olkin (1999) notes that this is not always the case. Livneh (1991) further noted that certain personality traits may predispose some persons to possess negative attitudes; however, Yuker (1994) warned against conducting such studies due to the futility in being able to change one's personality. Nevertheless, several studies have suggested that persons who were ethnocentric possessed poorer attitudes (Wright, 1960), as do persons with higher levels of anxiety in ambiguous or uncertain situations (Cloerkes, 1981; Fichten & Bourdon, 1986; Marinelli & Kelz, 1973). Further, nondisabled persons with a higher self-concept appear to possess more positive attitudes than those with a lower

self-concept (Jabin, 1966; Yuker, 1962). Finally, persons with a more positive body image and scoring high on ego strength also possessed more positive attitudes toward disability than those with low ego strength and poor body image (LeClair & Rockwell, 1980; Noonan et al. 1970; Siller, 1964).

3. *Perceptions of burden*: Without any prior knowledge or experience, many nondisabled persons automatically assume that disability connotes a "burden." Olkin (1999) noted how many researchers studying disability in families are biased from the onset regarding their findings and look for the burdening and stressing aspects of caring for someone with a disability. She cited numerous studies with the word *burden* in the title and suggested that the simple repetition of these ideas permeates consciousness. Olkin further noted that many parent–child studies where the child is born with a disability are conducted sometime shortly after the birth of the child, when parents are most distressed. Such findings, she argues, are negatively skewed as the parents attempt to come to terms with the situation. In opposing research discussed in Chapter 10, many caregivers do not perceive their loved one as a burden, are less depressed or stressed than was previously hypothesized, feel a sense of purpose in caring for their loved one, and overwhelmingly would choose to care for their disabled loved one at home rather than placing the person in a nursing home (Bogdan & Taylor, 1989; Lawrence et al., 1998; Smart, 2009). Marini et al. (2013) found that among Caucasian and Hispanic undergraduate students asked about establishing an intimate relationship with someone with a physical disability, "perceived it would involve 'too much caregiving,'" which was cited as the number one reason why they would not consider such a relationship. Recently, Kalargyrou et al. (2021), studying attitudes toward persons with physical disabilities in relation to other disabilities with 395 undergraduate students in Austria, found the students had more positive attitudes in terms of working with persons with disabilities but not more intimate situations such as dating or marriage. This was particularly the case in singling out potential marriage partners with persons with physical disabilities.

4. *Environmental factors*: Environmental barriers (inaccessible establishments) that exclude persons with disabilities from fully participating in society and the community can also indirectly lead to negative attitudes (Graf et al., 2009; Hammel et al., 2015; Hastbacka et al., 2016). An unwelcoming environment can, in turn, negatively impact those with disabilities in terms of how they perceive their disability, their self-concept, and their self-esteem (Graf et al., 2009; Hergenrather et al., 2005). When persons with disabilities are not employed or find social establishments where contact with others is still inaccessible after the Americans with Disabilities Act (ADA), it diminishes the likelihood of social networking and relationship building. Numerous studies (see Yuker, 1988) suggest that contact with persons with disabilities generally enhances positive attitudes; therefore, if that contact is unable to occur, educating or enhancing others about disability cannot ensue.

Positive Attitudes or Traits Ascribed to People With Disabilities

Although studies of positive attitudes toward persons with disabilities are much fewer in number than those dealing with negative attitudes, the findings nevertheless are consistent with other studies in that people without disabilities often make assumptions about groups they have little knowledge about. As such, these perceived positive stereotypes about people with disabilities are no more accurate than are the negative traits ascribed to them.

Persons with disabilities are sometimes ascribed angelical traits, despite the apparent paradox of attitudes that disability is a punishment for having sinned. Mitchell (1976) had respondents rate counselor effectiveness by viewing videotaped interviews of counselors who were wheelchair users versus counselors who had no disability. The counselors who used wheelchairs were rated more effective and positively by both male and female respondents; however, female respondents rated the counselors in wheelchairs significantly more effective in areas of empathic understanding, level of regard, and congruence.

Comer and Piliavin (1975) compared the attitudes of a group of persons without a disability versus persons who were disabled for some time versus those who had acquired a disability within the past year. Participants were asked to rate three photographs: one of a White male using a wheelchair, one individual with an amputation, and a third of a nondisabled Black male. The nondisabled participants rated the two persons with disabilities as more intelligent, sensible, and admirable. Conversely, respondents who were disabled for a long time rated the nondisabled person more positively than respondents who became recently disabled. The authors suggested that those who were injured for a long time realized that there were no saintly qualities to being disabled, as are sometimes bestowed on persons with disabilities for assumedly being courageous in dealing with adversity.

As noted earlier, pity and admiration are common emotions expressed toward those with disabilities. One might initially think that inspirational stories in which persons with disabilities have accomplished some goal would enhance development of positive attitudes toward disability. Zola (1991), however, described the double message meaning after watching media reports on Franklin Delano Roosevelt and Wilma Rudolph. He explained how the message that is directly conveyed to the general public is that people with disabilities can accomplish great things (e.g., become president or an Olympic runner). Unfortunately, the indirect double message conveyed is that if others with disabilities are not successful, it is their own failure, weakness, or lack of motivation. This concept of blame relates back to how the majority culture tends to blame the individual, whereas persons in minority cultures often tend to attribute blame to external causes (Sue & Sue, 1999). Smart (2009) refers to disabled heroes as "super crips," a term used primarily by persons with disabilities to describe those who have overcome insurmountable odds to succeed.

It has become apparent that more contemporary writers addressing the psychosocial issues of persons with disabilities have philosophically approached the topic from a *social constructivist* viewpoint (Chan et al., 2009; Chubon, 1994; Hammel et al., 2015; Hastbacka et al., 2016; Mackelprang & Salsgiver, 2009; Smart, 2009). Social psychologists and sociologists have been addressing disability from this viewpoint for some time. The social construct model of disability (aka the minority or environmental model) posits blame for the handicapping elements of a disability with faults in the environmental and attitudinal barriers imposed by society (Blackwell et al., 2001; Graf et al., 2009). Situations such as employment discrimination or opposing the building of a halfway house for persons with mental illness in residential areas are examples of attitudinal barriers, whereas being unable to enter a restaurant with stairs if you use a wheelchair exemplifies an environmental barrier to social participation. The World Health Organization (WHO, 1980) defines *disability* as the consequences of impairment in terms of functional performance, while *impairment* refers to abnormalities of body structure and appearance with organ or system function resulting from any cause. This, in turn, may or may not lead to a *handicap*, defined as disadvantages experienced by the individual as a result of impairments and disabilities. Handicap thus reflects an interaction with, and adaptation to, an individual's surroundings or environment. In other words, an individual may have a disability (spinal cord injury) caused by an impairment (paralysis), but is not otherwise handicapped in crossing a street if there are curb cuts. He does, however, become handicapped from crossing the street if there are no curb cuts.

Are People Really Ambivalent Toward Disability?

Several researchers argue that the general public's attitudes toward disability are mainly ambivalence because they essentially have not formed an opinion one way or another (Makas, 1988). Persons who have little or no contact with persons with disabilities likely do not give the issue much thought (out of sight, out of mind) until a situation presents itself. Makas (1988) argued that many nondisabled persons misunderstand what even constitutes a positive attitude. She developed a 37-item multidimensional attitude survey, the *Issues in Disability Scale* (IDS, formerly titled Modified Issues in Disability Scale), where the questions are worded in such a neutral way that the survey taker is unable to answer in a socially desirable manner. In one study, comparing the responses of persons with disabilities versus those without disabilities, nondisabled respondents scored significantly differently in their response to the question, "If a person with epilepsy becomes angry with people over little things, it should be overlooked because of his/her disability." Respondents with disabilities expressed essentially not feeling sorry for someone with epilepsy, whereas those without a disability perceived the anger and frustration someone having epilepsy might feel (making the disability salient), thereby believing that such behaviors are acceptable considering the circumstances. Another example is the question, "For a severely disabled person, the kindness of others is more important than any educational program." Once again, respondents with disabilities viewed education as a means to earn equal status and likely interpreted the kindness of others as paternalistic, whereas those without disabilities viewed being kind as a sign of compassion. On a more subconscious level, in viewing the importance of kindness over education, persons without disabilities may be expressing the negative belief that persons with disabilities are unlikely to complete an educational program, and therefore, kindness and charitable donations are indeed more important.

Katz et al. (1988) opined that attitudes toward disability are ambivalent due to conflicting cognitions of wanting to help and wanting to avoid an encounter. Although there exist a number of studies indicating the anxiety many nondisabled persons have in interacting with someone with a disability (wanting to avoid), some studies indicate that where there is a clearly defined need to provide assistance, the likelihood of an interaction increases (Stephens et al., 1985). Stephens et al. (1985) found that nondisabled persons spent more time and gave more assistance in helping a wheelchair-using female look for a lost earring when compared with a female without a disability. Stephens et al. concluded that the social obligation toward helping someone who is perceived as not being able to help himself or herself overrides interaction anxiety, or the desire to avoid the situation. It may be that we are so conditioned to offer some sort of assistance toward those with disabilities (e.g., open the door, give to charity, volunteer time) that when an opportunity to simply interact with someone with a disability occurs, many nondisabled persons basically do not know what to say or do. Another potential barrier to interacting with individuals regardless of having a disability or not is simply the perception of not having anything in common with the other person and basically little to talk about (Leary, 1990).

Overall, it is likely that attitudes toward persons with disabilities depend on many of the factors discussed earlier. Measuring attitudes is too complex to generalize the results of any one study or combination of studies and relate them to the general population (Antonak & Livneh, 1988, 2000). Indeed, some people with and without a disability do possess negative attitudes to varying degrees, ranging from blatant prejudice to simple ignorance and misinformation. Similarly, some persons with and without disabilities possess positive attitudes toward those with disabilities. Research indicates that in many instances, such persons have had previous contact with or exposure to someone with a disability that was a positive experience (Chan et al., 2009; Yuker, 1988). Finally, people without disabilities who have had limited or no exposure to those with disabilities may not harbor any preconceived positive or negative attitudes because they have not given the topic much thought. These individuals are simply ambivalent or apathetic to the subject and may be influenced by education and exposure to persons with disabilities. The next section focuses on improving the social consciousness toward disability.

Improving the Social Consciousness Regarding Attitudes Toward Disability

Havranek (1991) has indicated that although we can mandate legislative changes to improve access and equal rights for persons with disabilities, we unfortunately cannot mandate people's attitudes. Bowe (1978) further claimed that the greatest barrier facing persons with disabilities today is societal attitudes. Despite the numerous civil and human rights laws, discrimination and indifference still exist. As such, and having reviewed the common reasons how and why people possess negative attitudes toward disability, it becomes important to explore what factors and conditions are necessary to potentially enhance people's attitudes. Research findings essentially delineate such studies into three general categories: (a) increased contact and familiarity with persons with a disability; (b) providing accurate education and information that minimize misconceptions about disability; and (c) mixing contact with education, or essentially having the educator be a person with a disability.

Contact

Within the realm of exploring attitudes toward disability lie a number of studies pertaining to the influence of contact with or exposure to someone with a disability. Yuker (1988) found that of the 274 studies relating to contact between someone with and without a disability, 51% of the studies suggested that participants' attitudes became more positive, 39% of the studies were inconclusive, and 10% of the studies reported that participants had a more negative attitude after contact. Yuker believed that certain factors must be present for a positive change in attitude to occur. He surmised from his analysis that persons with disabilities must be perceived as possessing good communication and social skills, be perceived as competent, and be willing to self-disclose some information about their disabilities in an unemotional manner. Yuker further concluded that the interaction must be reciprocal and not a one-sided conversation, where each participant gains some reward from the interaction.

The concept of each participant gaining something from the interaction was discussed earlier concerning Leary's (1990) research on social anxiety. Leary believed that we regularly cognitively assess whether we have something to gain from an anticipated social interaction, regardless of whether someone has a disability. If the individual perceives nothing can be gained from the interaction, he or she will tend to avoid the situation. When a disability is then entered into the equation, we know from other studies that many nondisabled persons feel anxious in not knowing what to say or how to behave, and therefore are likely to avoid the interaction altogether (Albrecht et al., 1982; Kleck, 1968; Marinelli & Kelz, 1973; Piliavin & Piliavin, 1972). Wright (1988) described the stranger phenomenon (we may avoid first-time interactions with nondisabled persons for the same reasons) and that researchers must be careful in analyzing such findings so as to not make the disability salient.

Albrecht et al.'s (1982) finding that some people feel anxious in not knowing what to say or how to behave has also been linked to an irrational fear that many nondisabled persons have: namely, the myth that a person with a disability may become emotional about his or her situation. Evans (1976) concluded from his review of previous attitude studies that nondisabled persons likely have conflicting thoughts of not wanting to offend, wanting to approach due to curiosity while concomitantly wanting to avoid due to discomfort, and trying not to stare or say the wrong thing. He recommended that it is largely up to the person with a disability to put others at ease about the disability. This is accomplished by explaining a little bit about the disability and how it was acquired. In addition, if the person with the disability can talk about the disability in an unemotional manner, this conveys that the person is "okay" with his or her situation. This strategy serves to minimize the curiosity many nondisabled persons may have about the story behind the disability as well as indicating that the person with the disability can talk about it without becoming emotional. Sagatun (1985) found, however, that although nondisabled persons liked it better when the person with the disability initiated contact first and acknowledged his or her disability, persons with disabilities preferred the nondisabled person to initiate contact and ask about the disability rather than having to volunteer that information. Persons without disabilities seem to prefer those with disabilities to acknowledge their situation, to more or less get it out of the way, whereas many persons with disabilities do not like volunteering such information if it does not "fit" into the flow or context of the conversation. These findings are further supported in studies by Belgrave (1984), Belgrave and Mills (1981), and Evans (1976).

Children's attitudes toward disability can be positively influenced at an early age based largely on contact and regular exposure to those with disabilities (Armstrong et al., 2016). Armstrong et al. (2016) assessed 1,881 children regarding their self-reported contact with persons with disabilities, the children's attitudes, social anxiety in interacting, and empathy for persons with disabilities. The authors found that those students with more contact had more positive attitudes toward disability, less anticipated anxiety in interacting, and greater empathy for persons with disabilities.

Barr and Bracchitta (2015) similarly measured younger individuals' contact with persons of varying disabilities (physical, developmental, and behavioral disabilities). The authors found that contact overall helped to reduce misconceptions and stereotypes. Participants held the most positive attitudes toward contact with those with physical disabilities and moderately so for behavioral disabilities. The least favorable contact and attitudes were expressed for those with developmental disabilities. The authors opined that as younger individuals learn to develop empathy for others, positive attitudes through greater exposure will occur.

Finally, as noted by Yuker (1988), Donaldson (1980) concluded that in order for positive attitudes to ensue from social contact, the individual with the disability must be perceived as having "equal status" in relation to age, education, competence, and occupation. It should be noted that these same qualities, as well as the factors Yuker (1988) cites regarding possessing good social skills, are basically the same factors necessary for anyone to decide whether he or she is interested in becoming acquainted with someone, regardless of disability status. Ison et al. (2010) conducted two disability awareness groups for 147 children ages 9 to 11, placing them in either a three-session group or eight-session group concerning topics surrounding environmental and contextual factors. Someone with a disability copresented. Students in the eight-session awareness program demonstrated improved knowledge, attitudes, and acceptance of disability. Showing the nondisabled students that persons with disabilities were much like them served to minimize stigma and misconceptions about persons with disabilities and view them as equal-status individuals.

Environmental factors may also be related to changing attitudes. Stewart (1988) placed two students with physical disabilities in a weight training class and pre–post tested the class after 10 weeks regarding their attitudes toward disability, compared with a control group class without any students with disabilities. Findings were significant in that attitudes became more positive for the class with the two students with physical disabilities. Conclusions drawn from this study indicate that regular contact in an equal-status environment where similar interests are perceived and engaged in is likely to enhance attitudes toward disability.

Education

Newspaper, television, and movie coverage regarding disability has traditionally conveyed more misinformation and stereotypes than accurate information (Black & Pretes, 2007; Marini, 1992). News stories about disability are typically human interest stories that depict persons with disabilities as victims of some tragedy or, conversely, stories of courage in which the individual with the disability has accomplished something "in spite of" the disability.

Aside from pure media entertainment or human interest stories that have done little to educate the public about disability, rehabilitation researchers have used attitude surveys after having participants view films to determine whether educational films regarding disability can enhance participants' attitudes. Researchers have found that when participants viewed an educational or humorous film regarding disability designed to change attitudes, participants' attitudes statistically were more positive following the film when compared with a control group (Elliott & Byrd, 1984; Matkin et al., 1983). Sadlick and Penta (1975) found similar significant results after rehabilitation nursing students were shown a film of 10 former patients with tetraplegia who were employed and doing well compared with a no-film control group. The film group scored a more positive attitude on Osgood's Semantic Differential Scale (Osgood et al., 1957) both immediately after the film and again 10 weeks later. Antonak (1982) also conducted a similar study with similar results using lay persons who viewed a slide presentation of persons with disabilities performing various activities of daily living independently in their homes. Researchers of these studies recommended avoiding pretesting attitudes, as it can invalidate findings by tipping participants off and having them answer in a socially desirable fashion at posttesting (Antonak, 1982; Matkin et al., 1983).

There are unfortunately still other researchers or therapists at universities, colleges, and rehabilitation centers who continue to use experiential sensitivity exercises, such as the disability-for-a-day or class period activities in which students/employees must ambulate in a wheelchair, wear earplugs, or use a blindfold. Although seemingly a good exercise for students to experience and better empathize with persons with disabilities, some researchers arguably have found that this exercise creates more negative attitudes than positive for several reasons. Wright (1978) was the first to criticize these activities by arguing that such exercises make the disability salient and demonstrate the initial frustration anyone in a new situation would experience. Participants are often not informed about how someone with a disability generally grows accustomed and adapts to their situation and eventually learns to problem-solve everyday barriers without a second thought. The exercises by themselves, however, focus on the daily frustrations and "contribute to disabling myths about disabilities" (Wright, 1980, p. 174). Wilson and Alcorn (1969) had students simulate being blind, deaf, or paralyzed via wheelchair and found no significant change in attitude toward persons with disabilities.

Grayson and Marini (1996) conducted a wheelchair-using exercise for an experimental group of rehabilitation counseling graduate students in which they were required to wheel a quarter-mile to the cafeteria, order and drink a beverage, then wheel back to the main building. A control group did not participate. Both groups completed a qualitative survey about disability. A significant *t*-test finding showed that the experimental wheelchair-using group perceived greater differences between persons with and without disabilities, indicating that persons with disabilities must have a harder time in society. Another significant difference between groups was that the sensitivity group further indicated that "persons with disabilities must get frustrated often . . . must feel different from being stared at so much . . . and, must be preoccupied with how accessible certain places must be" (p. 128). Without correcting such beliefs, counselors are likely to have preconceived notions regarding such clients and spend unnecessary time probing these otherwise irrelevant issues. If such exercises are to be utilized in training, debriefing is highly recommended. Instructors need to acknowledge how participant feelings of frustration are most common during the first several months following a trauma as the individual learns to adapt to his or her situation, but that most persons with disabilities learn to cope with and minimize daily hassles over time (Grayson & Marini, 1996; Silver, 1982; Wright, 1980). Leo and Goodwin (2016) found similar results and argued that persons with disabilities must be included in designing simulation activities. They noted the shortsightedness of simulation activities that do not represent real life, as some of their participants laughed at the novelty of the experience.

A major contributor to individuals' educational information is through the media. We have already seen how the inaccurate and stereotypical portrayals of persons with disabilities in the media actually create more negative attitudes, be it fear, pity, or sympathy. Chen et al. (2014) studied the content messages of media portrayals of disability with Chinese children. The authors found that when fear or pity was evoked in the media messages, negative attitudes were more prevalent. Conversely, when persons with disabilities were portrayed as having normal capabilities but needing some assistance, positive attitudes were more prevalent.

Education and Contact

Perhaps the strongest method of enhancing attitudes toward disability is to have the messenger or educator be a person with a disability. Aside from being perceived as a more credible source of information, the exposure or contact with someone perceived as having "equal status" facilitates attitude change (Yuker, 1988, p. 27). Scheiderer et al. (1995) pre–post tested two separate classes using the Modified Issues in Disability Scale (Makas, 1988) at the beginning and end of the semester. One class was taught by a professor who used a wheelchair, and the other was taught by a nondisabled instructor. Although there were no differences between groups at pretest, results were significant at posttest, indicating more positive attitudes in the class that had the instructor with the disability. Chesler and Chesney (1988) further discuss the benefits of self-help groups regarding persons with disabilities educating and assisting other persons with disabilities. Overall, these authors cite the benefits of networking, sharing emotional experiences, gaining access to information, learning new coping skills and resources, contributing to the welfare of others, and mobilizing to advocate for change. Finally, Chan et al. (2009) delineate several other methods of attitude change, including persuasion, disability simulation, affirmative action, and impression management. Persuasion becomes most effective when the message contains strong and cogent arguments that are similar to the attitudes held by the individual. Disability simulation exercises discussed earlier must have a built-in debriefing component after the simulation to be effective; otherwise, participants' perceptions may become more negative due to first-time frustrations attempting to negotiate the physical environment (Flower et al., 2007; Grayson & Marini, 1996). Such debriefings must include an acknowledgment that the majority of persons with disabilities generally adapt to their environment and circumstances over time. Regarding affirmative action, although mandated by laws such as the ADA, laws themselves in all likelihood have mixed results regarding positive or negative attitude change. Positive changes can occur because more persons with disabilities have access to the social environment, therefore increasing contact with others, which often leads to more positive attitudes. Conversely, for individuals who are not in favor of federal mandates regarding disability rights, this may facilitate even greater negative attitudes (McMahon et al., 2008). Finally, protests have been shown to be somewhat effective in changing behaviors (e.g., government legislation, damaging media portrayals); however, research is lacking regarding whether positive attitude change necessarily follows (Corrigan et al., 2001).

CONCLUSION

With the 1990 ADA allowing for greater social and employment interaction between persons with and without disabilities, nondisabled persons continue to be exposed to persons with disabilities in a variety of situations every day. As researchers have found in more than 50% of instances, this daily exposure or contact is likely to enhance attitudes and minimize interaction strain (Corrigan et al., 2001; Yuker, 1988). Depending on the circumstances of the interaction, however, a nondisabled person's attitudes could become more negative or not change demonstrably. Researchers have found that when the interaction is more structured, such as someone with a disability asking for assistance, there is a greater likelihood that an interaction will take place, especially because the behavior of helping persons with disabilities is engrained in our culture. If, however, there is no clear reason or cause for someone without a disability to approach and initiate a conversation with someone who is disabled, then the likelihood of such an interaction becomes less likely. This is due not only to the stranger phenomenon (Wright, 1988) but also to anxiety over not knowing what to say, how to behave, and irrational fears that the person with the disability may become emotional, causing further awkwardness (Albrecht et al., 1982; Evans, 1976; Leary, 1990; Marini, 1992). In a potential interaction situation, we cognitively weigh the rewards and costs of the interaction consciously and/or subconsciously. If we perceive there is nothing to gain from an anticipated interaction and experience anticipatory anxiety thinking about the encounter, we will likely avoid the situation.

When initial contacts between persons with and without disabilities do occur, it often is up to the person with the disability to place the nondisabled person at ease during the interaction (Evans, 1976; Marini, 1992). This may be accomplished by voluntarily self-disclosing a little information about how one came to be disabled and doing so in a matter-of-fact, nonemotional way. This not only satisfies the nondisabled person's curiosity but also suggests that the person with the disability is comfortable with his or her situation. Unfortunately, many persons with disabilities would rather not self-disclose particulars about their disability unless specifically asked about it or if it seems relevant to the conversation. Allport (1954) noted a number of conditions that generally facilitate positive attitudes when contact occurs. These factors include the following: (a) perceived equal status (e.g., education, occupation); (b) the contact is necessary to achieve a desired goal; (c) the contact is promoted by some authority or social climate; (d) the contact is intimate; (e) the contact is pleasurable; (f) the contact is by choice; (g) the contact is selected over other rewards; and (h) the contact is to complete some functional goal or activity.

Despite the numerous suspected origins regarding negative attitudes toward persons with disabilities, nondisabled persons who are not blatantly prejudiced and unwilling to change their attitudes may only require greater exposure and accurate information regarding disability. With the 1990 ADA representing the greatest civil rights legislation for persons with disabilities in U.S. history, persons with disabilities now enjoy greater access to employment, education, and social participation than ever before. This increasing exposure and contact with persons with disabilities of equal status or similar interest situations over time have seemingly continued to enhance positive attitudes toward those with disabilities, but still is perceived by many with disabilities to have a long way to go (Graf et al., 2009).

Hammel et al. (2015), for example, held focus groups with 201 persons with diverse disabilities regarding environmental barriers and supports to participation in society. Respondents expressed that physical barriers (inaccessible establishments) and societal barriers (negative attitudes) represented major obstacles to their full participation in society in which many felt socially isolated and disenfranchised, negatively impacting their quality of life. The authors describe how the *micro* (an individual's finances, accessible home, social support, access to assistive technology, and transportation), *mesa* (community factors such as social networking, information, universal design, and transportation), and *macro* (societal factors such as attitudes, political influence, civil rights legislation, and systems such as health and social service care) all intertwine. This environment–person interaction then shapes in part how persons with disabilities perceive their self-concept and well-being. If they perceive they are excluded from society and devalued, this can ultimately negatively impact self-esteem (DiTomasso & Spinner, 1997; Li & Moore, 1998).

Similarly, Hastbacka et al.'s (2016) literature review regarding barriers and facilitators to social participation of persons with disabilities found that exclusion from participating in society was facilitated by financial barriers, unemployment, lack of power, negative attitudes, and poor health. Social injustice through inequitable treatment and employment opportunities leads to oppression, lack of finances, and poor transportation access to the community; this ultimately leaves many persons with disabilities out of the public view. This resulting restricted ability to participate in public life further exacerbates the stigma surrounding those with disabilities if exposure and education are unable to take place.

DISCUSSION QUESTIONS

1. What types of social interactions make you nervous? Recall an individual you were with the last time this occurred, and describe how you felt, behaved, and what your thoughts were during the interaction.

2. Which type of disability do you believe you would feel *most and least* comfortable socially interacting with? Describe your reasons why.

3. Discuss common stereotypes of various disabilities and where or how such views originate.

4. Have students discuss who their circle of friends includes and what their friends have in common with them.

CLASS ACTIVITIES

1. Ask students to discuss what they believe are common misconceptions and prejudice that some Americans have toward one another, including those with disabilities, Anglos, African Americans, Hispanic Americans, Native Americans, and Middle Eastern populations.

2. Break the class up into two groups. Have one group discuss the misconceptions noted in question 1, and have the other group discuss what they know of to be more accurate descriptions of each of these populations and why.

3. Have students select and watch three movies over the course of the semester, then write a two-page reaction paper for each about how the person with the disability was portrayed. They should address whether the disability was made salient, whether the person was a hero or victim, whether he or she was sexually active, and whether he or she was employed; how the person was treated by others; and if there was a happy ending for the individual.

Movie List: 1. *Children of a Lesser God*; 2. *Whose Life Is It Anyway?*; 3. *Coming Home*; 4. *The Waterdance*; 5. *One Flew Over the Cuckoo's Nest*; 6. *Edward Scissorhands*; 7. *If You Could See What I Hear*; 8. *Born on the Fourth of July*; 9. *My Left Foot*; 10. *Without Warning: The James Brady Story*; 11. *Forrest Gump*; 12. *Rain Man*; 13. *Scent of a Woman*; 14. *Nell*; 15. *Lorenzo's Oil*; 16. *Philadelphia*; 17. *What's Eating Gilbert Grape?*; 18. *At First Sight*; 19. *Mask (with Cher)*; 20. *The Other Sister*; 21. *Frida*; 22. *I Am Sam*; 23. *There's Something About Mary*; 24. *As Good As It Gets*; 25. *Door to Door*; 26. *Gattaca*; 27. *Hunchback of Notre Dame*; 28. *Powder*; 29. *A Beautiful Mind*; 30. *Girl Interrupted*; 31. *Pumpkin*; 32. *The Ringer*; 33. *Murderball*; 34. *The Doctor*; 35. *Reign Over Me*; 36. *Home of the Brave*;

37. Million Dollar Baby; 38. Passion Fish; 39. Ray; 40. The Sea Inside; 41. Vanilla Sky; 42. Awakenings; 43. Sling Blade; 44. The Music Within.

4. Have students participate in a disability sensitivity exercise (e.g., wear a blindfold, use earplugs, use a wheelchair) and perform some activity around campus; then have them discuss their experience as well as the strengths/weaknesses of such activities.

KEY REFERENCES

Only key references appear in the print edition. The full references appear in the digital product on Springer Publishing Connect™: https://connect.springerpub.com/content/book/978-0-8261-5111-7/part/partI/chapter/ch02

Antonak, R. F. (1982). Development and psychometric analysis of the scale of attitudes toward disabled persons. *Journal of Applied Rehabilitation Counseling, 13*(2), 22–29. https://doi.org/10.1891/0047-2220.13.2.22

Antonak, R. F., & Livneh, H. (1988). *The measurement of attitudes toward people with disabilities*. Charles C. Thomas.

Barr, J. J., & Bracchitta, K. (2015). Attitudes toward individuals with disabilities: The effects of contact with different disability types. *Current Psychology, 34*, 223–238. https://doi.org/10.1007/S12144-014-9253-2

Bogdan, R., & Taylor, S. (1989). Relationships with severely disabled people: The social construction of humanness. *Social Problems, 36*, 135–148. https://doi.org/10.2307/800804

Chan, F., Livneh, H., Pruett, S., Wang, C. C., & Zheng, L. X. (2009). Societal attitudes toward disability: Concepts, measurements, and interventions. In F. Chan, E. De Silva Cardoso, & J. A. Chronister (Eds.), *Understanding psychosocial adjustment to chronic illness and disability: A handbook for evidence-based practitioners in rehabilitation* (pp. 333–367). Springer Publishing Company.

Dembo, T., Leviton, G. L., & Wright, B. A. (1956). Adjustment to misfortune: A problem of social-psychological rehabilitation. *Artificial Limbs, 3*(2), 4–62. https://doi.org/10.1037/H0090832

DiTomasso, E., & Spinner, B. (1997). Social and emotional loneliness: A re-examination of Weiss' typology of loneliness. *Personality and Individual Differences, 22*, 417–427. https://doi.org/10.1016/S0191-8869(96)00204-8

Havranek, J. E. (1991). The social and individual costs of negative attitudes toward persons with physical disabilities. *Journal of Applied Rehabilitation Counseling, 22*(1), 15–21. https://doi.org/10.1891/0047-2220.22.1.15

Li, L., & Moore, D. (1998). Acceptance of disability and its correlates. *The Journal of Social Psychology, 138*(1), 13–25. https://doi.org/10.1080/00224549809600349

Livneh, H. (1991). On the origins of negative attitudes toward people with disabilities. In R. P. Marinelli & A. E. Dell Orto (Eds.), *The psychological & social impact of disability* (pp. 111–138). Springer Publishing Company.

Marini, I. (1992). *The use of humor to modify attitudes, decrease interaction anxiety and increase desire to interact with persons of differing abilities* (Unpublished doctoral dissertation). Auburn University.

Vash, C. L., & Crewe, N. M. (2004). *Psychology of disability* (pp. 288–299). Springer Publishing Company.

Wright, B. A. (1988). Attitudes and the fundamental negative bias: Conditions and corrections. In H. E. Yuker (Ed.), *Attitudes toward persons with disabilities* (pp. 3–21). Springer Publishing Company.

Yuker, H. E. (1988). *Attitudes toward persons with disabilities*. Springer Publishing Company.

CHAPTER 3

HISTORY OF TREATMENT TOWARD PERSONS WITH PSYCHIATRIC DISABILITIES

KIM L. NGUYEN-FINN

LEARNING OBJECTIVES

After reading this chapter, you should be able to:

- Understand the significant events in the history of treatment of psychiatric disabilities
- Explain the effects of stigma against psychiatric disabilities throughout history
- Describe the evolution of classification systems of psychiatric disabilities
- Summarize the vulnerabilities of those with psychiatric disabilities throughout history

PRE-READING QUESTIONS

1. In what ways did the general population's views of persons with psychiatric disabilities change over time?
2. Which key historical figures were instrumental in reducing stigma against psychiatric disabilities?
3. How did deinstitutionalization affect individuals with psychiatric disabilities?
4. How have the wars the United States have been involved with affected mental health-care for those with psychiatric disabilities?
5. How did the COVID-19 pandemic affect psychiatric treatment?

MENTAL ILLNESS TREATMENT SINCE THE MIDDLE AGES

The premodern era and early modern period, specifically from the Middle Ages to the 1800s, saw much cruel and inhumane treatment toward people with mental, intellectual, and developmental disabilities. Those who were viewed as mentally ill were often labeled as witches and burned at the stake (Dix, 1904; Gilman, 1988; Rosen, 1968; Shorter, 1997). Many were accused of demonic possession and subjected to exorcism, beaten, flogged, ridiculed, chained, or otherwise treated with fear and derision (Dix, 1904; Gilman, 1988; Rosen, 1968; Shorter, 1997). However, to view the treatment of those with mental illness during the Middle Ages solely through the modern lens would be unduly harsh. One must be mindful of the historical and cultural context of the general population and their knowledge, or lack thereof, of mental illness. People during the Middle Ages knew little in terms of the causes and treatment of diseases and even less so about mental illness. Physicians of this period viewed disease and disability as often being caused by an imbalance of humors in the body, a belief inherited from the ancient Greeks. The theory was that the body is composed of four humors—blood, phlegm, yellow bile, and black bile. For instance, "madness" and "melancholy" were often viewed as caused by an excess of black bile (Gilman, 1988; Thachil, 2021). One possible treatment for imbalanced humor was bloodletting (Thachil, 2021)—a process of drawing blood from a patient to balance the humors and restore health. That which could not be explained by an imbalance of humors was believed to be an evil brought forth by sin committed by the sufferer, demons, or Satan or a spell cast by a witch and thus requiring to be cured by the Church or with magical herbs and incantations (Obermann, 1965).

The *Canon Episcopi,* a document that received a great deal of attention in the early medieval period, asserted that a belief in witches and sorcery, especially the idea that women rode on animals in the night, was a satanic delusion (Hansen, as cited in Rosen, 1968). A later document of the Middle Ages, the *Malleus Maleficarum* (*Hammer of Witches*), revised the notion that a belief in witchcraft was brought about by Satan to assert that witches indeed carried out Satan's orders and espoused procedures for identifying, putting to trial, and forcing confessions out of witches (Dimitrijevic, 2015; Rosen, 1968). These two documents show a shift in societal beliefs about mental illness. The *Canon Episcopi* asserted that those who believed in witchcraft had a mental illness; later, the *Malleus Maleficarum* stated that the accused likely were the ones with mental illness. In reality, accusations of witchcraft were often the result of petty jealousy, social or familial conflicts, spurned sexual advances, suggestion, delusions, and mental illness. Indeed, some accused witches seem to be described in accounts during the period of the Inquisition as elderly women afflicted with dementia. In cases of demonic possession, one may find symptoms of the accused that are consistent with dysthymia, dementia, paranoia, mania, compulsive disorders, epilepsy, and schizophrenia (Yang et al., 2016). Care for the mentally ill was essentially the responsibility of relatives so long as the individuals did not cause a disturbance or were deemed too dangerous to be cared for at home (Rosen, 1968; Shorter, 1997). If they could not be cared for, authorities would confine the person viewed as insane to an asylum, a hospital, a prison, or a workhouse (Rosen, 1968; Shorter, 1997). Cases have been noted of accused witches being recognized as actually mentally ill and transferred to hospitals (Lea, as cited in Rosen, 1968). One of the oldest hospitals to treat people with psychiatric disabilities was the Priory of Saint Mary of Bethlehem, or Bethlem, which was founded in the 13th century in Europe. As centuries passed, the institution began to focus almost entirely on those with mental illness, and its name gradually morphed from Bethlem to "Bedlam"; the hospital remained in use as an asylum until 1948 (Shorter, 1997). Institutions of this time often did little more than warehouse people with psychiatric disabilities to keep them away from the public.

Much of the treatment for this population during the Middle Ages was often moral or religious in nature and sometimes included fasting, prayer, and pilgrimages to shrines; for the latter, financial assistance was often provided by religious groups (Rosen, 1968). Two stained-glass windows from this period found in the Canterbury Cathedral illustrate a man suffering from mental illness and depict prayer as a treatment; one window caption states, "Mad he comes," whereas the other reads, "He prays. Sane he goes away" (Torrey & Miller, 2007). Ibn Sīnā, or Avicenna, as he was known in the Western world, was a Persian physician who lived in the late 1st century or early 2nd century and promoted treatments for ailments such as melancholia and "lovesickness." These included moisturizing the body, assisting with good sleep hygiene, promoting good nutrition, giving laxatives to reduce the toxins accumulated in the colon (which was believed to drive a person to madness; Shorter, 1997), and assisting in focusing on other matters and activities as a healthy distraction (Ibn Sīnā, 12th century/2010). Some of these treatments are like those espoused by mental health professionals of today.

COLONIAL AMERICA

Conditions for people with psychiatric disabilities did not fare much better in the American colonies. Similar to the circumstances during the Middle Ages, care for this population was the family's responsibility, if they had a family to care for them (Torrey & Miller, 2001). Those less fortunate who were held in institutions were often subjected to extremely unhygienic conditions, flogged, jeered at, confined to workhouses, and manacled and chained to walls or floors. In extreme cases, people with psychiatric disabilities were shackled for years until they lost use of their limbs and gradually died from lack of food (Shorter, 1997). Shackling individuals with a psychiatric disability remains in use in some parts of the world to this day, such as parts of Africa and Asia (Patel & Prince, 2010; Widodo et al., 2019).

Occasionally, if a family could not adequately care for or control what they deemed a "distracted person," a colonial town would construct a small house (generally approximately 5′ × 7′) to confine the individual (Shorter, 1997). Eventually, asylums began to be built in the United States to house those with psychiatric disabilities. In 1729, Boston's governing board began discussions of separating the Almshouse to keep those with mental illnesses in a separate ward from those who were there for being in poverty (Golembiewski, 2017). However, it was nearly 45 years before the first psychiatric hospital was opened in 1773 in Williamsburg, Virginia, with 30 beds where individuals with mental illnesses were housed separately from others (Golembiewski, 2017; Torrey & Miller, 2001). This psychiatric hospital was partly modeled after Bethlem in England (Scull, 1981).

By contrast, although not a belief shared by all American Indian tribes, some looked on those with possible mental illness with high regard, believing them to possess "special gifts," especially those with psychoses (Grandbois, 2005; Thompson et al., 1993). Other tribes viewed mental illness similarly to European Americans, as resulting from supernatural possession, soul loss (the loss of part of the soul or life force due to trauma or substance abuse), or internal or external imbalance (Grandbois, 2005; Thompson et al., 1993). In other tribes, those who displayed behavior outside of their cultural norm because of a mental or physical disability were treated as if they had misbehaved and were punished accordingly (Thompson et al., 1993). Yellow Bird (2001) asserts that First Nations do not generally have a word for *mentally ill*; what is translated as *crazy* means a humorous person or someone too angry to think clearly. With the expansion of the territory of the "White man," Western views and standards of practice in addressing mental illness also spread. The first asylum for a specific ethnic group was established in 1899 for the Northern Plains tribes, the Hiawatha Asylum for Insane Indians in Canton, South Dakota (Yellow Bird, 2001).

MENTAL ILLNESS IN 19TH-CENTURY AMERICA

In the 1800s, there was a huge rise in the number of those confined to asylums. The number of beds in each of the institutions increased to the low hundreds (Shorter, 1997). Braslow (1997) states that as more asylums were being built, still more were needed. Physicians of this time had scant training in diagnosing and treating mental illness (Caplan, 1969), but believed that they would be able to cure 80% of all such cases (Yanni, 2003). Indeed, they were so confident in their work that in 1853, psychiatrists who formed the American Organization of Asylum Physicians refused any association with the American Medical Association, as they held other physicians in lower regard (Shorter, 1997).

The asylums of the early 19th century were largely therapeutic institutions providing moral treatment (Yanni, 2003). This treatment modality emphasized a positive change in environment (including staying within the asylum), an avoidance of immoral behavior and temptations, living a healthy lifestyle through exercise and proper nutrition, and abiding by a consistent daily schedule. Attendants were also instructed to show respect to patients, refrain from chaining them, and encourage supervised vocational and leisure activities. Proponents of moral treatment also founded the *American Journal of Insanity,* a publication that aimed to educate citizens about mental illness and disability, as well as combat stigma and the abuses of those with a psychiatric disability (Caplan, 1969). However, in reality, moral therapy in its truest form was practiced in only a few institutions.

Patients of this period were still being treated with physical therapies, including those designed to balance the humors. Records show that even up to the 1830s blistering, by which a patient's skin was burned with caustic substances to extract poisonous humors, was still being performed (Shorter, 1997). Treatment also used laxatives, bleeding, opiates, and hydrotherapy, or therapeutic baths, which came into vogue during this period (Shorter, 1997; Yanni, 2003).

Physicians tried to link disorders with treatments, but were limited in their scope of understanding. Phrenology became a popular diagnostic and predictive tool and was developed through the belief that a direct relationship existed between the shape and size of the skull and mental illness and disability (Crocq, 2013). Categorizing mental illness as chronic or curable was of paramount importance, as it enabled physicians to focus only on the few patients they believed could be successfully treated (Caplan, 1969). During this period, diagnosing illness could also be viewed as a way of identifying and compartmentalizing people who appeared different from the rest of society. Common diagnoses included melancholia, mania, idiocy, and paresis (a condition with symptoms of dementia, seizures, and muscle impairment resulting from syphilis; Braslow, 1997). Shorter (1997) writes of one doctor from Albany, New York, who described what he termed "insane ear," or bloodied blisters within the ear, to be a symptom of mental illness. In reality, the blisters were the result of asylum workers clubbing patients' heads.

MENTAL ILLNESS AND TREATMENT AT THE TURN OF THE CENTURY

Moral treatments began to decline in the second half of the 19th century in favor of somatic therapies and behavioral control techniques (Braslow, 1997). Behavior that was deemed loud, offensive, or otherwise obnoxious by hospital staff was frequently managed by restraint, punishment, or sedative. Patients were physically restrained through the use of straitjackets, strapped to their beds—sometimes for years—confined in cells, and wrapped tightly in wet sheets (Braslow, 1997; Dix, 1904). Criticized as another form of restraint, medications were administered to sedate patients and control symptoms of mental illness (Braslow, 1997; Shorter, 1997). Drugs in use during the 19th century included narcotics and the sedatives bromide, chloral hydrate, and hyoscine (Ackerknecht, as cited by Braslow, 1997). The most popular drug in use in the majority of asylums at this time was chloral hydrate (Caplan, 1969). Chloral hydrate, an addictive sedative related to chloroform, was especially popular among women, whose families were too embarrassed to commit them to an asylum, as a home remedy for psychosis, anxiety, and sleeping difficulties (Shorter, 1997). Physicians and psychiatrists often diagnosed females with hysteria.

Forced sterilization to control reproduction began to be employed and continued through the 1940s (Braslow, 1997). The eugenics movement has been likened to Nazi Germany's efforts to control the quality of future generations and involved the mass sterilization of those deemed to have a mental illness or hereditary-linked disability. Patients were often considered incurable, and their offspring were at risk of inheriting the disease. Originally, however, laws allowing for forced sterilization made no mention of offspring. For example, the original 1909 California law known as the "Asexualization Act" stated that patients could be involuntarily sterilized if it benefited the physical, mental, or moral condition of any inmate. Nearly 10 years later, an amendment was introduced that stated involuntary sterilization may be performed on persons confined to an asylum if they had a disorder or disability that might be inherited and could be transmitted to descendents. This law broadened physicians' ability to decide about patients' reproductive capabilities. Many viewed forced sterilization as an economic issue. One such individual, Horatio M. Pollock, a statistician for the New York State Hospital Commission, wrote in 1921 that the United States loses over $200 million each year as a result of mental illness and less than a quarter of those afflicted are curable. Pollock (1921) further stated that mental illness heredity is an accepted fact, and thus the limitation of reproduction by "defective stock" should be employed to reduce the burden on taxpayers.

Sterilization was not only used to control the population of those with a psychiatric illness, but some physicians believed it to be therapeutic. In the case of men, physicians asserted that by severing the vas deferens, the testicles compensated by increasing the production of a hormone that was thought to make the patient feel physically and mentally invigorated (Money, 1983). For women, sterilization was often an ill-guided, but more socially acceptable, attempt at reducing the psychological strain of having more pregnancies than desired (Braslow, 1997). Research at this time also posits that genital abnormalities were seen as common among those with mental illness or disability—a way of nature ensuring that these individuals did not reproduce—while physicians believed that vasectomies could provide a cure (Gibbs, 1923).

Hydrotherapy, based on the idea that water had healing properties, became a widely used mode of treatment that remained in use until 1940 (Braslow, 1997). Hydrotherapeutic techniques were modeled after hot or cold mineral spring spas, long used as a curative, and consisted mainly of wet-sheet packs and hours of hot continuous baths. Patients who underwent wet-sheet packs were tightly wrapped in either cold or hot water-drenched sheets in which they had to remain until the treatment administration was deemed completed. Continuous bath treatments required patients to remain in a bathtub with limbs bound until they appeared to be more tranquil (Winslow, as cited in Braslow, 1997).

THE SHIFTING PUBLIC VIEW OF PSYCHIATRY

Although treatments were changing through the end of the 19th century, so was the public's perception of psychiatry. By the 1900s as therapy and treatment reverted back to confinement, physicians who were specialized in mental illness were deemed in poor light (Shorter, 1997). The profession was considered to be dangerous, and quality entrants into the field were scarce (Caplan, 1969). There was a huge increase in the number of patients in mental hospitals in the United States (150,000 in 1904, or 2 for every 1,000 in the population; U.S. Bureau of the Census, 1975, as cited in Shorter, 1997). Psychiatrists in the United States lacked the education to address the mental health needs of their patients, as less than 10% of psychiatrists graduated from a respected medical school and 20% had never attended a medical school lecture (Stevens, as cited in Shorter, 1997). Mental hospitals also struggled to hire attendants and other staff who were even minimally qualified (Caplan, 1969). Further, the negative perceptions of those with mental illness persisted. The "us versus them" attitude against those perceived to have a psychiatric illness increased with the rise in the number of immigrants in America and its asylums, particularly against Irish immigrants, whom psychiatrists claimed were prone to mental illness because of their irascibility and excessive indulgence in alcohol (Torrey & Miller, 2001).

Not surprising, the quality of mental health care in the United States had reached a new low during this time. Physicians who did not know how to treat mental illnesses and disabilities resorted to simply warehousing patients; reformers and former patients began to speak publicly about the treatment of those in mental institutions, which they viewed as little more than prisons. One early mental health reformer, Dorothea Dix, traveled throughout New England in the early 1840s investigating the treatment of the "insane poor" and prisoners (Novicoff, 2018). Dix was spurred to activism in 1841 after teaching a class of female prisoners at a jail near Boston, Massachusetts, and was exposed to the unheated and squalid conditions in which the women presumed to be insane were confined (Torrey & Miller, 2001). Dix spoke in 1843 to the Massachusetts legislature and described how the "insane poor" were kept naked, chained, beaten with rods and whipped, and appeared filthy and disheveled. Dix (1904) also reported about those confined to cages, cellars, stalls or pens in stables, and closets. In her speech to the legislature, she related how she visited an almshouse and met a woman who was kept for years in a cellar and had wasted down to bone. Dix was told the woman had to be kept there because of violent tendencies. Dix's impassioned descriptions of the suffering of prisoners and those with mental illness helped raise the public's awareness of the needs of the "insane poor" and convinced states' legislatures across the country to increase funding for mental health needs (Novicoff, 2018).

Others spoke of their personal experiences in the nation's mental institutions. Packard (1868) wrote *The Prisoners' Hidden Life, or Insane Asylums Unveiled* in 1868 after being freed from an asylum following being involuntarily committed by her husband after a disagreement with him about religious beliefs (Eghigian, 2010). Lawsuits were being successfully brought forward against asylums for false imprisonment (Caplan, 1969). A few newspapers had reporters committed in mental institutions so that they could investigate patients' treatment firsthand and report on it. In 1889, the *Chicago Times* sent a reporter into Jefferson Asylum in Cook County. The newspaper reported abuses ranging from verbal abuse, to assault, to murder, which spurred public outrage and an investigation by authorities.

Another former patient, Clifford Beers, who wrote *A Mind That Found Itself* in 1907 (Beers, as cited in Clifford W. Beers Guidance Clinic, Inc., 2009), spent 798 days in confinement after a failed suicide attempt. Rosen (1968) argues that Beers's work played a tremendous part, if not the most important part, in the development of the modern mental health movement. Recounting his nearly 3-year confinement in a state mental institution, Beers describes witnessing beatings, days spent in cold cells wearing only underwear, and being restrained so tightly that his hands went numb. The story of how a Yale-educated man could be degraded with shockingly brutal treatment resonated with the public. Beers founded the National Committee for Mental Hygiene in 1909 to improve the care of patients in mental institutions, promote research, and disseminate information on the prevention and treatment of mental illnesses (Caplan, 1969; Rosen, 1968).

The work of Beers and other reformers helped make substantive changes in the field of mental health. For example, *asylum* would no longer be used to refer to mental hospitals, a sign of the change in focus from confinement to treatment (Caplan, 1969). In addition, patients were afforded the opportunity to appeal the decision to commit them, and institutions were directed to keep up with the latest knowledge through the purchase of updated medical books and subscriptions to scientific medical journals.

Initially, however, psychiatrists responded to critics indignantly and with charges of ignorance and hypocrisy. They accused reformers of unjustly frightening the public away from receiving care and tarnishing psychiatrists' reputations (Caplan, 1969). Reformers were dismissed as ill-educated concerning proper behavioral management techniques and treatment modalities for mental disorders, and accused of hypocritically refusing to care for those with mental illness or disability themselves. Other physicians, including neurologists, were cast as jealous individuals who lacked the qualifications to work in a mental hospital.

DEVELOPMENT OF TREATMENTS IN THE 20TH CENTURY

Although psychiatrists initially scoffed at the notion that the quality of the care they provided in mental hospitals was subpar, research was conducted in the treatment of mental illness that brought about improvements. Physicians continued to develop and work toward improvement of somatic treatments for psychiatric disabilities in the early part of the 20th century. Physicians of this period largely believed that fevers could treat a wide range of psychiatric illnesses (Braslow, 1997). Fevers were also believed by many physicians to kill the bacteria that causes syphilis, and fever therapy for paresis was in use until the early 1960s (Braslow, 1997). Interestingly, Wagner-Jauregg (1927), a winner of the Nobel Prize in Physiology and Medicine for his work in the development of this treatment, states that fever alone does not destroy the spirochetes in that, sometimes, it will return once the fever has passed.

Other treatments included shock therapies. In the 1930s, some physicians used insulin to induce hypoglycemic coma in patients as a treatment for mental illness after noticing that patients who were difficult to manage became sedate and more cooperative with insulin (Braslow, 1997; Shorter, 1997). Insulin had previously been used to relieve depression and stimulate the appetite, as well as relieve diabetic symptoms (Shorter, 1997). Researchers could not agree why producing physiological shock through the use of insulin seemed to produce a positive effect (Braslow, 1997), but its use gradually rose in popularity. More than 100 mental hospitals in the United States usedinsulin units by the 1960s (Shorter, 1997).

Metrazol injections, which produced seizures or convulsions, began to be administered (Braslow, 1997). Thus began the start of convulsive therapies. Physician–researchers have been unable to definitively state why convulsive therapies work but continue to use the procedure in specific cases. Some theorize that fear of the treatment itself induced improvement. Shorter (1997) reports that physician–researchers of the 1920s noted that when patients who had epilepsy developed schizophrenia, they experienced fewer epileptic seizures. They posited that there must be a correlation; thus, by inducing epileptic-like seizures, symptoms of schizophrenia might be reduced (Shorter, 1997). Initially, camphor, a naturally produced chemical that was sometimes used to treat psychosis in the 18th century, was used to shock the body to convulse. The drug metrazol was developed and used in place of camphor. The use of metrazol was fraught with problems, however, because physicians could not predict the onset or the intensity of the convulsions, which were reported to be agonizingly painful for the patients who experienced them and the hospital staff who witnessed them.

Later, seizures were induced in patients by passing electrical currents through electrodes on each of the temples and deemed to be safe (Braslow, 1997; Shorter, 1997). The use of electroshock therapy or electroconvulsive therapy (ECT) soon expanded from treating symptoms of schizophrenia to treating a wide array of mental illnesses such as depression, senile psychosis, melancholia, and alcohol abuse (Braslow, 1997). Although ECT remains in use today as an acceptable psychiatric intervention for mental illness, it is not without critics. A large portion of the criticism lies in the fact that more women than men are administered ECT (Braslow, 1997; Karanti et al., 2015). Another criticism is that ECT alters the physician–patient relationship to one of control and discipline.

Psychosurgery, based on the viewpoint that the cause of mental illness or disease originated in the frontal lobe, began to gain ground in the 1930s (Caruso & Sheehan, 2017). Prefrontal lobotomy or leucotomy entails cutting the white matter in the frontal lobes of the brain, thought to be associated with insight, and severing its connection with the thalamus, thought to control emotion, and thereby reducing mental pain (Freeman & Watts, 1947). Surgery initially involved pouring alcohol onto the white matter of the frontal lobe through two holes that were drilled into the skull (Caruso & Sheehan, 2017). The neurologist Egas Moniz developed the prefrontal leucotomy based on observations of wartime head injuries, autopsies, and animal experiments for which he later received the Nobel Prize (Eghigian, 2010). Moniz's procedure utilized an instrument called a *leukotome*, which is a rod affixed with a steel loop at one end that was inserted into the skull through holes drilled to cut the brain's white matter (Caruso & Sheehan, 2017). Freeman and Watts, two American physician–researchers, developed the transorbital lobotomy in which an ice pick is inserted into the eye socket of the patient and then the brain tissue is destroyed by tapping the ice pick with a hammer. Freeman and Watts (1947) assert that prefrontal lobotomy is most successful with those patients whose mental illness may be anxiety disorder, depression, or excitability with schizophrenia, but is not successful for those with substance-use disorders, epilepsy, organic brain disease, and criminality. They also relayed doubts about the benefits of lobotomy with severe schizophrenia (Grob, 1991a). Moniz also questioned the effectiveness of leucotomy on schizophrenia, believing the surgery to be most successful on those with affective disorders (Grob, 1991a). Mahli and Bartlett (as cited in Juckel et al., 2009) reported that of those with certain psychiatric disabilities who underwent prefrontal leucotomy or lobotomy, approximately 67% had schizophrenia and 20% had an affective disorder. Shorter (1997) notes that lobotomies did indeed tend to calm patients with management problems. Psychosurgery, however, is also not without its hazards. It is not only dangerous to perform this surgery, but side effects of this treatment include a decline in social skills and judgment, loss of mental capacity, avolition or apathy, and a change in personality, such as loss of interest in previously enjoyed activities and changes in temperament (Juckel et al., 2009).

With the advent of talk therapy, psychological practice began its shift from being solely hospital based and became office based (Shorter, 1997). Outpatient psychiatric clinics were started in the 1920s, and by 1934 the practice of group psychotherapy began to be conducted (Shorter, 1997). Psychotherapy became the preferred treatment for middle and upper socioeconomic class individuals who were relatively high functioning, while somatic therapies tended to be used more often on those of the lower classes (Grob, 1991a).

The early 20th century witnessed the development of psychoanalysis, or the "talking cure." Sigmund Freud, a Viennese psychiatrist, developed an insight-oriented method of therapy (Shafti, 2019). According to Freud, neuroses are caused by repressed childhood memories, especially those of a sexual nature, as well as subconscious conflicts (Shorter, 1997). The goal of psychoanalysis is to bring the subconscious to consciousness and have the patient address the psychic conflict in a safe environment (Freud, 1910). Freud's theory of psychoanalysis conflicted with his contemporaries' views. Freud's focus on the individual unconscious thoughts and urges and childhood sexual development was in direct contradiction and thus ripe for criticism (Oberndorf, 2012). Despite its criticisms and limitations, Freud's work continues to have a major influence on contemporary therapeutic theories and practices (Corey, 2016). A significant assertion of psychotherapeutic theories is that the decision to undergo treatment rests with the patient.

Psychotherapy has also continued to evolve. Carl Rogers's client-centered therapy represented a fundamental shift in working with patients from Freudian and Jungian psychoanalysis. Rogers asserted that it is the client who has the ability and insight to know his or her problems and how to put forth the issues, thus making the client the expert. The psychotherapist is simply there to be a sounding board and reassure the client's progress (Rogers, 1961). Psychotherapy also does not discount the benefits of somatic treatments, but it affirms a combination with appropriate drug therapy as the most effective treatment modality for mental illness today (Huhn et al., 2014).

Gains in understanding brain chemistry and more effective psychotropic medication for the treatment of mental illness were being made as well. The first neurotransmitter was isolated in the early 1920s, and soon thereafter the chemical acetylcholine was found to have an effect on nerve impulse transmissions between neurons (Tansey, 2006). Chlorpromazine, an antihistamine that would have a major impact on psychiatry, was developed in 1951 and initially was used as a sedative for psychiatric patients but was found to also reduce psychosis (López-Muñoz et al., 2005). Today, chlorpromazine is more commonly known as an antipsychotic medication under the brand name Thorazine. Soon, other antipsychotic medications along with antidepressants and mood stabilizers were being developed and marketed. The success of psychotropic medications in reducing once-debilitating symptoms of mental illness has allowed more and more individuals to lead productive lives outside institutions.

THE SECOND WORLD WAR AND ITS INFLUENCE ON MENTAL HEALTH

Psychiatrists' wartime experiences expanded knowledge about mental health and the importance of the environment in both disorder development and treatment (Grob, 1991b); they applied what they learned during World War II (WWII) to their rehabilitation and therapeutic efforts (Grinker & Spiegel, as cited in Grob, 1991b). The war necessitated that those unfit for military service for physical and mental reasons be screened out and those serving and who required rehabilitation as psychological casualties receive treatment (Grob, 1991a). The screening out of recruits aroused controversy and was not wholly successful. Approximately 1.75 million potential recruits were rejected by the Selective Service (Grob, 1991a) and an additional 500,000 were discharged for mental reasons (Pickren, 2005). These high numbers raised questions about the prevalence of mental illness, the screening criteria's validity, and personal privacy (Grob, 1991a). The problems with screenings, however, did successfully highlight the need for additional research in the field and the importance of prevention of mental health problems. The U.S. government began to assist the funding of psychological research on a large scale, which further shaped public perception of mental illness and treatment (Pickren, 2005). Psychiatrists serving during the war successfully utilized a more holistic approach to treatment, providing supportive counseling in conjunction with prescribing adequate sleep, good nutrition, and rest close to the patient's unit and support system (Grob, 1991b).

The successful treatment of psychiatric issues for returning veterans helped elevate the profession, and, in 1944, psychiatry was designated as a medical specialty within the Office of the Surgeon General (Grob, 1991b). Additional physicians were recruited into its ranks—at the outbreak of WWII, there were 35 psychiatrists serving in the military; the number swelled to 2,400 by 1945. Psychiatrists who were transitioning to civilian life at the end of the war began to enter academia, government, private practice, and public service and carried with them their unique knowledge and approaches (Grob, 1991a). Indeed, the end of WWII brought with it a renewed sense of hope within the mental health field and the intellectual and institutional means to effect substantive changes. It also produced fresh challenges that needed to be addressed. One year after the end of hostilities, 60% of the Veterans Affairs (VA) hospital patients were WWII veterans presenting with mental disorders (Brand, 1965). The rising number of those in need of quality mental health services spurred the VA, along with the American Psychological Association and several universities, to work together to develop a doctoral clinical psychology program (Miller, 1946). Of significance, the National Mental Health Act was passed in the same year, which assisted states in the implementation of services for the diagnosis, prevention, and treatment of mental illnesses, as well as provided for research, training, and the formation of the National Institute of Mental Health (NIMH; Pickren, 2005).

CLASSIFICATION OF MENTAL ILLNESS

The American Psychiatric Association (APA) started to devise a standard nosology for mental disorders in 1948 (Shorter, 2015), but the first standardized nosology for mental illness, *The Statistical Manual for the Use of Institutions for the Insane,* was developed in 1918 by the American Medico-Psychological Association in collaboration with the National Committee for Mental Hygiene at the request of the U.S. Bureau of Uniform Statistics (APA, 1918/2018; Fischer, 2012). This first nosology included instructions on recording clear and accurate in-patient intake and discharge information. Categorizing mental illnesses was found useful in that the public health statistical data regarding disorders could be collected and used in public policy development to uncover future trends and to show recidivism and recovery rates with different treatments or hospitals. The use of diagnoses in the development of treatment plans was not as important at this time. Over time, the inadequacy of the earlier classification systems was made increasingly apparent. In 1952, the APA published the *Diagnostic and Statistical Manual of Mental Disorders*. This volume is now referred to as the *DSM-I* (APA, 1952), which, like previous classification systems, reflected the intellectual, cultural, and political viewpoints on mental illness of its day (Fischer, 2012). Since its initial publication, there have been several revisions, and the *DSM* continues to be used as the standard diagnostic tool by a wide array of mental health researchers and clinicians in a variety of settings (*DSM-5-TR;* APA, 2022). Critics of the *DSM,* however, have cited that the resource fails to fully capture a holistic picture of an individual's circumstances. As such, in coordination with the World Health Organization (WHO), the APA has endorsed a more holistic resource that can be cross-referenced with almost any disability and that takes into account an individual's external environment and medical and psychological problems (Peterson, 2011). Specifically, the International Classification of Functioning represents the most contemporary source available to mental health professionals in holistically assessing an individual's situation.

DEINSTITUTIONALIZATION

There were 131 state-funded mental hospitals at the turn of the 20th century to house 126,137 patients; by 1941, there were 419,374 patients, but the number of hospitals had increased by only 181 (Braslow, 1997). With the overcrowding of mental hospitals, the need for an alternative to institutions became apparent. The increase in the use of drug therapies gave rise to the notion that individuals with mental illness could integrate back into the community if their symptoms were managed (Shorter, 1997). In addition, WWII evidenced how successful treatments outside of institutions were and psychiatrists who served worked to incorporate mental health care into community treatment and prevention efforts of mental illnesses (Kelly, 2005). The antipsychiatry movement further drove the shift to deinstitutionalization. The movement in large part comprised mental health professionals themselves who were critical about overuse of psychotropic medications, the viewpoint that behaviors simply outside of the norm implied mental disorders, and what they considered inferior institutional practices (Eghigian, 2010; Grob & Goldman, 2006). Deinstitutionalization also appeared to be strongly influenced by financial reasons, as Medicaid payments gave states impetus to move patients to nursing homes (Mechanic & Rochefort, 1990).

Programs and centers with a community health focus began to rise. The Menninger Clinic in Topeka, Kansas, was started by William and Karl Menninger, brothers who served as psychiatrists in WWII; their model became a respected form of mental health care (Kelly, 2005). In 1955, Public Law 84–182 established the Mental Health Study Act, which examined mental health care in the United States. The final report contributed to the development of the Community Mental Health Centers Act of 1963 (Stockdill, 2005). This Act required community mental health centers to provide inpatient and outpatient services, partial hospitalizations, emergency services, training and education, and consultation services. Thousands of institutionalized patients were placed with their families for care at home; however, the difficulty of patient monitoring and the lack of case management and coordination of care plagued the community mental health clinics (Grob & Goldman, 2006). New York recognized that patients needed a transition period between hospitalization and reintegration into the family and community and developed aftercare clinics in 1954 (Carmichael, as cited in Grob & Goldman, 2006). Halfway houses, which were either linked to hospitals or founded by mental health professionals or laypeople, were created to also help patients' transition back into the community (Grob & Goldman, 2006). Underfunding and what many perceived as disinterest by professionals for the rehabilitation and support of the reintegration into the community of those with severe mental illness posed major problems for halfway houses. As an alternative, independent living communities for those with mental illnesses, called "Fairweather Community Lodge Programs," were developed in California in the 1960s (Kelly, 2005). George Fairweather created his lodges believing that those with severe psychiatric illnesses can remain deinstitutionalized if they live and work together collaboratively. Other treatment facilities started, and still in use today are supervised apartments, board and care facilities, and group homes. Outpatient programs such as Assertive Community Treatment (ACT) have also come into use to serve the needs of those with severe and persistent mental illness living in the community (National Alliance on Mental Illness [NAMI], 2006). ACT programs provide highly intensive, multifaceted care available 24 hours a day/7 days per week with a low service provider-to-consumer ratio and have been shown to reduce the number of hospitalizations (NAMI, 2006). Between 1965 and 1975, the number of patients in state mental hospitals decreased an average of 8.6% per year (Mechanic & Rochefort, 1990). As the population in state mental hospitals reduced, general hospitals experienced a dramatic rise in the registration of patients with mental illness, necessitating the development of specialized psychiatric units as these hospitals were forced to house patients in surgical or emergency wards.

Reintegration into the community occurred on a large scale during the late 1960s; most of those released had been admitted to the hospitals in later life or had a lengthy confinement (Grob & Goldman, 2006). Disability and health insurance provided financial assistance and mental health benefits for individuals so that they may remain with their families (Mechanic & Rochefort, 1990). Moreover, the introduction of Medicaid and Medicare in 1966 gave states the incentive to transition patients from hospitals to nursing homes, as these social programs provided for the care of elderly patients with mental illness or dementia in nursing homes. In addition, Medicaid often provided funds for short-term inpatient care in general hospitals.

DISILLUSIONMENT WITH THE PROMISES OF DEINSTITUTIONALIZATION

In time, deinstitutionalization produced less-than-positive results. The concepts of using the least restrictive method of care and that those with severe and persistent mental disorders would be treated in the community rather than the psychiatric institution meant that an increasing number of individuals would receive inadequate care, as the community clinics were not poised to address their needs (Grob & Goldman, 2006; Mechanic & Rochefort, 1990). Many of those who would have been institutionalized in the past were forced to function independently in the community, and these individuals were frequently cited as being noncompliant with treatment, denying their mental illnesses, taking their medications irregularly, being aggressive, self-medicating with alcohol or drugs, and lacking social skills.

The massive slash of funding for welfare programs in the 1980s further hindered mental health care efforts and precipitated a rise in the number of those with mental illness among the homeless and prison population (Mechanic & Rochefort, 1990). Although a direct correlation with the cuts to social programs is difficult to make, roughly one-third of the nation's homeless population and 14% of county inmates in the 1980s were documented to have a psychiatric diagnosis (Torrey, as cited in Shorter, 1997). These figures contrast radically with the prevalence of severe mental illness in the general population at that time, which was about 2.8% (National Advisory Mental Health Council, 1993). According to the U.S. Department of Justice (DOJ), more than half of all inmates in 2005 had either a diagnosis of a mental disorder or met the criteria for one based on symptoms; these included psychotic disorders, major depressive disorders, and symptoms of mania (James & Glaze, 2006). In contrast, about 11% of adults in the general population met the criteria for a mental disorder two decades later according to the National Epidemiologic Survey on Alcohol and Related Conditions, 2001 to 2002.

MENTAL ILLNESS AND THE CRIMINAL JUSTICE SYSTEM

According to the U.S. DOJ, inmates with mental health problems are more likely to have violent records and are generally given longer sentences (James & Glaze, 2006). Although those with severe and persistent mental illness may and do commit criminal acts, many encounter law enforcement during mental crises or because they are exhibiting bizarre and/or disturbing behaviors in public (Lamberti & Weisman, 2004). Definite gains have been made in raising awareness of the unique needs of those with mental illness among law enforcement professionals. The Crisis Intervention Team (CIT) of the Memphis, Tennessee, Police Department is a model jail diversion program used in other communities as well. CIT officers volunteer to be educated about signs and symptoms of mental disorders and are trained in de-escalation techniques, community mental health and social service resources, and empathy of those with mental illness (Slate et al., 2013). CIT programs have resulted in fewer arrests of those with severe mental illness, as well as fewer officer and detainee injuries (Lamberti & Weisman, 2004). Other police departments have experimented with using mental health professionals or social workers in crisis response. The Law Enforcement and Mental Health Project Act of 2000 authorized funding for the development of "mental health courts" as an alternative for those with severe mental illness and to promote treatment and supervision for the accused. They were also designed to curb reoffending among those with severe mental illness and divert them into community-based treatment (Redlich et al., 2006).

Despite these improvements, the treatment of those with mental illness within the criminal justice system remains a concern. Suicide is the leading cause of death among inmates in jails and the third leading cause in prisons (Lamberti & Weisman, 2004). Some studies on inmates document that more than half of those who died by suicide had a history of mental illness. Inmates with mental illness are also more likely to have disciplinary problems and be involved in altercations with other inmates while incarcerated (Hafemeister et al., 2001). As many view prisons and jails as a source of punishment rather than treatment, psychotherapy and medication management are lacking for many inmates. Depending on the facility type (local jail, state or federal prison), only 17% to 35% of inmates with mental disorders are provided mental health services (James & Glaze, 2006). To prevent recidivism, prisons and jails face the challenging task of coordinating with community mental health and social services on release of inmates with mental illness for employment, housing, and mental health assistance (Lamberti & Weisman, 2004).

ABUSE OF PERSONS WITH MENTAL ILLNESS

Not only do a high number of prisoners have a psychiatric disability, but those with mental illness also appear to be more vulnerable to sexual and physical abuse. Those incarcerated in prisons or jails were two to three times more likely to have been sexually or physically abused than other inmates (James & Glaze, 2006). Although causality cannot be stated, O'Hare et al. (2010) found that of those they interviewed with severe mental illness, 51.8% reported physical abuse, 41.7% reported sexual abuse, and a greater number of women than men reported they were abused. Those with severe mental illness also may engage in high-risk behaviors such as running away and substance abuse, which puts them at greater risk for repeated abuse. In addition, people with severe mental illness are more likely to live in high-crime areas that can further expose them to risk of decompensation (Schwartz et al., 2005). Those with severe mental illness are particularly vulnerable to revictimization from the judicial system, given the difficulty in prosecuting based on a witness statement from someone with delusions, a history of engaging in multiple episodes of unprotected sex while having a manic episode, or having been severely impaired as a result of self-medication with drugs or alcohol (O'Hare et al., 2010). This also illustrates the negative public perceptions those with mental illness continue to face.

SOCIAL SECURITY BENEFICIARIES

The number of persons diagnosed with a psychiatric disability continues to grow rapidly, and psychiatric disability is the number-one disability on Social Security benefit rolls (Marini et al., 2004). Psychiatric disability continues to be the disability with the fastest-growing percentage of beneficiaries, currently estimated to be approximately 28% of disabled workers and 41% of those on Supplemental Security Disability Income plus those on Social Security Income (Vercillo, 2011). Of more than 75% of beneficiaries with this diagnosis, half are younger than 30 years and the other half are aged between 30 and 39, thus representing the youngest population among beneficiaries (Marini et al., 2004). This is an alarming increase considering more than 69 million individuals receive benefits from Social Security Administration (SSA) programs (SSA, 2020), and less than 1% of them ever return to gainful employment (Marini et al., 2004).

CONTINUED STIGMA AGAINST PEOPLE WITH MENTAL ILLNESS

Link et al. (1999) conducted a systematic literature review of people's perceptions of mental illness and their thoughts on causes of mental disorders, the dangerousness of those with mental illness, and preferred social distance. Link et al. (1999) found that Americans at that time generally perceived individuals with mental illness to be dangerous and desired minimal contact with them. In terms of causality of mental illness, though, more people shared the views of contemporary mental health professionals that disorders are caused by a variety of complex factors, including environment, biology, and social experiences. A study by Corrigan et al. (2000) a year later found that among their participants, physical illness such as cancer was viewed benignly and depression was the only mental illness seen as nonthreatening and more acceptable. Those with cocaine addiction, psychotic disorders, and what was then termed mental retardation were perceived negatively and discriminated against in the study.

One classic study focused on the stigmatizing attitudes against people with mental illness among mental health professionals. Rosenhan (1973) studied normal and abnormal behaviors, noting that differences existed among cultures. From this, he wondered whether the symptomatic criteria for diagnoses are met solely because they are exhibited by the individual or based on the environment or context. Eight healthy individuals were admitted to 12 different mental hospitals across the United States as pseudopatients. Each pseudopatient falsely reported only his or her name, employment, and psychosocial history and proffered fake symptoms of hearing voices such as a "thud" sound. Further, while in the wards, the pseudopatients behaved as they normally do, were compliant, and reported to the hospital staff that they no longer experienced symptoms when asked. Although the individuals were very high functioning in their daily lives, and the group included a graduate student in psychology, a psychiatrist, three psychologists, a pediatrician, a housewife, a painter, and Rosenhan himself, each was discharged with a diagnosis of schizophrenia in remission, implying that all members of the group were perceived as having schizophrenia throughout their hospitalization. In addition, the pseudopatients were treated dismissively by hospital staff; their questions were ignored completely and, in one instance, a nurse adjusted her bra in front of male patients as if they were not present. At other times, they were verbally and physically abused. It is interesting to note that it was other patients who detected the pseudopatients as being sane. The Rosenhan study demonstrated that behaviors of the pseudopatients were judged in the context of the diagnostic label they were given and the hospital setting they were confined to (Hock, 2019).

The Rosenhan study also illustrated how dangerous stigmatized beliefs about mental disabilities are, as the beliefs lead to prejudicial behaviors. This association of beliefs and behaviors regarding mental illnesses was supported by the findings of the systematic review of 36 articles in various populations by Parcesepe and Cabassa (2013). Stigma against those with mental disabilities include more difficulty finding employment, housing, and adequate healthcare (Overton & Medina, 2008; Stier & Hinshaw, 2007). Stigma can also cause one to be more prone to bullying and violent victimization and problems with the legal system, including voting and parental rights. More recently, Seeman et al.'s (2016) study on stigma and mental illness for both developed and developing countries worldwide found that 45% to 51% of individuals from developed countries view mental health issues similarly to physical health issues. However, 93% of these respondents believe that rehabilitation from mental illness is not possible and 7% to 16% believe that those with a mental illness are more violent than others, illustrating the need to continue to work toward attitudinal change amongst the general population.

CURRENT ISSUES REGARDING MENTAL ILLNESS AND ITS TREATMENT

In their effort to raise awareness, reduce stigma, and encourage help-seeking behaviors, NIMH organized the now-annual National Depression Screening Day in 1991 (Pickren, 2005). Each year since its inception, approximately half a million individuals are screened annually (Screening for Mental Health, Inc., 2011). The U.S. Surgeon General released a landmark publication, *Mental Health—A Report of the Surgeon General*, in 1999 (cited in Grob & Goldman, 2006), emphasizing that mental illnesses are valid conditions and treatments have been shown to be effective (Grob & Goldman, 2006). In addition, the report included the importance of reducing stigma and attitudinal barriers to help-seeking behaviors, tailoring intervention to the individual's cultural background, and the need for more clinicians to be trained in research-based treatments such as cognitive behavioral therapy (Office of the Surgeon General, 2011).

Another government agency, the Department of Veterans Affairs, is making promising efforts on treatment and preventative measures for mental illness. The global war on terrorism (GWT) and its fronts in Afghanistan and Iraq have highlighted the need for improved mental health services as an increasing number of psychiatric casualties are returning to civilian life. For example, the VA disseminates to healthcare providers and mental health clinicians evidence-based clinical practice guidelines for mental and physical health issues (U.S. Department of Veterans Affairs, 2011). Furthermore, taking into account the stigma against disclosing emotional concerns among service members and their resulting hesitancy to go to a mental health center, the VA expanded its primary care services to be better equipped to address veterans' clinical mental health needs (Committee on Veterans Affairs, 2007). According to the U.S. Department of Defense (DOD), as of July 2011, there were close to 45,000 servicemen wounded in action in the GWT, many of whom were diagnosed with a mental disability such as posttraumatic stress disorder (DOD, 2011). As veterans are returning to civilian life with service-related emotional disabilities, greater protections have been placed to help ensure they are provided equal treatment and opportunities.

In 1990, the Americans with Disabilities Act (ADA) was passed by Congress to provide equal opportunity and protection against discrimination on the basis of physical and mental disabilities (DOJ, 1990). For veterans and other individuals diagnosed with a mental illness, the ADA means that they have a right to reasonable accommodations, such as having a service dog trained to ease heightened anxiety and for the dog to be allowed to accompany them, flexible work schedules that enable them to attend counseling sessions, to have instructions provided in writing, to have tasks broken down to more manageable increments, extended deadlines, and additional breaks for those with memory impairments or difficulty focusing (DOJ, 2010).

Chamberlin (1993) noted that the ADA's inclusion of mental disabilities aroused controversy at the time and exposed some prejudices. Some of those who debated the bill questioned whether individuals with mental illnesses are reliable employees or whether they are dangerous, unstable, undependable, and lazy. Despite the controversy, the ADA was passed into law and individuals with mental disabilities were afforded the same protections as those with physical disabilities. Since its inception, the ADA has undergone several revisions to strengthen its language and enforceability (DOJ, 2009).

Although those with mental illness still face multiple challenges, such as discrimination, stigma, lack of access to treatment, and disability (Mechanic & Rochefort, 1990), barriers are being reduced and treatments are being improved. Individuals and organizations, both public and private, continue to strive to raise public awareness and lobby for the needs of those with mental illness. A growing number of treatment options are available, including psychiatric hospitals (long- or short-term inpatient), emergency services (short-term acute care), private practice psychotherapists and psychiatrists, community mental health centers (comprehensive and state funded), community support services (halfway houses, quarter-way houses, day treatment centers), medication management, and self-help. Holistic treatment approaches are also being used as a way of improving the quality of mental health care, combining skills training, a social support system, environmental and behavioral modification, vocational assistance, and medication. With the variety of options available, more Americans are receiving mental health treatment than ever before (Shorter, 1997). Although gaps remain, the definite gains in efforts to prevent and effectively treat mental illness through the years are worthy to note.

Successful efforts are being made through public policy, advocacy organizations, and private individuals to raise awareness of mental illness, reduce its stigma, and combat discrimination against those with the disability. For example, more Americans are seeking treatment for mental health and emotional issues; 46.2% of adults with any mental illness received inpatient, outpatient, or prescription medication treatment in 2020 (NIMH, 2022). The costs for mental health care, however, have been increasing. Mental health treatment was estimated to cost $225 billion in 2019 (Open Minds, 2020) and was projected to grow 4.6% in subsequent years (SAMHSA, 2014). The cost in 2019 was a 52.1% growth from 2009 (Open Minds, 2020).

FUTURE TRENDS IN THE TREATMENT OF PSYCHIATRIC DISABILITIES

The emergence of the COVID-19 pandemic in 2020 brought unique challenges to individuals worldwide. While some subsets of individuals have experienced improved functioning, many others have experienced increased challenges during this traumatic period of time (Mancini, 2020). Cutler and Summers (2020) reported that the proportion of the U.S. population who had symptoms of depression or anxiety was approximately 11% in early 2019. However, by mid-2020, the number had risen to approximately 40%, which translates to roughly 80 million additional people with mental health conditions as a result of the pandemic. The increase in those needing mental health treatment in a time where many were losing their jobs and healthcare insurance while being quarantined posed unique challenges to mental health professionals.

Various strains related to COVID-19 negatively affected the global population, and in particular those with disabilities and other chronic conditions, who were at greater risk for increased complications due to their conditions (Umucu & Lee, 2020). Past research had demonstrated that the greater the perceived stress, the greater the probability of lower quality of life, depression, anxiety, and general health (Bishop-Fitzpatrick et al., 2018; Park et al., 2019; Umucu & Lee, 2020). For those with disabilities, greater perceived stress may increase functional limitations. In their rapid review of 11 research articles conducted on the impacts of COVID-19 for people with physical disabilities, Lebrasseur et al. (2021) found that service barriers encountered were the discontinuance of home healthcare, halting of physiotherapy, lack of available ambulances and public transportation, and medication shortages. Individuals were not only afraid of health complications from their disabilities but were fearful of going to the hospital and contracting COVID-19 there. In addition to elevated stress and anxiety levels, respondents reported anger, frequent mood changes, and poor sleep hygiene. Satisfaction with sexual functioning, however, was found to increase during the pandemic. Health outcomes for those with intellectual, developmental, and mental disabilities during the pandemic were likewise poor. One study on nearly 65 million individuals found that an intellectual disability was the strongest risk factor for presenting with a COVID-19 diagnosis and second to age for mortality from COVID-19, independent of any other risk factor (Gleason et al., 2021).

For those with spinal cord injuries (SCIs), the challenges faced were exacerbated by the disability. The common effects of the pandemic for those with *any* disability—such as social isolation (including from providers) and loss of access to medical services—cause a level of distress that intensified pain and spasms experienced by individuals with SCI (Hearn et al., 2021). Respiratory complications were already a frequent concern for those with SCI prior to the pandemic (Sánchez-Raya & Sampol, 2020). The devastating respiratory effects of COVID-19 presented individuals with a new layer to their already heightened anxieties about their health. This is coupled with the lack of healthcare and rehabilitation services specific to SCIs that were the most commonly reported issue among this population during the pandemic (Hearn et al., 2021; Sánchez-Raya & Sampol, 2020). Even when health and rehabilitation services were available, individuals with SCI reported being much less inclined to attend outpatient appointments, much less the hospital, for necessary care due to concerns that they would increase their risk of contracting COVID-19. The gains many had made in their rehabilitation pre-COVID were greatly diminished post-COVID, which in turn had a negative impact on mental well-being. Other issues unique to those with SCIs that had increased feelings of fear and vulnerability are proneness to respiratory ailments, immunosuppression, and the need for caregivers.

While technology had been utilized for the decades preceding COVID-19, the arrival of the pandemic spurred many professionals, wary and slow to adopt telehealth technology into their practice, to do just that. The adoption of telehealth was necessary to connect with clients who were otherwise isolated due to lockdown measures and would not have been able to receive services. As aforementioned, telecommunication with clients was not new and evolved as technology improved. Methods include counseling by telephone, text messaging, and videoconferencing. Letter writing between patient and psychiatrist was not uncommon at the turn of the 20th century (Everett, 1999). Sigmund Freud was said to correspond with patients via letters, one of which to survive was a letter requesting dream analysis and his reply in 1927 (Benjamin & Dixon, 1996). An early professional organization promoting the use of online communications for mental health provision is the International Society for Mental Health Online (ISMHO, 2022), which was formed in 1997. Conducting all of its business online, the organization provides a forum for professionals to discuss and collaborate on issues related to online mental health services.

Despite its early start, therapists were slow to adopt the technology. A prevalent concern was confidentiality and informed consent. Therapists and clients alike did not fully trust that online data remained private from hackers and government surveillance (Hertlein et al., 2015; Lustgarten & Colbow, 2017). Therapists were also concerned about whether or not they could identify the identity of the individual they were conversing with online or via telephone and who else might be in the client's vicinity during the telehealth session (Hertlein et al., 2015). Another ethical concern cited by professionals was the risk to patient–provider relationship. The therapeutic relationship is the bedrock of the work that is done in counseling, and many therapists wondered if they would not be able to fully connect to clients or read nonverbal cues. Therapists were especially concerned about their ability to assess and care for clients who present with active suicidal or homicidal ideation. Competency in providing online therapy services, whether licenses allowed clinicians to provide services to individuals in other states, and which online platforms were considered secure were other ethical concerns. Most psychiatric and counselor training programs did not educate on utilizing technology for service provision, and thus many did not feel confident that they would be able to provide ethical and competent treatment (MacMullin et al., 2020). For a sizeable portion of mental health providers and those with psychiatric disabilities, the concerns outweighed the benefits. Despite this, research had consistently demonstrated that online therapies were as effective as traditional face-to-face therapies (Amichai-Hamburger et al., 2014). Proponents countered criticisms by providing suggestions on how to enhance assessment procedures, gather as many client cues as possible, maximize client outcomes, and meet with clients who are unable to travel for an in-person session. Online proponents also pointed out that telephone hotlines had long intervened in crises and these procedures could translate to online counseling provision.

Resistance to the adoption of telehealth by providers was effectively ended after the COVID-19 pandemic hit in early 2020. The options were to not see clients or see clients willing to come in person and risk contracting the disease. Professional organizations, training organizations, and educational institutions assisted in alleviating discomfort by providing easily accessible trainings and informational materials on providing technology-based counseling services (MacMullin et al., 2020). Online videoconferencing platforms worked to address confidentiality concerns and make their platforms were compliant with the Health Insurance Portability and Accountability Act (HIPAA). Procedures were promoted to address the ethical concerns of telehealth delivery. Providers were able to meet with clients who were already more difficult to meet with prior to the pandemic, such as persons with disabilities and refugees and found that they were able to provide quality mental health services to their clients (Dores et al., 2020). Acceptance of telehealth counseling for both providers and clients is evidenced by many choosing to continue to provide online remote therapy despite lockdown restrictions being lifted, changing the landscape of treatment for persons with psychiatric disabilities.

CONCLUSION

By analyzing past issues, we are better able to understand and address present concerns. Much like understanding our own personal histories enables us to identify goals and plan our future trajectory, a historical literacy of the treatment of psychiatric disabilities enables us to work toward continued best practices and policies for persons with such disabilities. From its inception, the field has witnessed new and evolving waves of thought regarding psychiatric disabilities, and that process continues. The Middle Ages, the starting point for this chapter, was a time when mental illness was viewed through superstitious and religious lenses. Those with mental illnesses did not fare much better in Colonial America, where warehousing or incarceration of individuals in inhumane conditions were commonplace, which carried over into the Industrial Age. The exception to this occurred within generally unacculturated indigenous populations, who often viewed those with psychiatric disabilities as having "gifts." The mid-20th century and the end of WWII brought us a more modern, evidence-based view of psychiatric disabilities and their treatments, including the development and refinement of psychotherapy or "talk therapy." While mental illness continues to be stigmatized, improvements in public policies and continued refinement and evolution of treatment practices present a promising future. This revised chapter includes an analysis of how the 2020 COVID-19 pandemic impacted future trends in the treatment of persons with psychiatric disabilities.

CLASS ACTIVITIES

1. Design a group discussion around the topic of "what if" everyone who had a severe psychiatric illness had to wear a sign indicating their diagnosis around their neck. How would their family, friends, and the public think, feel, and likely interact with them?

2. Conduct a take-home assignment to read about, then write a two-page double-spaced paper about the Willowbrook psychiatric hospital scandal in New York.

3. Newspaper Assignment: Working in groups of four, students create the front page of a newspaper complete with stories and images of key events during a period of time relating to psychiatric disabilities.

4. Mini Lecture Assignment: Each student will choose one key historical figure in the evolution of the treatment of psychiatric disabilities highlighted in the chapter or elsewhere and develop a mini lecture on that individual explaining their significance to the class.

KEY REFERENCES

Only key references appear in the print edition. The full references appear in the digital product on Springer Publishing Connect™: https://connect.springerpub.com/content/book/978-0-8261-5111-7/part/partI/chapter/ch03

American Psychiatric Association. (2018). *Statistical manual for the use of institutions for the insane*. Franklin Classics Trade Press. (Original work published 1918).

American Psychiatric Association. (2022). *Diagnostic and statistical manual of mental disorders* (5th ed., text rev.). https://doi.org/10.1176/appi.books.9780890425787

Dix, D. (1904). *Memorial to the legislature of Massachusetts*. https://archive.org/details/memorialtolegisl00dixd

Lebrasseur, A., Fortin-Bédard, N., Lettre, J., Bussiéres, E., Best, K., Boucher, N., Hotton, M., Beauliei-Bonneau, S., Mercier, C., Lamontagne, M., & Routhier, F. (2021). Impact of COVID-19 on people with physical disabilities: A rapid review. *Disability and Health Journal, 14*(1), 101014. https://doi.org/10.1016/j.dhjo.2020.101014

Marini, I., Feist, A., & Miller, E. (2004). Vocational expert testimony for the Social Security Administration: Observations from the field. *Journal of Forensic Vocational Analysts, 7*(1), 25–34.

Obermann, C. E. (1965). *A history of vocational rehabilitation in America* (2nd ed.) [Electronic version]. T.S. Denison & Company. https://www.bjs.gov/content/pub/pdf/mhppji.pdf

Shorter, E. (2015). The history of nosology and the rise of the *Diagnostic and Statistical Manual of Mental Disorders*. *Dialogues in Clinical Neuroscience, 17*(1), 59–67. https://10.31887/DCNS.2015.17.1.eshorter

Social Security Administration (SSA). (2020). *Fast facts & figures about Social Security, 2020*. https://www.ssa.gov/policy/docs/chartbooks/fast_facts/2020/fast_facts20.html#:~:text=69.1%20million%20people%20received%20benefits,beneficiaries%20in%202019%20were%20women

CHAPTER 4

DISABILITY IDENTITY AND DISABILITY CULTURE

CARLYN MUELLER, ERIN E. ANDREWS, AND BRADLEY J. MINOTTI

LEARNING OBJECTIVES

After reading this chapter, you will be able to:

- Define disability identity and disability culture
- Explain the importance of models of disability and their application to theories of disability identity development
- Evaluate usage of disability language in clinical settings and its impact on disability identity
- Apply appropriate counseling techniques, activities, and strategies to disability identity as integrated into counseling and psychotherapy

PRE-READING QUESTIONS

1. What do you think of when you hear the term "disability identity"?
2. Is identity development mostly an individual or social process?
3. Where have you seen examples of disability culture in your community or work settings?

In our broader cultural conversation about disability, individuals with disabilities are often depicted as passive recipients of clinical interventions designed to erase or minimize disability and its impact on the body and mind (Andrews, 2019). These passive depictions of individuals with disabilities not only minimize the role and importance of disability in embodied experiences; they also dismiss essential internal and social processes of developing disability identity and culture that are fundamental to understanding a holistic picture of the individual with a disability. In this chapter, we discuss a growing body of scholarship focused on exploring the processes of identity and cultural development around disability, toward a new understanding of people with disabilities themselves as agentic and involved in co-creating, defining, and growing disability as an identity and cultural category.

DISABILITY IDENTITY

One way people with disabilities understand their disability labels is through the development of disability identity. Disability identity development is a psychological, social, and cultural process of understanding and making meaning out of disability labels, embodied experiences, and participation in the disability community. It includes internal and external influences and processes, including positive senses of self, alongside feelings of connection with the disability community more broadly (Dunn & Burcaw, 2013; Forber-Pratt & Zape, 2017). Mpofu and Harley (2006) note that disability identity as a construct is built from three assumptions that individuals hold: First, disability status is an important and significant way to define themselves; disability identity acceptance is essential to improving psychosocial functioning; and awareness of disability identity necessarily leads to greater consciousness and connection to disability community discrimination, marginalization, and prejudice. Disability identity, then, includes many aspects and facets that often relate to self-concept, including aspects of self-esteem, group identity, and self-efficacy (e.g. Bandura, 1977). As a social group identity with internal meaning-making about impairment, it also includes facets of solidarity and affinity with the disability community, disability pride, disability activism, and the meaning and value in disability experiences (Bogart, 2014).

History of Disability Identity and Scholarship

Disability identity has been described, defined, and explored across a variety of fields and methods interested in the life experiences of people with disabilities. Disability identity development is also relevant across all fields that serve people with disabilities, and each field has a different approach to studying and understanding the process. This is evident even in the beginnings of this field of research. Though people with disabilities have always formed identities and relationships to understand their impairments, the mid-1990s saw an increased amount of academic work describing this phenomenon. Kathy Charmaz and Arthur Frank, both sociologists, and Carol Gill, a clinical and developmental psychologist, are credited among the earliest scholars to describe the social phenomenon of disability identity (Forber-Pratt et al., 2017). Importantly, all three had personal experience with disability and illness, including chronic illnesses and cancer, that informed and animated their research to consider disability as not solely a clinical experience but a deeply personal, internal, and communal one. This approach led both Frank (1993) and Charmaz (1994, 1995) to center their analysis on illness narratives and longitudinal qualitative analyses that focused on individuals' understandings of acquired disability. Frank (1993) described a period of critical reflection essential after the acquisition of a disability that results in major changes to the individual's understanding of themselves. Charmaz (1995) emphasized the importance of "identity synthesis" in understanding and making meaning out of disability; if an individual acquires a disability after undergoing this process, there is a marked difference compared with an individual still in the process of forming their identity. In contrast, Gill (1997) noted the importance of developing the self in relation to others with disability, suggesting not only the importance of others in the disability identity development process but also the role of isolation and separation inherent in many individuals' understandings of disability as a phenomenon.

Disability identity in rehabilitation psychology is an important feature of identity with real-life impacts. Recent research on disability identity suggests that identification with disability predicts higher collective and personal self-esteem (Nario-Redmond et al., 2013) and lower depression and anxiety in people with specific disabilities (Bogart, 2015). These kinds of positive outcomes suggest that disability identity can act as a counternarrative to the stigma and negative associations that many also experience, given the larger social and societal context of disability and ableism. As Gill (1997) suggested, disability identity as an internal experience involves more than just identification or "overcoming" negative societal ideas. It involves community connection, participation, and affiliation as a feature of identity development (Putnam, 2005). As an internal and external experience, disability identity can act as an important way for individuals to understand their personal experience with impairment, as well as the larger societal response to disability and potential affiliation with the disability community.

DISABILITY CULTURE

Disability culture is the celebration and reappropriation of a traditionally negative identity and consists of expressions of disability pride (Andrews, 2019; Andrews & Forber-Pratt, 2022). Because people can become disabled at any point in their life span, disability is a unique group identity, but it shares commonalities with other stigmatized groups such as the LGBTQIAP+ community (Mona et al., 2017). A disabled person may come from a long line of disabled people or, conversely, may be the only person in their family with a disability.

Brown (2002) described disability culture as the creation of artifacts, beliefs, and expressions of disabled people themselves as a reflection of their own life experiences. Gill (1995) reasoned that the purpose of disability culture is the cross-disability promotion of connection, camaraderie, and shared purpose to advocate from within the disability community. She developed arguably the most well-known model of disability culture, which she states has four functions: fortification, unification, communication, and recruitment (Gill, 1995). Gill (1995) postulated that disability culture brings people with disabilities together and helps them energize one another toward common goals and values. Both Gill (1995) and Brown (2002) point out that the shared experience of oppressive treatment alone is not the sole basis for disability culture, but rather that it goes beyond that to universally transmitted characteristics and preferences, that Gill (1995) noted even cross international boundaries. Gill (1997) identified eight values inherent in disability culture; among them are an appreciation of human differences, interdependence, tolerance of unpredictability, problem-solving skills, use of disability humor, and an adaptive and nontraditional approach to tasks.

One of the most important core values of disability culture noted by Gill (1995) is interdependence. Longmore's (1995) work on the shift from disability rights to disability culture similarly noted the disability community's values around the importance of personal connection over functional separateness and self-determination over self-sufficiency that are "markedly different from, and even opposed to, nondisabled majority values" (p. 147). This value of being able to accept care and assistance, whether from others or from devices or technology, is in stark opposition to the heavy Western emphasis on independence as a value. Within disability culture, autonomy, or the ability to make choices and have a sense of control over one's life, is crucial, but not the ability to independently carry out all tasks of everyday living (Andrews & Forber-Pratt, 2022). In disability culture, disabled life is not devalued the same way that it is by outsiders, and in fact disability is celebrated and considered a source of pride (Grue, 2016).

History of Disability Culture and Scholarship

Disability culture is not a new phenomenon, but one that has received increasing attention in recent years (Andrews, 2019). However, it historically has not received the same degree of attention as other cultures, despite the fact that disability is the largest minority group in the United States. This is largely an artifact of disability being most commonly conceptualized as a medical rather than a cultural experience (Brown, 2002; Gill, 1995). Gill (1995) noted that this medicalized context, which often results in marginalization, poverty, isolation, lack of education, silencing, imposed immobility, and encouragement to separate from other people with disabilities, has not simultaneously stamped out the existence of disability culture. In fact, disability culture has always existed; "any time people with disabilities have been able to come together," through activism, peer support groups, camps, congregate settings such as jails and nursing homes, and other ways people with disabilities opt in or are forced to be together, "culture flourishes." (Gill, 1995, p. 166).

Disability culture is also often associated with certain sociopolitical stances, including a social justice orientation and at times an anticapitalist view (Sins Invalid, 2017). It can also include a position against physician-assisted suicide and eugenic abortion (based on disability status) along with promotion of emancipation from nursing homes and general deinstitutionalization. These views are not universally held, but for those involved in disability rights advocacy groups such as American Disabled for Attendant Programs Today (ADAPT) and Not Dead Yet, these issues are important tenets.

MODELS OF DISABILITY AND DISABILITY IDENTITY DEVELOPMENT

Models of disability can help frame the way we consider the notion of disability identity development and disability culture. Older models such as the moral model frame disability as a distinctly negative concept, associated with sin and shame (Andrews, 2016). More contemporary models such as the medical model position disability as a problem residing within the person, in need of healthcare services for amelioration or compensatory strategies (Andrews, 2016). These models are focused on fixing the person and aim for maximum assimilation with the nondisabled population (Haegele & Hodge, 2016). The social model of disability, however, postulates that disability is a problem of interaction between the person and the environment and therefore does not inherently consider disability to be a problem in and of itself (Andrews, 2017). The onus is on society to make changes to become more accessible (Haegele & Hodge, 2016). The diversity model goes even further to suggest that disability is a normal human state and can even be celebrated (Andrews, 2016). It is these two latter models, then, that are most consistent with the construct of disability identity, of the development of an integrated positive sense of self to include one's disabled identity.

Medical Model of Disability

The medical model views disability as an individual problem for a disabled person to address through the use of medical treatments and other interventions to treat the impairments that stem from a person's disability (Haegele & Hodge, 2016). Furthermore, disability is often viewed through the lens of a diagnostic label given by medical professionals. Subsequently, the person's disability is seen as a set of symptoms that exist within the individual that are unrelated to broader societal or environmental factors. Therefore, this paradigm positions disability as a medical problem that can only be addressed through the alleviation of symptoms in order to fit into the norms of a society built for nondisabled people (Dunn & Andrews, 2015).

Research has suggested that the medical model of disability has had a negative impact on the lives of people with disabilities. This is particularly true for those with chronic illnesses and disabilities who report that they face prejudice and discrimination due to the long-term nature of their disabilities, which discourages them from seeking care from a medical or mental health care provider (Earnshaw & Quinn 2012). Additionally, belief in the medical model predicted more negative attitudes toward those with disabilities among college students (Bogart & Nario-Redmond, 2019). Furthermore, one experimental study found that those exposed to beliefs central to the medical model were less likely to support legislation to improve accessibility for disabled people (Dirth & Branscombe, 2017). Taken together, these research findings indicate that the medical model of disability may contribute to negative attitudes toward people with disabilities, which can have a negative impact on their quality of life.

Social Model of Disability

In contrast with the medical model of disability, the social model of disability proposes that the environment imposes barriers on people with disabilities that lead to difficulty with full participation in society (Barnes, 2019; Haegele & Hodge, 2016). Therefore, the focus of the social model is on removing barriers in the environment that impede a disabled person's ability to live as they choose in society. This can take the form of societal changes to support people with disabilities through laws to promote accessibility and prevent discrimination against people with disabilities. Some examples include the Americans with Disabilities Amendments Act (ADAA; 2008) and the Individuals with Disabilities Education Act (IDEA, 2004), which provide accommodations for students with disabilities. However, it is important to note that medical treatment, adaptive equipment, and other personalized supports can be a part of the social model to support disabled people, but the emphasis remains on removing environmental barriers for students with disabilities in the K–12 education system.

The social model of disability is focused on the environmental barriers faced by disabled people and shifts the person's disability to a condition that is caused by an inaccessible and ableist society. Therefore, disability can be viewed as a part of an individual's lived experience (Haegele & Hodge, 2016). The social model enables disabled people to advocate for their needs in order to dismantle the barriers present in their lived environments. Additionally, those who work with disabled people, such as psychologists, medical doctors, and others, can also work to address inequities disabled people face due to societal inaccessibility and the negative stereotypes and perceptions that exist about disabled people (Goering, 2015).

Diversity Model of Disability

The diversity model of disability positions disability as a social identity and postulates that people with disabilities have a sense of community through shared experiences due to being disabled (Andrews, 2016). Furthermore, the diversity model of disability recognizes that social networks of disabled people have created a disability community in which many disabled people have developed a strong sense of disability identity. This model focuses on how ableism and relationships with both disabled and nondisabled people shape the experiences of those with a disability. In contrast to the categorization of disability as a negative construct, as in the medical model, disability is seen as an integral part of a person's identity similar to other social identities such as race and ethnicity, sexual orientation, and gender identity (Andrews & Forber-Pratt, 2022).

Given that disability is viewed as a social identity, having a disability is no longer determined solely by impairment due to medical symptoms or environmental barriers (Andrews, 2016). Moreover, this allows for the unique experiences of each disabled person to be heard and understood. Furthermore, this model enables an intersectional analysis of how a person's disability interacts with their other identities to shape their individual experience due to the intersection of ableism and other forms of oppression (e.g., sexism, homophobia, racism; Artiles, 2013; Crenshaw, 1989). Therefore, the diversity model recognizes the multifaceted identity of individuals with disabilities in order to center their experiences. This model may support the development of disability identity, which has been linked to lower levels of some forms of mental health distress among disabled people (Bogart, 2015).

Models and Components of Disability Identity Development

Inside a broader understanding of disability comprising different models (including medical, social, and diversity models), there are also various models specific to disability identity that theorize and describe various external and internal factors which comprise this process of identity development

(Forber Pratt et al., 2017). The Gill (1997) model of disability identity development was one of the first models to examine the various facets of disability identity development. In this model, people with disabilities defined "who they are and where they belong" based on four types of status integration, which people with disabilities move through sequentially: coming to feel we belong (integrating into society), coming home (integrating with the disability community), coming together (internally integrating our sameness and differentness), and coming out (integrating how we feel with how we present ourselves; Gill, 1997, p. 42). Importantly, this is a process that builds from a desire for acceptance in society into a focus on disability community and appreciation of disability in relation to a larger sense of self; the community affiliation with disability is an essential component in this model toward this integration process.

Similarly, Putnam (2005) emphasizes the role of political activism and awareness of the importance and consistent fight for disability rights as significant in the development of *political* disability identity development. In this model, the fundamentally political nature of disability as a minoritized identity bridges some complicated terrain between individual and collective notions of disability as an identity category (e.g. Caldwell, 2011; Schur, 1998). To understand this terrain, Putnam (2005) identified six domains that together shape political identification with disability as an identity category: self-worth, pride, discrimination, common cause, policy alternatives, and engagement in political action. Internal aspects of these domains, like self-worth or pride, represent ways individuals can relate to their identity. External aspects, like discrimination, develop as a result of interactions with ableism and inaccessible public and social structures. Together, this model suggests the importance of collective action and participation for development of disability identity and awareness of the ways individuals might vary in their understanding of this community.

Some more recent models of disability contend with the internal aspects of disability identity and awareness. Gibson (2006) identified three stages of identity development, across birth to adulthood (though the stages do not necessarily move sequentially). The first stage, Passive Awareness, can occur in the first part of life into adulthood and includes a lack of role models of disability and denial of the social aspects of disability. In stage two, Realization, which occurs in adolescence or early adulthood, people with disabilities begin to see their relationship to disability and often experience self-hate, anger, and concerns over appearance and perception from others. As a result, they may develop what Gibson (2006) terms the "superman/woman complex," and has also been described as the "supercrip," where people with disabilities work hard to overcome their disability and are depicted by others as inspirational and heroic (Martin, 2017). In the final stage, Acceptance, adults with disabilities are able to progress from this negative and difference-based understanding of disability into something more holistically positive. Often, people at this stage participate in the disability community, develop as advocates and activists, and embrace their identities as a whole.

The Darling and Heckert (2010) model of disability examined the internal views of those with disabilities toward their disability, interaction with the disability community, and a sense of disability pride. Importantly, they examine these views based on an understanding of "orientation toward disability," which they consider broader than disability identity development as a construct, though related. Similar to Putnam, Darling and Heckert (2010) position disability activism, models or perspectives on disability, internal definitions, evaluative understandings, and behavioral commitments as aspects of orientation to disability. They found that older individuals over the age of 65 reported higher medical model beliefs and lower levels of disability pride than younger disabled people.

Forber-Pratt and Zape (2017) proposed a four-status model of disability identity. These statuses include acceptance of disability, which is when a disabled individual accepts that they are disabled and shares this with others; the relationship status, where the person meets other disabled people; the adoption status, where the individual views themselves as a part of the disability community; and the engagement status, where disabled individuals give support to others with disabilities. This model uses statuses to highlight that disabled people can be in multiple statuses at the same time and that a person's sense of their disability identity can change over time (Forber-Pratt & Zape, 2017). The aforementioned models and most of the current literature are focused on disabled adults. However, recent research suggests that disabled teenagers may also be engaging in complex processes internally (understanding their disability) and externally with both disabled and nondisabled peers as they work to build a sense of disability identity (Forber-Pratt et al., 2021).

In sum, while scholars have proposed different theories about disability identity and its components, most models contain both an internal individual component and an external component of connection to other disabled people and the wider disability community (Forber-Pratt et al., 2017). This highlights that disability identity development is shaped by a person's view of their disability and their interaction with disabled people as well as their experience of ableism from society. This is closely linked to the models of disability. The medical model stigmatizes disability and views disability as an individual problem to be treated (Andrews, 2017). This paradigm may make it challenging for disabled people to accept their disability and begin to develop their own disability identity. Conversely, the social and diversity models seek to mitigate disability stigma, which may help disabled people to explore their disability identity. Lastly, it is important to note that the disability community is diverse and that each disabled person may view their disability from any of the models presented earlier and have vastly different ideas about whether and in what way they identify as disabled, due in part to life experience and the intersectionality of other identities.

HIGHLIGHTING THE IMPORTANCE OF IDENTITY DEVELOPMENT FOR PEOPLE WITH DISABILITIES

Role of Disability Self-Concept in Adaptation to Congenital or Acquired Disability

While models of disability and disability identity development emphasize the importance of a collective sense of disability community and membership, there are important differences in disability experiences that impact disability identity development as well. Adaptation to acquired disability has been an important ongoing conversation in rehabilitation psychology research, where individuals undergo a variety of internal changes in relationship to their impairment and understanding of their new lived reality (Livneh & Antonak, 1997; Livneh & Martz, 2012). Disability identity development is similarly impacted by the distinction between acquired and congenital disability experiences, and there are important subgroup differences that inform our broader understanding of the larger community experience of disability identity. For example, people with congenital disabilities are more likely to consider disability an important aspect of themselves (Smart, 2008). In contrast, people with acquired disabilities contend with sudden membership in a group that experiences social stigma and report a significant sense of loss of identity (Smart, 2008). The development of disability identity is impacted significantly by the onset and type of disability and by the way the person integrates (or does not) into the disability community.

Extant research on adaptation of people with congenital and acquired conditions reports a difference between the groups. People with congenital disabilities are generally "better adapted" than people with acquired disabilities (Bogart, 2014, p. 5). This adaptation includes better acceptance of disability (Li & Moore, 1998) and usage of compensatory strategies (Bogart et al., 2012). In a landmark study on the differences between congenital and acquired disability, Bogart (2014) similarly found that people with congenital disabilities had higher disability self-concept and satisfaction with life than people with acquired disabilities and that disability identity and self-concept themselves were significant predictors of satisfaction with life.

How can rehabilitation psychologists and other clinicians support positive disability identity development of people with acquired disabilities? Baldridge and Kulkarni (2017) suggest that people with acquired severe hearing loss engage in a meaning-making search for answers such as "Who am I?" and "Am I still successful?" as part of a redefinition of themselves in relation to their disability. Dunn and Burcaw (2013) encourage this meaning-making process with individuals' disability stories, suggesting that the search for meaning-making itself can result in positive "silver linings" that motivate and sustain the redefinition process. Later in this chapter, we discuss specific strategies for use in clinical and therapeutic settings that open conversations about disability identity across both acquired and congenital disabilities and specifically focus on the importance of personal stories about disabilities. As part of this clinical process, it is also important to consider tools and measures that engage the identity development process in a more quantitative way.

Existing Disability Identity Measures

Because disability identity is a complex social and cultural phenomenon, it can be understood through a variety of methods. Often, and most frequently in existing identity research across different fields, disability identity is described qualitatively. This may include interviews, individual reflection, and longitudinal methods (Forber-Pratt et al., 2017). Qualitative methods of understanding the disability identity method afford an in-depth, detailed, and complex description of the process based on a typically small number of participants, who describe their experiences, histories, memories, and current understandings of themselves and their broader connections to the disability community. While this is an important and widely used strategy in both research and clinical settings, it is not the only way of understanding disability identity.

More recently, researchers and clinicians have also explored quantitative methods appropriate to understand and "measure" disability identity for use in counseling and clinical practice. Quantitative measurement tools, such as scales and batteries, allow for an examination of disability identity with a larger and more varied scope and number of participants. Disability identity quantitative measures afford clinicians a statistical examination across different disability labels and components of disability identity; it also can include an understanding and comparison of the impacts of identity on other constructs, such as disability pride (e.g., Nario-Redmond et al., 2013). Quantitative measurement tools, like qualitative measurement tools, are grounded in theoretical and empirical definitions of disability identity (such as the ones discussed earlier in this chapter) that inform the validation and usage of the tool for everyday practice. In this way, an underlying theoretical understanding of disability identity as a phenomenon guides all of the ways psychologists and clinicians might assess and understand this with their clients.

To date, there are five quantitative disability identity measures for potential use in clinical and counseling settings (Darling & Heckert, 2010; Forber-Pratt et al., 2022; Gibson et al., 2018; Gill, 1997; Hahn & Belt, 2004). Each measure defines and explores the construct of disability identity across a wide range of disability experiences, includes item and scale development information, and some state the internal validity of the items in the measure. For further discussion of the importance of construct validation in disability identity development measures, see (Forber-Pratt et al., 2017). Importantly, each of the mentioned scales and measurement tools have differing and individual subscales, subconstructs, or ways of conceptually defining disability identity.

The earliest quantitative measurement tool was developed by Gill (1997). The Disability Identity Scale includes 17 statements consisting of attitudes about disability, which correspond to a Likert scale and Gill's (1997) model of disability integration. The model of disability integration has been used with populations across disability and other intersectional identities, including lesbians and bisexual women with chronic illnesses (Axtell, 1999); women with hidden disabilities, including muscular dystrophy, arthritis, and epilepsy (Valeras, 2010); and queer women with disabilities, including arthritis, chronic pain, and mental health issues such as posttraumatic stress disorder (PTSD), depression, and social anxiety (Whitney, 2006).

Another influential and broadly utilized quantitative measurement tool is Hahn and Belt's (2004) Personal Identity Scale. The Personal Identity Scale measures two constructs through an eight-item Likert scale: affirmation of disability, or immersion in the common disability community experiences and positive feelings about membership in the disability community, and denial of disability, or feelings of worthlessness or uselessness to other disabled people. These constructs are both conceptualized as separate and independent facets of disability identity. The Personal Identity Scale was adapted by Zhang and Haller (2013) in their Self-Identity Scale and utilized to demonstrate associations between disability identity and satisfaction with life for people with multiple sclerosis (Bogart, 2014), self-efficacy for people with retinitis pigmentosa (Zapata, 2018), and relationship between disability affirmation and employment status for people with physical disabilities (Zapata, 2020).

Darling and Heckert's (2010) Questionnaire on Disability Identity and Opportunity (QDIO) explores two dimensions of disability through a 30-item Likert scale: participation and orientation. Participation includes both mainstream society and disability community, where people with disabilities have access to both communities and engage in activities (Darling & Heckert, 2010). Orientation includes constructs of identity (including pride and stigma or shame), model (social and personal), and role (activism versus passivity; Darling & Heckert, 2010). The QDIO pride subscale has been utilized by Bogart et al. (2017) to discuss the mediating relationship between disability pride and stigma.

More recently, Gibson et al. (2018) developed the Gibson Disability Identity Development Scale, based on an earlier conceptual model of disability identity development. This model includes three developmental stages: Passive Awareness, Realization, and Acceptance. These stages correspond to ages from birth to adulthood, but can also occur across the life span (Gibson, 2006). Importantly, this is the only current identity scale that is developed for potential use with children and adolescents. The scale contains 12 Likert-scale statements that represent each developmental stage. In an application of the Gibson Disability Identity Development Scale for people with visual disabilities, Gibson et al. (2018) found that the majority of adult participants with congenital visual disabilities scored in the Acceptance range.

A final disability identity measurement tool is the Disability Identity Development Scale (DIDS; Forber-Pratt et al., 2020, 2022). This scale identifies four components of disability identity that collectively make up the construct: internal beliefs about an individual's disability and the disability community, anger and frustration with disability experiences, adoption of disability community values, and contribution to the disability community (Forber-Pratt et al., 2022). The scale results in a total score that reflects the salience of disability identity at a given time.

Alongside other counseling techniques and strategies described in the next section, measuring disability identity quantitatively provides clinicians and researchers with tools to open up conversations with people who have disabilities and to allow those measurements to inform their practice. Importantly, regardless of the strategy or tool used, the person with the disability should still be seen as the expert in their own identity, awareness, and relationship to disability. Measurement tools are one way of strengthening the individual's efficacy and autonomy around these constructs.

SUPPORTING IDENTITY DEVELOPMENT WITH COUNSELING

In addition to the usage of measurement tools like the ones described in the previous section, there are many ways in which the concept of disability identity development can be integrated into counseling and psychotherapy. It is important, first, however, to acknowledge that our understanding of how disability identity can be applied in clinical settings is not yet well understood (Forber-Pratt et al., 2019). It is also important to underscore that disability may not be the reason that a person seeks counseling, nor the most salient aspect of their presentation, and that it is important to view disability through the lens appropriate to the context so that other personal factors are not overshadowed (Olkin, 2017). Disability identity concepts can be used broadly to assist clients in improving their well-being, rather than applied in a linear or rigid fashion (Forber-Pratt et al., 2019). Similarly, it is important for clinicians not to directly challenge a given person's lived experience of disability. There are ways of challenging ableism without invalidating the client's own experiences. Clinicians are advised not to attempt to try to persuade disabled patients about the reality of ableism or the positive possibilities of disabled life, but rather work alongside clients to collaboratively explore their experiences and beliefs (Forber-Pratt et al., 2019). Techniques such as motivational interviewing, a client-centered approach, can be used to help clients explore ambivalence without being directive or prescriptive (Miller & Rollnick, 2012).

Counselors can attend to the ways in which clients use disability language (Dunn & Andrews, 2015). A significant proportion of disabled people, despite the presence of objective impairments, do not consider themselves disabled at all, and in fact identify themselves as able-bodied or nondisabled (Bogart et al., 2017; Nario-Redmond et al., 2013). Those who avoid identifying themselves with the term *disability* may have a negative disability identity. This is likely a result of significant stigma associated with disability in society. It is normal, based on disability identity research thus far, for disabled people to have periods in their lives where they may reject disability identity and avoid others with disabilities; it is important not to pathologize that stance (Forber-Pratt et al., 2019). Rejection of disability as an identity is an inevitable consequence of societal ableism and the proliferation of the medical model of disability. Other clients may identify themselves as persons with disabilities and acknowledge their disability identity (Bogart & Nario-Redmond, 2019). They may use person-first language such as "person with a disability" to signify that disability is part of their experience but not necessarily a core part of who they are. Some others may use language that identifies disability as a core part of their identity, including identity-first language such as "disabled person." Attending to the language used by clients and explicitly asking them about preferred terminology is one way to obtain an initial assessment of the individual's disability identity development.

It may be helpful for clinicians to gain a greater understanding of the messaging clients have received about disabilities throughout their life span. Olkin (2017) notes that those with congenital or childhood-onset disabilities may have disability-adjacent experiences that color their perceptions, such as medical trauma, social exclusion, negative body image, and experiences of abuse. Further, disabled people are often very limited in their exposure to role models with disabilities (Olkin, 2017). This can result in a lack of positive disability influences. Other experiences with disability may have left a negative impression, such as seeing a family member in a nursing home or hearing others talk about how they would never want to be dependent on others for their care.

Disabled people may exhibit feelings of anger and resentment. These are also a result of ableism and have historically been pathologized as maladaptive (Forber-Pratt et al., 2019). It is important for clinicians to understand that these feelings, too, can be a normal part of a healthy disability identity and may in fact be adaptive (Caldwell, 2011). Clinicians can acknowledge the harmful ways in which ableism has impacted the lives of people with disabilities, including from within their own disciplines (Andrews et al., 2019).

One important area of exploration is the experience of microaggressions (Sue et al., 2007). Microaggressions are indirect, subtle, or unintentional discrimination against members of marginalized groups, which can include everyday slights, insults, put-downs, invalidations, and offensive behaviors that people of marginalized groups experience in daily interactions with usually well-intentioned people who may be unaware of their impact (Sue et al., 2007). These may be reflections of implicit bias or prejudicial beliefs and attitudes (usually) beyond the level of conscious awareness. Disability microaggressions are prominent in everyday disability life. Keller and Galgay (2010) found several themes of microaggressions perpetuated toward those with disabilities, including denial of personal identity, denial of disability experience, denial of privacy, helplessness and infantilization, secondary gain, spread effect, patronization, second-class citizen, and desexualization. Denial of personal experience occurs when aspects other than disability are ignored or overshadowed and the person's disability is seen as the other salient and overshadowing characteristic. Denial of disability experience is when disability-related experiences are minimized or denied, such as being told "we all have a disability of some sort." Denial of privacy occurs when others are intrusive and require personal information about a disability, such as asking "what happened to you?" Helplessness and infantilization take place when outsiders assume the disabled individual needs assistance, for example, when they frantically try to help a disabled person even when assistance has been rejected. This can even have dangerous consequences or cause unintentional harm. Secondary gain is the notion that others obtain gratification for assisting a disabled person; they may expect to be praised for their efforts. Spread effect is a concept coined by Wright (1983) wherein the effects of disability are assumed to apply to other aspects of the person; for example, others often assume persons with physical impairments also must have cognitive impairments. Patronization occurs when disabled people are praised for nearly any ordinary task, such as being called brave or inspiring. Second-class citizen is the idea that a disabled person's right to equality is denied because they are considered to be bothersome; expensive; and a waste of time, effort, and resources. Desexualization occurs when the disabled person's sexuality is denied or feared.

Olkin et al. (2019) found three additional domains of microaggressions: the need for the disabled person to manage interpersonal affect, blame, and denial of the reality of symptoms. Management of interpersonal affect is the onus placed on disabled people to put others at ease and manage their discomfort. Blame occurs when disabled people are directly or indirectly held responsible for their disabilities, such as others questioning whether they may have been at fault in a motor vehicle accident or if they smoked prior to being diagnosed with cancer. Denial of the reality of symptoms is the tendency to assume that a disabled individual's symptoms are an overreaction to or a manifestation of psychological concerns. Olkin (2017) postulates this may occur more often toward disabled women. Experiencing these chronic microaggressions can leave individuals with disabilities psychologically exhausted and lead to dysphoria and anger (Olkin, 2017). Focusing on microaggressions in counseling can help clients understand the origin of associated negative affect and allow them to externalize the ableism that perpetuates these incidents. It can also enable disabled clients to problem-solve which microaggressions to address constructively once they are identified and others that they may choose to ignore to conserve emotional energy.

Another important concept is assessing the individual's connection to, or lack thereof, with the disability community. Some individuals are the only people with disabilities in their families and immediate social circles and may have no connection whatsoever to other people with disabilities. This may be by choice, or it also might be a result of disability-related barriers such as segregation, poverty, and lack of accessible transportation. Again, it is to be expected that societal ableism has been internalized and that clients at times may not be ready to engage with the disability community or receive peer support from others with the lived experience of disability. Other people may express a strong connection to the broader disability community and specific subcommunities based on disability type or other shared experiences. these individuals are more likely to endorse a positive disability identity, as they intentionally expose themselves to other disabled people. It is within these contexts that disability culture is likely to be found in terms of shared experiences, language, terminology, and beliefs

(Gill, 1997). People who identify themselves as disability advocates may be the most likely to report a strong sense of positive disability identity and a fuller integration of disability into their core sense of self. Clinicians must not impose the disability community onto clients, but rather follow their developmental lead with appropriate offerings of peer support or other connection as indicated by the client's natural progression (Forber-Pratt et al., 2019). Furthermore, clinicians should build an awareness of community resources from which they can refer clients who would benefit from being linked to the disability community (Olkin, 2017). For example, peer support groups, nonprofit organizations, Centers for Independent Living, advocacy groups, and other community resources can be rich sources of disability-affirmative social support. These are also the ways in which individuals become exposed to and immersed in disability culture.

Narrative approaches can be useful for clinicians to assist their clients in exploring and telling their own stories of the lived experience of disability, allowing them to structure meaning-making related to disability, which has been found to be associated with greater well-being (Dunn & Burcaw, 2013). Again, it is important that clinicians not attempt to influence the story, but rather to facilitate, through reading, writing, and other forms of communication, the client's own evolving self-reflection related to their disability experience (Forber-Pratt et al., 2019). Another approach to assessing disability identity is to use the Disability-Identity Circle activity wherein clients are asked to place an X to demonstrate where her or his disability "falls" in relation to their core selves, revealing the extent to which an individual feels disability is or is not a part of their self-identity (Forber-Pratt et al., 2019). Similarly, there are a number of starter questions suggested by Forber-Pratt et al. (2019) that can be used to elicit discussion about one's disability identity and relation to the disability community, listed in Class Activity. All of these approaches must be used from a client-centered standpoint in order to be culturally relevant and appropriate.

CONCLUSION

Disability identity development is an emerging concept related to the ways in which individuals with disabilities come to understand and recognize their disabilities and their connection to the disability community. Although a separate concept from that of adaptation or adjustment to disability, disability identity development can impact adaptation to disability. Those with a positive disability identity development have been shown to have high levels of satisfaction with life. Thus, it is important to promote the development of positive disability identities through counseling as well as advocacy. Advocacy efforts individually may include linking clients with disability organizations and ties to the disability community, while systemic efforts could include identifying and combatting incidences of ableism, inequity, or inaccessibility. All of these efforts should promote the development of healthy, positive disability identities.

CLASS ACTIVITY

Instructions: For starter questions about disability identity, see Forber-Pratt et al. (2019). Disability identity negotiation may be an important focus in counseling. The following is an example of questions that might be repeated with a client periodically throughout the counseling relationship so the client can explore their ideas about disability identity over time.

A. IN-CLASS ACTIVITY:

With a partner, role play addressing the following questions with a client.

1. When you hear the word disability, what are the first words that come to mind? These words may be positive or negative.

2. What messages have you heard from others (family, friends, the media, etc.) about disability?

3. Do you identify as disabled? How does the thought of identifying as disabled make you feel?

4. Ask the client to write a short narrative or draw a picture of their feelings about having a disability.

Then, ask the client to share what they drew or wrote, if they feel comfortable.

B. OUT OF CLASS ACTIVITY:

Write a response about the above activity. What questions came up for you? What feelings or concerns did the questions raise?

KEY REFERENCES

Only key references appear in the print edition. The full references appear in the digital product on Springer Publishing Connect™: https://connect.springerpub.com/content/book/978-0-8261-5111-7/part/partI/chapter/ch04

Andrews, E. E., & Forber-Pratt, A. J. (2022). Disability culture, identity, and language. In M. L. Wehmeyer & D. S. Dunn (Eds.), *The positive psychology of personal factors: implications for understanding disability* (pp. 27–40). Lexington Books.

Andrews, E. E., Forber-Pratt, A. J., Mona, L. R., Lund, E. M., Pilarski, C. R., & Balter, R. (2019). #SaytheWord: A disability culture commentary on the erasure of "disability." *Rehabilitation Psychology, 64*(2), 111–118. https://doi.org/10.1037/rep0000258

Bogart, K. R. (2014). The role of disability self-concept in adaptation to congenital or acquired disability. *Rehabilitation Psychology, 59*(1), 107–115. https://doi.org/10.1037/a0035800

Bogart, K. R., & Nario-Redmond, M. R. (2019). An exploration of disability self-categorization, identity, and pride. In D. S. Dunn (Ed.), *Understanding the experience of disability: Perspectives from social and rehabilitation psychology* (pp. 252–267). Oxford University Press.

Forber-Pratt, A. J., Lyew, D. A., Mueller, C., & Samples, L. B. (2017). Disability identity development: A systematic review of the literature. *Rehabilitation Psychology, 62*(2), 198. https://doi.org/10.1037/rep0000134

Forber-Pratt, A. J., Price, L. R., Merrin, G. J., Hanebutt, R. A., & Fairclough, J. A. (2022). Psychometric properties of the Disability Identity Development Scale: Confirmatory factor and bifactor analyses. *Rehabilitation Psychology, 67*(2), 120–127. https://doi.org/10.1037/rep0000445

Gill, C. J. (1997). Four types of integration in disability-identity development. *Journal of Vocational Rehabilitation, 9*, 39–46. https://doi.org/10.3233/JVR-1997-9106

Putnam, M. (2005). Conceptualizing disability: Developing a framework for political disability identity. *Journal of Disability Policy Studies, 16*(3), 188–198. https://doi.org/10.1177/10442073050160030601

Zapata, M. A. (2020). Disability affirmation and acceptance predict hope among adults with physical disabilities. *Rehabilitation Psychology, 65*(3), 291–298. https://doi.org/10.1037/rep0000364

CHAPTER 5

RECOGNIZING, UNDERSTANDING, AND CONSTRUCTIVELY RESPONDING TO ABLEISM

DANA S. DUNN

Everybody just needs to chill and understand that disability is just a variable, like height or skin color or weight. We don't need to correct it, we need to correct society's responses to it.

—Person with a physical disability (2015, cited in Nario-Redmond, 2020, p. 221)

Because the world sets people with conspicuous disabilities apart as different, we become objects of fascination, curiosity, and analysis. We are read as avatars of misfortune and misery, stock figures in melodramas about courage and determination. The world wants our lives to fit into a few rigid narratives and templates. . . . Instead of letting the world turn me into a disability object, I have insisted on being a subject in the grammatical sense: not the passive "me" who is acted upon, but the active "I" who does things. . .

—Harriet McBryde Johnson (2005, pp. 2–3)

LEARNING OBJECTIVES

After reading this chapter, you will be able to:

- Identify ableism as a reaction to disability
- Describe some social and behavioral consequences of ableism for disabled people
- Explain the different perspectives and experiences of *insiders* (people with disabilities) and *outsiders* (nondisabled people)
- Value opportunities to be an ally for people with disabilities and an advocate for disability justice

PRE-READING QUESTIONS

1. How does ableism operate as a form of prejudice and discrimination aimed at people with disabilities?
2. When ableism occurs, is it intentional, unintentional, or can it be either?
3. Why do you think disability is not usually recognized as a form of diversity like gender, race, sexuality, social class, and other similar characteristics?

It is relatively easy to recognize that the built environment we live in was designed almost exclusively with nondisabled people in mind. This may not have been a truly intentional decision, but it is relatively certain that the needs of disabled people were not considered when most town and city streets, buildings, and homes were planned—not to mention public venues, like restaurants, some parks, and theaters. To be sure, times have changed and many streets have curb cuts, and new buildings must comply with building codes as well as the Americans with Disabilities Act (1990) that dictate accessibility and ready egress for people with disabilities. But everyday indignities that block the progress of rights of disabled people still occur—often representing structural problems of a different sort.

On the day I began writing this chapter, an online article posted by a colleague detailed a much-heralded attempt to make the Emmy Awards stage more accessible for disabled actors, writers, and directors. In fact, co-director James LaBrecht of the highly praised film *Crip Camp* (Neman & LaBrecht, 2020) was told that a ramp would be available so that wheelchair users like himself could take the stage with ease. No ramp was apparent during the awards show, and LeBrecht took to Twitter immediately afterward to complain that the CBS Network and the Television Academy lied to him and others about the venue's accessibility (Lopez, 2021). Stories like this one are not surprising and illustrate the extent of everyday ableism aimed—intentionally or not—at disabled individuals.

Ableism is not new, but recognizing and reacting to it constructively is still a somewhat novel enterprise. The term *ableism* encompasses stereotyping processes, prejudicial attitudes, social oppression, and discriminatory behavior aimed at disabled people (e.g., Bogart & Dunn, 2019; Nario-Redmond, 2020). While most scholarship on ableism is linked with disability studies (Bogart & Dunn, 2019), social and rehabilitation psychologists, among others, have shown great interest in this form of negative social behavior. What makes ableism egregious, problematic, and widespread is its ubiquity due to intersectional ties; people with disabilities constitute the largest minority group in the United States (as well as about 15% of the world's population; WHO, 2011). These facts mean that disability crosses, connects to, and involves numerous people and even groups due to gender, race, sexual orientation, social class, ethnicity, and religion, among other factors. In short, disability represents a form of diversity about which people, particularly professionals, should become culturally competent (Andrews, 2020; Dunn & Hammer, 2014).

Yet ableism persists, in part, because a nondisabled majority—sometimes knowingly, other times without apparent intention—pushes a social agenda where whole and able-bodies represent a desired standard or norm, so that people with impairments or apparent differences should either be "repaired" (i.e., seek to be like the nondisabled "ideal") or simply accept a lesser place in the sociocultural pecking order. Ableism is based on ideas, expectations, cultural beliefs, institutional practices, everyday social relations, and, admittedly, misunderstandings between nondisabled and disabled people (whether the disability is physical, intellectual, psychological, or due to some chronic disease or other health issue) that create an "us" versus "them" dynamic. The "us" are outsiders or the nondisabled majority, while the "them" are insiders or the disabled minority who know the actual, lived experience of disability, its positive as well as negative qualities (see Dunn, 2015; Dembo, 1964).

The goals of this chapter are to provide an overview of ableism as a reaction to disability as well as a discussion of its consequences for people with disabilities. Stigma and the distinction between insiders and outsiders will be considered, as well as examples of intentional and unintentional ableism. I then turn to issues of disability advocacy and justice. Topics to be considered include disability as diversity, advocacy for self or from others, a COVID-19 case study on medical rationing and disability, activism and allyship, and the utility of rehabilitation psychology's foundational principles.

DEFINING ABLEISM AS A REACTION TO DISABILITY

Ableism is often a response to a disabled person or to thinking about or discussing disability and related issues. Ableist behavior and language appear when disability is perceived to represent a stigma, as well as when some nondisabled people encounter disabled individuals.

Stigmatization

As a reaction to disability, ableism is tied to a larger literature on stigma (Bogart & Dunn, 2019). Considerable research in mainstream social psychology, the social psychology of disability, and sociology demonstrates that social perceivers are drawn to and often curious about how people differ from one another (e.g., Dunn, 2015; Goffman, 1963; Jones et al., 1984; Kelley, 1967, 1973; Wright, 1983). When a difference (or differences) present in one group creates negative interest in another group, then the former group is likely to be stigmatized. A stigma, then, is a mark or quality that sets one group of people apart from another or from other groups. Where disability is concerned, greater visibility of an impairment as well as the age at its acquisition trigger both interest and judgment (usually negative, sometimes ambivalent, occasionally favorable; e.g., Barker, 1948; Katz, 1981; Kleck, 1969; von Hentig, 1948).

Stigma creates psychological and sometimes physical distance between some people and others. According to Phelan et al. (2008), for instance, a stigma satisfies three socially related functions: exploitative intent on the part of the observer(s), the enforcement of (possibly arbitrary but still established) social norms, and avoiding some perceived disease. Disability is seen as a stigmatized condition because those affected are—depending on the nature of their impairment—seen as imperfect, less-than-whole people, or damaged in some way (and disabilities are viewed hierarchically—some more negatively than others viz. psychiatric disability, compared to intellectual disability, compared to physical disability; Chan et al., 2002), especially if one is deemed responsible for a condition's onset (e.g., choosing to engage in a risky behavior that leads to permanent impairment; see Corrigan & Watson, 2002). Once stereotyped by stigma, a person's individual characteristics are ignored and then replaced by negative attitudes that promote prejudiced feelings and discriminatory behaviors. Worse still, awareness of being recognized as a member of a stigmatized group can cause individuals to internalize and even privately accept the negative social judgment (Earnshaw & Quinn, 2012) or fall prey to other psychosocial processes, such as stereotype threat (e.g. Desombre et al., 2018; Silverman & Cohen, 2014).

However, when disability is stigmatized and ableism results, the response directed at disabled individuals may not always be superficially negative (e.g., shunning, name calling, inappropriate questions). Ableism can masquerade as a positive response, as when disabled people are unduly, even inappropriately, praised for accomplishing normal daily activities (e.g., being employed, raising a family, having a job or a career) thought to be beyond their abilities. As we will see later, such insidious ableism is still a source of prejudice and discrimination.

Insider Versus Outsider Perspectives

Of course, being stigmatized does not mean the target always accepts the judgment of observers, but admittedly it may be difficult to ignore. Disabled persons frequently encounter ableist behavior from nondisabled others. Indeed, many nondisabled people often think nothing of asking a disabled person very "personal" questions about the nature, origins, and even potential consequences of the impairment (e.g., "Have you always been like this? Can't you seek medical treatment for it?"), often in an inquisitive manner that many nondisabled people themselves would resent if asked about aspects of their private lives (e.g., "How much money do earn each year? Then why don't you have children?"). Situations like this—real or imagined—highlight the aforementioned *insider–outsider distinction*.

Identified and labeled by the Lewinian social and rehabilitation psychologist Tamara Dembo, this distinction explains the divergent perspectives of so-called insiders—disabled people—and outsiders—that is, nondisabled people. The latter often assume the former lead limited lives due to their disabilities. Dembo (1964) memorably wrote that:

> The role of the outsider is that of an observer, and the role of the insider is that of a participant . . . because the observer is an outsider, the impact of the situation affects him little. (p. 231)

The "situation" here refers to the Lewinian "life space," or the psychological environment (real and imagined) that insiders inhabit (Dunn, 2015; Lewin, 1935). The social psychological problem posed by the insider–outsider distinction is that outsiders generally believe they know what having a disability *must* be like—that is, an ongoing preoccupation that must be a source of pain, humiliation, embarrassment, distraction, and dysfunction. In short, disability must disrupt the disabled person's daily life, so that a sense of normalcy, let alone happiness, is not achievable. When these perceptions occur, outsiders fall prey to what social psychologists refer to as *naïve realism*, where *their* particular perspective on reality must represent the *only* objective reality possible rather than the imagined interpretation of another's (unknown and subjective) experience (e.g., Ross & Ward, 1996; see also, Pronin et al., 2004).

In actuality, of course, having a disability does not necessarily predict the quality of a person's lived experience (nor does *not* having one), which is influenced by numerous factors (e.g., stress, coping abilities, physical and mental health, income, social support; Duggan & Dijkers, 2001). The subjective and self-reported experience of disabled individuals is often favorable and positive, as disability is only one facet among many of a person's ongoing experience. Indeed, for some people with disabilities, it is only when they are asked about their disability that they focus on it or when some environmental or situational constraint impedes them. We might expect that people with a recently acquired disability due an accident or the onset of a chronic health condition might focus on their impairment, but those with a congenital disability are unlikely to do so, as their condition has always been there—quite literally, they know no other way to be. In effect, "becoming" disabled is usually a distinct state from "being" disabled (see, for example, Kahneman, 2000). Indeed, as the late disability lawyer, author, and activist, Harriet McBryde Johnson (2003), noted, disabled individuals frequently live with limits they would never elect to have—but they create abundant and rewarding lives in any case.

Nonetheless, insiders intuit that the insider–outsider distinction guides their social relations with outsiders and how the latter perceive and interact with them. Outsiders, in turn, are often unaware that they send negative social cues to insiders by speaking too loudly, for example, or in a patronizing or overly familiar manner (e.g., "Honey, do you need my help?"). Others infantilize insiders by speaking very slowly to them or by using "baby talk," and some outsiders ignore the disabled person altogether by speaking only to a companion (if one is present), who may be an attendant or a relative or friend. For their part, most outsiders remain unaware that their presumed objective discernment of insiders' experiences is wholly subjective, as the possibility that disabled individuals enjoy a good quality of life rarely occurs to them. This ableist gulf poses consequences for both perceivers (outsiders) and the perceived (insiders).

ORIGINS AND CONSEQUENCES OF ABLEISM

Like many stereotypes, ableism affects both the observer and the observed. Very often, however, the latter experiences the consequences of ableist attitudes and acts, while the former (often) obliviously performs them, as the presence of a disability leads nondisabled people to perceive some difference that can influence subsequent social relations. As we will see, perceived disability leads outsiders to treat insiders as different, though the outsiders may not realize this is so. Similarly, outsiders see nothing wrong in praising insiders who "accomplish" typical everyday outcomes. Ableism is sometimes intentional and sometimes not, but it usually has an adverse effect on insiders. One explanation for the occurrence of ableism is that it promotes particular privileges for outsiders. The ongoing evolution of language for disability has identified some heretofore unrecognized forms of ableism. And, as already acknowledged, one of the perils tied to ableism is that it can be accepted and internalized by some disabled individuals. We begin with the basic dynamics of how people categorize people into groups and why ableism can result in the case of disability.

Disability and Mere Difference

A ready but basic source of ableism may be linked to the phenomenon known as ingroup favoritism. The classic work of Tajfel et al. (1971; see also, Brown, 2020) found that the mere categorization of people into groups can lead to behavioral discrimination—even when there is no intergroup conflict or any evidence of competing interests. Studies of the so-called *minimal group paradigm* show that merely being labeled as the member of one group or being arbitrarily assigned to another leads to more favorable attitudes toward group members and a predilection to discriminate against nongroup members. What makes the effect both interesting and egregious is that it occurs when individuals are placed into groups by the flip of a coin (i.e., at random) or due to some trivial quality (i.e., the purported preference for the work of one modern painter—say, Klee—over that of another—say, Kandinsky). When asked to allocate some resources (e.g., money, points) between their own ("ingroup") members and those in the other ("outgroup"), more resources are routinely allocated to the former but not the latter (e.g., Mullen et al., 1992). This imbalance results despite the fact that participants cannot allocate any of the resources to themselves, they neither know nor have met the others who will receive the resources, and they will experience no subsequent interactions with the members of either group. The key—and causal—factor is knowledge of the group membership of the respective sets of targets.

Tajfel and Turner's (1986) social identity theory posits that such *ingroup favoritism* results from a socio-motivational process, one where the resource allocators wish to maintain favorable distinctiveness by increasing the status of the group tied to their own self-concept (however arbitrary that tie may actually be). Replicating the original effects has been something of a challenge (for one review, see Mullen et al., 1992). Some scholars have suggested a more parsimonious explanation for the effect that is tied to group norms (an account that was once stipulated by Tajfel, 1970). Perhaps people simply favor ingroup members because doing so represents a basic social norm. Supporting this interpretation, Wilder (1986) suggested that people are endorsing a social script that promotes the favoritism or loyalty to one's group as an anticipated and sanctioned social act. Perhaps, then, such instances of ingroup favoritism indicate that people are following a normative social script—to wit, "I reward others who are somehow like me but not those who are not like me" (see Hertel & Kerr, 2001).

In the context of disability, it would seem that nondisabled people (the "ingroup") see themselves as similar and perceive that disabled others (whether due to physical, intellectual, psychological, or some other known or apparent quality) constitute an "outgroup." Once group differences are identified by nondisabled people, other biases can emerge (for a review, see Dunn, 2019a). In-group members, for example, often see themselves as displaying varied moods, personality traits, and behaviors, but they see out-group members' characteristics, like those possessed by disabled persons, as being much more stable and predictable (Kammer, 1982). This *trait ascription bias* is attributable to the fact that one's own internal states seem more accessible than those found in others, pointing to the origin of many stereotypes and prejudices, as well as triggering discriminatory acts.

At the group level, such projections represent an example of the *outgroup homogeneity effect* (Rubin & Badea, 2012), where all the members of a given outgroup are believed to have the same (usually negative) characteristics (e.g., "All disabled people are needy"). At the same time, one's own ingroup is construed in heterogeneous terms ("We have such diverse skills, interests, and outlooks"). The outgroup homogeneity effect, like the trait ascription bias, can be rolled out when ingroup members reflect on race, gender, social class, and disability, among other factors. Thus, once an ingroup and an outgroup are identified via some recognized or imagined difference or differences, these intergroup processes and their consequences can manifest themselves.

Intentional and Unintentional Ableism

When mere differences lead to ingroups and outgroups, the "us" and "them" dynamic develops, and, where disability is concerned, ableism may occur. Ableism can be either intentional or unintentional. The only saving grace of intentional ableism is that it is straightforward and obvious, as when a nondisabled person pokes fun at someone who is disabled or refers to people with disabilities using cruel slurs or other vulgar comments. Intentional ableism emphasizes that disability is a deviation from some supposed "normal" way of being and that, if uncorrected, the disabled person will never be "right" or "whole" in the world.

Oddly, unintentional ableism leads to the same conclusion and message: Something is not right with anyone with a disability. Unintended ableism is much subtler than the intentional variety, however, but often just as offensive or hurtful to a recipient. Inappropriate, personal questions were already identified as ableist, as are spoken musings about whether an impairment can be "fixed" with surgery. Some people are intrusive and happy to share that "If I had to live like you, I think I'd kill myself" (from Johnson, 2005, p. 2). Unintended ableism also occurs when:

- Social gatherings or business meetings are held in inaccessible venues
- Posted signage or elevator buttons lack instructions in Braille letters
- Requests for reasonable accommodations in classrooms are refused because "it's too much trouble"
- Disability must be visible in order to be seen as being a "real" thing
- Accessible bathroom stalls are used by nondisabled people when nonaccessible stalls are available
- A person's disability is viewed as sad or tragic—or seen as being somehow inspirational (more about this later)

Unintentional ableism also occurs when people commit what are known as *microaggressions,* a subset of ableist acts (though microaggressions also occur in response to gender, race, religion, weight, and height, among other factors; see Sue & Spanierman, 2020, for a recent review). Microaggressions occur when nondisabled people are confronted with a disabled person or group of disabled people and they respond with verbal or behavioral expressions that convey understated insults, slights, or other negative messages to their targets (e.g., "It must be nice to get to board the airplane first just because you use a wheelchair" or "Funny, you don't seem disabled"). Though supposedly positive comments can also qualify as microaggressions (e.g., "God only gives you what you can handle!" or "I'll be praying for you and your condition!"). Ignoring a disabled person by speaking to his or her attendant is a behavioral microaggression, as is being extremely solicitous or "overhelping," thereby implying the disabled person has low or even no autonomy (Gilbert & Silvera, 1996).

A slightly different but equally ableist outcome occurs when nondisabled people or outsiders judge the actions of some disabled insiders to be noteworthy or surprising; generally this occurs when a nondisabled person, often a child or teen, performs some feat that nondisabled persons assume should be beyond their abilities (e.g., playing well in a basketball game, doing a gymnastics routine). Disabled athletes, for example, are placed on metaphorical pedestals and celebrated for doing something that would go unremarked if done by any nondisabled peer. Other times, a disabled youth might serve as a team mascot or an honorary team manager and receive public accolades as a result.

Some members of disability culture label such responses to be indicative of *inspiration porn* (Andrews, 2020; Grue, 2016). The late Australian disability activist, Stella Young, coined the term to refer to representations that objectify and "sensationalize" people with disabilities (Andrews, 2020). The main point is that the resulting social media images of inspiration (*YouTube*, for example, is replete with examples of disabled people doing common activities like drawing, taking part in a sport, or running a race) do three things: They encourage nondisabled spectators to feel better about themselves (i.e., "I'm grateful I'm not disabled") while simultaneously triggering pity reactions toward disability (e.g., "If she can do it, then so can I!") while holding typical disabled individuals' actions up to a ridiculously high bar (Serlin, 2015). Young (2012) observed that when disabled folks reject these sorts of characterizations, nondisabled onlookers view them as bitter and unappreciative—the reality of their actual objectification by the nondisabled is ignored.

Disabled adults going about their routine daily lives are not immune from inspiration porn–like judgments either. Some are singled out for casual praise for being able to do everyday activities, like grocery shopping, child care, holding down a job, or performing household maintenance activities. While such praise may not seem ableist, it is to the extent that similar accolades would not be offered by one nondisabled adult to another. Whenever a disabled person is admired for engaging in normal responsibilities ("You just keep trying, don't you? You never give up."), ableism is likely present. It may seem churlish to complain about such "well-intentioned" compliments—after all, who doesn't like to be recognized on occasion—but not if you consider that such remarks reinforce the idea that a disabled person's efforts are always being evaluated by nondisabled observers—as if the former's autonomy is always suspect or even probationary.

What about ableism on a more institutional level? The past placement—really, segregation—of students with disabilities in separate schools from nondisabled students qualifies as ableist, as did putting adults and children with disabilities into institutions (a practice sometimes referred to as "warehousing"). Any unwillingness to comply with disability rights laws, such as the Americans with Disabilities Act (1990), not incorporating accessibility into a building's design plans, or creating inaccessible or digitally difficult-to-navigate websites are also examples of institutionalized ableism.

Disabled persons, too, are often at an educational disadvantage. They are twice as likely to have less than a high school education by age 25 than their nondisabled counterparts, just as only slightly over 10% of disabled students will have completed a college degree by that age (compared to over 21% of nondisabled students, who will have more than a 4-year degree by the same age; Lauer & Houtenville, 2018). The resulting economic consequences are pronounced and profoundly troubling, as Nario-Redmond (2020) observed:

> In 2016, 76.8% of people (18-64 years old) without disabilities were employed compared to only 35.9% of people with disabilities; and only 23% of these disabled people worked full-time year round (Lauer and Houtenville, 2018). This 40% employment gap has remained constant for the past 10 years across economic

downturn and recovery (Kraus et al., 2018). In 2016, median work earnings were over $10000 lower for those with disabilities while their poverty rate was more than twice as high (26.7%) as those without disabilities (11.6%). (p. 7)

Whether intended or not, ableism touches the lives of people with disabilities in most areas of their daily lives and livelihoods. What motivates nondisabled people to engage in ableism?

Ableism as Outsider Privilege

Earlier, we touched on some possible reasons that might motivate nondisabled people to engage in ableism. One motivation we have not considered is what can be called *outsider privilege*, which occurs when nondisabled people feel, think, and behave so that their desires or needs take precedence over those of disabled individuals (Dunn, 2019b). A column in a Sunday edition of *The New York Times* provides a simple but telling example (Galanes, 2022). A mother wrote to the advice columnist of "Social Q's" regarding whether her recent requisitioning of a wheelchair in an art museum was justified. Suspecting her healthy 8-year old child might become weary while walking from exhibit to exhibit, the mother took a wheelchair from the coat checking area and had the child sit in it. They enjoyed their tour of the galleries, returning the wheelchair a few hours later. The mother wrote to ask if borrowing the chair was an acceptable act—by no means did they truly need it but it made the experience a happier one for her and her daughter.

The columnist replied that borrowing the chair for a child who had no mobility issues was not a reasonable course of action. Wheelchairs available for public use are there for people, especially disabled individuals, who actually do need them. In fact, it's possible someone needing the chair in question was compelled to wait until it or another became available. Although the columnist did not identify the situation as ableist, he closed with a key point tied to outsider privilege: The mother's actions might have suggested to the child that the needs of people with disabilities are not as important as the convenience of able-bodied others (Galanes, 2022). Convenience—here, conveyance via a wheelchair—illustrates how the privilege presumed by nondisabled outsiders can override the potential needs of real or imagined disabled insiders.

Dunn (2019b) described a hypothetical but common example of outsider privilege affecting a disabled individual. A woman using a wheelchair made her way toward a bank of elevators in a hotel lobby. At the same time, a nondisabled man observed her progress and met her at the elevator—he "helped" by pressing the call button for her, holding the elevator doors open, and asking, "Which floor?" despite the fact the woman did not ask for any help (she may very well be tired of such aid, feeling frustrated by it or even infantilized). Many disabled people frequently encounter strangers who want to help them; few ask in advance if such help is needed or, more pointedly, desired. In other words, nondisabled observers often believe that people with disabilities *must* need or want assistance, so they proffer it without considering whether people are capable of taking care of themselves or, in fact, prefer to do so.

Such interventions contain a subtle but prejudicial message (e.g., "people like you can't do things for yourselves") while also advancing the interests of the nondisabled (Goodley, 2014; Wolbring, 2007; see also, Perrin, 2019). Indeed, the nondisabled helper has a vested interest in this situation— he feels good about "doing good for the less fortunate" (e.g., Isen, 1987; Steger et al., 2008) in a very public way—by performing a good deed that other nondisabled people can witness and admire, and even feel vicariously good about themselves. Where affect is concerned, the nondisabled man who helped the woman in the wheelchair has actually "helped" himself and collected the respect and warm feelings (whether real or imagined) from other outsiders. Ableist encounters of overhelping like this one are all too common in the lives of disabled individuals (Hebl & Kleck, 2000).

Finally, the expression or withholding of empathy by nondisabled people can also be ableist. Wu and Fiske (2019) discussed how the warm-but-incompetent stereotype discerned by the stereotype content model (SCM) guides empathy in selective ways. Briefly, the SCM demonstrates that nondisabled persons see people with disabilities as warm (friendly, trustworthy) but also incompetent (neither assertive nor capable; Fiske et al., 2002). Like older people, disabled individuals are to be pitied, leading to a mixed stereotype of being likeable but still necessarily disrespected (see also, Cuddy et al., 2009). Emotional prejudice like this example often occurs because the elicited stereotype allows nondisabled observers to express pity and sympathy, which are variations of empathy. Additionally, however, the social status of the disabled is viewed as one of inferiority and powerlessness, which leads (as already discussed) to patronizing actions by nondisabled persons.

Empathy is attributionally dependent on whether any perceived fault (i.e., responsibility via personal control) is tied to the presence of disability (Weiner et al., 1988). If a disabled person is discovered to have been somehow responsible for an acquired disability (e.g., falling off a steep ledge while inebriated), then less empathy will be directed at that individual. If a disability is congenital or acquired due to genuine accident (e.g., falling badly on an icy walkway) or the fault of another (e.g., a drunk driver hits a pedestrian who becomes disabled), then higher levels of empathy likely will be expressed. Wu and Fiske (2019) also note that investigators should be sure to explore whether such fault finding is due to causing one's own disability (pointing to rightful or karmic punishment; see also, the just world hypothesis; Lerner, 1980) or for continuing to sustain a disability (neglecting to do something about an impairment, such as a facial blemish, that might be "corrected"). In the latter case, empathy may be withheld from the affected person—as may any offer of aid.

Since ableism is familiar to many, if not all, disabled people, what are the consequences for them? One large risk is clearly internalized ableism.

Internalized Ableism

Simply put, *internalized ableism* occurs when insiders accept—either implicitly, explicitly, or both— outsider perspectives regarding their disabled status (e.g., Dunn, 2019b). Some insiders may decide to try to overlook, cover up (i.e., "passing"), or even overcome their impairments by mimicking or becoming more like outsiders. Others stay clear of other disabled people so as not to socialize with them or to hazard being exposed or "outed" by them (Dunn, 2015; Olkin, 1999). Others cope by behaving consistently with the lifestyles of the nondisabled, who view them as role models or even "heroes" for not allowing disability to affect their lives (i.e., a variant of inspiration porn).

All of these responses are problematic because by acting like outsiders, such insiders are behaviorally confirming the belief that being nondisabled is the normative and desired way to live (Campbell, 2009). That is, they "buy into" the ableism spread by outsiders, failing to realize it corrupts an authentic way to live and denies solidarity with other disabled individuals (Gill, 1997). Any pride tied to the disability community or being disabled is suppressed due to the social press caused by ableism, so that "Disability is then cast as a diminished state of being human" (Campbell, 2001, p. 44).

Not surprisingly, the prejudice and discrimination tied to ableism have potentially negative influences on insiders' stress levels, health (mental and physical), achievement efforts (e.g., education, employment), and trait and state self-esteem, among other challenges. Many disabled individuals lack contact or fellowship with other people with disabilities (Olkin, 1999); being the sole disabled person in many settings sometimes leads to tokenism, which is a distinct problem (Roberson et al., 2003; Steele, 2010). For a more detailed discussion of internalized ableism and its socioemotional consequences, see Nario-Redmond (2020).

Now that some of the consequences of ableism are recognized, we will consider ways that people with disabilities and their allies can challenge ableism when they encounter it.

NAVIGATING ABLEISM: RESISTING, COPING, AND CHANGING MINDS

Ableism is clearly a widespread problem, one that has been documented and studied in a variety of ways within psychology and outside of it (e.g., disability studies; Albrecht et al., 2001; Davis, 2006). The obvious question remaining to be addressed is what can be done to ameliorate its effects on individuals with disabilities while also informing or even educating nondisabled people about its pernicious influence. The last section of this chapter focuses on ways to navigate ableism, including claiming disability as a form of diversity, promoting disability culture and disability identity, attending to language use for disability, considering activism and allyship, advocacy efforts, and considering some ways to concretely cope with ableism.

Promoting Disability as Diversity

Having a disability is a characteristic that represents diversity, one that needs to be recognized alongside other diverse qualities (e.g., Andrews, 2020; Dunn, 2015; Dunn & Hammer, 2014). The rationale is simple: Whether aimed at professionals who work with disabled individuals or simply lay people in everyday settings, doing so is a means to develop necessary cultural competence in our increasingly multicultural world. Disabled people represent a "heterogeneous group" of people; one form of disability is distinct from another or others (Andrews, 2020), as are the life experiences of those involved. Diversity education and workshop opportunities need to include disability alongside race and ethnicity, gender, social class, sexual orientation, religion, and other factors or qualities. Disability in all its myriad forms, whether visible or invisible or congenital or acquired, must be considered. Further, its intersectionality with other factors must be introduced so that nondisabled persons recognize its ubiquity. One approach to doing so is to consider how disabled people create their own culture or even cultures, as well as identities.

Disability Culture and Disability Identity

As Andrews (2020) claims, "People with disabilities have rich traditions in history, language, aesthetics, and sociopolitical stances that make up a distinct cultural experience" (p. 57). Disability culture is real, and it represents an opportunity for connections and fostering positive perspectives among people with disabilities. Such positive perspectives include comradeship and developing shared purpose (e.g., advocacy efforts) as a means to counter negative stereotypes of ongoing dysfunction and presumed unhappiness due to the presence of impairments. Gill (1995) highlighted four main goals of disability culture:

- *Fortification* – energy and strength aimed at targeting oppression and promoting equal rights
- *Unification* – elimination of splintering in the disability community in order to stress belongingness and a shared future
- *Communication* – creating connection and discourse among disabled people so that a distinct but shared disability identity takes root
- *Recruitment* – inviting disabled people to have pride in themselves and their larger community, embracing and bringing younger and recently disabled people to participate

More on disability culture and its positive utility can be found in Andrews (2020).

Disability identity is important to disability culture but also to the development, growth, and outlook of individuals with a disability, as they can form their own distinct disability identities. As a standalone construct, disability identity refers to favorable and possibly advantageous self-views linked to one's own disability while sustaining positive connections to other people who are members of the disability community (Dunn, 2015; Dunn & Burcaw, 2017; Forber-Pratt et al., in press; Gill, 1997; Nario-Redmond, 2020; Olkin & Pledger, 2003). Disabled individuals vary in terms of how much or even whether they have a disability identity. Some play down, hide, ignore, or even fail to realize they have a disability, while others make it clear that their disability is part and parcel of who they are as individuals, so that this quality leads to pride in and connection to other disabled people. Obviously, then, there are multiple dimensions of disability identity that lie between these two extremes, and disabled people may or may not develop more distinct disability identities across time, experience, and their individual life spans.

Various models have been proposed to capture and describe the nature of disability identity and its utility for people with disabilities (see Forber-Pratt et al., in press, for a recent and detailed review). Most of these models share the view that positive identification is indicated by recognizing and accepting one's own disability as an important part of the self as well as a means to forge connections to other disabled people. There is some evidence, for example, that those with congenital disabilities are likely to report greater identification than those with acquired disabilities (Bogart, 2014). One study using an international sample found that identification with disability was highest among individuals who had been living with impairments for a greater proportion of their lives (Nario-Redmond & Oleson, 2016). In another study, people with more visible disabilities had higher identity scores on measures compared to those whose disabilities were "invisible" unless they had been disclosed to others (Nario-Redmond et al., 2013).

How can disability identity research challenge ableism? Disability activists are likely to have well-developed disability identities that can guide their protest and advocacy efforts on behalf of the educational, social, economic, and political needs of the disabled community. Other disabled individuals, including the newly disabled, who come to learn about the importance of disability identity via counseling or rehabilitative therapy, may choose to join in the collective struggle to obtain both civil rights and equality. One of the most important fronts for identity concerns what language is used to refer to or to portray disability.

Language for and About Disability

There has been something of a sea change regarding how disabled and nondisabled people refer to and talk about disability. Within psychology, practitioner-researchers, notably Beatrice A. Wright (1983), had long argued for using person-first language. *Person-first language* is designed to emphasize the person first rather than his or her disability. For example, a person-first construction would be "she is a person with a disability" rather than a "disabled person." The goal is to make disability a secondary concern and to remind people to always put the person ahead of the impairment. Since disability is often construed as an "either/or" proposition, so that one is or is not disabled (Dunn, 2015), the risk of such automatic categorization is not only stereotyping but also *essentializing* the disability (Bogart & Dunn, 2019). Essentializing occurs because the disability itself takes precedence over whatever other qualities (good or bad) a person possesses—in effect, when present, the disability represents the person's essence (Bloom, 2010; Dunn et al., 2013). Person-first language, which has long been embraced by rehabilitation psychology, is an attempt to de-essentialize discourse about disability. In fact, for many years, the American Psychological Association's *Publication Manual* advocated its use for writing and presenting research on disability.

However, like culture, language, too, evolves. For some time, disability advocates and scholars in disability studies argued that although it was well-intentioned, sole reliance on person-first constructions creates some problems. First, these constructions seem to deny or even attempt to obscure the presence or reality of a disability. Second, such labored constructions rarely occur elsewhere in everyday language: With the possible exceptions of "people of color" or "person of color," English speakers do not say things like "people who are African American" or "person who is female." Rather, they say "African Americans" and "female"—and by doing so, the individuals' identities come first (Bogart & Dunn, 2019; Dunn & Andrews, 2015). And in point of fact, many people with disabilities prefer to be called disabled (i.e., "I am a disabled person" or "I am an amputee"). Identity-first-language does not render disability ambiguous; rather, it highlights an important part of someone's sense of self (Bogart & Dunn, 2019). After all, Deaf people tend to prefer being called Deaf or even the Deaf, just as blind people resonate to being called blind people.

Third, use of identity-first language is a means to confront ableism by making disabilities salient in daily life. Disability, then, becomes a statement of identity and a point of pride and connection among disabled people. An important distinction between person-first and identity-first language is that the latter allows a disabled individual or group to claim that disability is a key aspect of their identities (Dunn & Andrews, 2015; recall, too, the earlier discussion of disability culture and dynamics of disability identity). Some readers may wonder how or when to use either formulation. Generally, the best course to follow is to refer to people as they themselves prefer to be labeled. When uncertainty arises, revert to person-first language until it is clear identity-first options are viewed as valid. Using a mix of person-first and identity-first constructions when speaking or writing is also acceptable. More detailed guidance can be found in the most recent edition of the *Publication Manual* (APA, 2020).

Although adopting appropriate language for disability is good way to counter ableism, another is to be an intentional ally of the disability community.

Allyship as Activism

Being a disability ally or displaying allyship entails using one's own group's sociopolitical influence and social capital to aid or advocate on behalf of individuals in a group with less sociopolitical influence and social capital (Mio & Roades, 2003). To be an effective disability ally, one must be aware of biases often aimed at disability (Dunn, 2019a), including reflecting on one's own potentially narrow understanding of disability and chronic diseases. During the COVID-19 pandemic, for example, a group of disabled and nondisabled psychologists joined together to draw attention to medical rationing (chiefly of ventilators) unfairly aimed at people with disabilities, whose conditions were presumed to be immune from such interventions (Andrews et al., 2021; see also, Lund & Ayers, 2020).

Forber-Pratt et al. (2019) offer a list of ways that rehabilitation and other psychology professionals can exhibit allyship. Beyond educating oneself, these include learning about intersectionality, relying on principles of universal design, appreciating current disability rights issues affecting the disability community, rooting out objectifying beliefs and responses tied to sensationalizing the experiences of disabled people or inspiration porn, and accepting cross-cultural solidarity among different disabled groups. Both professionals and lay people alike need to proverbially "show up" to offer active assistance to disabled individuals where civil rights and equality are concerned. By doing so, everyday ableism can be reduced.

Advocacy Activities

Researchers and practitioners from the field of rehabilitation psychology (Division 22 of the American Psychological Association) have codified seven foundational principles tied to clinical and research efforts (e.g., Bentley et al., 2019; Dunn, 2022; Dunn et al., 2016). Drawn in part from the work of Beatrice A. Wright (1983), notably her list of value-laden beliefs and principles (Wright, 1972; see also, Wright, 1973), the foundational principles articulate ways for disabled individuals and their families, rehabilitation and medical professionals, and other allies to understand disability while constructively responding to challenges, including ableism. The original six principles are the person–environment relation, the insider–outsider distinction, adjusting to disability, the importance of psychological assets, construing the self-perception of bodily states, and maintaining human dignity (see, for example, Dunn et al., 2016). The recent seventh principle is based in advocacy efforts, including self-advocacy by people with disabilities themselves. Such efforts are aimed at enhancing the health and well-being of disabled individuals, on their own and with the help of allies. One goal for the foundational principles is to encourage the development of positive disability cultures and identities while organizing resilience designed to overcome social, psychological, and environmental obstacles.

The bulk of most advocacy activities are probably aimed at educating nondisabled people about the actual nature and experience of disability; that is, to change minds in ways that move away from ableist tendencies. For example, *The New York Times* recently introduced an inaugural disability reporting fellow (Morris, 2022). The new fellow, Amanda Morris, delineated her advocacy goal in her first article, where she described how some of her friends were excited to tell her about a Starbucks where all the employees use sign language. Morris, who is hard-of-hearing, viewed the situation a bit differently: Though she was delighted that Starbucks was seeking to be more diverse, hiring disabled people was not a special event, nor was creating one accessible store for Deaf or hard-of-hearing coffee drinkers. Morris was much more interested to learn that many of the new workers possessed master's degrees—yet they still struggled to find other sorts of jobs because of their disabilities. Combatting ableism, however well-intentioned it may be, is and will be an ongoing process. Advocacy efforts from within and outside of the disability community are necessary in order to alter long-existing attitudes in new directions.

Attitudes and Ableism

Ableism is largely due to erroneous attitudes held by nondisabled people toward disabled persons. The attitude literature concerning disability is voluminous and generally characterizes those aimed at disabled people to be negative (Dunn, 2015). One clear antidote to changing such attitudes is known as the *contact hypothesis*, where diverse groups of people encounter one another during sessions of meaningful contact (e.g., Pettigrew & Troop, 2006, 2008). There is evidence that such intergroup contact can lead to favorable attitude change toward race and ethnicity, mental health issues, aging, AIDS, LGBTQ issues, and disability (Pettigrew & Troop, 2011). Favorable intergroup contact and subsequent attitude change are dependent on personal social interaction, being of equal status, using established social norms, and engaging in cooperative activities. The real challenge, of course, is creating opportunities where disabled and nondisabled people can meet face to face and learn from one another.

As Dunn (2015) also noted, there a numerous measures (i.e., scales, questionnaires) of attitudes toward disability and disabled that were developed over the last several decades. A problem shared by virtually all of them is that the vernacular used to refer to or discuss disability has changed radically and, as noted earlier, continues to evolve. While most of them are psychometrically validated, many of these scales used outmoded terms (e.g., "crippled," "handicapped") and concepts. To use them with contemporary samples of people would be problematic (some of the terms in them would be deemed offensive today), and updating the scales with newer language would be psychometrically unwise unless (re)test development was conducted properly. Nonetheless, many of these scales are likely worth updating for research and clinical uses and, in any case, doing so might be much more expedient than beginning from scratch. Like evidence from the contact hypothesis, revised and updated versions of these scales could be quite helpful where reducing ableism is concerned.

CONCLUSION

Ableism itself is not new, but it is more likely to be recognized, critiqued, or even called out than in the past. Yet the real challenge remains in educating nondisabled individuals that ableism is all too often a form of prejudice or even discrimination aimed at the disability community. This chapter offered some ways to recognize, understand, and constructively deal with ableism. But it is only a beginning, as much more research and advocacy work need to be done.

DISCUSSION QUESTIONS

1. Ableism is often unintentional but still harmful to people with disabilities. What can be done to educate or inoculate nondisabled people from expressing ableist attitudes or performing ableist behaviors?

2. When disability is seen as a form of stigma, why do outsiders view those who are stigmatized (i.e., insiders) as being similar to one another? Can anything be done to counter this form of social judgment?

3. Can you identity some other situations in everyday life where ableism operates as a form of outsider privilege? What can be done to counter, reduce, or even eliminate this form of outsider privilege?

4. Why does disability identity serve as a positive element in the lives of many people with disabilities? How does disability identity relate to person-first language and identity-first language?

5. How can the *contact hypothesis* be enacted in everyday life in order to potentially reduce ableism?

CLASS ACTIVITIES

Thinking About Ableism

Reflect on what you learned about ableism while reading this chapter. Review some of the theoretical and social psychological reasons that ableism and ableist behavior occur. Have you ever relied on one (or more) of these reasons for how you think about disability and disabled people? Which one(s) do you think you use or may have used in the past? Why did you do so? Can you point to any experience(s) you've had or sources (e.g., television, advertising) that may have led you to associate disability with negative feelings or thoughts? Were you concerned that your feelings and beliefs were disapproving? Why or why not?

Developing a Perspective for the Future

Ableism is common and, for most of us, unavoidable unless we work to change how we think, feel, and act toward people with disabilities. Write down a list of reasons why you or others might engage in ableist thinking. Once you do, reflect on this: How can you go about changing how you think the next time you encounter a disabled person or something that reminds you of disability?

Psychologists draw a distinction between fast and slow thinking. When we are in a fast thinking mode, we rely on shortcuts, including stereotypes, to make sense of our experience. These admitted biases save time and mental energy—they allow us to think quickly and easily—but we risk drawing false conclusions, especially where people who may be different from us are concerned.

Slower, more careful cognition requires us to engage in critical thinking in order to revisit and to perhaps revise our earlier conclusions. By slowing down and questioning our assumptions and conclusions about disability, we may be able to reduce the likelihood that we will engage in ableist thinking.

Take some time and reflect on the reason or reasons you may have engaged in ableist thinking in the past. How can you try to avoid doing so in the future? What (slower) alternative views or beliefs can you identify now to counter previous (faster) conclusions about disability?

How will you remember to think more carefully and slowly the next time you encounter something or someone who makes you think about what you believe and feel about disability?

KEY REFERENCES

Only key references appear in the print edition. The full references appear in the digital product on Springer Publishing Connect™: https://connect.springerpub.com/content/book/978-0-8261-5111-7/part/partI/chapter/ch05

Andrews, E. E. (2020). *Disability as diversity: Developing cultural competence.* Oxford University Press.

Bogart, K. R., & Dunn, D. S. (2019). Ableism special issue introduction. *Journal of Social Issues, 75*(3), 650–664. https://doi.org/10.11112/jos.12354

Dembo, T. (1964). Sensitivity of one person to another. *Rehabilitation Literature, 25,* 231–235.

Dunn, D. S. (2015). *The social psychology of disability.* Oxford University Press.

Dunn, D. S. (2019). Outsider privileges can lead to insider disadvantages: Some psychosocial aspects of ableism. *Journal of Social Issues, 75*(3), 665–682. https://doi.org/10.1111/josi.12331

Dunn, D. S., & Andrews, E. (2015). Person-first *and* identity-first language: Developing psychologists' cultural competence using disability language. *American Psychologist, 70,* 255–264. https://doi.org/10.1037/a0038636

Johnson, H. M. (2005). *Too late to die young: Nearly true tales from a life.* Picador.

Nario-Redmond, M. R. (2020). *Ableism: The causes and consequences of disability prejudice.* Wiley-Blackwell.

Wright, B. A. (1983). *Physical disability: A psychosocial approach.* Harper & Row.

CHAPTER 6

THE EVOLUTION OF LAWS AND POLICIES IN THE UNITED STATES AND THEIR IMPACT ON DISABLED PEOPLE

ALLISON R. FLEMING, SARAH M. ROUNDTREE, AND K. LYNN PIERCE

LEARNING OBJECTIVES

After reading this chapter, you will be able to:

- Understand how historical views on disability and entrenched ableism influence current policy
- Recognize how disabled people have advocated for rights and access in U.S. history
- Question laws regarding accessibility and civil rights and the impact on disabled people
- Evaluate limitations in our medical system, across access, quality, and availability that negatively impact disabled people
- Identify directions in allyship and advocacy to support goals of disabled people and community

PRE-READING QUESTIONS

1. What constitutes civil rights? What civil rights do adults in the United States have?
2. What does it mean for a space to be accessible? Why is it important for all spaces to be accessible to people with disabilities?
3. Why is it important as a counselor to be familiar with disability law and policy?
4. When were civil rights granted to disabled people in the United States? How did that happen? What rights are still not available to adults with disabilities in the United States?

HISTORICAL VIEWS ON DISABILITY

Both person-first language and identity-first language are used in this chapter. Our choice reflects the recognition of preferences among disabled persons as well language used in academia and rehabilitation counseling (typically, person-first). Many in the disability community disagree with person-first language and prefer identity-first language for themselves and their communities, as a way of reclaiming their identity as a disabled person. We acknowledge that the issues raised in this chapter are far reaching and complex and are impacted by so many different laws, policies, and social norms that they are difficult to comprehensively explain and capture. We focus on the historical context and current situation across the key policy areas of accessibility, individual rights, and healthcare as areas that we believe are critical to the well-being of disabled people but are typically only sparsely covered in other rehabilitation counseling training materials. We will finish the chapter with a presentation of points of allyship and advocacy that align with the needs and priorities of disabled people and topics emphasized in the community.

The construct of disability has biopsychosocial roots, and notions of how disability is considered have changed over time (Rembis et al., 2018). Disability, in all its forms and definitions, intersects with other aspects of identity such as race, gender, sexuality, socioeconomic status, and age. Historical treatment of disabled people in the United States is riddled with violence, abuse, maltreatment, erasure, exclusion, and confinement (Nielsen, 2012). Some historians refer to this inhumane treatment as a "hidden history," which encompasses violations including systemic and state-sponsored segregation, coercion with medical experimentation, eugenics and forced sterilization, and exclusion from education, employment, and community living (Rembis et al., 2018). Ableism and oppression are closely intertwined in U.S. history, with disability used to rationalize racism, sexism, and many other forms of injustices. For example, laws created to prevent female and Black Americans from voting because of a perceived lack of cognitive ability or a declaration of mental illness or defectiveness of enslaved Black people who tried to escape (Nielsen, 2012).

All areas of life for disabled people continue to be impacted by laws, policies, and cultural norms entrenched with ableist ideas. In this chapter, we review the connection between historical context and current policies and the treatment of individuals with disabilities in the United States. This history includes how disabled people were identified, defined, and treated and how individual differences in physical, cognitive, and emotional functioning reflected the "value" of a person. Disability was seen as a reason to exclude people from full citizenship, including both the rights and the responsibilities therein (Nielsen, 2012). As a result, disabled people were made dependent, either being placed in state care (i.e., institutions and prisons) or supported by public welfare to meet their basic needs. Immigration laws barred disabled people from emigrating to the United States under the rationale that the person would not be able to financially support themselves and become a burden or a public threat (Longmore & Goldberger, 2000).

Industrialization and the labor movement had occupational health and safety and disabled workers at its crux, with organizers demanding safer working conditions and a safety net that would provide some measure of financial security for injured workers and their families (Jennings, 2018). Trade organizations had privately funded aid societies for injured and disabled workers and their families as early as the 18th century to fill the gap in financial security that families experienced when the primary earner became injured or incurred chronic health conditions preventing work or was killed (Jennings, 2018). Social safety net legislation, associated with the New Deal, positioned disabled Americans among the "deserving poor" that needed welfare because they are unable to work (Burke & Barnes, 2017). It was during this time that the first rehabilitation professional, Regina Dolan, led a study of injured workers in Wisconsin and emphasized the potential for injured workers to return to work with accommodations and retraining if necessary. In her report, she included individuals' descriptions of their efforts to hide their physical disabilities as they sought employment post-injury, and the different experiences based on visibility of their disability. For example, people with injuries to fingers or hands were able to pass as nondisabled more easily than people with injuries to legs or feet (Ayers, 1969; Obermann, 1966).

Scholars have marked the early 20th century as the time when policy makers and professionals across helping professions and charitable organizations coalesced around the medical definition of disability that would go on to dominate policy and professional practice and privileged the authority of medical "experts" and other professionals in terms of treatment of people with disabilities (Longmore & Goldberger, 2000). Disability was recognized as both an individual and a social problem, constructing the identity of disabled people and setting up a dichotomy of "normal" versus "disabled" as an organizing concept in society (Longmore & Goldberger, 2000). At the same time, medical experts, policy makers, rehabilitation professionals, and program administers had to recognize the relative independence of the concepts of impairment and disability and the potential for "social contexts to create, mitigate, or eliminate disability" (Longmore & Goldberger, 2000, p. 892). This social context is critical to disability rights activists, who argue that the solution to disadvantage associated with disability is to enact civil rights legislation and remove structural and attitudinal barriers that exclude disabled individuals from participating in all parts of public and private life (Bagenstos, 2009).

Disability Rights Movement

The disability rights movement, led by disabled people, achieved significant legislation that codified rights to physical access, education, and employment opportunities for disabled Americans (Heumann & Joiner, 2020). While many people are familiar with the Americans with Disabilities Act of 1990 (ADA), disabled people were fighting for rights and access in the United States long before then. It is important to note that some of their advocacy efforts were aimed at addressing ableist and exclusionary policies and practices of public services, such as rehabilitation agencies and higher education. An example of such efforts is the American Federation of the Physically Handicapped (AFPH) in 1942, who organized against employment discrimination and advocated for greater availability to federal services for disabled people to support employment, education, healthcare access, and economic sustainability for those who were unable to work. The AFPH focused on the State-Federal Vocational Rehabilitation Program (VR), demanding that the agency be more consumer-focused (Jennings, 2018). One major victory for the AFPH came in the form of the President's Committee on the Employment of the Physically Handicapped, convened in 1947, as a place for activists, business leaders, veterans, and service professionals to convene and promote changes to policy. Famous disability rights activists such as Ed Roberts and Fred Fay attended meetings and continued to organize more accessibility legislation rooted in this committee's work.

Another example of disabled people organizing to gain access to educational spaces is found in a group of disabled veterans who used their G.I. Bill benefits to attend a branch of the University of Illinois that was housed in a former hospital in the late 1940s. When the branch campus closed, the students wanted to transfer to the main campus, which was inaccessible to wheelchair users. The veterans staged a protest at the governor's mansion and were granted access shortly thereafter (McCarthy, 2003). In 1962, Ed Roberts began studies as an undergraduate at the University of California-Berkley, despite his use of a wheelchair for mobility, need to sleep in an iron lung, and need for personal care attendants to accomplish most of his activities of daily living. Roberts would go on to organize a group of other students with disabilities, called the "rolling quads," to advocate for greater access and autonomy for disabled students on the Berkley campus (McCarthy, 2003) and to establish the first Center for Independent Living in Berkley, California, in 1972 (Pennsylvania Statewide Independent Living Council [PASIL], n.d.).

Disability activism gained visibility and momentum in the early 1970s with the adoption of the Rehabilitation Act of 1973, including sections that barred employment discrimination within the federal government and by contractors, mandated architectural and transportation compliance in terms physical access, barred disability discrimination by programs receiving federal assistance (including institutes of higher education), and provided access to communication and technology (Wilcher, 2018). The Rehabilitation Act was the first legislative effort to address the issue of equal access for disabled Americans, with efforts to remove barriers to access including transportation and to address discrimination and other societal barriers experienced by individuals with disabilities. The Rehabilitation Act was passed via congressional override of President Nixon's veto (Wilcher, 2018). However, regulations for enforcement were significantly delayed under the Ford and Carter administrations and were not signed until disability activists staged several lengthy and highly public demonstrations. Leaders from Centers for Independent Living (CILs) coordinated the demonstrations and collaborated with the media to make sure they were seen and heard by the public. The regulations were finally signed on May 4, 1977 (Wilcher, 2018).

Disabled people continued to organize, forming several more advocacy groups concerned with issues and barriers to specific disability groups. This included People First, a group formed by individuals with intellectual disabilities to lobby for deinstitutionalization and community living; "psychiatric survivors" who lobbied for similar movements and freedom from being forced to take medication; and American Disabled for Attendant Programs Today (ADAPT), advocating for independent living and radical deinstitutionalization and freedom from forced living in nursing homes and other noncommunity spaces for those with significant physical disabilities (Bagenstos, 2009). Individuals who are culturally Deaf, Blind, and representing other factions of disabled people put forth their own desired changes to policy and practice as it pertained to their lives. As a result of continued advocacy, additional legislation was passed to ensure access for children with disabilities to a free and appropriate education (PL 94-192, 1975), voting accessibility (1984), and access to air transportation (1988). The ADA (1990) was the first comprehensive civil rights protection for disabled Americans, modeled after section 504 and Title V of the Rehabilitation Act and the Civil Rights Act of 1964 (PASIL, n.d.). The ADA broadly prohibited disability discrimination and codified reasonable accommodations and accessibility in a world that was not designed for persons with disabilities (Bagenstos, 2009).

Disability Policy and Access in the United States Post-Americans with Disabilities Act

The United States post-ADA is much different than before this landmark legislation. However, the law itself has not had the impact that many had hoped for when it was passed. There is no office or agency charged with enforcement, putting the responsibility for challenging violators on individuals who can make complaints through a variety of channels. This creates a situation where a person must sue if they are denied access or are the target of discrimination (Bagenstos, 2009). In the years following the ADA's passage, it became clear that the Supreme Court was narrowly interpreting the definitions of "qualified individual with a disability" and "reasonable accommodations" in ways that have excluded many people from legal protections and limited the potential for addressing structural barriers for disabled workers (Bagenstos, 2009). The ADA Amendments, passed in 2009 and implemented in 2011, sought to broaden the protections under the ADA as were initially intended, rejecting standards imposed by the Supreme Court that narrowed protections under the law (United States Equal Opportunity Commission, 2008).

A noted tension in disability policy is the way disability is defined. Burke and Barnes (2017) argue that the underlying issue in U.S. disability law and policy is the layering of legislation guided by civil rights (the ADA) on top of existing disability services and insurance programs based on the medical model without an effort to coordinate or integrate approaches. The two leading opposing views are considered this way: Activists promote civil rights, access, and equity, while professionals and systems view disability through a medical model lens, mandating diagnosis or proof of condition to "qualify" for services, supports, and accommodations under the law. The result of this layering of policies that represent different social views is a complex existence, encompassing many different laws, policies, and social norms. We will highlight accessibility, civil rights, and access to quality medical treatment as containing specific laws, policies, and practices that continue to marginalize disabled people, with explanations of the issues and areas for advocacy.

ACCESSIBILITY AND THE AMERICANS WITH DISABILITIES ACT

Despite legislation mandating accessibility to public services and structures and public transportation, inaccessibility is still a major barrier for disabled people. The aging infrastructure of the United States is problematic when it comes to access and usability. Bagenstos (2009) argued that the root cause of access issues is related to historical ableism, where people with disabilities were hidden, ignored, and excluded, leading to the creation of the physical and social environment without considering disabled people as typical users. Since people with disabilities were not considered as those who would need to access stores, schools, and health facilities, they were not thought of in design choices and construction. This means that post-ADA, older buildings must be retrofitted for accessibility. Limitations associated with what can be modified and the costs are considered in decisions on how and where accessibility may be granted and when it is considered too costly or burdensome. Additionally, compliance with the law does not necessarily make a building usable or easy to navigate. When physical spaces are not accessible and usable for people with a variety of disability-related impairments, it means they cannot fully participate in communal life and are limited in a way that nondisabled people are not.

The Architectural Barriers Act (1968) and the ADA (1990) are the two pieces of legislation that guide much of the present system of standards guiding physical accessibility. The Architectural Barriers Act "requires certain Federal and Federally funded buildings and other facilities to be designed, constructed, or altered in accordance with standards that ensure accessibility to, and use by, physically handicapped people" (Cornell Law School, n.d.). The ADA expanded areas covered by accessibility requirements to public services (i.e., hotels, restaurants, recreation facilities, healthcare facilities, banks), transportation (excluding some rail service and air travel), telecommunications, and miscellaneous services such as historical sites and wilderness areas (Parker & Szymanski, 1998). Facilities and services must be usable by individuals with disabilities, with requirements to modify existing structures and services and set new standards for those built after January 26, 1993 (Cornell Law School, n.d.).

The ADA has five titles: Employment, Transportation, Public Accommodations and Services, Telecommunications, and Miscellaneous. Other resources clearly outline each title, and readers are directed to the ADA National Network (www.adata.org) for more information. See Table 6.1 for federal agencies responsible for enforcement of discrimination under the ADA.

A limitation of the ADA is that it is largely incumbent on individuals with disabilities to report discrimination or inaccessibility when they encounter it to one of several federal agencies. For example, a person who would like to eat dinner in a restaurant but cannot get a wheelchair through the door would need to pursue a complaint to compel the business owner to make the adjustments. If no one reports inaccessibility, the structure will simply remain unusable. The result is that people with disabilities continue to move about spaces in their daily lives that are inaccessible to them, sending the message that they are not valued or welcomed. While civil rights legislation has created new opportunities for people with disabilities, Parker and Szymanski (1998) noted that "legal mandates do not, of themselves, change the attitudes of society or increase societies awareness of the individual's needs" (p.

TABLE 6.1: **Enforcement Entity and Purview**

ENFORCEMENT ENTITY	PURVIEW
U.S. Equal Opportunity Commission (EEOC)	Title I: Employment and Title V: Miscellaneous; complaints related to disability discrimination in hiring, firing, compensation, job requirements, promotion, or other employment aspects, disability-related harassment, and reasonable accommodations; this includes coercion or retaliation under Title V
U.S. Department of Justice (DOJ)	Title II: Public Services and Title III: Public Accommodations; complaints of disability discrimination resulting in lack of access to public services, including websites, polling sites, restaurants, educational institutions, medical facilities, and public spaces
Federal Communications Commission (FCC)	Title IV: Telecommunications, is enforced by the Federal Communications Commission, and individuals may report complaints regarding accessibility of communications services or equipment (e.g., phones, email, or texting), video programming on television or other equipment (i.e., internet streaming), and other services such as those made available to individuals who are Deaf and Blind
U.S Department of Transportation (DOT)	Title II: Public Services, specifically complaints related to discrimination in the provision of public transportation services; this generally includes fixed-route buses, complimentary paratransit, and rail, air, and water transportation, including ferries
Department of Housing and Urban Development (HUD)	Title II: Public Services addresses complaints of discriminatory housing practices, including denying housing or an accessible living space because of disability status

Source: ADA National Network. (2015). *An overview of the Americans with Disabilities Act.* Author. https://adata.org/factsheet/ADA-overview; Federal Communications Commission (n.d.). *Accessibility complaint filing categories.* https://consumercomplaints.fcc.gov/hc/en-us/articles/204231424-Accessibility-Complaint-Filing-Categories; U.S. Department of Justice, n.d. Disability Rights Section. www.justice.gov/crt/disability-rights-section

20) and, alone, do not create equity for disabled people. Unfortunately, inaccessible spaces continue to exist and negatively impact the activities and participation of disabled people.

CIVIL RIGHTS

Historically, biases toward people with disabilities have influenced what individual rights they are permitted through various forms of state and federal legislation. The United States' dark history regarding the treatment of people with disabilities included several measures that limited basic human rights. From medical abuse during institutionalization in the 1800s to the eugenics movement in the early 1900s leading to forced sterilization and Ugly Laws (Fox & Marini, 2018; Rembis et al., 2018), people with disabilities in the United States have always had limited autonomy. This fact is increasingly true for disabled people of color; advocates such as Brad Lomax worked to blend goals of the disability rights movement with those of the civil rights movement with the goal of amplifying both. These movements had a large impact on the shift toward legislation that protected people with disabilities. Throughout the 1960s and 1970s, disabled advocates fought to move away from the medical model of disability and toward the social model of disability, which includes values such as empowerment and human rights protections (Charlton, 1998; Tucker, 2017). The United States currently has more disability rights cases than any other country and continues to influence disability legislation across the globe (Burke & Barnes, 2017).

Despite the establishment of civil rights protections, disabled people still struggle to receive equitable treatment. The situation is complicated by a lack of cohesion in policies guiding accessibility and individual rights. For example, organizational policies such as attendance, financing, and documentation regulations have the potential to support or oppose civil rights granted in other forms of legislation (Ordway et al., 2021). Sometimes, such as the case in disability law, these new laws exist in contradiction with the previously enacted laws and rely on individuals to pursue litigation when their rights are violated (Burke & Barnes, 2017). The following sections overview relevant laws and policies impacting disabled people in the areas of financial wellness, autonomy and decision-making, community living, parenting, and voting access.

Financial Wellness

Financial wellness is an important aspect of community life, as self-sufficiency is highly valued in U.S. culture. People with disabilities experience financial exploitation and extortion at a higher rate than nondisabled people (Findley et al., 2016; Fisher et al., 2012) with strong associations with social vulnerability (Fisher et al., 2012). Disabled people are also five times more likely than nondisabled people to live in poverty, with greater risk for those with an additional minoritized identity (McDonald et al., 2015; McGarity et al., 2020). Despite the link between financial education and financial wellness, standardized financial education is minimal, if nonexistent, for disabled people (McGarity et al., 2020).

Historical views of disabled people as unable to work and in need of financial support have created a tension between need for social welfare benefits for survival and the cost to freedom and citizenship associated with dependence on these benefits. Social Security Disability Insurance (SSDI) and other disability-related financial sources of support (i.e., supplemental security income [SSI]; public medical insurance, housing supports) integrate the definition of disability with an inability to work, making them functionally equivalent. In these programs, if you can work, you do not meet the definition of disabled and do not qualify for any assistance (Burke & Barnes, 2017). However, the financial support available through these programs is minimal; the listed maximum monthly SSI payment for an individual person is $841 per month or $1,261 for an eligible couple (Social Security Administration [SSA], 2021). The SSA maintains formulas to reduce benefits if an individual should receive any other forms of income or support. The result is a system that is seen as highly bureaucratic, stigmatizing, and uncompassionate. Individuals may endure extreme poverty during the waiting period of application for benefits while they cannot work and are only provided minimal financial sustenance if their application is approved (Whittle et al., 2017).

For individuals who do qualify for benefits, policies in place that are designed to prevent "abuse of the system" or "malingering" may actually impede employment progress. For example, some disabled individuals need personal assistance for activities of daily living. These services may or may not be covered under private insurance that is available through employment and are prohibitively expensive to pay out of pocket. For a worker who needs to maintain personal assistance to get to work each day, they may need to decline raises or promotions to stay within income caps to qualify for public insurance to keep their access to this critical resource. When people with disabilities who have received benefits consider entering or re-entering the workforce, they also must consider whether they are willing to lose their SSDI, Medicaid, and/or Medicare eligibility in the process (Bagenstos, 2009). Exercising other political rights, such as running for office, may jeopardize SSI payments (The Advocacy

Monitor, 2021). Regulations surrounding disability benefits also may influence the choice to get married. Many benefits across SSDI, SSI, and Medicaid cease to exist when one is legally married or, at a minimum, are significantly decreased, depending on state regulations (Belt, 2015).

Autonomy and Decision-Making

Efforts to provide legal protection for people with disabilities who are considered vulnerable have been complicated by trying to appropriately balance autonomy and protection. Assisting individuals to maintain their rights is important, but this power has often been abused. Researchers have coined the term *overprotection* to describe the tendency to limit people with disabilities because of assumptions of what individuals are capable of (Hollomotz, 2011; Lindsey, 2020). This phenomenon is not exclusive to the United States and has been demonstrated in other countries (Callus et al., 2019). Laws have the power to affect both material and intangible protections, as they can limit what someone with a disability is allowed to do, as well as impact larger societal biases and individual autonomy:

> *the pattern that consistently comes into view is of adults with intellectual disability being held back from being included in society, from participating in mainstream activities, and (most importantly) from living their own life on their own terms, in the name of keeping them safe from harm.* (Callus et al., 2019, p. 358)

Although perhaps well-intentioned, overprotection reinforces dangerous societal stereotypes that people with disabilities cannot make autonomous decisions and can be considered a form of discrimination, impacting self-esteem (Callus et al., 2019; Sanders, 2006).

Overprotection is particularly prominent for people with intellectual and developmental disabilities. The reasons for this may include perceived or actual vulnerability and dependence on the support of caregivers (Callus et al., 2019). Hemm et al. (2017) found that participants with intellectual disabilities were nearly twice as likely as participants without intellectual disabilities to identify decisions that their parents regularly made on their behalf. One participant reported, "Sometimes they [my parents] make decisions and I'm like, do I not even get a say in it?" (Hemm et al., 2017, p. 366). Instead of continuing to further restrict the autonomy of people with disabilities, the focus should be put on the perpetrators of abuse. A relevant term to address issues of abuse, manipulation, and advantage-taking is called underprotection (Lindsey, 2020). Overprotection and underprotection often stem from a lack of understanding of the actual needs of people with intellectual and developmental disabilities (Callus et al., 2019).

Laws around financial and other forms of decision-making for people with disabilities have changed throughout history and continue to vary by state. For example, a durable power of attorney is a written document that grants another individual the ability to make decisions for a person if they can no longer make decisions for themself due to disability, without having formal guardianship (Buckner, 2018). This can be helpful if the decisions are made in the best interest of the person with a disability. Two challenges with a power of attorney are determining whether (a) the individual with a disability is accurately deemed unable to make decisions for themselves and (b) the trustee of their finances is exploiting them.

Guardianships, otherwise called conservatorships, are another method designed to ensure the needs of people with disabilities and other vulnerable populations are adequately met while retaining as much autonomy as possible (National Council on Disability, 2019). Full guardianship is commonly assigned by courts to grant full decision-making power for someone who is deemed "incapable" to another individual, typically a family member or closest living relative (Buckner, 2018; National Council on Disability, 2019). While there are alternatives to guardianship or conservatorship, it is often offered as the first and sometimes only support for decision-making (Buckner, 2018). It is estimated that 1.3 million people with disabilities are under conservatorship in the United States (National Council on

Disability, 2018). For clinicians, it is imperative to avoid assuming what decisions are best for a family and to increase awareness of other possibilities that provide the greatest autonomy for persons with disabilities (e.g., supported decision-making or power of attorney; Buckner, 2018; National Council on Disability, 2019).

Supported decision-making removes or limits legal arrangements designed to protect disabled people by putting others in charge of important life decisions. Instead, supported decision-making balances input from all stakeholders, but retains ultimate decision-making power with the disabled person (Buckner, 2018; National Resource Center for Supported Decision-Making, n. d.). Currently, only 12 states have supported decision-making as a legal option (National Resource Center for Supported Decision-Making, n.d.). The United Nations Convention on the Rights of Persons with Disabilities (UNCRPD) encourages supported decision-making as the "preferred response" for increasing autonomy (Gooding, 2013). Emerging research demonstrates that supported decision-making has been effective in the United States for maintaining greater decision-making rights for people with disabilities (Center for Public Representation, 2016).

Community Living

The Fair Housing Act of 1968 was designed to prohibit housing discrimination. However, the act did not include disability until 20 years later, when the Fair Housing Amendments Act was authorized in 1988 (Friedman et al., 2018; Schwemm, 2020), despite the knowledge that disabled people are likely to encounter inaccessible housing and ableist assumptions from landlords (Hammel & Smith, 2017). The impact of the lack of recognition of disability in housing regulations is still apparent; people with disabilities continue to live in lower-quality housing compared to those without disabilities (Friedman et al., 2018). In 2021, 54.56% of all housing discrimination complaints made to the Department of Housing and Urban Development were based on disability (Augustine et al., 2021). With the onset of COVID-19 in 2020, housing discrimination complaints based on disability harassment increased by 40% (Augustine et al., 2021).

Particularly for individuals with visible disabilities or need accommodations, there are significant barriers to searching for housing, communicating with renters and sellers, finding accessible units, and receiving reasonable accommodations (Aranda, 2015). Two types of claims are typically filed in relation to disability and housing: disability-impact claims, which are claims against disability discrimination, and reasonable accommodations claims, which are claims against the lack of adequate accommodations (Schwemm, 2020). Since 1992, the Department of Justice (DOJ) has supported a Fair Housing Testing Program that focuses on bringing lawsuits for demonstrated patterns of unlawful housing discrimination (U.S. DOJ, 2022).

Parenting and Disability

Legal barriers present a unique set of challenges for parents with disabilities. Disabled parents are subject to additional layers of scrutiny for "fitness" and "capability" far beyond the experience of nondisabled parents. These laws and policies may exist under the guise of protecting children and families but are overshadowed by biased views of disability. Kaye (2011) reported that roughly 4.1 million parents have disabilities, which was 6.2% of all parents in the United States at the time. In 32 states, disability is still considered in custody and visitation determinations (Belt, 2015; Francis, 2019; Powell, 2014). Difficulty in determining whether the ADA applies to custody cases has left many disabled individuals subject to discrimination. Only recently (2015), the U.S. Department of Health and Human Services (HHS) and the U.S. DOJ specifically addressed the civil rights of disabled parents (Belt, 2015). There is a strong bias toward parenting ability of people with intellectual and developmental disabilities in determining who is deemed a "fit" or "unfit" parent (Francis, 2019). Furthermore, enacted laws have the power to affect wider societal perspectives of the disabled community. This can, in turn, impact internalized ableism, where individuals apply oppressive beliefs onto themselves because of harmful societal messages. Slice (2020) describes her experience as a disabled parent and her feelings of devaluation: "My disability limits me in performing the mundane physical acts of caregiving that I associate with 'real' parenting" (p. 130).

Further complicating the relationship between disability and parenting are abortion laws. With the recent overturn of *Roe v. Wade*, the case that set the precedence for protected access to abortion, this landscape is quickly changing. Regardless of how this decision by the Supreme Court will be implemented in each state, efforts to restrict access to reproductive healthcare will most greatly impact minoritized populations, including people with disabilities (Center for Reproductive Rights, 2021). We will highlight two main areas within this broad topic that are most discussed within the context of disability: bodily autonomy and reproductive healthcare and disability-selective abortion.

Bodily autonomy, particularly as it relates to reproductive healthcare rights, has long been a fraught issue in the disability community and remains a highly valued human right. Historically, disabled people have not been granted control over their bodies, making this a high-stakes issue for those in the disability community. Forced sterilization laws are typically discussed as a historical artifact. However, forced sterilization continues to be allowed in most states and is only banned in North Carolina (National Women's Law Center, 2022). Forced sterilization arose in tandem with the eugenics movement in the United States with the hope of eliminating disability from humanity, and later influenced Nazi tactics (Rembis, 2010; Thomson, 2012). Indiana was the first state to pass a forced sterilization law in 1907 (Rembis, 2010; Thomson, 2012). Forced sterilization has not been banned in part because historical case law (i.e., *Buck v. Bell*, 1927) has yet to be overturned. Another aspect of reproductive healthcare concerns people who are at high risk for pregnancy complications or death and for these reasons may not want to carry a pregnancy to term (Gleason et al., 2021).

Some disabilities can be identified before birth through genetic and chromosomal testing; disability-selective abortion is the termination of a pregnancy based on results from testing conducted before birth that indicate the child will be born with a disability (Fox & Griffin, 2009). Down syndrome, for instance, can be diagnosed as early as 11 weeks. An issue becoming increasingly relevant with the overturn of *Roe v. Wade* is whether prenatal nondiscrimination acts should be enacted or if increased healthcare support for people with disabilities would make having a disabled child more accessible (Denbow, 2020). A report from the American College of Obstetricians and Gynecologists revealed practitioner perception of counseling patients on genetic issues as highly important; however, knowledge and awareness of appropriate sources of information is inadequate (Adjei et al., 2017). These limitations in legislation and education are a direct result of the societal value, or lack thereof, for the lives of disabled children. Within the disability community, laws regarding reproductive care continue to be a charged discussion.

Political Access and Voting

Voting is a critical aspect of participation in the U.S. political system. If disabled individuals do not participate in the political process, they do not have the same opportunity as nondisabled voters to elect public officials who align with their own interests to create laws and policies that they feel would benefit them. The term *social inaccessibility* as it refers to political participation describes whether the space is welcoming to people with disabilities and whether the political interests of people with disabilities are represented, both identified as problems by disabled people (Schur et al., 2017; Schur & Adya, 2012). Andrews et al. explained the necessity of political involvement by highlighting the need for activism: "Disability advocates face impending legislation meant to weaken, de-fund, or eliminate services that are relied upon disproportionately by people with disabilities" (Andrews et al., 2019, p. 115). Involvement of people with disabilities in developing voting access has been shown to be beneficial in voting structures across the globe (Atkinson et al., 2014; Schur et al., 2017). Yet educational materials to inform about political issues are not necessarily made to be accessible to people with disabilities, especially people with intellectual disabilities (Agran et al., 2016). Some states also have specific limitations on voting for people under guardianship arrangements or those deemed "incapable" (Disability Justice, n.d.). For those eligible, voting is a powerful way to participate in the selection of public officials who shape policy affecting all aspects of community life; therefore, it is critical for voting and all political advocacy efforts to be accessible to disabled people (Erkulwater, 2018).

Within the current system, polling site access is often not physically accessible to people with disabilities (Agran et al., 2016; Schur et al., 2017), despite voting rights being covered by several pieces of legislation, including Title II of the ADA, the Voting Rights Act of 1965, and the Help America Vote Act (2002). The Help America Vote Act was specifically enacted to make polling places accessible to disabled persons to enhance privacy and independence of casting a ballot, reducing the need for disabled voters to rely on others (Matsubayashi & Ueda, 2014). Barriers for people with physical disabilities may include having to wait in line for polls or a lack of accessible transportation. Other disability-related barriers concern the form of the ballot (print-only versus electronic or Braille), comprehension of the ballot questions, and manual dexterity required to create a signature that matches a file to ensure the ballot will be accepted (Agran et al., 2016; Schur et al., 2017).

Voters with disabilities report difficulty with voting at much higher rates than of voters without disabilities, and disabled people are much less likely to vote overall (Butler & Johnson, 2022; Schur et al., 2017). Analysis of population data in the United States from 1980 to 2008 revealed a consistent gap in voting participation between disabled and nondisabled people. Voting trends noted increased voting participation by both groups starting after the 1996 election, with no change in the gap during the time examined. Individuals with cognitive and mobility impairments were the least likely to vote, and the likelihood of voting by mail was higher than voting in person for individuals across disability groups. Researchers concluded that voting by mail is effective in increasing participation for persons with disabilities (Matsubayashi & Ueda, 2014). However, many disabled people report that they prefer to vote in person (Schur et al., 2017), placing a high priority on ensuring accessibility of voting through multiple methods.

HEALTHCARE

Healthcare for disabled people is a complex issue, encompassing systemic barriers to care that is accessible, high quality, and affordable. The laws that shape the U.S. medical system as it relates to care for disabled people are rooted in ableism and a lack of recognition of humanity. This system of care is tainted by a history of violence, forced medical treatment, and "therapeutic approaches" that were barbaric, ineffective, and harmful. Examples of some of the violations and devaluations of disabled people incurred by the medical community include forced sterilization, removal of children with disabilities from their families to be placed in institutions, inhumane treatment in institutional settings, and the euthanasia movement (Rembris et al., 2018). Other more recent professional movements that devalued disabled people included the "oralist" movement, insisting that Deaf people move from using sign language to communicate to learn speech and speechreading (Longmore, 1995), and applied behavior analysis (ABA), designed to train autistic people to behave in a more socially acceptable way according to the priorities of the therapist (Shyman, 2016).

Activists argue that ongoing devaluation of disabled lives is connected to nondisabled people's perception of quality of life and their assumption that a person who has a disability cannot possibly be happy, thriving, fulfilled, or contributing to society. This results in the denial of appropriate treatment because of devaluation and discrimination (Longmore, 1995). This observation is well explained by Tamara Dembo's insider-outsider dynamic, where insiders (disabled people) understand what life with a disability or chronic condition is like and are more likely to incorporate positive aspects of their experience and outsiders (nondisabled people) do not and thus make assumptions, often negative, about what it must be like (Dunn et al., 2016). Individuals who are close to a disabled person are also more likely to consider strengths and positive aspects and have a more favorable impression of quality of life (Wright, 1988).

As previously discussed, the disability rights movement rejects the medical model espousing the view that disability is the result of a condition that must be cured to function in society. This conflict has resulted in somewhat of a culture clash (Longmore, 1995) and an adversarial relationship between disability rights activists and the medical community on topics such as medical ethical issues (i.e., decision-making, healthcare access and rationing) and impacts relationships between disabled people and healthcare providers (Longmore, 1995).

Healthcare inequality is a significant issue for the disabled population, with observed consequences for those with intellectual and developmental disabilities, mental illness, mobility issues, and chronic conditions and those whose conditions come with multisystemic implications. While some health consequences of disability are unavoidable because they are directly related to an underlying health condition, many are avoidable because they are a direct result of social, economic, and environmental disadvantages (Krahn et al., 2015). Disabled people fare far worse on health indicators and social determinants of health when compared to nondisabled people, including keeping up to date on preventative care; rates of obesity, smoking, and sedentary lifestyle; rates of diabetes and cardiovascular disease; and access to social support and safety (Krahn et al., 2015). Unfortunately, civil rights law has not been effective at addressing healthcare disparities for people with disabilities (Ordway et al., 2021). Additional attention to addressing ableism and inaccessibility within our healthcare system is needed. The following sections expand on the existing barriers to healthcare for disabled people in the key areas of affordability, quality, and accessibility.

Affordability

Health insurance in the United States was not widely available until the 1940s, when employers started offering coverage as a benefit to attract highly qualified employees when wages were capped by federal regulations (Blumenthal, 2006). This combined with other policy changes that occurred over the next two decades fueled an expansion of employer-sponsored health coverage such that, by the 1960s, employer-based health insurance served as the primary source of coverage (Blumenthal, 2006). Public insurance programs Medicaid and Medicare were signed into law in 1965, authorized by Title XIX of the Social Security Act (Centers for Medicaid & Medicare Services, n.d.). In 2014, the Affordable Care Act (ACA) provided states the authority to expand Medicaid eligibility to individuals below the age of 65 who meet income guidelines and standardized the eligibility and benefit rules for Medicaid and other public programs, recognizing that eligibility was traditionally built on highly restrictive income limits. The ACA also included several other program changes, including program and funding improvements to ensure availability of long-term care in the individual's home or community, focus on wellness and health promotion, and program transparency and quality improvements at the individual and provider level (Centers for Medicaid & Medicare Services, n.d.).

Specific to individuals with disabilities, Medicaid provides unique access to home and community-based services such as personal and attendant care, durable medical equipment, and supportive housing services. These services are often not covered under private insurance and are prohibitively costly. Medicaid also provides access to employment services and supports, including assessments, job development and coaching, and vocational training (Center on Budget Priorities, 2017). Forty-five states expand Medicaid to working adults with disabilities who exceed the income and/or asset limits for the other eligible pathways (Musumeci et al., 2019). This pathway to Medicaid allows individuals who qualify to retain access to medical and long-term supports that are rarely available through private insurance.

Quality Care

Disabled people report significant barriers to receiving quality care, stemming from attitudinal barriers such as prejudice, stigma, and discrimination when interacting with healthcare professionals (World Health Organization [WHO], 2021). Providers lack sufficient training on disability, and particularly for individuals with rare medical conditions or those whose manifestations mimic a variety of conditions, it may take a long time to find an accurate diagnosis with a treatment plan that meets medical needs.

Descriptions of negative medical experiences of disabled people take several forms, but typically are centered around invalidation, minimization, and indignity (Berglund et al., 2010; de Vries McClintock et al., 2016; WHO, 2015). Common examples include instances where a provider addresses a person other than the disabled person for information or questions even when the disabled person is the one leading communication and dismisses clear accessibility needs, such as calling a patient name out loud in a waiting room when the person has explained that they are not able to hear (de Vries McClintock et al., 2016). Additional examples of poor treatment include providers dismissing reports of pain or symptoms, ignoring healthcare needs such as reproductive healthcare for women with disabilities because they are assumed to be asexual or not able to parent, blaming the person for the manifestations of their condition, and redirecting individuals to psychiatric services when physical evidence of pain or dysfunction is not initially found (Berglund et al., 2010; WHO, 2015). The consequences of these experiences are considerable. Individuals may develop mistrust of medical professionals, change providers until they can find one who takes them seriously (delaying diagnosis and treatments in cases where clinical impressions are needed), and avoid seeking care when they need it because they have little faith that it will result in a satisfactory experience (Berglund et al., 2010; Senai, 2019).

For individuals with intellectual disabilities, severe and chronic mental illness, and communication barriers, assumptions about capabilities and quality of life may impede high-quality care or even lead to a situation where care is withheld. A recent example is found in the state of Oregon when a woman with an intellectual disability was brought to the hospital with COVID-19 symptoms in March 2020. A doctor denied the woman a ventilator when she needed one because he judged her quality of life to be poor. He instead asked her to sign a legal document (a do not resuscitate order, or DNR) agreeing that providers should not revive or intubate her if she lost consciousness. She was alone in the hospital due to pandemic restrictions, and it was not clear that she understood what she was being asked to sign. The hospital also sent DNRs to the group home where the woman lived to fill out in advance for other residents if they were to need medical attention (Shapiro, 2020). A complaint was filed, and lawyers working for Disability Rights Oregon became involved. As a result of their inquiries, the woman was moved to a different facility where she was provided appropriate treatment and recovered. This violation is only one example of several nationwide, where medical professionals make treatment decisions based on perception of poor quality of life due to disability status. These cases in Oregon resulted in advocacy for a state law (Senate Bill 606), prohibiting hospitals from withholding care pending agreement to a DNR order and requiring that persons with certain disabilities be allowed to have a trusted person accompany them to explain their medical choices (Shapiro, 2020).

Accessibility

Despite the ADA mandates regarding accessibility of public services and entities, physical accessibility of medical facilities and treatment continues to be an issue. Inaccessibility poses the greatest limitations to people with mobility impairments and communication barriers. In 2005, the U.S. Surgeon General proposed a "Call to Action to Improve the Health and Wellness of Persons with Disabilities" (Office of the Surgeon General, 2005), outlining some of the leading barriers to care for disabled Americans. Some issues were related to architectural barriers and lack of appropriate equipment, such as small examination rooms that do not have enough space for wheelchairs; stairs, examination tables, scales, or chairs that do not adjust for height or allow for transfer; inaccessible bathrooms; and lack of accessible parking (Krahn et al., 2015; Office of the Surgeon General, 2005). Ensuring effective communication is also a concern, particularly for individuals with visual, hearing, or speech impairments and people with intellectual or developmental disabilities who may need assistance in understanding information and making informed choices about their care. Examples of common communication needs include access to a qualified sign language interpreter, digital versions of printed materials, phone relay services, and digital accessibility of health records, kiosk systems, and telehealth (ADA National Network, 2020). Finally, policies may serve as barriers to quality care for disabled persons, necessitating accommodations such as priority scheduling of appointments to match when transportation is available, allowing service animals, helping complete forms or intake questionnaires, or allowing a person to accompany the patient to provide personal care during the appointment time (ADA National Network, 2020).

FUTURE DIRECTIONS FOR ADVOCACY AND POLICY CHANGE

As we reflect on the historical treatment of disabled people in the United States and celebrate the 33rd anniversary of the ADA, the advances disabled activists have won are evident, as are the areas that are still in need of change to promote human rights, inclusion, and equity of disabled people. In this final section, we will summarize and highlight areas of advocacy and policy change commonly highlighted in the disability community and discuss strategies for counselors to be effective allies and supporters of policy change.

It is key for nondisabled people wishing to be allies to the disability community to be aware of and engage with their own ableism and bias. This is important for potential allies to be advocating alongside disabled people, rather than unintentionally pushing their own bias on the community. One example of this has been the gap between use of language in disability spaces and in nondisability spaces. Despite the well-established preference for many subcommunities to use identity-based language (Mairs, 1986), able-bodied caregivers, academics, and medical and rehabilitation professionals have often enforced person-first language. This has limited the expression of disabled people and their autonomy in choosing their own expression of identity. In general, those seeking to be allies would benefit from spending time in community spaces, seeking education and resources designed by and for disabled people, and listening carefully with cultural humility, rather than acting on biases and assumptions.

While disabled people experience ableism in many forms, experiencing ableist microaggressions or discrimination from a provider is particularly harmful because counselors and other professionals are supposed to be there to help. As noted by Forber-Pratt et al. (2017), "Rehabilitation practitioners hold immense power in settings that serve disabled individuals, including providing access to services, particular tools or resources, and overall knowledge about disability" (p. 122), and this inherent power differential means that allyship and examination of internalized ableism are critical for effective and ethical practice (Melton, 2018). Allyship demands active engagement, and an ally can be described as a person who "demonstrates consciousness of issue(s) as well as understanding and commitment to a particular position and acts accordingly. Furthermore, the active ally publicly demonstrates a supportive stance, even when not popular or politically expedient" (Melton, 2018, p. 84). At times, a counselor acting as an ally may find themselves having to speak up against internal agency policies or systems in support of equitable treatment of clients.

Throughout history, disabled people have always been their own most effective advocates. They have demonstrated again and again that they know best what they need. A famous phrase within the disability rights movement, "nothing about us without us," reminds nondisabled people, including professionals, that the community needs to be centered in any advocacy efforts (Charlton, 1998). Rehabilitation counselors and disability service professionals need look no further than the disability community to identify initiatives to join to support disabled people. Consult Exhibit 6.1 for some national and international, cross-disability organizations with a common vision on promoting civil and human rights for disabled people. Other organizations may be disability-specific, for example, primarily focused on issues affecting a particular disability group (i.e., Blind people, autistic people). Allyship and effective advocacy demand understanding and aligning with the priorities of individuals in the community.

CONCLUSION

Civil rights for persons with disabilities in the United States have expanded greatly in the last century, culminating with the ADA in 1990, amended in 2008. However, laws, policies, and social conventions continue to marginalize disabled people, impacting their participation and community living opportunities. While much of our disability policy and services are based on the medical model, the social, political, and biopsychosocial models of disability are thought to encompass a more holistic view on disability and the experiences of disabled people. Disabled people continue to advocate for greater access to housing, community life, employment, legal standing, and voting, among other priorities. Counselors and allies need to listen to the disability community to understand the priorities of individuals to best align with and support their goals.

EXHIBIT 6.1. Disability Advocacy Organizations

Here, we will highlight a few examples of organizations to consult to learn more about disability advocacy and public policy. This list is not meant to be exhaustive, and certainly will not reflect the great diversity of views and opinions within the community. All three selected example organizations provide methods for learning more and getting involved.

ADAPT (American Disabled for Attendant Programs Today), www.adapt.org, is an activist organization with a rich history of nonviolent political activism demanding civil and human rights for disabled people. The main priorities of ADAPT include the rights of disabled people to live freely in the community, without surveillance, with adequate supports (https://adapt.org/adapts-community-for-all-platform/, 2022). ADAPT proports that disabled people should have full access to everything a community offers, with respect and valuation for disabled lives, including equitable access to disaster relief services (ADAPT, 2022).

The National Council on Independent Living (NCIL) is the "longest-running national cross-disability, grassroots organization run by and for people with disabilities" (NCIL, 2022, "About"). NCIL's mission and vision are to advance rights, standing, value, and participation of people with disabilities. NCIL publishes the *Advocacy Monitor*, their newsletter focused on policy and news topics relevant to the human and civil rights of disabled people. Common topics include voting rights, healthcare, housing, transportation, community living, employment, youth issues, veterans issues, and aging (NCIL, 2022; https://advocacymonitor.com/).

TASH (www.tash.org) is another cross-disability organization focused on advocating for human rights and inclusion of disabled people, particularly those with significant support needs. Fundamental principles of TASH are inclusion, full participation, self-determination, and self-advocacy. Priorities include providing access to communication, education, employment, high-quality and individualized services and supports, and ensuring that people can live where they choose (TASH, 2022).

DISCUSSION QUESTIONS

1. Consider the concepts of *physical accessibility* and *social accessibility*. How are they different? How are they similar?

2. What is implicit bias? How might implicit bias interfere with counseling or other professional relationships with disabled clients who are seeking supports?

3. What learning experiences are effective in helping us identify and address our biases?

4. How is supported decision-making distinct from other legal arrangements for important decisions? How does it work?

5. What does it mean to be an ally versus an advocate?

CLASS ACTIVITIES

1. Counseling organizations are possibly groups that can lobby for policy change. As an active ally, these are some organizations with which you can participate in policy change with other counselors. These resources will vary state by state, so similar organizations will likely also be found in the state in which you practice. Within these organizations, you can also consider if these spaces in and of themselves are accessible for disabled people to be advocates and, if not, this is an area you can encourage change. The state of Oregon, for example, has COPACT: https://copactoregon.com

   Reflect on the following questions:

   a. How does COPACT explain their advocacy priorities? How do these priorities align with the needs of clients?

   b. How can professional counseling associations align themselves with the priorities of disabled people?

   c. Consider how organizations can approach accessibility or self-audit for accessibility to be inclusive.

2. Identify one disability activist in the chapter and research them. What do you find out about their life experiences and leadership journey? What impact did they have on the community?

   a. Other suggested individuals to research: Frances Perkins, Johnnie Lacy, Anita Cameron, and Marca Bristo.

3. Visit the website of a disability activism organization. It can be international, national, statewide, or local. How does the organization explain its vision and mission? What are their main priorities?

4. Compare and contrast the Americans with Disabilities Act with the United Nations Convention on the Rights of Persons with Disabilities.

   a. Are there areas of life mentioned in the chapter that are covered by one but not the other?

   b. What is the difference between "prohibiting discrimination" and "ensuring equal participation"?

   c. How are they enforced?

KEY REFERENCES

Only key references appear in the print edition. The full references appear in the digital product on Springer Publishing Connect™: https://connect.springerpub.com/content/book/978-0-8261-5111-7/part/partI/chapter/ch06

Bagenstos, S. (2009). Law *and the contradictions of the disability rights movement.* Yale University Press. https://doi.org/10.12987/9780300155433

Burke, T. F., & Barnes, J. (2017). Layering, kludgeocracy and disability rights: The limited influence of the social model in American disability policy. *Social Policy and Society*, *17*(1), 101–116. https://doi.org/10.1017/S1474746417000367

Dunn, D. S., Ehde, D. M., & Wegener, S. T. (2016). The foundational principles as psychological lodestars: Theoretical inspiration and empirical direction in rehabilitation psychology. *Rehabilitation Psychology*, *61*(1), 1. https://doi.org/10.1037/rep0000082

Melton, M. L. (2018). Ally, activist, advocate: Addressing role complexities for the multiculturally competent psychologist. *Professional Psychology: Research and Practice, 49*(1), 83. https://doi.org/10.1037/pro0000175

Nielsen, K. E. (2012). *A disability history of the United States* (Vol. 2). Beacon Press.

THE PERSONAL IMPACT OF DISABILITY

Part II offers insights into the personal impact of illness and disability by looking closely at several unique psychosocial life experiences. This section blends a focus on the issues with theory and practice for rehabilitation professionals in exploring the intrapersonal and interpersonal impact of disability on the individual. The current authors discuss various theories of adaptation to disability, the unique experiences faced by women with disabilities, gender differences regarding sexuality and disability, the psychosocial impact micro-aggressions, and quality of life (QOL) issues for those with disabilities.

MAJOR HIGHLIGHTS IN PART II

- The processes of psychosocial adaptation to chronic illness and disability (CID) are, and have historically been, a defining focus of rehabilitation counseling and rehabilitation psychology. The broader counseling profession is increasing-ly awakening to the awareness that CID impacts clients and families across the spectrum of counseling issues and disciplines. Chapter 7 provides an update and expansion of Livneh and Antonak's 2005 classic primer on the psychosocial adaptation to CID process for counselors. The authors provide an overview of the dynamic process of psychosocial adaptation to CID, including a review of basic concepts, CID-related responses, coping models and strategies, methods and approaches commonly used to assess psychosocial adaptation to CID, and counsel-ing interventions in working with people in the psychosocial adaptation process.

- Chapter 8 explores the differences in psychosocial adjustment between persons with a congenital disability and those who sustain an adventitious disability later in life. It summarizes seven major theories of psychosocial adaptation to disability—the stage model, chaos theory, ecological model, disability centrality model, somatopsychological model, recurrent or integrated model, and transac-tional model—that offer different but ultimately overlapping explanations. This comparative view is a highlight of the book, synthesizing the author's previous writings on this topic.

- The authors of Chapter 9 examine issues of abuse and intimate partner violence (IPV) among women with disabilities, one of the largest and most marginalized populations in the U.S., and one whose members face high risk of abuse. The physical and mental health consequences of abuse and IPV, barriers to intervention and escape, and resulting psychosocial disparities are explored through the lens of intersectionality. The authors present evidence-based counseling approaches for working with women with disabilities to reduce vulnerabilities and disparities in their psychosocial adjustment and health outcomes and call for increased professional awareness and cultural competence.

- Chapter 10 deals with sensitive issues relating to sexuality and disability. It explores the definition of sexuality as well as common myths and misconceptions regarding the impact of disability on a person's sexuality. The author examines sexuality from a social model perspective, noting that traditional ideas of what constitutes sexuality have been replaced by a new "normal," representing a broader spectrum of preferences and displays of sexuality.

- Chapter 11 is an overview of disability-related microaggressions. Microaggressions are understood as the daily slights, insults, and indignities experienced by minoritized people, communicating hostile and derogatory messages about the oppressed group. In Chapter 11, the author outlines disability microaggressions, and centers the experiences of disabled people. A common feature of Ableist microaggressions is that through words, actions, or environmental cues- individuals are expressing their implicit bias related to disability by communicating that disabled people are less valuable, less desirable, and outside of the "norm" as compared to nondisabled people. In this chapter, the author provides strategies for interrupting microaggressions from the perspective of the target or as a bystander. She also provides guidance for counselors who have unintentionally committed microaggressions during client interactions, including steps to take responsibility for their behavior and repair the relationship.

- Chapter 12 defines quality of life (QOL) and related constructs, and explores the changing definitions and applications of these constructs in rehabilitation, with a focus on their application in the area of psychosocial adaptation to chronic illness and disability. The ways in which QOL has been defined and utilized has changed considerably in the 50 years since it was first identified as an important outcome in the rehabilitation counseling and rehabilitation psychology literature. As views on both rehabilitation and disability are currently in a period of significant transition and change, the authors explore the current and potential future utility, meaning, and application of QOL and related constructs in rehabilitation.

CHAPTER 7

PSYCHOSOCIAL ADAPTATION TO CHRONIC ILLNESS AND DISABILITY: A PRIMER FOR COUNSELORS

MALACHY BISHOP, SARA PARK, HANOCH LIVNEH, AND PHILLIP RUMRILL

LEARNING OBJECTIVES

After reading this chapter, you will be able to

- Define the process of psychosocial adaptation to chronic illness and disability (CID)
- Articulate how each of the key concepts contributes to the dynamic process of psychosocial adaptation for individuals with CID
- Identify psychological responses that may be experienced with the onset of CID
- Conceptualize coping strategies with CID through different coping models
- Match the assessment scales to a specific construct within the psychosocial adaptation
- Apply theory-driven, psychosocial, reaction-specific counseling interventions and self-management strategies to practice

PRE-READING QUESTIONS

1. What are some biopsychosocial factors related to the dynamic process of psychosocial adaptation to chronic illness and disability?
2. How are CID acceptance, adjustment, and adaptation different?
3. What constructs are commonly assessed with psychosocial adaptation to CID?
4. Why is understanding psychosocial adaptation to CID of critical importance to all counselors?

Globally, over 1 billion people are currently living with a disability (World Health Organization [WHO], 2022). In the United States, it is estimated that 61 million adults have a disability, representing 26% of the U.S. population (Centers for Disease Control and Prevention [CDC], 2022a). Chronic diseases (defined as conditions that last 1 year or more and require ongoing medical attention and/or limit activities of daily living) affect 60% of adults and are the leading causes of death and disability in the United States (CDC, 2022b). Given the high prevalence and broad health, economic, and psychosocial impacts of chronic illness and disability (CID), counselors of all backgrounds and specializations will work with growing numbers of persons with disabilities and chronic illness (Chapin et al., 2018). Effective counseling practice requires that counselors have awareness and knowledge about CID, understand the issues and psychosocial barriers that may be experienced by those living with CID, and develop the skills and knowledge required to evaluate and incorporate CID in the counseling process as appropriate (Emir Öksüz & Brubaker, 2020; Peterson, 2022; Rivas, 2020). Our purpose in this chapter is to contribute to counselors' understanding of one specific aspect of the experience of living with CID, described as psychosocial adaptation.

Psychosocial adaptation to CID incorporates the wide variety of biopsychosocial processes by which people adapt, adjust, or function in the context of the experience of living with a chronic illness or disability. These processes are and have historically been a defining focus of rehabilitation counseling and rehabilitation psychology (Bishop et al., 2023; Livneh & Antonak, 2005). The broader counseling profession is increasingly recognizing that CID impacts clients and families across the spectrum of counseling issues and disciplines. As a result, nascent steps are being taken toward broader disability inclusion (Peterson, 2022). In 2018, the American Rehabilitation Counseling Association (ARCA) board of directors approved a set of Disability-Related Counseling Competencies (Chapin et al., 2018), which were subsequently approved by the American Counseling Association (ACA) governing council in 2019. The adoption of these competencies recognized the necessity of disability-related counseling competencies for all counselors, regardless of professional background and specialty (Peterson, 2022). Despite the long neglect of disability and disability-related training in the counseling profession (Peterson, 2022; Rivas, 2020; Smart, 2018) inclusion of disability-related counseling competencies will likely be increasingly integrated in the training curricula across accredited counselor educational programs in the future (Emir Öksüz & Brubaker, 2020; Peterson, 2022). Consistent with this important trend, the purpose of this chapter is to provide counselors with an overview of psychosocial adaptation to CID.

The purpose in this chapter is to offer a primer-level overview. This chapter is patterned after the 2005 article by Livneh and Antonak that had the same purpose. As in that article, we provide readers with an overview of (a) the dynamic process of psychosocial adaptation to CID, including a review of basic concepts, CID-triggered reactions, and CID-related coping strategies; (b) current models and theories; (c) methods and approaches commonly used to assess psychosocial adaptation to CID; and (d) counseling interventions in working with people in the psychosocial adaptation process. The nature of this chapter limits the depth of the exploration of these topics, each of which is individually associated with an extensive research literature. We encourage interested readers to increase their understanding through further exploration, particularly of the key references highlighted throughout with asterisks.

Historically, psychosocial adaptation to CID research has primarily focused on the period around the onset of CID, though the term has been defined more broadly to include the ongoing process of adapting to changing experience and responses associated with living with a CID over time (Bishop, 2005). Psychosocial adaptation to genetic or congenital disabilities has historically received relatively less research attention than acquired CID (Bogart, 2014; Livneh, 2022). Hence, the research reviewed in this chapter is focused primarily on psychosocial adaptation to acquired CID.

KEY CONCEPTS FOR COUNSELORS

We begin by emphasizing two related and fundamental concepts, foundational in rehabilitation counseling, of which all counselors should be aware. The first concerns the fluid nature of psychosocial adaptation research and the reason for this fluidity. Disability results from and exists in the interaction between individuals with a health condition and the social and structural environments in which they live (WHO, 2022). The processes involved in psychosocial adaptation to CID, which are the focus in psychosocial adaptation to CID research, must also be understood not only in terms of the individual but in terms of the individual in the context of their social and built environments (Livneh et al., 2019; WHO, 2022). Because social and structural environments change and evolve over time, the experience of disability, and professionals' understanding of and clinical responses to psychosocial adaptation are also continually evolving. As with any area of study or research, some historical assumptions, understandings, and perspectives endure, while others either require updating or else become irrelevant as social constructs, experiences, and structures change.

Second, disability and nondisability-related factors intersect and compound to affect the personal and psychosocial experiences of individuals living with CID. These intersections are evident, for example, in the fact that rates of disability are consistently higher among older people and members of marginalized populations (Courtney-Long et al., 2017; Livneh & Antonak, 2005). Statistically, Americans with disabilities are more than twice as likely to live in poverty, twice as likely to have less than a high school education, and half as likely to have a 4-year college degree compared to those without disabilities (Paul et al., 2021). The labor force participation rate of people with disabilities is perennially lower than that for people without disabilities. This chronic and persistent fact results in continued exclusion from full community participation and has lasting impacts on physical well-being, psychosocial health, and quality of life (U.S. Senate Committee on Health, Education, Labor and Pensions, 2014). These and other complex social relationships affect psychosocial adaptation processes and outcomes, and although frequently overlooked from a research perspective, should not be neglected in the process of psychosocial adaptation counseling.

BASIC CONCEPTS

In this section, the concepts of stress, trauma and crisis, loss and grief, body image, self-concept and disability identity, stigma, uncertainty and unpredictability, and quality of life (QOL) are reviewed. Specifically, we focus on the relevance and integration of these topics in the psychosocial adaptation research. Here, and throughout this chapter, we emphasize that none of the experiences described are universally experienced and that every individual's experience is unique.

Stress

Stress is generally defined as a negative experience; a response to an internal or external situation that is perceived as taxing or exceeding one's resources, that disrupts psychosocial equilibrium, and can threaten health (Lazarus & Folkman, 1984; Martz, 2015). The onset of CID is, for many people, extremely stressful (Martz, 2015). Individuals with chronic illnesses generally report higher levels of depression, anxiety, and psychological distress relative to those without (Helgeson & Zajdel, 2017; Jang & Kim, 2018; Martz & Henry, 2016). People with CID frequently experience an increase in both the frequency and severity of stressful situations surrounding the onset of CID (Falvo & Holland, 2018; Finkelstein-Fox & Park, 2019) and the effects of CID may "remain for a lifetime and require continuous attention and self-management" (Martz, 2015, p. 379).

The experience of increased stress may be associated with a variety of experiences, including initial functional impairment or loss related to CID; diagnosis and the diagnostic process; treatment and healthcare-related stressors (Devins & Deckert, 2018); changes in body image; financial changes and economic instability; changes in social, familial, and vocational roles and relationships; and alterations in future goals and plans (Livneh & Antonak, 2005).

Psychological response to the stressful nature of CID influences psychosocial adaptation outcomes (Bishop et al., 2023; Helgeson & Zajdel, 2017; Mullins et al., 2001). Acute illness stressors, such as onset or initial diagnosis of CID, and ongoing illness stressors together may impact motivation, coping, and self-management, thereby impacting the psychosocial adaptation process (Dekker & de Groot, 2018). Self-efficacy, hope, optimism, resilience, social support, and effective coping strategies have been found to positively influence and mitigate the impacts of stress in psychosocial adaptation to CID (Helgeson & Zajdel, 2017; Jang & Kim, 2018; Martz & Livneh, 2016; McKenna et al., 2022).

Trauma and Crisis

The sudden onset of many chronic health conditions and disabilities (e.g., myocardial infarction, spinal cord injury [SCI], traumatic brain injury [TBI], amputation) or the diagnosis of a condition that is life-threatening (e.g., cancer, Parkinson disease) or that will affect valued functions can be highly traumatic and constitute a psychosocial crisis (Livneh & Antonak, 2005; Moos & Holohan, 2007). Trauma is a psychological and physical response to the threat or experience of overwhelmingly harmful experiences to self or a loved one. Trauma may occur in response to a single, acute event such as a diagnosis of CID or as a reaction to long-term, prolonged exposure, such as progressive physical deterioration, burdensome treatments, and repeated discrimination. Therefore, traumatic response to CID is complex and enduring (Martz, 2005). Furthermore, individuals with acute traumatic onset of disabling conditions such as amputations, SCI, or TBI may experience polytrauma, which is defined as "as two or more injuries to physical regions or organ systems, one of which may be life threatening, resulting in physical, cognitive, psychological, or psychosocial impairments and functional disability" (Chronister et al., 2021, p. 113). Polytraumatic injuries may also co-occur with secondary health conditions, such as posttraumatic stress disorder (PTSD), diabetes, and high blood pressure (Chronister et al., 2021).

In mental health parlance, crisis is defined as a situation in which a person is either unable to function effectively or is at a risk of hurting self or others due to overwhelming negative emotions (Chronister et al., 2021). Crisis, by definition, is time limited. The psychological consequences of crisis may, in contrast, be lasting. The results of several meta-analyses suggest the prevalence of PTSD after CID is around 10% (Arnaboldi et al., 2017; Martz & Cook, 2001; Swartzman et al. 2017). Studies among people with breast cancer and SCI suggest higher prevalence rates (Boyer et al., 2000; Vin-Raviv et al., 2013). The severity of the crisis response may depend on event-related factors, such as anticipation, intensity, duration, and previous experiences of trauma, as well as person-specific factors such as sociodemographic variables and use of coping strategies (Chronister et al., 2021; Martz, 2005) as well as sociocultural and environmental resources.

Loss and Grief

Grief "refers to (a) an emotion, generated by an experience of loss and characterized by sorrow and/or distress, and (b) the personal and interpersonal experience of loss" (Humphrey, 2009, p. 5). Grief can have physical, emotional, behavioral, cognitive, and social components (Cicchetti et al., 2016; Humphrey, 2009). The onset of a traumatic or progressive CID may trigger feelings of loss (e.g., for a body part or function, valued role, or identity) or grief (Parkes, 1975; Smart, 2016; Wright, 1983). Although this reaction is not universal in response to the onset of CID or CID-related changes over time, it is important to be aware of and prepared to validate and respond effectively to grief in response to loss when present. Cicchetti et al. (2016) and others (e.g., Doughty Horn et al., 2013; Ober et al., 2012) noted that although grief and loss are universal in the human experience, there is a relative lack of attention to and preparation for these topics among counselors. These authors further suggested that the lack of knowledge and understanding of grief among counselors and other health professionals can compound the experience for clients and negatively affect clients' QOL.

Historically, loss and grief have been viewed as a part of a linear progression of psychological stages that may be experienced following the onset of CID (Chronister et al., 2021; see further discussion of stage models later). Some linear models of adaptation arose out of Kubler-Ross's (1969) stage model of coping with dying. Because coping with CID frequently involves dealing with loss, it is important to briefly point out that Kubler-Ross's stage model, based on extensive interviews with hospitalized individuals with terminal illness, is not an appropriate model of psychosocial adaptation to CID or a description of grief and loss in the context of disability (see e.g., Bishop et al., 2023).

Body Image

The experience of changes in body image have long been recognized as an important component of the psychosocial adaptation to the CID process. Body image, defined as the unconscious mental representation or schema of one's own body (Schilder, 1950), is a personal and social construct influenced by environmental factors (Shpigelman & HaGani, 2019). Body image emerges and is modified through interaction with sensory (e.g., visual, auditory, and kinesthetic), interpersonal (e.g., attitudinal), environmental (e.g., physical conditions), cultural (e.g., social norms, values, and standards), and temporal factors. When illness or disability affects physical appearance, functional capabilities, experience of pain, and social roles, body image and self-concept may be altered (Bramble & Cukr, 1998; Falvo, 1999).

Ongoing changes in body image have been found to be associated with feelings of anxiety and depression, psychogenic pain, chronic fatigue, social withdrawal, and cognitive distortions (Livneh & Antonak, 1997). Assessing and responding to the individual's unique experience is a critical but often overlooked element in psychosocial adaptation counseling.

Sociodemographic factors, such as gender, age, visibility of disability, and type of disability, influence body image perception (Shpigelman & HaGani, 2019). Tam et al. (2003) found that adults with visible physical disabilities reported lower levels of self-concept compared to those without disabilities and those with nonvisible physical health conditions. However, Shpigelman and HaGani (2019) reported that those with invisible disabilities, such as serious mental illness (SMI), reported significantly poorer body image and self-concept compared to those with physical disabilities. Persons with invisible disabilities, such as psychiatric disabilities, may face high levels of social and self-stigma as well as the emotional burden of needing to disclose or "pass" (Bogart & Nario-Redmond, 2019; Shpigelman & HaGani, 2019).

Self-Concept and Disability Identity

The relationship between self-concept and CID has been described in terms of the various ways in which CID may challenge existing ideas about the self (identity) and the individual's typical response to change (Morea et al., 2008). The onset of CID may present situations that challenge one's sense of self (i.e., self-identity). Kelly (2001) suggested that interactions in which others respond to the person as "disabled" first, for example, may affect one's sense of self. The implications of this dynamic are perhaps particularly evident in healthcare settings. Both healthcare access and health service utilization are disproportionately lower for people with disabilities (Kennedy et al., 2017). Diminished healthcare access results from both disability-based disparities in health insurance coverage and stigmatized and biased treatment of individuals with disabilities (Kennedy et al., 2017). Self-esteem, representing the evaluative component of the self-concept, and self-perceptions are likely to be challenged in such encounters.

The relationship of both congenital and acquired disability to self-concept and identity has increasingly been recognized as salient to the adjustment process (Bishop et al., 2023; Irvine et al., 2009) and has received increased research attention in recent years, particularly in the context of disability identity research. Disability identity, described as positive self-concept as a person with a disability, incorporates self-concept and feelings of connection to, or solidarity with, members of the disability community (Dunn & Burcaw, 2013; Zapata, 2018). Disability identity has been identified as helping individuals adapt to disability, including navigating negative social interactions and social stresses (Dunn & Burcaw, 2013). Zapata suggested that the degree to which individuals with CID "maintain beneficial self-beliefs regarding their disability and have positive connections to other members of the disability community" results in higher or lower disability identity (2018, p. 512).

Recent research on disability identity identifies disability group identity as having an important role in the formation of a positive view of one's disability (see the Mueller et al. chapter in this text). Disability group identity is associated with well-being, coping response to stigma, and support for social change through advocacy and activism. Positive disability group identity is referred to as disability pride. Those identifying as members of the disability community were also more likely to value their experience, have higher self-esteem, and be less likely to minimize, deny, or conceal their disabilities (Bogart & Nario-Redmond, 2019). Neurodiverse communities and Deaf and hard of hearing communities are examples of disability communities that have established affirmed group identities by subverting the dominant values, redefining and celebrating their disabled identities (Bogart & Nario-Redmond, 2019).

Stigma

People with disabilities continue to experience stigmatization on both interpersonal and structural levels (Wang & Ashburn-Nardo, 2019). Stereotypes, prejudice, and discrimination are components of stigma. Stereotypes are collective negative notions about a group of people. Stereotypes are schemas of the public that categorize and label people. Stereotypes become prejudice only when these negative beliefs are endorsed and cause a negative emotional reaction toward the stigmatized group. Finally, discrimination occurs when behavioral response accompanies the cognitive and affective responses that arise from a prejudice (Corrigan & Watson, 2002).

Stereotypes and prejudice act to increase stigma toward people with CID (Corrigan, 2000). Deviations from societal norms and expectations may be viewed negatively by society and result in stigmatizing perceptions and discriminatory practices (Livneh & Antonak, 2005). When internalized, stigmatizing social encounters may result in increased life stress, reduced self-esteem, and withdrawal from social encounters, including treatment and rehabilitation environments (Wright, 1983). Internalized stigma may lead to feelings of rejection and negatively influence psychosocial adaptation (Cataldo et al., 2011). Kang et al. (2020), for example, reported that stigma was the strongest predictor of psychosocial adjustment among cancer survivors, followed by social support and coping strategies.

People with conditions such as diabetes, lung cancer, and liver cancer frequently experience high levels of public stigma due to a stereotype that their individual behaviors are responsible for the development of the conditions. People with accident-related disabilities, such as SCI and TBI, may experience similar stigma when blame is attributed to the individuals' risk-taking behavior (Kang et al., 2020). Mental and psychiatric illnesses are also highly stigmatized, leading to discrimination and disparities in employment, safe housing, and healthcare access (Corrigan & Watson, 2002). Furthermore, these disparities disproportionately impact minorities with disabilities (Stuber et al., 2008), which is partly attributable to the more than additive effect of being subjected to stigma, prejudice, and discrimination on the basis of more than one minoritized characteristic (Smart, 2016).

Uncertainty and Unpredictability

Although the course of some CIDs (e.g., amputation and cerebral palsy) is generally stable, most conditions may be regarded as neither stable nor predictable (e.g., epilepsy, cancer, multiple sclerosis [MS], diabetes mellitus). These conditions may be characterized by intermittent periods of exacerbation and remission, unpredictable complications, alternating experiences of pain or loss of consciousness, and alternating pace of progression. The concept of "perceived uncertainty in illness," or illness uncertainty, was coined by Mishel (1981, p. 258) to depict how uncertainty, or the inability to structure personal meaning, results if the individual is unable to form a cognitive schema of illness-associated events. Medical conditions such as cancer and MS, which are associated with heightened levels of perceived uncertainty regarding disease symptoms, diagnosis, treatment, prognosis, and relationships with family members, have been found to be associated with decreased psychosocial adaptation (Mishel, 1981; Wineman, 1990).

Illness uncertainty describes perceived ambiguity regarding the diagnosis and prognosis of CID, including predictability and availability of treatment. Illness intrusiveness (Devins, 1989; Devins et al., 1992; Devins et al., 1993; Devins & Deckert, 2018) is defined as the degree of interference with individuals' valued activities due to illness-induced impairments. Both of these cognitive appraisal mechanisms are hypothesized to impact QOL and have been found to be salient predictors of adjustment, even after controlling for demographic and illness-related variables such as age, education, and physical and cognitive impairment (Mullins et al., 2001).

Quality of Life

Over the past half-century, QOL has become one of the most prominent and central concepts in the field of rehabilitation (Bishop, 2005; Crewe, 1980; Frain et al., 2009; Livneh, 2022). In the context of psychosocial adaptation to CID, QOL has been actively applied and explored in multiple capacities, including as a framework for describing and understanding adaptation processes, as a measurement, as a goal, and as an outcome (Bishop, 2005; Crewe, 1980; Fabian, 1991; Herschensohn, 1990; Livneh, 2022; Mullins et al., 2001; Roessler, 1990). As a global and multidimensional construct, QOL can be used to incorporate and assess coinciding positive and negative experiences of living with CID and psychosocial adaptation outcomes (Bishop, 2005; Livneh, 2022). Several current theories and models of psychosocial adaptation processes incorporate QOL as a structure or framework for portraying psychosocial adaptation experiences and processes (Bishop et al., 2023).

CHRONIC ILLNESS AND DISABILITY-TRIGGERED RESPONSES

As suggested thus far, with the onset of CID, a wide range of psychological responses may be experienced. Martz (2015, 2018) grouped these in terms of negative affectivity (e.g., depression and anxiety) and positive affectivity (e.g., acceptance and adjustment, posttraumatic growth, benefit finding). In this section we review the responses most frequently described in the specific context of sudden, acute, or traumatic onset, as cited in the rehabilitation research and disability studies literature. It is important to clarify that although many models of adaptation have described such responses in terms of stages or phases of adjustment (e.g., Dunn, 1975; Fink, 1967; Livneh, 1986; Roessler & Bolton, 1978; Shontz, 1978), suggesting a predictable, linear ordering of responses, this conception has been criticized as having several significant limitations. Livneh and Antonak (1997) noted that the existence of a universal, progressive, phaselike, orderly sequence of predetermined psychosocial reactions to disability has not been supported by empirical research. The responses described in such models are not universally experienced and do not universally follow a linear, sequential pattern (Livneh, 1986,

2001; Smart, 2016). Despite the problematic descriptions of the manner in which these responses have been experienced, research continues to support the prevalence of these commonly identified responses to sudden, acute, or traumatic-onset CID (Livneh & Antonak, 1997; Livneh & Martz, 2012; Martz, 2018; Smart, 2016; Wright, 1983).

Shock and Anxiety

Shock may occur at the onset or initial awareness of the injury or condition and be accompanied by disbelief, a sense of physical and emotional numbness, disorganized thinking, confusion, or feeling overwhelmed (Chronister & Fitzgerald, 2021; Smart, 2016). Shock has been identified as an early self-protective response (Chronister & Fitzgerald, 2021). Anxiety, associated with feelings of fear and worry, may arise when threat is perceived or expected (e.g., to life, functioning, roles, goals, relationships, financial stability, and other forms of security). Particularly acutely, anxiety may manifest in physiological responses, such as rapid heart rate, sweaty palms, and/or in cognitive responses such as rumination and worrisome thoughts and fears (Chronister & Fitzgerald, 2021; Livneh & Antonak, 2005). Providing information and ensuring shared decision-making can be helpful in reducing anxiety (Chronister & Fitzgerald, 2021).

Denial

This reaction, also regarded as a defense mechanism employed to avoid anxiety and other threatening emotions, involves the minimization or negation of the chronicity, extent, and future implications of the onset of CID. Denial, harboring both conscious and unconscious elements, has been perceived as an inability to process threatening information and may involve selective attention to one's physical and psychological environments, unrealistic expectations of recovery, and disregarding medical advice and therapeutic or rehabilitation recommendations (Livneh & Antonak, 2005; Bishop et al., 2023). Although denial may successfully alleviate anxiety and depression during the initial phases of adaptation, its long-term impact is often considered potentially harmful (Livneh & Antonak, 2005).

Depression

Depression, feelings of sadness, or hopelessness and despair may occur as an individual struggles with the uncertainty, permanence, magnitude, or future implications of their condition (Katon et al., 2010; Livneh & Antonak, 2005; Smart, 2016). Although this response may be prevalent around the period of onset/diagnosis, not all individuals experience depression, and among those who do, depression may be temporary. However, because prolonged depression may result in self-destructive behaviors (Falvo & Holland, 2018), it is important to evaluate and monitor its progression.

Anger/Hostility

The reactions of anger or hostility may be experienced and have been divided in terms of internalized danger (i.e., self-directed feelings and behaviors of resentment, bitterness, guilt, or self-blame) and externalized hostility (i.e., other-directed or environment-directed anger; Livneh & Antonak, 1997). Internally directed anger may reflect self-attributions of responsibility for the condition's onset or failure to achieve successful outcomes (Livneh & Antonak, 1997). Anger may be characterized by low frustration tolerance, aggression, irritability, antagonism, arguing, and complaining (Chronister & Fitzgerald, 2021; Livneh & Antonak, 2005). Chronister and Fitzgerald (2021) noted that anger may provide a sense of control and help to ward off feelings of despair, helplessness, or sadness; as such, help individuals to regain a sense of control and express anger in appropriate ways.

Acceptance and Adjustment

Acceptance in the context of adaptation to CID is generally defined as a change in the value structure associated with (a) the person's awareness of the permanence of disability-related change (Bishop, 2012) and (b) "personal reconciliation that these changes do not determine or reduce their self-worth" (Bentley et al., 2019, p. 81). Researchers have identified that disability acceptance predicts a variety of psychosocial outcomes, including QOL, satisfaction with life, well-being, and mental health (e.g., Aaby et al., 2020; Elfström et al., 2005; Kennedy et al., 2012; Sanchez et al., 2019; Smedema et al., 2010; Wollaars et al., 2007; van Leeuwen et al., 2015; Yehene et al., 2020).

Acceptance was originally described in the context of adaptation to CID by Dembo et al. (1956), Wright (1983), and Wright and Remmers (1960) as the process of adjusting or realigning one's value system to accommodate disability-related changes. Specifically, these researchers (primarily based on research focused on adjustment to physical disabilities) described acceptance in terms of four distinct value changes, including (a) enlarging the scope of values, in which a person is able to see values other than those that conflict with having a disability; (b) subordinating physique relative to other values, in which a person is able to deemphasize physical ability and appearance and physical attributes are reconceptualized; (c) containing disability effects, in which a person realizes and finds meaning in areas of life not affected by disability, and the individual limits the spread of the disability beyond actual physical limitations; and (d) transforming comparative values into asset values, in which a person does not compare himself or herself to others, but is able to recognize and focus on personal strengths and abilities (Dembo et al., 1956; Wright, 1983). This particular conception of acceptance is the most frequently used in the rehabilitation literature; however, many other definitions have been described (see, e.g., Martz, 2004; Vash & Crewe, 2004). In acceptance and commitment therapy (ACT), acceptance has been broadly defined as "the active and aware embracing of private events . . . without unnecessary attempts to change their frequency or form" (Hayes et al., 2006, p. 7). From the ACT perspective, disability acceptance may be viewed as a two-part process that involves (a) a willingness to experience disability and (b) the engagement in values-based life activity despite disability (Bond & Bunce, 2003; McCracken et al., 1999).

Adjustment is closely tied to acceptance in the CID research (Bentley et al., 2019; Chronister & Fitzgerald, 2021) and has been defined in the literature in terms of reorganization, reintegration, or reorientation and movement toward psychological equilibrium (Livneh, 2001; Livneh & Antonak, 1997, 2005). Adjustment is described in terms of several components incorporating acceptance, including (a) cognitive reconciliation of the condition, its impact, and its chronic or permanent nature; (b) an affective acceptance, or internalization, of oneself as a person with CID, including a new or restored sense of self-concept, renewed life values, and a continued search for new meanings; and (c) an active negotiation of obstacles and pursuit of personal, social, vocational, and other goals (Livneh & Antonak, 2005).

Posttraumatic Growth

Also identified in the positive affectivity category of responses to CID onset are posttraumatic growth and related constructs, such as (a) benefit finding (reducing stress by identifying positive outcomes) and (b) meaning-making (searching for meaning and finding meaning or purpose in or from CID; Livneh, 2021). Tedeschi and Calhoun (2014) define posttraumatic growth as positive change resulting from the struggle with a major life crisis or a traumatic event. These leading researchers on the topic describe posttraumatic growth as potentially occurring or being recognized in several areas, including the awareness of newly emerged opportunities; closer relationships or increased connection with others; an increased sense of strength; a greater appreciation for life; and a deepening of one's spiritual life or a significant change in one's belief system (Tedeschi & Calhoun, 2014). Research on these constructs in the context of CID is active and rapidly expanding (Martz, 2015).

CHRONIC ILLNESS AND DISABILITY-ASSOCIATED COPING STRATEGIES

Coping is a psychological response to "circumstances that are new, require special efforts, or are unusually taxing" (Costa et al., 1996; Lazarus & Folkman, 1984, in Martz, 2015, p. 381). As suggested by Livneh and Antonak in 2005, and is even more true at the time of this update, the research related to coping with CID is vast. It continues to grow rapidly as researchers explore questions related to the form, nature, structure, process, and measurement of coping in the evolving context of changing experiences with and perceptions of CID (Cheng et al., 2019; Livneh et al., 2019). In this section, the concept of coping is briefly discussed and its relevance to CID is illustrated, followed by a cursory overview of commonly identified coping strategies related to coping with CID and an introduction to three of the many coping models (for more extensive and comprehensive reviews, we refer readers to Martz & Livneh, 2007).

Appraisal and coping inform how individuals respond to stress within their environment (Lazarus & Folkman, 1984). Appraisal describes the ways individuals interpret stressors. Individuals may interpret situations based on the potential for harm, the difficulty of the experience or task, the anticipation of growth from the experience, and the perceived significance of stressful life events on health and well-being. Coping is defined as conscious efforts to regulate appraised stressors by using available personal and social resources. Lazarus and Folkman (1984), pioneering coping researchers, defined coping as "constantly changing cognitive and behavioral efforts to manage specific external and internal demands that are appraised as taxing or exceeding the resources of the person" (p. 141).

Although coping is related to similar constructs, such as adjustment and adaptation, characteristics that define and distinguish coping from related constructs include (a) the temporal element, in that psychosocial adaptation is a longer-term outcome (reflecting psychological equilibrium, reintegration, active participation, etc.) and coping reflects more immediate, shorter-term responses and strategies; (b) a hierarchical organization that spans the range from macroanalytic, global styles of coping (e.g., locus of control and optimism) to microanalytic, specific behavioral acts; and (c) that coping efforts may include a range of cognitive, emotional, and behavioral strategies directed at both internal and external stressors (Krohne, 1993; Livneh, 2016; Livneh & Martz, 2007; Martz, 2015; Zeidner & Endler, 1996).

In the context of coping with CID, coping has been defined and conceptualized in various ways. In the context of CID, Dembo et al. (1956), Wright (1983), and Wright and Remmer (1960) described the "coping versus succumbing" framework. The former is characterized by a worldview that emphasizes positive aspects and abilities inherent in the person with CID (e.g., what the person is capable of doing, areas in which the person can participate, the belief that one's difficulties and limitations are manageable), whereas in the latter worldview the focus is on impairment and physical limitations (e.g., what the person is incapable of doing, areas in which the person cannot participate, and emphasizing one's difficulties and limitations (Dembo et al., 1956; Wright, 1983).

More broadly, coping strategies have also been categorized in multiple ways. Lazarus and Folkman (1984) organized these in two overriding categories in terms of function, including problem-focused and emotion-focused. Chronister and Chan (2007) summarized a tripartite taxonomic structure, including (a) emotion-focused strategies, aimed at reducing distress by changing or managing emotions; (b) problem-focused approaches, aimed at modifying the problem that is creating distress; and (c) appraisal-focused approaches, involving reducing stress by altering one's appraisal, assumptions, or perception of the stressor. Bishop et al. (2023) similarly described a tripartite model of coping strategies, including (a) engagement/approach coping (including approach-based, problem-focused, task-oriented coping strategies); (b) disengagement or avoidance approaches, including emotion-focused strategies; and (c) seeking and using social support, including efforts to mobilize emotional, social, and instrumental support from family members and social networks.

Due to variations in research methods and in coping definitions and measurement, it would be inaccurate to suggest that universal conclusions can be made about the relationships among categories of coping strategies (e.g., engagement or avoidance approaches) and particular psychosocial outcomes (Cheng et al., 2019). However, some generalizations and trends in the coping and CID research have been noted. For example, research generally supports a positive relationship between engagement coping strategies (such as problem-solving, planning, and cognitive restructuring) and positive psychosocial outcomes such as increased psychological well-being and life satisfaction and lower psychological distress (Bishop et al., 2023; Kennedy et al., 2009; Livneh & Martz, 2012). Social support–seeking strategies have also generally been found to be related to positive psychosocial adaptation outcomes (Livneh et al., 2019). Alternatively, disengagement or avoidance coping approaches, such as the use of wishful thinking, avoidance, escapism, and substance and alcohol use, have more frequently been associated with negative adaptation outcomes, including higher levels of depression, anxiety, and psychological distress (Bishop et al., 2023; Livneh et al., 2019). It is important to note again, however, that these are generalizations about an extensive and diverse body of research and these relationships vary situationally, contextually, and by type of CID and its experienced functional limitations.

As noted earlier, many models of coping have been proposed and applied in the context of coping with CID. Three specific models of coping are briefly introduced in this section: (a) Lazarus and Folkman's stress-appraisal coping model, Moos's crisis and coping model, and the conservation of resources theory.

Stress-Appraisal-Coping

The central tenet of the stress-appraisal-coping model is the cognitive appraisal of one's coping resources as the primary mediator between stress (related to a crisis) and perceived well-being. Coping resources can encompass a broad range of personal and environmental factors, such as emotional stability, problem-solving skills, social networks, natural supports, individual beliefs (e.g., self-efficacy and locus of control), and access to health and monetary resources (Folkman, 2010; Kelso et al., 2005). Furthermore, the stress-appraisal-coping model acknowledges individual differences in their appraisals of similar events and circumstances. Depending on their appraisal and available resources, people can engage in flexible coping strategies (i.e., modify coping strategies adaptively to meet the demands of different stressful situations) or disengaging coping strategies (i.e., denial, wish-fulfilling fantasy, self-and-other blame, and substance use; Tobin et al, 1989). In this model, coping is viewed as process-oriented, not to be confounded with outcomes or successful mastery of one's environment. The focus of coping is on the moment-to-moment attempts to balance one's resources according to their cognitive appraisal of the stressful event (Livneh & Martz, 2007).

Crisis and Coping Model

Moos and colleagues (Moos & Schaefer, 1984, 1986; Holahan et al., 1996; Moos & Holahan, 2007) offer another comprehensive model of coping with life crises and CID. In summary, Moos's crisis and coping model is a biopsychosocial model consisting of three major groups of components. The first set of components, known as the interacting factors, addresses personal resources, health-related factors, and the social-physical environment. The personal resources include sociodemographic (e.g., age, gender, education level) and personality characteristics (e.g., emotional stability, cognitive functioning, achievement orientation, resiliency). Health-related factors include factors such as the severity or stage of CID, body parts and functions, and the nature of CID (progressive versus static). The sociophysical environment includes social support networks and access to one's community, including work, leisure, and healthcare. The second set of components highlights the individualized coping process by including cognitive appraisal, adaptive tasks, and coping skills. Cognitive appraisal influences and informs adaptive tasks and coping skills. Adaptive tasks refer to many CID-related tasks, such as managing symptoms, treatments, and relationships. The third component of the model is health-related outcomes. Health-related outcomes are viewed as both the final element and the outcome within the model. The model recognizes the cyclical nature of coping in that the health-related outcome, at any point, influences the first two sets of components, thereby altering the longer-term health outcome.

Moos and Holahan (2007) also described eight categories of specific coping strategies classified along a two × two (approach versus avoidance × cognitive versus behavioral) grid. For example, logical analysis coping strategy is an approach × cognitive coping strategy. Seeking support is an approach × behavioral coping strategy. On the other hand, avoidance or denial is an avoidance × cognitive coping strategy, while emotional venting can be classified as an avoidance × behavioral coping strategy.

Conservation of Resources Theory

Along with the pioneering theory of Lazarus and Folkman (1984) and Moos's crisis and coping model, the conservation of resources (COR) theory (Hobfoll, 1989) has become a leading coping theory, especially in terms of chronic and traumatic stress, in the last 30 years. A basic tenet of the COR theory is the assumption that people are motivated to acquire and protect the resources they value (Hobfoll, 1989). At the same time, COR theory acknowledges that certain situations, especially where valued resources are threatened or lost, are universally and objectively stressful (Holmgreen et al., 2017). Many instances of acquired CID can be seen as being objectively stressful. Furthermore, building on Lazarus and Folkman's model of stress-appraisal-coping, COR also emphasizes the importance of individual perception of balance between available coping capacity and the environment.

Ultimately, COR theory provides a theoretical framework for how one prevents resource loss, maintains existing resources, and acquires new resources to sustain well-being. These resources are classified into four major categories: condition, energy, object, and personal.

Condition resources encompass interpersonal relationships (e.g., being married) and statuses (e.g., having a stimulating job) that affect QOL. Energy resources are exchangeable "things," including money and time, that can be deployed to obtain more resources. Object resources entail amenities in the physical environment (e.g., housing, transportation). Lastly, personal resources are personal attributes and identities (e.g., gender identity, socioeconomic status, severity of injury/illness; Hobfoll, 1989).

COR proposes that individuals seek to create an environment that protects and promotes their integrity within their family and community (Hobfoll & Schumm, 2009). Individuals are viewed within their social environment, and individuals act to protect and preserve their valued resources. COR theory proposes that (a) resource loss is a more powerful influence than resource gain and (b) resources must be first invested before they are preserved or gained. These proposals acknowledge that people already lacking in resources are more vulnerable to loss of additional resources, while those with ample resources have more opportunities to gain other resources. Roessler et al. (2019) applied the COR theory to predict variability in perceived stress and coping for individuals with MS. People with more difficulties meeting their financial obligations, poorer housing satisfaction, and lower levels of community engagement (lacking in existing resources) reported experiencing higher levels of stress.

ASSESSMENT OF PSYCHOSOCIAL ADAPTATION TO CHRONIC ILLNESS AND DISABILITY

Psychosocial adaptation is a multifaceted construct and has been measured using numerous instruments and indicators, both positive and negative in nature (Bishop et al., 2023; Livneh & Antonak, 1997; Stanton et al., 2007). Whereas earlier efforts to measure adaptation in the context of CID focused almost exclusively on unidimensional and negative indicators, more recently, the importance of including both multidimensional and positive indicators of adaptation has been recognized, affording researchers a more balanced, realistic, and accurate perspective (Bishop et al., 2023).

Livneh and Martz (2012) and Bishop et al. (2023) suggested that measures of psychosocial adaptation may be grouped in terms of several broad categories (modified here), including (a) QOL-based measures, including comprehensive, multidimensional measures of various life domains, health-related QOL measures, and measures of related constructs, such as life satisfaction and subjective well-being; (b) unidimensional or multidimensional clinical measures, focused, for example, on depression or anxiety; (c) CID-specific measures that assess acceptance of or adjustment to CID; and (d) physical or functional capacity measures. A large and growing number of measures of psychosocial adaptation have also been developed that are specifically designed for assessment among persons with a specific condition or disability. In this section, we review a selection of representative, psychometrically sound measures frequently reported in the literature. This necessarily restricted selection provides an indication of the conceptual breadth of assessments used and is by no means meant to represent a comprehensive review.

Psychosocial Adjustment to Illness Scale and Psychological Adjustment to Illness Scale-Self Report

The Psychosocial Adjustment to Illness Scale (PAIS; Derogatis, 1986; Derogatis & Derogatis, 1990) is a 46-item multidomain, semistructured interview designed to be conducted by a trained interviewer. A self-report version, the Psychological Adjustment to Illness Scale-Self Report (PAIS-SR), is also composed of 46 items, designed to match the items of the PAIS interview. Versions of the PAIS are frequently used in the psychosocial adaptation research. Both instruments measure psychosocial adjustment to illness in terms of seven domains as well as a total adjustment score. The domains include healthcare orientation, vocational environment, domestic environment, sexual relationships, extended family relationships, social environment, and psychological distress. The strengths of the PAIS include the psychometric robustness of its scales, having both self-report and clinician interview forms, and the availability of condition-specific norm scores (Livneh & Antonak, 2005).

Acceptance of Disability Scale and Revision

The Acceptance of Disability Scale (ADS; Linkowski, 1971) and Revised ADS (ADS-R; Groomes & Linkowski, 2007) are among the most frequently used measures of CID acceptance in the rehabilitation literature. The ADS is a 50-item, 6-point, summated rating scale developed to measure the degree of acceptance as theorized by Dembo et al. (1956) and further expounded by Wright (1983) and Wright and Remmers (1960), including (a) enlarging the scope of values, (b) subordinating physique relative to other values, (c) containing disability effects, and (d) transforming comparative values into asset values. This particular conception of acceptance remains the most frequently cited in the rehabilitation counseling literature (Bishop, 2012). The ADS-R contains 32 items rated on a 4-point Likert-type scale and includes four subscales that parallel the earlier four value changes. Major strengths inherent in the ADS and its revision include extensive use in rehabilitation research internationally, their theory-driven rationale, and established reliability (Livneh & Antonak, 2005).

Reactions to Impairment and Disability Inventory

The Reactions to Impairment and Disability Inventory (RIDI; Livneh & Antonak, 1990; 2008) is a 60-item, multidimensional, self-report summated rating scale. Its intended use is to investigate eight clinically reported classes of psychosocial reactions to the onset of CID, including shock, anxiety, denial, depression, internalized anger, externalized hostility, acknowledgment, and adjustment. The strengths of the RIDI include its comprehensive psychometric development, established reliability, and multidimensional perspective (Livneh & Antonak, 2005).

The Profile of Mood States

The Profile of Mood States (POMS; McNair et al., 1981) is a 65-item multidimensional scale originally developed for assessing response to pharmacological and psychotherapeutic treatment. The POMS, the 37-item POMS short-form (SF; Shacham, 1983), and several additional brief and alternative forms (Searight & Montone, 2017), have frequently been used in psychosocial adaptation research. The POMS and the POMS-SF include six subscales assessing tension-anxiety, depression, anger-hostility, fatigue, confusion-bewilderment, and vigor-activity and can provide a composite score representing overall mood disturbance or distress.

RAND Medical Outcomes Study 36-Item Short-Form Health Survey

The Medical Outcomes Study (MOS) 36-Item Short-Form Health Survey (SF-36; Hays et al., 1993) assesses health-related QOL and is well represented in the psychosocial adaptation to CID literature. The SF-36 is a brief, multidimensional QOL scale that assesses the impact of health on QOL in the following eight domains: physical functioning, bodily pain, role limitations due to physical health problems, role limitations due to personal or emotional problems, emotional well-being, social functioning, energy/fatigue, and general health perceptions, as well as a single item evaluating perceived change in health (Ware & Sherbourne, 1992). The strengths of the scale include its comprehensive psychometric development, established reliability, multidimensional perspective, and extensive use in the rehabilitation research.

Note that under the umbrella of QOL-based assessments, measures of life satisfaction and subjective well-being are also frequently used in the psychosocial adaptation research. These may serve in a variety of capacities, including as subjective proxies for psychosocial adaptation to CID.

INTERVENTION STRATEGIES FOR PEOPLE WITH CHRONIC ILLNESS AND DISABILITY

Psychosocial adaptation is an immensely complex process and as has been highlighted throughout this chapter, individual responses to the onset of CID vary considerably. The timing, setting, and role of counselors in working with individuals during the psychosocial adaptation process are also extremely varied. It is challenging, therefore, and particularly given the purpose and scope of this chapter, to discuss counseling interventions in a comprehensive and meaningful way. In this section, therefore, we briefly review at a conceptual level, theory-driven and reaction-specific intervention strategies in working with individuals during the psychosocial adaptation to CID process. We include a brief discussion of self-management, which is increasingly recognized as an important component and perspective in adaptation to CID.

Theory-Driven Interventions

These interventions focus on the clinical applications of widely recognized personality theories and therapeutic models to persons with CID in the context of psychosocial adaptation. When adopting theory-driven interventions, clinicians typically follow a three-step sequence. First, core concepts from a particular theory are identified and examined. Second, the usefulness of these concepts within the context of psychosocial adaptation to CID is evaluated. Third, the benefits derived from these concepts for practical counseling interventions, for people with CID are assessed and, if deemed appropriate, applied in practice. Researchers have explored and described matching theoretical approaches with specific responses to CID in the adaptation process (e.g., Livneh & Antonak, 1997; Livneh & Sherwood, 1991), coping strategies (e.g., Martz, 2015), and populations (see, e.g., Chan et al., 2015).

As noted by Martz (2015), modern psychotherapeutic and counseling approaches tend toward brief, time-limited, highly structured, and evidence-based approaches. Livneh and Martz (2012) and Martz (2015) provide reviews of theory-based counseling interventions to promote coping, suggesting, for example, that person-centered and gestalt approaches can target emotion-focused coping (providing interpersonal support, validation, and encouragement); cognitive behavioral therapy (CBT) interventions to promote active coping strategies or problem-focused coping (e.g., modeling, challenging irrational beliefs, exploring cognitive processes, role-playing); or to promote emotion-focused coping through the development of stress management skills (e.g., relaxation, mindfulness, meditation).

Psychosocial Reaction-Specific Interventions

These interventions aim at offering a logical match between specific psychotherapeutic strategies and those responses or experiences evoked during the process of adaptation to CID (e.g., anxiety, depression, denial, anger). It is generally argued that strategies regarded as supportive, affective-insightful, or psychodynamic in nature (e.g., person-centered therapy, gestalt therapy, Adlerian therapy) may be more useful during earlier phases of the adaptation process. In contrast, strategies viewed as more active-directive, goal-oriented, or cognitive behavioral in nature (e.g., cognitive therapy, behavioral therapy, coping skills training) may be more beneficial during the later stages (Livneh & Antonak, 1997, 2005; Mainella & Smedema, 2019).

To illustrate this rationale, Mainella and Smedema (2019) noted the efficacy of the evidence-based practice of CBT in addressing depression and anxiety and suggested that CBT techniques have been associated with reduced depression and increased QOL. Long-term depression can be further managed by reinforcing social contacts and activities and by practicing self-assertiveness, self-determination, and independent living skills. Anger and hostility may be addressed through the interruption and challenging of irrational beliefs, role-playing, and behavior modification (Mainella & Smedema, 2019).

The selection of counseling interventions should be informed by an understanding of evidence-based practice principles and current research evidence (Turner & Bombardier, 2019). Recent reviews and meta-analyses (e.g., Akyirem et al., 2022; Graham et al., 2016; Helgeson & Zajdel, 2017; Kiropoulos et al., 2016; Turner & Bombardier, 2019) highlight the breadth of counseling and therapeutic interventions evaluated at early stages of the adaptation process or for specific mental health conditions (e.g., depression and anxiety) and specific populations of individuals with CID.

Self-Management

Self-management is increasingly recognized as an important component in adaptation to CID and in long-term health and QOL among people living with a CID (Chronister & Fitzgerald, 2021). Self-management has been defined as learning and practicing the skills necessary to carry on an active and emotionally satisfying life in the face of a chronic condition and has as a central philosophy that the responsibility for day-to-day health and symptom management lies with the person, rather than medical providers (Lorig & Holman, 2003). Self-management has been found to be associated with a wide range of positive health and coping-related outcomes, including, for example, people with MS, improved coping, enhanced decision-making, autonomy, increased use of health-promoting behaviors, increased perceived control over both illness and nonillness aspects of life, reduced depression, and reduced psychosocial role limitations (see Bishop & Frain, 2018).

Highly compatible with active coping models described earlier in this chapter, self-management may involve such tasks as learning about and staying knowledgeable about one's health condition or disability; making healthy lifestyle choices with respect to nutrition, exercise, and self-care; maintaining psychological health; establishing and maintaining effective and supportive social networks; managing changes in personal, familial, vocational, and community participation roles; and managing healthcare relationships and coordinating multiple healthcare services (Bishop & Frain, 2018; Ghahari et al., 2014). Interventions to promote self-management are primarily based on education and support, and may include helping clients to develop and practice self-advocacy skills and health behaviors and plan for effective healthcare interactions (Bishop & Frain, 2018). A comprehensive exploration of self-management theory and research, including content specific to a range of CIDs, is available in Martz (2018) and Cuthbert et al. (2019).

CONCLUSION

People with CID often encounter physical, psychological, social, educational, financial, and vocational barriers that interfere with their QOL. In this chapter, we have attempted to provide counselors with useful and pragmatic concepts, processes, assessment tools, and intervention strategies related to psychosocial adaptation to CID. When working with individuals with a CID, counselors are commonly called to draw on their expertise in the areas of (a) stress, trauma, crisis, and coping; (b) self-concept, body image, and QOL; and (c) the effects of disability-linked factors (e.g., uncertainty and unpredictability) and societal reactions (e.g., stigma and prejudice) to psychosocial adaptation to CID.

Counselors must also be cognizant of clients' psychosocial reactions to their conditions and the social and structural environment. Several CID responses have been discussed. These include (a) reactions commonly experienced earlier in the adaptation process (e.g., anxiety); (b) reactions that normally suggest distressed and unsuccessful coping efforts (e.g., depression and anger); and (c) reactions associated with adaptation and renewed homeostasis (adjustment). Of the many measures available for assessing psychosocial adaptation to CID in the counseling context, several have been reviewed in this chapter. Assessment of clients' levels of psychosocial adaptation should inform selection of intervention strategies. To this end, the chapter concludes with an overview of strategies commonly applied in counseling people with CID and a brief overview of self-management.

CLASS ACTIVITIES

1. Consider: Quality of life (QoL) is a prominent outcome measure of psychosocial adaptation to chronic illness and disability. The World Health Organization (WHO) defines QoL as "individuals' perception of their position in life in the context of the culture and value systems in which they live and in relation to their goals, expectations, standards, and concerns" (WHO, 1997, p. 1). QoL can mean many different things depending on individuals' values and expectations. How would you define and measure a person's QoL in the context of psychosocial adaptation?

2. Several CID-triggered responses are discussed in this chapter, including (a) generally short-lasting responses that are more commonly experienced earlier in the psychosocial adaptation process (e.g., shock, anxiety, denial); (b) responses that are associated with distress or unsuccessful coping (e.g., depression, anger); and (c) reactions that suggest acceptance and value changes (adjustment). For each of the CID-triggered responses, identify and discuss some specific coping strategies associated with the response (e.g., shock and denial are associated with avoidance coping strategies such as escapism or wishful thinking).

3. In small groups, discuss: How are CID acceptance, adjustment, and adaptation different? Is it important to distinguish these, and if so, why?

4. Write a brief argument in favor of or against this proposition: Understanding psychosocial adaptation to CID is of critical importance to all counselors. Defend your answer. Discuss with the larger group.

KEY REFERENCES

Only key references appear in the print edition. The full references appear in the digital product on Springer Publishing Connect™: https://connect.springerpub.com/content/book/978-0-8261-5111-7/part/partII/chapter/ch07

Bogart, K. R. (2014). The role of disability self-concept in adaptation to congenital or acquired disability. *Rehabilitation Psychology, 59*(1), 107–115. https://doi.org/10.1037/a0035800

Livneh, H. (2022). Psychosocial adaptation to chronic illness and disability: An updated and expanded conceptual framework. *Rehabilitation Counseling Bulletin, 65*(3), 171–184. https://doi.org/10.1177/00343552211034819

Martz, E. (2018). Defining self-management on the individual level. In E. Martz (Ed.), *Promoting self-management of chronic health conditions: Theories and practice* (pp. 10–30). Oxford University Press.

Smart, J. F. (2016). *Disability, society and the individual* (3rd ed.). PRO-ED.

Wright, B. A. (1983). *Physical disability—A psychosocial approach.* Harper & Row.

CHAPTER 8

THEORIES OF ADJUSTMENT AND ADAPTATION TO DISABILITY

IRMO MARINI AND LAURA A. VILLARREAL

LEARNING OBJECTIVES

After reading this chapter, you will be able to:

- Understand the seven common theories of adjustment and adaptation to acquired disabilities
- Differentiate the nuanced conceptual differences between the models of adaptation
- Identify potential value and potential shortcomings to certain stage models of adjustment
- Examine additional concepts regarding responding to one's disability
- Explore the commonalities and overlapping concepts within the theories

PRE-READING QUESTIONS

1. How do persons with acquired disabilities adapt to their situation?
2. How might mourning following a disabling injury be more of a projected value judgement by others rather than a requirement for the person with the disability?
3. Would linear models or complex models of adaptation be best suited to help understand adjustment to disability?
4. What do all seven theories of adaptation have in common?

Perhaps one of the most profound and important empirical questions that researchers have regarding the psychological and sociological impact of disability is: How do persons with disabilities react to their situation, and why do some actually excel, whereas others become indefinitely incapacitated both mentally and physically? To begin with, there is some debate regarding appropriate terminology. Some experts, such as Olkin (1999), do not agree with the term *adjustment* to disability. Olkin argues that the concept of *adjusting* is a pathological term presuming something is wrong and implies persons with disabilities must successfully negotiate or transition through a series of stages to finally accept their situation. She is not a proponent of the stage model of disability, but rather believes that individuals "respond" to their disability throughout their lives and that final adjustment or acceptance does not exist. Other experts, such as Livneh (1991), do support a stagelike model and believe that persons with later-onset or adventitious disabilities often do transition through stages and reach a level of final adjustment or acceptance; however, they may experience setbacks. Still other experts, such as Vash and Crewe (2003), describe how some persons with disabilities may actually "transcend" beyond their disability once they acknowledge or come to terms with their situation, accept the implications, and embrace the experience.

In this chapter, the terms *adjustment, adaptation, reaction,* and *response* are used interchangeably; despite the fact that they may be different concepts, they have overlapping definitions. When used, they essentially refer to individuals with disabilities in their attempts to come to terms with their disability. Certain terms like *adjustment* and *adaptation* also have a temporal or time component to them (Livneh & Antonak, 1997). In other words, one would typically need to be adapting before he or she can reach final adjustment. Livneh and Antonak describe psychosocial adaptation as:

> An evolving, dynamic, general process through which the individual gradually approaches an optimal state of person-environment congruence manifested by (1) active participation in social, vocational, and avocational pursuits; (2) successful negotiation of the physical environment; and (3) awareness of remaining strengths and assets as well as existing functional limitations. (p. 8)

The concept of *adjustment,* however, is defined as:

> a particular phase (e.g., set of experiences and reactions) of the psychosocial adaptation process. As such, adjustment is the clinically and phenomenologically hypothesized final phase—elusive as it may be—of the unfolding process of adaptation to crisis situations including the onset of chronic illness and disability. It is alternatively expressed by terms such as (1) reaching and maintaining psychosocial equilibrium; (2) achieving a state of reintegration; (3) positively striving to reach life goals; (4) demonstrating positive self-esteem, self-concept, self regard, and the like; and, (5) experiencing positive attitudes toward one's self, others, and the disability. (p. 8)

Also, as discussed in Chapter 2, each and every day we experience thoughts, emotions, and behaviors that may or may not be in congruence with each other (e.g., we can be emotionally upset about something but behaviorally smile and pretend nothing is wrong). Each of the aforementioned concepts involves an emotional, cognitive, and behavioral response. When Olkin (1999) states that individuals respond to their disability, it means that they actually feel and think something while they are responding. Likewise, when individuals accept their circumstances, this again involves certain cognitions, behaviors, and emotions that accompany successful adaptation. Therefore, persons who are believed to have genuinely adapted to their disabilities should otherwise experience congruent feelings of contentment, thoughts of self-confidence with their disability identity, and some type of overt accompanying measurable behaviors such as socializing more, developing assertiveness, being employed, volunteering, attending school, and having the desire and confidence to date, if relevant.

Overall, seven common theories of adaptation to a traumatic physical disability are explored in this section. Some proposed theories have stronger evidence-based empirical support, whereas others rely on more qualitative and case study accounts, as well as clinical observation. This chapter first explores persons born with a congenital disability and questions whether such individuals actually experience any type of adjustment process since they have no preinjury, nondisabled experience with which to compare their situation. Olkin (1999) shares her life experience as an individual born with polio and prefers to describe her experience as "in response" to life circumstances she interfaces with in her external environment. Yet others born with a disability report different developmental experiences. As this phenomenon of adaptation to a congenital disability is less understood or written about in the literature, we lead off with this investigation. The remainder of the chapter explores the following seven theories of adjustment: stage models (Livneh, 1991), somatopsychology (Lewin, 1935; Trieschmann, 1988; Wright, 1983), the disability centrality model (DCM; Bishop, 2005), ecological models (Livneh & Antonak, 1997; Trieschmann, 1988; Vash & Crewe, 2004), recurrent or integrated model (Kendall & Buys, 1998), transactional model of coping (Lazarus & Folkman, 1984b), and chaos theory (Parker et al., 2003).

RESPONSE TO DISABILITY FOR PERSONS WITH CONGENITAL DISABILITIES

Although there is a plethora of conceptual and empirical literature regarding the adjustment or adaptation to an acquired disability, far less attention has been directed toward the psychosocial impact of a congenital disability, or those disabilities people have at birth (Varni et al., 1989). Some researchers anecdotally believe that as individuals born with a disability have no predisability background to compare with or a loss of function to grieve, they generally do not have any apparent difficulties adjusting (Olkin, 1999). In actuality, the available literature is inconsistent in these findings (Cadman et al., 1987; Olkin, 1999; Trask et al., 2003; Varni et al., 1989; Wallander et al., 1989; Witt et al., 2003).

From a psychosocial development standpoint, theoretically, we all generally pass through a number of critical life cycle stages of development (Erikson et al., 1986). Erikson et al. unfortunately did not take into account when a disability occurs; however, as he was a former student of psychodynamics, he would likely view the individual as experiencing some pathology at various stages. Statistically, data from the 1994 to 1995 National Health Interview Surveys, Disability Supplement population study (Witt et al., 2003) indicates that psychological maladjustment was 10% to 15% higher among children with chronic illness and disability (CID) as opposed to otherwise healthy children in the early 1970s (Pless et al., 1972). As previously indicated, however, the level of severity of the disability has little impact on response (Wallander & Varni, 1998). In the 1994 to 1995 national health survey of biological mothers, the psychosocial statuses of 3,362 disabled and nondisabled children and adolescents aged 6 to 17 years were assessed. Children with psychiatric disabilities were excluded. Poor maternal health or mental health, child-perceived family burden (scored by answering yes to one or more of three questions asking whether family disruptions in work status, sleep patterns, or financial problems occurred), and living in poverty were all positively associated with reported maladjustment of the children. Mothers of children with disabilities were more likely to be divorced, separated, or never married, as well as in poorer health and depressed, as opposed to mothers with a nondisabled child. In addition, children with communication or learning limitations also were positively associated with poor adjustment. Conversely, Varni et al. (1989) found that family cohesion, organization, and moral-religious emphasis were all predictors of positive psychological and social adaptation in 42 children with congenital or acquired limb disabilities. Researchers also found that increased parental distress, such as wishful thinking and self-blame, were associated with an increased distress among children and adolescents with cancer. It appears that environmental or external influences such as emotionally stable family support and cohesion are key factors that predict child adaptation.

Olkin (1999) notes that even among well-meaning or well-intended parents, children with disabilities can still run into adjustment problems. Specifically, Olkin discusses the "conspiracy of silence," where well-meaning parents intentionally withhold information or ignore discussing important topics with their child regarding their prognosis, sexuality, and so forth, because the parents perceive that it upsets their child. Similarly, some parents overprotect them by not allowing opportunities for their child to compete or attempt new experiences for fear of him or her failing. This undermines the child's ability to handle stress and be exposed to new experiences, ultimately hurting the child as he or she becomes an adult (Hogansen et al., 2008). By being sheltered, some children with disabilities are often less physically independent, having had everything done for them; as a result, they may experience low self-esteem and greater social anxiety and immaturity (Holmbeck et al., 2002; Levy, 1966; Thomasgard, 1998). Seligman (1975) uses the concept of "learned helplessness" to describe instances where individuals repeatedly have things done for them over time, essentially learning to be helpless and unable to perform tasks or activities they could otherwise be capable of performing had they been taught or empowered to learn.

In reverting back to the Erikson et al. (1986) theory of psychosocial development, some children with congenital disabilities might otherwise experience psychosocial difficulties with shame or self-doubt (Erikson's *autonomy versus shame*) at an early age as a result of not being allowed, or physically able, to explore their environment (Kivnick, 1991). This can carry over during school-age years (Erikson's *industry versus inferiority* stage) where children with severe disabilities are unable to master their environment, and at times come under ridicule from fellow students (Connors & Stalker, 2007; Kivnick, 1991). Adolescents with disabilities can experience a particularly awkward and difficult time (Erikson's *identity versus identity confusion*). Generally believed to be a time when they develop a sense of identity, Kivnick (1991) notes how adolescents' general acceptance of their disability and mastery over their environment dictates the strength of their identity. If adolescents have been unable to master and/or explore their environment, they may theoretically succumb to societal expectations about disability. Other potentially problematic areas during teenage years include body changes like puberty and body image, peer relations, sexuality, and rejection (Davis et al., 1991; Gordon et al., 2004; Hofman, 1975; Rousso, 1996). Livneh and Antonak (2007) cite the importance of body image on one's self-esteem and note how persons with disabilities may be particularly vulnerable to poor body image perceptions. Not being viewed as "different" becomes critically important to the psychosocial well-being of adolescents, as the alternative, rejection and ridicule can be devastating to their self-esteem (Bramble, 1995; Connors & Stalker, 2007; Davis et al., 1991; Gordon et al., 2004; Howland & Rintala, 2001; Rousso, 1996).

Despite what appears to be a number of societal attitude barriers for persons growing up with an acquired or congenital disability, overall reports of happiness, contentment, and life satisfaction are mixed, but generally positive (Albrecht & Devlieger, 1999; Allman, 1990; Cohen & Napolitano, 2007; Connors & Stalker, 2007; Freedman, 1978; Lucas, 2007; Marinic & Brkljacic, 2008). Connors and Stalker (2007), for example, in interviewing 26 children aged 7 to 15 years found that despite the children citing public reactions of sometimes being stared at, condescended to, harassed, and pitied, they otherwise reported seeing themselves in a positive way and basically as similar to nondisabled children. However, as Thomasgard (1998) and others have found, parental perceptions and projections of their child's psychosocial well-being are frequently viewed much more negatively than the child views their own circumstances (Holmbeck et al., 2002; Trask et al., 2003), sometimes leading to parental guilt.

Marinic and Brkljacic (2008) surveyed 397 persons with varying types of disabilities compared to 913 nondisabled Croatians regarding levels of happiness and well-being. Of the group with disabilities, approximately 22% were either born with their disability or acquired it before the age of 7 years. The authors correlated happiness among both groups with life satisfaction by measuring happiness with the Fordyce scale (1988) and subjective well-being (SWB) using the Personal Wellbeing Index (Cummins, 2006), which measures satisfaction with life domains. The results indicated that both groups showed positive happiness and satisfaction with the majority of life domains; however, happiness levels of persons with disabilities were lower than the control group in several areas. Less than 15% of persons with disabilities rated themselves as "extremely happy" compared to 40% of the nondisabled control group. Overall happiness score means on a 10-point scale, with 10 being extremely happy, showed the disability group ($M = 6.14$) scored slightly lower compared to the control group ($M = 7.8$). In contrast, Myers and Diener (1996) conducted a meta-analysis of 916 research projects from 45 countries with over 1 million participants, finding that people on average are moderately happy and score a mean of 6.75/10 on the same scale. Participants in the Marinic and Brkljacic (2008) study also scored moderately satisfied regardless of the disability. The disabled group, however, scored significantly different in the areas of happiness and physical safety and community acceptance. The authors opine that safety of the physical environment and positive or negative societal attitudes had an impact on their happiness, whereas this generally is not a consideration for persons without disabilities.

Overall, persons born with a disability are statistically at a greater risk of substance abuse problems, twice as likely to drop out of school, and more likely to be living in poverty than children without disabilities (Helwig & Holicky, 1994; Olkin, 1999). Research indicates that family and community support are critical in the positive psychosocial development of children and adolescents. When family cohesion, stability, and nurturing are dysfunctional, the likelihood increases for children to grow up with greater levels of adjustment problems. In addition, the person–environment interaction has time and again in numerous studies proved to be critical regarding individual self-concept and adaptation to disability. There is, however, what Freedman (1978) describes as the "disability paradox," whereby persons with disabilities who otherwise perceive themselves as having successfully coped with environmental and societal barriers and believe that they have emerged even stronger than others generally report a very high quality of life (QOL) and level of happiness (Weinberg, 1988).

THEORIES OF ADJUSTMENT AND ADAPTATION TO ACQUIRED DISABILITIES

A Brief History of Adjustment Theories

This section addresses seven various models of adjustment, adaptation, or reaction to an acquired disability sometime later in life. Again, some models have stronger evidence-based empirical support, while others are supported by clinical observation or qualitative self-report methods. As this line of academic study has evolved, some of the earliest theories on adjustment to disability were postulated by Dembo et al. (1956), and later expanded upon by Wright (1960, 1983). Successful versus unsuccessful adjustment was initially conceptualized within a "coping" versus "succumbing" framework. Essentially, Dembo et al. (1956) theorized that successful coping involved assisting clients to recognize what they functionally could do as opposed to dwelling on what they no longer could do, emphasizing personal accomplishments, taking direct control of one's life, successfully negotiating physical and social access barriers, enjoying and expanding on social activities that one enjoys, and appropriately dealing with negative life experiences. Conversely, poor adjustment was described as succumbing to one's disability by dwelling on the past, focusing on one's limitations rather than assets, and passively accepting the disabled role as defined by society (e.g., helpless, pitied, incapable).

Wright (1983) refined her earlier theory by equating adjustment or acceptance to disability by emphasizing the values and beliefs individuals ascribe to their condition. Wright distinguished between successfully reevaluating one's disabling circumstances as opposed to devaluing or denigrating oneself with the onset of a physical disability. She proposed four reevaluation changes that must occur for successful adaptation. Specifically, (a) subordination of physique or placing less self-worth emphasis on one's physical appearance, (b) containing or minimizing the "spread" effect of the disability to other unaffected functions and activities, (c) enlarging one's scope of values and interests consistent with our abilities, and (d) transforming from comparative to asset values. In other words, instead of comparing oneself to those without disabilities, it is better to focus more on the remaining abilities and qualities one can engage in rather than the functions one can no longer engage in. Wright's thinking on adjustment to disability went through a transformation as well. In her 1983 classic, *Physical Disability: A Psychosocial Approach*, Wright affirms the significance of the social environment and interpersonal relationships on adjustment, whereas in her 1960 book titled *Physical Disability: A Psychological Approach*, she focused mostly on the psychodynamics of adjustment and the individual. Although psychologists have been criticized for ignoring the impact of environmental barriers and negative societal attitudes on an individual's adjustment, Wright began to acknowledge this relationship early on.

Stage Models

Livneh (1986, 1991) provides a succinct summary and synthesis of more than 40 explicit and implicit stage models of adjustment, described as a reaction to a sudden and unexpected permanent physically disabling condition. The variations of this model range in theory from 3 to 10 stages, but most commonly 4 to 6 stages. Livneh cites several authors regarding a number of shared assumptions or rules of thumb applicable to these models. Several of the more pertinent assumptions are (a) adjustment is not a static, but rather a dynamic ongoing process, despite the concept that adaptation is considered to be the final outcome (Kahana et al., 1982); (b) the initial insult causes a psychological disequilibrium that typically restabilizes over time; (c) most individuals sequentially transition through time-limited stages by coming to terms psychologically with whatever trauma has occurred to them; (d) although most individuals experience most stages, others may not; (e) not everyone transitions through all stages sequentially; some individuals skip stages, some regress backwards to a previous stage, some can become stuck in a stage for long periods, and others may never reach the final adjustment stage (Gunther, 1969, 1971); (f) experiencing different stages separately and sequentially does not always occur, as some individuals may be observed to be in overlapping stages (Dunn, 1975) without any particular timeline, and often fluctuate based on individual circumstances and coping mechanisms; (g) observations at each stage can be correlated with certain cognitions, emotions, and behaviors; and (h) although stages are self-triggered, appropriate behavioral, psychosocial, and environmental interventions (counseling) can positively affect coping strategies to successfully transition toward adaptation (Livneh, 1991, pp. 113–114).

The five stages of adjustment to a sudden-onset physical disability postulated by Livneh (1991) are formulated as follows.

INITIAL IMPACT

This first stage generally involves individual and often family reaction during the initial hours and days following a sudden and severe bodily trauma such as a spinal cord injury, limb amputation, heart attack, or sudden onset of a life-threatening disease. Two substages are commonly identified: *shock* and *anxiety*. *Shock* is described as a surreal experience in which thought processes are disorganized, disoriented, and confused, as many individuals in shock have difficulty concentrating and are unable to make simple decisions (Gunther, 1971; Livneh & Antonak, 1997; Shands, 1955). *Anxiety* is described as overwhelming and can trigger a panic attack or hysteria-like behavior in extreme reaction cases. Some empirical support for these two reactions exists in the cross-sectional study by Livneh and Antonak (1991) with 214 rehabilitation facility inpatient and outpatient participants with various conditions, including spinal cord injury, cerebrovascular accidents, and multiple sclerosis. Participants distinguished between past and present reactions to their disability, indicating earlier adaptation phases were reported significantly more frequently in the past than in the present, including shock, anxiety, depression, internalized anger, and externalized hostility.

DEFENSE MOBILIZATION

This stage is characterized by two substages as well: *bargaining* and *denial*. Bargaining is described as a religious or spiritual attempt to negotiate with God or a higher power to be cured with the expectation of full recovery. In essence, the individual (and often the family) prays for survival and/or recovery with a promise to pay penance for any past wrongdoing (Livneh, 1991). In addition, in return for a cure or recovery, individuals may promise to donate to the church, do charitable work, and so forth. Livneh describes bargaining as being short term in nature, whereas denial is seen as lasting longer. Although bargaining and denial are seen as overlapping, denial is viewed as a more "extensive level of suppression or negation of the disability and its ramifications in order to maintain self-integrity" (p. 119). Related to this is the extensively studied and debated coping dimensions of problem- versus emotion-focused coping (Carver et al., 1989; Folkman & Moskowitz, 2004).

Problem-focused coping is described as a more task-oriented, constructive, and positive way of dealing with stressful events whereby an individual recognizes the problem, thinks of strategies to solve it, weighs the pros and cons of the decision, decides, and implements the chosen strategy (Cheng et al., 2010; Endler & Parker, 1990). *Emotion-focused coping* is described as a coping strategy to minimize or reduce the negative emotions associated with the stressor by denying, avoiding, or engaging in distracting activities (Folkman & Lazarus, 1980, 1985). The debate has centered around which coping strategy is more appropriate for alleviating an individual's distress. Typically, problem-focused coping has received greater support; however, emotion-focused coping appears best in instances where an individual experiences some emotionally overwhelming and extreme trauma for which he or she has little control over, and the problem cannot be solved. More recently, researchers suggested that both coping domains cannot be clearly distinguished from one another and may overlap and represent variations of one another (Endler & Parker, 1990; Folkman & Moskowitz, 2004). Cheng et al. (2010), in their study of 180 undergraduate students regarding problem- and emotion-focused coping strategies, defined *certainty emotions* (such as anger, disgust, happiness, and contentment) as eliciting problem-focused coping because they perceived being in control of the situation. "Uncertainty emotions" (hope, surprise, worry, fear, and sadness) most often elicited emotion-focused coping when the event was perceived as uncontrollable. These findings were originally supported by Folkman and Lazarus (1980) and have since been affirmed by Nabi (2003) and C. A. Smith and Ellsworth (1985).

Denial is the other major substage cited during this period (Livneh, 1991; Livneh & Antonak, 1997). Denial is a defense mechanism to protect the self from overwhelming fear and sadness by optimistically hoping things will get better and temporarily escaping the immense emotional sadness and fear of the unknown. Smart (2009) notes that denial can take three forms: denying the presence of the disability, denying the implications of the disability, or denying the permanency of the disability (p. 393). Livneh (1991) cites additional cognitions, behaviors, and emotions during this stage, including distorting facts and paying selective attention to good news, repressing unacceptable realities, constantly seeking information, setting unrealistic goals, having unrealistic expectations, refusing to modify the home or talk to persons with similar disabilities, and evading future planning with the belief that it will not be necessary (Dunn, 1975; Falek & Britton, 1974; Gunther, 1971; Naugle, 1991). Ironically, persons in denial have been observed with a range of emotions, including cheerfulness and happiness at one end as they unrealistically hope for recovery (Parker, 1979), to despair and anger during moments of realizing the permanency of their disability (Weller & Miller, 1977). Meyerowitz (1980), however, noted that denial can be adaptive as well, protecting the individual from overwhelming life-altering news. As Livneh and Antonak (1997) cite, denial continues to be debated by researchers regarding its relative value or hindrance in adjusting to a disability. Specifically, Livneh and Antonak (1997) cite denial in the literature as either a stage or phase of adaptation in dealing with traumatic loss or a defense mechanism that protects our ego to minimize or escape overwhelming anxiety. In this latter instance, denial is part of an emotion-focused response, which has arguably been viewed as temporarily helpful soon after injury, especially where the circumstances cannot be controlled (Meyerowitz, 1980). Theoretically, and for practical application purposes, should counselors confront patients and their family regarding the seriousness and/or grim permanency of the disability, or should these individuals be allowed to "hope"? This is debatable. The practical application may indeed be to assist individuals by never taking their hope away, but to encourage them to continue with their rehabilitation program, therapy program, and so forth, in the event that the disability may be with them for a while. This tangible compromise could then be viewed as "healthy denial," where the individual and their family continue to move forward, while not being denied their hope that a miracle or medical advances may exist in the near or distant future (I. Marini, personal communication, September 14, 2009).

INITIAL REALIZATION

The third stage is again also characterized by two major substages: *mourning and depression* and *internalized anger.* Mourning or grief is typically of shorter duration where the individual grieves the loss of body function and past way of life. Depression is generally longer and future oriented, where cognitions involve fear of an often uncertain and perceived grim future. Suicidal ideation is sometimes present during this stage, as well as asking "Why me?" of God or a higher power (Kübler-Ross, 1981). The theory of mourning and depression has encountered some debate among researchers as to whether all individuals actually go through a diagnosable clinical depression and whether going through a depression is mandatory to move on to acceptance (Trieschmann, 1988). Wortman and Silver (1989) reviewed the existing empirical evidence regarding bereavement following a physical disability and found that not all individuals report experiencing depression. Recently, Maciejewski et al.'s (2007) grief study with 233 individuals who had suffered the death of a loved one from natural causes found participants mourned the loss of a loved one more so than they reported becoming depressed. The temporal sequence reported by grieving loved ones included disbelief that peaked at 1 month, yearning at 4 months, anger at 5 months, and a depression plateau at about 6 months post-loss. Acceptance of the loss was observed to gradually occur as time went on over a 24-month observation period. Livneh (1991) and Livneh and Antonak (1997) cite common reactive depression observations during this stage as including feelings of hopelessness, despair, anxiety, intense sadness, withdrawal, and despondency .

Alternatively, Worden's (2009) task of mourning concept identifies four tasks that mourners can actively work through to adapt to their loss. The first task involves accepting the reality that the loved one has died and will not return. Some mourners see their loved one in a crowd, deny he or she is dead, keep the person's possessions ready for him or her to return, and so on. The second task Worden identifies is the process of experiencing the emotional and behavioral pain. Some mourners repress painful emotions and do not allow themselves to feel the pain. Burying or avoiding such emotions can eventually lead to clinical depression. The third task involves adjusting to a world without the loved one. External adjustments include taking on the activities (e.g., paying bills, shopping, house chores) the loved one performed, while internal adjustments involve being an independent person from your loved one concerning self-esteem, self-identity, and the like. Spiritual adjustments during this task involve making sense of the world and testing one's faith and beliefs as to why this happened. The final task is that of maintaining an enduring, healthy connection with the deceased loved one while moving on with a new life. Worden indicates that these tasks are not fixed stages and can be experienced and worked on simultaneously because grieving is a fluid and not a static process.

Smart (2009) differentiated between how the individual mourns and/or possibly becomes depressed following a disabling injury and the societal expectation of the "requirement to mourn" as hypothesized by Wright (1983). It is expected that persons with a disability should feel bad and constantly grieve their loss indefinitely because it is the presumed normal response to one's misfortune. This societal belief that an individual must mourn and continually grieve their loss is a common misconception, but a projected value judgment by others nonetheless regarding how they think they would feel if they became disabled. Despite studies showing that most persons with a traumatic-onset disability gradually adjust to their situation over time, the societal requirement to mourn continues to be perpetuated (Livneh & Antonak, 1991; Marini et al., 1995; Silver, 1982; Wright, 1983).

Internalized anger essentially involves self-blame, guilt, and shame. The individual blames himself or herself and often views the disability as a punishment from God for some alleged wrongdoing (Hohmann, 1975; Marini & Graf, 2011). This self-blame can be amplified if the individual was indeed the cause of their injuries (e.g., drunk driving), which can make adjustment much more difficult (Livneh & Antonak, 1997). Suicidal ideation, risk-taking, and self-injurious behavior can occur at this stage as well. Janoff-Bulman (1979) differentiated between behavioral and characterological self-blame attributions and their perceived impact on adjustment. Behavioral self-blame refers to individuals who believe their behavior caused their injury; in such cases, individuals can adjust more readily knowing that they were, and are, in control of events. Conversely, characterological self-blame refers to individuals who attribute blame to a flaw in their character or personality and hence believe their fate was unavoidable and deserving. Overall, research is mixed regarding self-blame attributions of disability, with some finding a positive relationship between coping and self-blame attributions (Janoff-Bulman, 1979) and others a negative relationship where individuals with a spinal cord injury were perceived as coping less well (L. Bordieri et al., 1989; Westbrook & Nordholm, 1986). J. E. Bordieri and Kilbury (1991) surveyed 84 rehabilitation counseling graduates using observer simulation regarding self-blame attributions. They found that characterological self-blamers were rated as coping less well, being more depressed, and having perceived less control of future life events than individuals who attributed blame to behavior.

RETALIATION

In Livneh's (1991) conceptualization of the five-stage model of adjustment, retaliation is the fourth stand-alone stage with no substages. In their 1997 description of this concept, Livneh and Antonak refer to retaliation as externalized hostility. This stage essentially involves "rebelling against a perceived dependency fate . . . anger is now projected onto the external world in the form of hostility toward other people, objects, or environmental conditions" (Livneh, 1991, p. 124). During this stage, individuals may blame and lash out at perceived incompetent medical professionals for not doing enough and/or significant others for no apparent reason because of frustration and anger. Behaviorally, individuals may become noncompliant with hospital rules, use profanity, make accusations, attempt to manipulate hospital staff and significant others, or physically strike others (Livneh & Antonak, 1997). Smart (2009) notes how some individuals may initially be angry with God about being unfairly punished. Marini and Graf (2011) surveyed 157 persons with spinal cord injury regarding their spiritual or religious beliefs and practices and found that whereas some respondents were initially angry with God postinjury, this tended to subside over time in the majority of, but not all, cases. Similar findings have been empirically supported when surveying persons with chronic pain conditions and those with multiple sclerosis (Chen et al., 2011; Graf et al., 2007).

FINAL ADJUSTMENT OR REINTEGRATION

This final stage delineates a cognitive, affective, and behavioral component. Livneh and Antonak (1997) note how acknowledgment is a cognitive reconciliation or acceptance of the disability and its permanency. A new disability self-concept is formed, and individuals seek to master their environment by problem-solving. Persons who reach this stage are able to "accept him or herself as a person with a disability gain a new sense of self-concept, reappraise life values, and seek new meanings and goals" (p. 22). Emotionally, individuals are "okay" with their disability and can talk about it without becoming upset. Behaviorally, persons in this stage begin to actively pursue social, academic, and/or vocational goals and learn to successfully navigate physical and social environmental barriers. Livneh and

Antonak (1991) found correlational support for acceptance among 214 rehabilitation patients during the temporal later phase of disability onset. Similarly, Marini et al. (1995) surveyed 63 persons with spinal cord injury during their first, second, or fifth year postinjury, finding that self-esteem increased over time as respondents became more comfortable and confident with their disability status.

Despite all the caveats to the stage model of adjustment, a number of criticisms have been cited (Kendall & Buys, 1998; Olkin, 1999; Parker et al., 2003). Some concerns relate to the dangers of counselors expecting and anticipating persons with a sudden onset of physical disabilities to go through specific stages (Kendall & Buys, 1998). Others cite the complexity of human behavior and the attempt to fit everyone through these stages when there are so many complex individual differences regarding people's coping mechanisms, environmental factors, and extenuating circumstances (Parker et al., 2003). Relatedly, some researchers argue that there exists little empirical support for the stage model of adjustment (Chan et al., 2009; Olkin, 1999).

Although many injured persons have been found to progress from initially experiencing higher to lower levels of distress over time, others do not show any signs of intense distress, and some remain in a heightened level of distress for longer periods (Wortman & Silver, 1989). As discussed later with the recurrent model, some researchers argue that persons with physical disabilities do grieve the loss of bodily function and preinjury lifestyle and that the permanency of the loss leads to recurrent and unpredictable periods of chronic sorrow (Burke et al., 1992; B. H. Davis, 1987; Kendall & Buys, 1998; Teel, 1991).

Somatopsychology

As briefly introduced in Chapter 4, field theory, postulated by Kurt Lewin (1935, 1936), centers around the belief that our self-concept or self-worth can be, and is, affected by the feedback we perceive from interacting with others in our environment, referred to as our "life space." Although Lewin's original theory did not include the impact a disability has on this reciprocal interaction, researchers since then have refined the hypothesis to include the impact of disability (Barker et al., 1953; Dembo et al., 1956; Trieschmann, 1988; Wright, 1960, 1983). The revised theory has been encompassed as follows: *Behavior* (B) is a function (*f*) of *Psychosocial* variables such as self-esteem and coping skills (P), *Organic* factors related to the disability such as paralysis or blindness (O), and *Environmental* or physical access and attitudinal factors (E), comprising the formula $B = f(P \times O \times E)$ summarized by Trieschmann (1988). Lewin's somatopsychology theory was the first to take a more social psychological view of human behavior as opposed to focusing exclusively on individual behavior in isolation. In essence, this formula showcases that a person's behavior is a function of the interaction between the internal and external factors mentioned earlier (Chan et al., 2020). More specifically, the field of somatopsychology, as argued by Wright (1983), can be described as what psychosocial factors impact people with CID and how these factors limit or help the adjustment to CID, personal functioning, and life activity involvement.

Specific to this theory, then, arises the central question: "How do persons with disabilities perceive themselves in Western society's mirror?" A synopsis of historical attitudes in general would suggest many persons with disabilities have been stigmatized, discriminated against, persecuted, devalued, dehumanized, and essentially treated as minorities (Chubon, 1994; Mackelprang & Salsgiver, 2009; Olkin, 1999; Smart, 2009). Arguably, for individuals who possess a more *internal locus of control*, many of these negative experiences would potentially not have as demoralizing an emotional effect as for persons who have a more *external locus of control* (Elfstrom & Kreuter, 2006; Frank & Elliott, 1989). Past research indicates that the link between locus of control and emotional well-being is mediated by coping strategies (Elfstrom & Kreuter, 2006; Frank & Elliott, 1989). These authors found that persons with spinal cord injuries who perceived that they were more in control of their life circumstances (internal locus) possessed greater levels of acceptance and emotional well-being than the group who believed their destiny was not in their hands (external locus). As Maltby et al. (2007) note regarding clinical depression and various illnesses and disabilities, persons who are internally located tend to attribute their self-worth to their own efforts and internal evaluation, whereas persons who are externally located are more likely to evaluate their self-worth based on how others respond to them and believe their circumstances are controlled more by environmental influences and not themselves. Wright (1983) would otherwise view those externally located individuals who regularly experience discriminating and demoralizing attitudes of others as more susceptible to "succumbing" to the societal limitations imposed by society, thereby adjusting less well. According to Wright (1980, 1983 as cited by Livneh et al., 2014), the behaviors of people with CID that are influenced by the environment are more readily discernable in a variety of settings. For example, a person who is hard of hearing may be able to communicate well in a quiet room; however, the same would not apply in a loud environment.

Some of the empirical support for this theory centers around assessing the attitudes of persons with disabilities in relation to their lived experience in the community. Li and Moore (1998) surveyed 1,266 adults with disabilities in relation to their experiences in the community. Aside from emotional support from friends and family playing a significant role in adjustment, perceived societal discrimination had a negative impact on accepting one's disability. DiTomasso and Spinner (1997) additionally found their respondents with disabilities reported greater levels of loneliness when confronted by the negative attitudes of others. Similarly, Hopps et al.'s (2001) sample of 39 adults with physical disabilities showed a high correlation between feelings of loneliness, social anxiety, and poorer social skills that they attributed to poor physical access in their community. Finally, in the qualitative survey by Graf et al. (2009) of 78 persons with spinal cord dysfunction who were asked to compose in 100 words or less what experience(s) best exemplified their living with a disability, most frequently reported anger and frustration from encountering physical access barriers in the community. Clearly, repeated negative experiences with others in society can, over time, impact how well someone adjusts to their disability.

Disability Centrality Model

The most recent adaptation model to CID has shown to have great promise theoretically, empirically, and with tangible clinical implications (Bishop, 2005). Drawing upon Devins's illness intrusiveness approach (Devins et al., 1983; Devins, 1994), Livneh's (2001) conceptual framework, and the value change concepts of Dembo et al. (1956) and Wright (1960, 1983), Bishop proposes the disability centrality model (DCM). He (2005) describes six tenets as the theoretical underpinnings for DCM that factor in subjective and objective QOL satisfaction and control over one's medical and environmental circumstances. These are summarized as follows: (a) The impact of a CID can be measured by a multidimensional subjective QOL measure; (b) QOL is an individual's overall perceived subjective satisfaction of life domains that are disproportional because of individual differences regarding which domains are more important (central) to us; (c) the onset of a CID results in an initial reduction in overall QOL and centrally important satisfying activities, as well as feelings of personal control; (d) the degree of QOL reduced is dependent on how many central domains are affected; (e) individuals seek to maintain and maximize overall QOL by minimizing gaps (distress) caused by the CID; and (f) people strive to close these gaps by either changing their values and interests commensurate with their disabled abilities, employ strategies to increase perceived control over their health and environment, or alternatively do nothing to improve control or change their values (p. 223; Bishop & Feist-Price, 2002; Devins et al., 1983).

Bishop (2005) incorporates the concept of domain satisfaction and importance described by Devins et al. (1983) and others (Frisch, 1999; Pavot & Diener, 1993) regarding the relative significance various QOL domains may have for each individual. For example, a construction worker with a grade 9 education who sustains a tetraplegia and has derived great satisfaction from work and playing sports preinjury likely experiences a poorer adjustment if he or she can no longer engage in either domain. In contrast, a professor with the same injury is likely able to retain employment and try to compensate (develop new interests) for being unable to play sports. In both instances, the former individual would likely experience a greater reduction in satisfaction and perceived control than the professor, and hence a greater reduction in overall QOL (Frisch, 1999). Although Bishop (2005) concedes there is never a universal agreement on what all the QOL life domains should include, there has been an increased agreement over the years on certain domains, including physical and mental health, social support, employment, or a satisfying or avocational activity and economic or material well-being (Bishop & Allen, 2003; Jalowiec, 1990). Cummins (2002) differentiated between objective and subjective QOL domains. Objective indicators include more tangible domains such as employment, wage earnings, marital status, and so forth, whereas a more subjective assessment of one's QOL includes what Roessler (1990) describes as an individual's private assessment or feeling about their life situation. As Cummins (2005) has noted, however, there is a weak relationship between objective and subjective measures of QOL. In other words, people can have what others may think is a great job, income, marriage, and so forth, and yet those who seem to have it all score poorly on life satisfaction, subjective well-being, and happiness (Dijkers, 1997; Myers & Diener, 1995). Bishop discusses more contemporary QOL studies later in this book.

In addition, incorporating Devins's illness intrusiveness model (Devins et al., 1983; Devins & Shnek, 2000) proposes that when individuals sustain a CID, the impact compromises psychological well-being by temporarily or permanently reducing positive or meaningful activities, as well as reducing real or perceived control to regain the positive activities or outcomes and avoid negative ones. The central question then becomes whether individuals can compensate for lost interests that once brought them enjoyment, but they can no longer engage in. With Bishop's DCM, the counselor must be able to assess what the "central" or most important life satisfaction domains are for clients and how these can be compensated for or replaced (Groot & Van Den Brink, 2000; Misajon, 2002). This concept is similar to Wright's (1960, 1983) "value change" theory, whereby individuals who perceive a loss in one area of their lives attempt to develop new interests within their capabilities (i.e., transitioning from enjoying jogging to reading for persons with a mobility impairment). This has also been termed "preference drift" (Groot & Van Den Brink, 2000) and "response shift" by Schwartz and Sprangers (2000).

Empirical support for DCM is building. Bishop (2005) assessed 72 college students with disabilities using the *Delighted–Terrible Scale* (Andrews & Withey, 1976), the *Ladder of Adjustment* scale (Crewe & Krause, 1990), and what Bishop (2005) describes as the *Domain Scale*, which assessed 10 domains like the QOL. Overall, the results indicated a positive correlation between QOL and psychosocial adaptation to CID. A second correlation was found between satisfaction and perceived control in relation to the impact of CID and QOL. Additional research has been conducted to assess the application of the DCM to persons with traumatic brain injury (TBI; Mackenzie et al., 2015). The research involved surveying 125 eligible participants by using the *Disability Centrality Scale (DCS)* to understand their needs. Results indicated that the measures of higher life satisfaction and greater perceived control over one's situation mediated the effects of TBI on QOL. Bishop also describes counseling interventions that empower clients to assert more control over their circumstances, developing new interests or response shift, and working through the loss of satisfying activities no longer accessible.

Bishop et al. (2007) conducted a follow-up DCM study with 98 persons with multiple sclerosis. In this study, Bishop et al. (2007) discuss subjective quality of life (SQOL) or subjective well-being relating to the previously described QOL domains (Johnson et al., 2004) and psychosocial adaptation. The assessments used were the *Delighted–Terrible Scale, Ladder of Adjustment,* and the *DCS* (Bishop

& Allen, 2003), the latter of which measures 10 life domains, including physical health, mental health (emotional well-being, happiness, enjoyment), work/studies, leisure activities, financial situation, relationship with significant other, family relations, other social relations, autonomy/independence, and religious or spiritual expression (p. 7). Results indicated a positive correlation between scores on the self-management scale and both perceived control and QOL. The second positive correlation was found between scores on the Ladder of Adjustment scale and overall QOL satisfaction across domains. Bishop et al. (2007) again cite similar tangible counselor intervention strategies that involve assisting clients in developing new interests and asserting more control over their situation. Livneh and Antonak (1997) view the DCM as an ecological model; however, it is treated separately here because of its emphasis on perceived control and satisfaction of life domains.

Ecological Models

Chan et al. (2009) make the observation that even within the ecological models of adjustment to disability, there is overlap representing the stage or phase theory of adjustment, including early reactions of shock, anxiety, and denial; intermediate reactions of depression, internalized anger, and externalized anger; and later reactions involving acknowledgment, acceptance, and adjustment (p. 58). As we conclude later, all of these proposed theories have overlapping and similar concepts.

Two theorists who summarize the complexity of ecological models best are arguably Trieschmann (1988) and Vash and Crewe (2004). These models involve a foundation of three major determining factors that consider the (a) nature of the disability, (b) characteristics of the person, and (c) environmental influences. Within each of these determining factors are subsets that require exploration by the counselor to assess what, if any, bearing each of these factors has on psychosocial adjustment. It is important to note that none of these factors may negatively influence poor adjustment; conversely, any one of these factors, in and of themselves, if deemed important by the individual, may delay or prolong adjustment. A brief summary of each is provided.

NATURE OF THE DISABILITY

This factor explores aspects of the disability itself and the implications of each. The first subfactor considers the *time of onset* regarding whether an individual was born with a disability or acquires it sometime later in life. Vash and Crewe (2004) discuss some potential implications for someone who is born with a disability, including being treated as an infinite child, isolated and overprotected, unable to engage in many childhood activities, and as (Olkin, 1999) describes, sometimes subjected to a "conspiracy of silence" where parents do not discuss their child's prognosis or treatment with him or her at the risk of upsetting their child. Conversely, as we explore in detail regarding the psychosocial aspects of an acquired disability, one can succumb to a whole host of other adjustment issues (Kendall & Buys, 1998; Livneh, 1991). The next subfactor, *type of onset,* concerns whether the disability had a sudden impact (spinal cord injury from a car accident) versus a prolonged onset (more gradual such as multiple sclerosis) and the implications of each. In the case of a sudden onset, perceived attribution of blame becomes a factor that influences adjustment. Specifically, research is mixed regarding the implications of self-induced versus other-induced attribution of blame on adjustment. Although findings indicate those who accept the responsibility of their injury may possess a more internal locus of control and therefore may adjust better, they may also be more self-critical and angrier at the fact that they could have possibly prevented their accident (Athelstan & Crewe, 1979; Bulman & Wortman, 1977; Reidy & Caplan, 1994). *Functions impaired* address the relative importance each of us places on our functional abilities. For example, some individuals are most terrified to lose their sight, while others fear becoming paralyzed or losing their hearing the most. Related to this factor is the significance these abilities play in our lives. An academic whose livelihood and intrinsic interests revolve around reading may be devastated by vision loss. Wright (1983), however, reminds us of the "insider" perspective, whereby those persons who have lived and adapted to their disability emphatically disagree that it is the worst thing (bodily function) they could lose. Unfortunately, many lay public mostly perceive any disability as a tragedy and one that they are not certain they could live with (Olkin, 1999). *Severity of the disability* essentially considers how severe the disability is, with the once-assumed belief that those with more severe disabilities were likely more maladjusted (Livneh & Antonak, 1991). Although some literature finds that this may indeed be the case, it is more commonly believed now that the severity of a disability has little or no impact on how someone adjusts (Livneh & Antonak, 1997; Wallander & Varni, 1998). *Visibility of the disability* considers the reactions individuals with visible disabilities sometimes experience (wheelchair users) such as discrimination, devaluation, and being ignored (Graf et al., 2009; Marini et al., 2009). Conversely, consider the plight of those with invisible disabilities unknown to the public (low back injuries) who may be thought of as lazy or unmotivated if unable to participate in certain activities, such as not wanting to find a job owing to ongoing chronic pain. *Stability of the disability* addresses whether the disability is stable and generally will not become worse (spinal cord injury) versus those that have an uncertain prognosis but become progressively worse over time (Parkinson disease; Cheng et al., 2010; Elfstrom & Kreuter, 2006; Folkman & Lazarus, 1980; Frank & Elliott, 1989). The uncertainty of waking up each morning not knowing whether one is still able to walk or see not only leaves an individual with no control over their situation but also compromises making any future plans. Finally, the concept of *pain* deserves a category unto itself in addressing psychosocial adjustment. As Vash and Crewe (2004) emphasized, unlike many of the other disabilities, chronic pain is a primary or secondary debilitating condition that can have a significant negative impact on an individual's thoughts, emotions, and behaviors. Cognitively, individuals can exhibit poor concentration and attention, suicidal ideation, and reduced problem-solving abilities. Emotions often include depression, feelings of hopelessness and helplessness, and despair (Banks & Kerns, 1996; Fishbain et al., 1997). Behaviors have been defined as social isolation; withdrawal from activities; and, in worst-case scenarios, addiction to pain prescription medications, substances, and drug abuse (Lewinsohn et al., 1990; Waters et al., 2004).

PERSONAL CHARACTERISTICS

These determining factors involve individualized traits or characteristics. *Gender* largely considers gender differences in coping with disability, as well as societal expectations of males and females (Hwang, 1997; Livneh, 1991; Marini, 2007; Tepper, 1997). There are mixed findings regarding which gender adjusts to a disability better; however, Western societal expectations of each gender are quite clear (Charmaz, 1995; Hwang, 1997). Males are supposed to be rugged, independent, breadwinners, stoic, athletic, dominant, and tough (Charmaz, 1995; Marini, 2007; Zilbergeld, 1992), whereas women are expected to be beautiful in physical appearance, passive, homemakers, and good nurturers (Hwang, 1997). Males and females with severe disabilities may not be able to live up to some or any of these expectations and may have difficulty adjusting if they rely on external cues (societal expectations) for affirmation of their self-concept/self-esteem (Charmez, 1995; Marini, 2007; Nosek & Hughes, 2007). *Activities affected* relates to the significance individuals place on their activities. A hockey player who becomes paralyzed and is no longer able to play sports may experience greater difficulty adjusting than a professor who has the same injury but can still perform academic activities. Similarly, *interests/ values/goals* pertain to the differing passions people have in their lives. Those who proverbially "put all their eggs in one basket" or have few, if any, interests and lose the ability to engage in them likely find adjustment more stressful than those persons who have multiple interests and are still able to return to some of them (Massimini & Delle Fave, 2000; Schafer, 1996). Lewinsohn et al. (1990) indicate that when people experience a loss and withdraw from engaging in what were once pleasurable activities, there is a greater likelihood of lengthening or exacerbating a reactive depression. *Remaining resources* are described by Vash and Crewe (2004) as the abilities and traits an individual retains regardless of their disability. These include intelligence, motivation, sense of humor, extroversion, social poise, resilience, emotional stability, and coping strategies, all of which have been implicated in positive adjustment (see Livneh, 1991). Finally, *spiritual and philosophical base* refer to one's spiritual or religious beliefs, particularly as to whether some people believe their disability is a punishment from God or a higher power, with the assumption that those who believe they are being punished have a more difficult time adjusting (Byrd, 1990; Gallagher, 1995; Graf et al., 2007). Conversely, individuals who believe their disability to be a divine intervention or calling for them to serve a higher purpose for God experience lesser adjustment difficulties (Eareckson, 2001, Graf et al., 2007).

ENVIRONMENTAL INFLUENCES

As extensively detailed earlier, environmental influences may have a significant impact on adaptation to disability (DiTomasso & Spinner, 1997; Graf et al., 2009; Hopps et al., 2001; Lewin, 1936; Li & Moore, 1998; Wright, 1983). In this determining factor, Vash and Crewe (2004) as well as Trieschmann (1988) describe several contributing factors. *Family acceptance and support* becomes significant in that if a disabled loved one is viewed as a contributing family member and not devalued, this generally correlates with a more positive adjustment to the disability (Li & Moore, 1998). In addition, those families that have been shown to possess positive coping strategies and support one another typically adapt well to the disability (Trask et al., 2003). *Income* plays an important role not so much as in overall happiness, but rather in overall QOL (Diener & Seligman, 2004; Inglehart, 1990; Lykken, 1999). Once people have their basic needs met, there is relatively little difference in happiness ratings between those who are extremely wealthy and those of more modest means (Diener & Seligman, 2004); however, a higher income and adequate healthcare positively impact one's ability to remain healthy, as well as purchase necessary accommodations and equipment/devices (modified van, accessible home) for a better QOL. *Available community resources* refer to support from local agencies, which could include Centers for Independent Living (CILs), Veterans Affairs services, Client Assistance Programs (CAPs), access to modernized hospitals, and so forth. Individuals with severe disabilities who live in rural settings with no resources may not only have to travel long distances for appointments but also be required to be away from home and family at times if having to remain in the city for several days (A. J. Smith et al., 2009). *Social support* is also critical for positive adjustment and fostering self-esteem in most, but not all, instances (Buunk & Verhoeven, 1991; Li & Moore, 1998). Schwarzer and Leppin (1992) define functional support by differentiating between instrumental support (offering financial aid), informational support (giving information and advice), and emotional support (caring, empathy, and reassurance). Functional support is further delineated by individuals' perceptions of the support they received (retrospective evaluation) and the perception of available support if needed (anticipation of getting the support; Lakey & Cassady, 1990; Symister & Friend, 2003). Much like Yuker's (1988) extensive review of the impact of contact regarding positive and negative attitudes toward disability, empirical findings are somewhat mixed regarding the benefits of social support (Barrera, 1981; S. Cohen, 2004; Heller & Rook, 2001; Hupcey, 1998; Lazarus & Folkman, 1984a; Li & Moore, 1998). On the positive side, social support is believed to be a buffer against stress, an appropriate coping strategy, and a regulator of negative emotions (S. Cohen et al., 2000). For example, persons who sustain a severe disability may have friends who give or loan them money, help them in finding community resources, and provide emotional support by empathizing and genuinely listening to their concerns. Conversely, having a social support system made up of people who are themselves dysfunctional; who have promised to help but always have excuses; or in the worst-case scenario, take advantage of the person with the disability by neglecting, abusing, or stealing from him or her are all clear examples of a potentially poorer adjustment process for the disabled individual. Finally, *institutionalization* becomes a concern for those persons with severe disabilities who are unable to physically take care of themselves, do not have the funding to hire an attendant, or have no family or friends who can perform a caregiving function. In such cases, individuals are faced with temporarily or permanently having to reside in a nursing home. Aside from most Americans not wanting to live in a nursing home, the U.S. General Accounting Office (2002) published a study indicating an approximate 25% abuse rate, which either resulted in death or serious injury of nursing home residents nationwide. The forms of abuse include neglect, physical abuse, sexual abuse, and malnourishment. Clearly, individuals who have no choice but to live in a nursing home may, in the worst-case scenario, be subjected to such abuse or minimally deprived of the freedom to control their environment and thus experience a resulting reduction in QOL (Bishop, 2005). In a best-case scenario of well-run nursing homes, persons with severe disabilities may be medically well cared for as well as having a resident support network that residents would not otherwise have if they lived alone.

Recurrent or Integrated Model of Adjustment

The recurrent or integrated model of adjustment following an acquired disability was essentially hypothesized as owing to perceived shortcomings of the stage or linear model of disability (B. H. Davis, 1987; Wikler et al., 1981; Wortman & Silver, 1989). One of the several criticisms of the stage model was its theoretical emphasis likening the stages of grief over a deceased loved one (Kübler-Ross, 1981) to that of acquiring a disability. The main argument is that persons with acquired disabilities continue to live with their disability every day; therefore, although the emotional upheaval subsides over time, those with acquired disabilities continue to periodically experience chronic sorrow throughout their lives. In this sense, there is never a final adjustment or adaptation stage where the disability no longer affects the individual (B. H. Davis, 1987; Kendall & Buys, 1998; Wortman & Silver, 1989).

Pertinent to this model are several key concepts. Beck's (1967) cognitive theory defines *cognitive schema* as our ingrained beliefs and assumptions regarding ourselves, others, and how the environment works (Beck & Weishaar, 1989). When a sudden and traumatic disability occurs, many individuals attempt to cling to the comfortable, old schemas because of an overwhelming anxiety and uncertainty that the disability brings. Wright (1983) refers to this as "as if" behavior, whereby individuals attempt to minimize anxiety by denying or distorting reality and pretending as if nothing (the disability) has happened. As the old schema no longer adequately works and the individual begins to realize the implications of the disability, depression may set in (Kendall & Buys, 1998). Yoshida (1993) uses the analogy of a wildly swinging pendulum to describe the initial injury phase of anxiety, fear, and grief. Over time, however, the pendulum gradually slows to a middle set point where individuals either develop a new positive or negative schema of life with a disability (Yoshida, 1993). Positive new schema are formed when individuals with traumatic disabilities can (a) search and find meaning in the disability and in postdisability life; (b) learn to master or control their environment, the disability, and their future; and (c) protect and enhance the self by incorporating the new disability identity (Barnard, 1990; Kendall & Buys, 1998, p. 17). Conversely, negative schema can also be formed about the disability, allowing stereotypical societal expectations about disability (helpless, incapable) to influence one's self-worth (Charmaz, 1983; Stewart, 1996). Wright (1983) would describe those who develop negative schema as otherwise having succumbed to their disability.

Undoubtedly, individuals with acquired disabilities who develop a more negative schema postinjury likely are more susceptible to self-pity, low self-esteem, and more frequent episodes of chronic sorrow. Regardless, according to the theory of recurrent periods of sadness, even individuals who have developed positive schema and have otherwise been successful in their lives still experience sorrow or sadness from time to time (Kendall & Buys, 1998). As some research has shown, it is quite likely that these periods of sorrow may be facilitated by environmental influences such as a relationship rejection, job rejection, or discrimination perceived by the individual because of their disability (Graf et al., 2009; Li & Moore, 1998; Marini et al., 2009). Overall, response to the disability varies for everyone depending on one's coping mechanisms (Lazarus, 1993; Lazarus & Folkman, 1984b).

Transactional Model of Coping

The most frequently cited and empirically supported theory of coping with stressful events is that of Lazarus and Folkman's transactional theory (1984a, 1984b). The authors define coping as "constantly changing cognitive and behavioral alternatives to manage specific external and/or internal demands that are appraised as taxing or exceeding the resources of the person" (1984a, p. 141). These appraisal efforts are constantly changing as the individual interacts with their environment back and forth like watching a tennis match. Central to transactional theory are two major components of a sequential appraisal process salient to when people encounter a stress-inducing event. The first component, referred to as *primary appraisal,* is an individual's assessment as to whether a situation is stressful or not. Key to this appraisal is the motivational strength attributed to various personal goals (goal relevance) the stressor may pose, otherwise called goal congruence or incongruence. Individuals assess whether the stressful event is deemed beneficial or harmful/threatening to the goal, specifically in the case of disability. Will the goal of maintaining optimal health be compromised by the stressful event? If not, no coping mechanisms are required and the individual returns to a state of emotional equilibrium. If, however, the situation is deemed harmful or threatening, the individual moves into the *secondary appraisal* component. At this level, individuals assess their options for coping and expectations about what will happen (Lazarus, 1993). The three subcomponents involved are (a) blame or who the event is attributable to; (b) coping potential as to whether the individual has any control to change the circumstances of the event and whether he or she can influence the person–environment relationship; and (c) future expectations regarding perceptions as to how the situation plays out. At both levels of appraisal, Lazarus and Folkman (1984a) discuss problem- versus emotion-focused coping strategies defined earlier. The authors suggest that emotion-focused coping is more likely when individuals perceive they have no control over the situation and that the stressful event (e.g., disability) is indeed harmful or threatening to achieving or blocking one's goals. Positive-focused coping has previously been shown to be more effective in the long run as far as adaptive coping strategies, particularly in situations where individuals can insert some control over their situation to minimize or eliminate the stressor (Carver et al., 1989; Cheng et al., 2010; Folkman & Lazarus, 1991; Folkman & Moskowitz, 2004; Groomes & Leahy, 2002; Nilsson, 2002; Provencher, 2007).

In the case of distress due to disability, the transactional theory is ideal in its attempt to explain the coping process as it focuses on the persons appraisal (Pande & Tewari, 2011). Individuals can participate in active reappraisals when coping with a physical disability. In a study conducted by Agarwal et al. (1995), researchers discovered that patients with high positive life orientation were more confident about their recovery from a myocardial infarction. This may suggest that persons with high positive life orientation also exhibit adaptive coping strategies. In effect, and as stated earlier, positive reframing gives the individual the opportunity to exert some control over their situation.

Overall, the transactional model of coping has excellent application in understanding how persons with CID react to and cope with a catastrophic injury resulting in significant functional loss and reduction in critical QOL domains (Bishop, 2005). In many such injuries, most individuals indeed do not have control over the situation, have initially little or no control over their health status, and, in the case of permanently disabling injuries such as a spinal cord injury or traumatic brain injury, are unable to perceive a positive future. Similarly, in cases where parents learn that their child is born with cerebral palsy, muscular dystrophy, or some other disabling condition, they too are likely to experience very similar emotions, cognitions, and behaviors as those with the disability (e.g., shock, anxiety, denial, anger, acceptance; Livneh & Antonak, 2005). Haspel et al. (2020), in another study using the transactional model to examine parents' perceptions of their children's adjustment following an acquired disability, surveyed parents of 140 children with an acquired disability. Specifically, these parents were asked about caregiver burden, adjustment, and their perception of their children's adjustment over time. Researchers discovered that changes in parents' adjustment was related to improvements in their perception of the child's adjustment to disability, thus supporting the transactional connection between caregivers and child functioning.

Chaos Theory of Adjustment

Chaos and complexity theory (CCT) of adjustment is essentially the human application response of a phenomenon originally hypothesized from the disciplines of mathematics, meteorology, engineering, physics, biology, geography, astronomy, and chemistry (Livneh & Parker, 2005, p. 19). Its origination appears to lie with mathematician and meteorologist Edward Lorenz back in the 1960s, when he famously coined the term *butterfly effect*, essentially explaining how a butterfly flapping its wings in Brazil could ultimately end up causing a tornado in Texas a month later (Gleick, 1987). This theory, in addition to Rene Thom's (1975) multidimensional and nonlinear catastrophe theory, forms the basis for its eventual application to human behavior.

An intriguing major concept about CCT is that, despite its complexity and initial perceptions of random, unorganized sets of behavior, there is indeed an ordered and deterministic set of rules (Chamberlain, 1998). Several concepts must first be understood and are briefly defined here. *Nonlinearity* is often referred to as "sensitive dependence on initial conditions" (Butz, 1997). Nonlinear behavior is described as a nonrepetitive, unpredictable, aperiodic, and unstable phase that experiences critical junctions of instability called *bifurcation points* (Capra, 1996). These bifurcation points might otherwise be analogous to watching ice crack on a lake. Specifically, there is no order to when the ice will cease in one direction and fork off to another. Bifurcation of behavior after an acute injury is representative of the anxiety, fear and shock, and individual experiences during a crisis, but with each critical bifurcation point (fork), it allows for growth, stability, and new behavior to result (Chamberlain, 1998). *Fixed-point attractors* are stable and predictable set points that Livneh and Parker (2005, p. 20) describe as synonymous with watching water approaching a drain. *Limited cycle or periodic attractors* are predictable open and closed loops, with donut-shaped trajectories where the system approaches two separate points periodically but is unable to escape the cycle (p. 20). *Strange attractors* are indicative of the unpredictable and unstable chaotic trajectories that demonstrate the sensitive dependence on initial conditions and bifurcate over time (Capra, 1996). The fixed point attractors, limited cycle attractors, and strange attractors all constitute the first-, second-, and third-order changes, respectively.

Dynamic systems are neither random nor determined systems interconnected with one another that depend on the system itself (the individual), the environment, and the interaction between the two (similar to somatopsychology). Complex systems are open systems in that they exchange and lose energy, information, and material through interacting with their environment (Cambel, 1993). In order to survive, the system must reduce internal disorder or entropy (decay), while drawing energy from the environment. The level of entropy (minimal versus extreme) represents the degree of chaos occurring within the system or individual in human application. There are, however, closed systems where the entropy cannot be dissipated and new energy cannot enter from the environment. In closed systems that are isolated from renewable environmental energy, maximum entropy continues (Kossmann & Bullrich, 1997). This may otherwise be a representation of what Livneh (1991) describes as "getting stuck" in a certain stage of psychosocial adjustment. *Self-organization* is defined by Livneh and Parker (2005) as open systems with nonlinear trajectories that experience dramatic changes following a stressor (injury), spontaneously develop new structures and behaviors (schema), and experience internal feedback loops that ultimately self-organize, stabilize, and develop new ways of adaptation (p. 21; Capra, 1996). *Self-similarity* involves similar patterns within chaotic systems such as the fact that no two snowflakes are alike; however, they all have six sides. Self-similar patterns are called "fractals," which are determined patterns essentially fixed inside of the chaos (Mandelbrot, 1977).

In aligning the hard science of chaos theory with human behavior, Livneh and Parker (2005) indicate that under everyday conditions, most persons without disabilities essentially function under a state of cognitive and behavioral equilibrium. When a crisis occurs, however, we generally react in a more complex and unpredictable manner. Chaos is described as an indication of this overwhelming anxiety, capable of facilitating emotions such as depression and anger (Butz, 1997). As a result of these distressing emotions, adaptation involves a series of bifurcation points that are unpredictable and may be observed with varying degrees of maladjustment in different people (Francis, 1995). There are, however, some "self-similar" observations (e.g., shock, anxiety, denial, anger) that can be observed in most individuals. As time goes on, the individual generally reorganizes their cognitions, emotions, and behaviors to restore preinjury equilibrium. Interactions with the environment (others) can have a positive or negative effect on the individual's adjustment that may either slow, stall, or facilitate adaptation. Chaos theory, as suggested by Bussolari & Goodell (2009), is "a current response to models of reductionism and determinism in the 20th century scientific community" (p. 99). Though it is a nonlinear process, it offers a more comprehensive and consistent perspective of how individuals experience a change process.

Chaos theory offers counselors a counseling model in which they are able to normalize unpredictability and stress responses (self-blame, internalized shame) in the face of significant life adjustment (Bussolari & Goodell, 2009). Livneh and Parker (2005) suggest that counselors can assist persons with acquired CID to shift their focus and energy from past and present thinking to the future, with goal-directed and community-oriented participation. Clients can be encouraged to look past their health and survival mentality and begin thinking about social, vocational, and environmental mastery activities. Finally, knowing that many individuals instinctively retrench (withdraw, succumb) following a traumatic injury, counselors can encourage clients to recognize their spontaneity and creativeness and begin taking risks again (p. 24).

Additional Adjustment Concepts

VALUE CHANGE SYSTEM

Although indirectly addressed previously, there are several additional concepts and/or theories regarding acceptance of loss and disability worthy of noting. The first stems from Dembo et al. (1956) and later Wright's (1960) theory of value system changes that are necessary regarding acceptance of loss. In her later conceptualization, Wright (1983) cites four value changes that may or may not occur in any particular order for the individual. The first is *enlargement of the scope of values*. This pertains to individuals needing to refocus or let go of preinjury activities or values they are no longer able to perform and instead expanding activities and interests to match their new abilities (e.g., an athlete who enjoyed playing sports becomes paralyzed and expands their values consistent with the limitations from the disability to enjoy reading). The second value change is *subordination of physique*, essentially cognitively reframing the significance of what is beautiful about oneself. Persons who place great importance on their physical appearance and ability must be able to redefine the remaining attributes (e.g., intelligence, personality) as becoming most important. The third value change, *containment of disability effects,* pertains to persons with disabilities not allowing the disability to "spread" to other parts of their being and assertively correcting those without disabilities who assume this to be so. For example, someone with a physical disability may be presumed as also being mentally retarded. Numerous personal reports exist regarding a waitress asking a nondisabled companion what their wheelchair-using partner would like to eat, based on the assumption that the individual is incapable of ordering for himself or herself. The fourth value change needing to occur for successful adjustment is *transformation from comparative to asset values*, involving cognitive reframing as well. Asset values are more intrinsic and personal regarding what the individual finds to be valuable and needs to change in their life to sustain asset values. Comparative values, however, are evaluations we make on comparing what we have with what is supposedly normal and in relation to what others have. Therefore, refocusing on one's own assets without comparing to what other nondisabled persons perceive as normal or standard needs to occur. Dembo et al. (1956) hypothesized in their coping with disability framework that, for persons with disabilities to successfully adapt and not ultimately succumb to the disability, they must be able to focus on the things they can do, take control of shaping their life, recognize personal accomplishments, manage negative life experiences, minimize physical and social barriers, and participate in activities that are pleasurable.

GOOD-FORTUNE COMPARISON

This concept refers to some sense of relief persons with CID experience when they meet and/or perceive other persons with severe disabilities are much worse off than they. This is referred to as the "downward comparison," whereby one's perceived good fortune is from the belief that he or she could have sustained a more severe disability (Shotton et al., 2007). In a Shotton et al. (2007) study of psychosocial adjustment, appraisal, and coping strategies of nine persons with TBIs, one of the significant findings was the comfort participants expressed in knowing their injuries could have been much worse. Psychologically, this realization assisted these individuals to enjoy what abilities they had remaining as opposed to what they had lost.

Conceptualized Synthesis of the Seven Theories of Adjustment to an Acquired Disability

Having explored both the old and contemporary theories and concepts of psychosocial adjustment (adaptation, response, or reaction) to disability, what then are the major overlapping areas that appear to be consistently supported empirically? In other words, what cognitions, behaviors, and emotions do most persons who acquire a CID go through immediately following, then long after sustaining, a disability? We attempt to synthesize the areas of agreement various authors have conceptualized in essentially explaining the same process. The references for these conclusions are found within this chapter and therefore not all are repeated here.

First, following a traumatic acquired injury with permanent long-term functional implications, all humans experience some type of reaction. They may or may not experience Livneh's (1991) five stages of adjustment in the exact sequential order initially proposed; however, the caveats Livneh noted with the stage theory make these cognitions, behaviors, and emotions more probable since he indicated some people skip stages, regress back to a previous stage, overlap stages, and can become stuck in a stage. In analyzing this initial period following injury, most people are overwhelmed with shock and anxiety, synonymous with Parker et al.'s (2003) chaos theory in describing bifurcation points. This also overlaps with Yoshida's (1993) analogy of a wildly swinging pendulum initially following a trauma to explain the response to overwhelming anxiety and shock as part of the recurrent model (Kendall & Buys, 1998). This type of response lasts differing lengths of time for different people, based on personality traits and strengths of coping strategies, family stability and support, and type of interactions with the environment or community.

Second, as Lazarus and Folkman (1984a) have hypothesized, in appraising whether a severe injury is harmful or a threat to the individual's well-being, unquestionably it is harmful and does threaten the individual's well-being. The disabling injury is largely not under an individual's direct control, and, as Cheng et al. (2010) found, we tend to levitate toward using emotion-focused coping because this is a situation, we are unable to problem-solve our way out of by self-repairing our bodily injuries. We therefore must rely on our physicians, and sometimes pray or bargain with God in the meantime, for a full recovery with or without medical intervention. Interestingly, Levin's (2001) analysis of more than 200 epidemiological studies regarding religion/spirituality and its impact on mental and physical health found positive relationships between religious participation and beliefs in relation to dealing with CID more positively.

Third, some or most individuals experience a clinical reactive depression of a mild, moderate, or severe nature from the loss of perceived and/or real preinjury functioning and QOL. Unquestionably, the majority of people grieve the loss of bodily function and previous way of life; however, whether these same people fall under the clinical diagnosis for depression varies from person to person. Again, synonymous with Parker et al.'s (2003) bifurcation points (Which way do the cracks in the ice go?), it depends on the personality traits and strengths in coping, family stability and support, and types of interactions with the environment regarding how one adjusts. The person–environment interaction is essentially the theoretical framework for somatopsychology as well as the "dynamic systems" concept of Parker et al.' explanation of chaos theory. The ecological model is a more complex model, but essentially is similar to somatopsychology, noting the interplay between aspects of the disability involving the person, personal characteristics and resources to cope, and the interplay with environmental forces (Trieschmann, 1988; Vash & Crewe, 2004). Basically, then, whatever occurs after what is considered a normal grief response (generally 3 to 6 months) may be classified as noteworthy to address in counseling (Livneh & Antonak, 1991; Silver, 1982). Suicidal ideation and suicide completion are statistically higher for persons with disabilities, so although not everyone becomes depressed, some disability groups are more likely to think about suicide as an option compared to the general public (e.g., spinal cord injury versus deafness).

Fourth, the occurrence of anger, be it internal or external, is a factor. Do most people with an acquired disability at some point after their injury become angry? Olkin (1999) discusses the contradictory societal perception of persons with disabilities are expected to be happy and grateful for the charitable crumbs thrown their way; however, conversely, they are also required to indefinitely mourn their loss as well. She further asserts that society does not tolerate, accept, or understand anger from people with disabilities, but that whatever negative emotion is displayed, it is somehow always thought to be related or salient to the disability. Clinical observation and empirical studies suggest anger is a response, whether a short-term transitional occurrence or long-term periodic state (Graf et al., 2009; Livneh & Antonak, 1991; Marini et al., 2009). Livneh (1991) initially described self-blame and anger at God or a higher entity for causing the injury or not being able to prevent it. When the higher entity or medical profession is unable to cure impairments from the disability, the anger is redirected outwardly toward medical staff, family, and God or a higher power (Graf et al., 2007; Graf & Marini, 2011). What few researchers have addressed, however, is not so much anger, but the combination of sheer boredom and frustration persons with acquired disabilities feel during their first weeks and months of recovery, and later when they encounter environmental barriers and negative societal attitudes (Graf et al., 2009; Marini et al., 2009). Initially, the boredom and frustration persons with an acute injury experience waiting for the few minutes every day to see the doctor can be aggravating for many. Once out in the community, people with disabilities periodically become angry and frustrated in their interactions with others in the community regarding wheelchair parking violators, inaccessible washrooms, rude or condescending medical staff, long waiting times to see a doctor, and so forth (Graf et al., 2009; Marini et al., 2009).

Fifth, and perhaps the most controversial, is whether persons with acquired or congenital disability eventually experience some type of final adjustment, adaptation, or transcendence to their disability (Livneh, 1991; Vash & Crewe, 2004). In defense of stage theory, Livneh (1991) noted the caveat that some individuals can regress back to an earlier stage. This is otherwise understood to mean that periodic setbacks can occur. Indeed, this is essentially very similar to the concept of periodic "chronic sorrow" that Kendall and Buys (1998) maintain in the recurrent model of adjustment. It is also synonymous with Parker et al.'s (2003) chaos theory concept of "self-organization," where individuals encounter a bad event and adapt or change what is necessary and within their control to adjust to the situation. The larger question becomes: What causes these periodic instances of chronic sorrow? Only two answers are plausible: (a) The individual experiences additional or recurrent health problems (e.g., loss of sight with diabetes, severe pressure sore requiring surgery for spinal cord injury) or (b) someone or something in the person's "life space" interacting with the environment upsets the individual. In the first instance, this potential health setback and subsequent sadness is an otherwise normal reaction. If these setbacks do not occur, it has already been demonstrated in various empirical studies that persons with disabilities revert to preinjury levels of emotions after roughly 2 months (Brickman & Campbell, 1971; Silver, 1982). The second instance concerns a negative experience with others or from encountering an environmental barrier; these causes are both socially constructed. A prejudicial or discriminatory attitude reminds the person with a disability that he or she not only has a disability but that he or she is even devalued by some people because of it (Li & Moore, 1998). Such interactions may well hurt the individual and can cause temporary sadness and/or anger as well. Similarly, when individuals with disabilities encounter an inaccessible restaurant or public place, it reminds them of their disability and the environmental barriers imposed on them that deny their civil rights (Graf et al., 2009; Marini et al., 2009). Regardless, many persons without disabilities in society automatically assume that when someone with a disability appears upset, it is somehow salient to the disability, and this may indirectly be so (e.g., requirement of mourning; Wright, 1983).

Finally, how do persons with disabilities reach any type of successful adjustment, adaptation, response, or reaction to their disability? For stage theory proponents, it is by successfully transitioning through the various stages over time and coming to terms with the disability. As with the grieving process, time heals. For somatopsychology proponents, it is that critical person–environment interaction where the individual possesses the personal characteristics and coping skills to succeed and learns to control and master their environment. Disability centrality proponents also postulate mastering one's environment and substituting new and interesting activities that are central for sustaining satisfaction and QOL in place of those pleasurable activities no longer accessible because of the limitations imposed by the disability. Ecological models are more complex, but again similar to somatopsychology in that psychosocial adjustment depends on the interplay of an individual's personal characteristics and coping abilities, aspects of the disability itself, and environmental influences including family and community support.

CONCLUSION

Overall, all models arguably converge into one at some point, or certainly overlap enough to provide counselors with some good insights as to what persons with disabilities may experience. For those with congenital disabilities, there does not appear to be a transitional stage of adjustment. It is more likely that this population experiences periodic sorrow if they allow themselves to sometimes wish that they could do all the activities someone without a disability supposedly can do. Such cognitions, however, from the literature appear to be rare (Connors & Stalker, 2007). In addition, it appears that emotional upsets may otherwise have an external cause such as being ridiculed or reminded of one's minority status. Again, this would hopefully be a rare occurrence, and the literature suggests that persons with congenital disabilities are otherwise generally happy and satisfied with their QOL. For those with acquired disabilities, there is for a time an emotional instability in grieving the loss of bodily function and preinjury lifestyle. This does appear to stabilize in most cases over time, and it does so when individuals can cognitively reframe (adapt new cognitive schema) their situation and what is important in life. This is accomplished by letting go of, and not dwelling on, what one used to be able to do, but instead focusing on new interests, values, and goals commensurate with remaining disability assets. The perception of being in control and mastering one's environment is central to reestablishing self-esteem. And, as discussed in the "disability paradox" theory (Freedman, 1978) and later in this text on positive psychology, persons who have not only survived their disability but become very successful in spite of it otherwise perceive themselves as stronger than most nondisabled persons. It therefore seems appropriate to end this chapter with Nietzsche's (1889) classic quote, "what does not kill me, makes me stronger," otherwise experienced as posttraumatic growth.

CLASS ACTIVITIES

1. In groups of four, use the following statement in your discussion: Some persons with disabilities thrive in their position, whereas others are rendered stuck and succumb to their medical condition and negative societal attitudes.

   a. Compare and contrast what you believe are the major factors as to why some individuals thrive and do well following a traumatic acquired disability, while others succumb to their condition and circumstances?

   b. Compare the various theories of adaptation to disability and discuss within the group which one or two theories you are inclined to agree with the most and why.

   c. Discuss with students how each of them believes they would adapt or adjust, as well as under what circumstances they would need regarding resources, support, and so on, in order to thrive with a disability.

KEY REFERENCES

Only key references appear in the print edition. The full references appear in the digital product on Springer Publishing Connect™: https://connect.springerpub.com/content/book/978-0-8261-5111-7/part/partII/chapter/ch08

Bishop, M. (2005). Quality of life and psychosocial adaptation to chronic illness and acquired disability: A conceptual and theoretical synthesis. *Journal of Rehabilitation, 71*(2), 5–13.

Chan, F., Da Silva Cardoso, E., & Chronister, J. A. (2009). *Understanding psychosocial adjustment to chronic illness and disability.* Springer Publishing Company.

Chubon, R. A. (1994). *Social and psychological foundations of rehabilitation.* Charles C Thomas.

Devins, G. M. (1994). Illness intrusiveness and the psychosocial impact of lifestyle disruptions in chronic life-threatening disease. *Advances in Renal Replacement Therapy, 1,* 251–263. https://doi.org/10.1016/S1073-4449(12)80007-0

DiTomasso, E., & Spinner, B. (1997). Social and emotional loneliness: A re-examination of Weiss' typology of loneliness. *Personality and Individual Differences, 22,* 417–427. https://doi.org/10.1016/S0191-8869(96)00204-8

Frank, R. G., & Elliott, T. R. (1989). Spinal cord injury and health locus of control beliefs. *Paraplegia, 27,* 250–256. https://doi.org/10.1038/sc.1989.38

Haspel, S. P., Benyamini, Y., & Ginzburg, K. (2020). Transactional model of parental adjustment and caregiving burden following a children's acquired disability. *Journal of Pediatric Psychology, 45*(10), 1177–1187. https://doi.org/10.1093/jpepsy/jsaa075

Hopps, S., Pepin, M., Arseneau, I., Frechette, M., & Begin, G. (2001). Disability related variables associated with loneliness among people with disabilities. *Journal of Rehabilitation, 67*(3), 42–48.

Kendall, E., & Buys, N. (1998). An integrated model of psychosocial adjustment following acquired disability. *Journal of Rehabilitation, 64,* 16–20.

Li, L., & Moore, D. (1998). Acceptance of disability and its correlates. *Journal of Social Psychology, 138*(1), 13–25. https://doi.org/10.1080/00224549809600349

Livneh, H. (2001). Psychosocial adaptation to chronic illness and disability: A conceptual framework. *Rehabilitation Counseling Bulletin, 44*(3), 151–160. https://doi.org/10.1177/003435520104400305

Livneh, H., Bishop, M., & Anctil, T. M. (2014). Modern models of psychosocial adaptation to chronic illness and disability as viewed through the prism of Lewin's field theory: A comparative review. *Rehabilitation Research, Policy, and Education, 28*(3), 126–142. https://doi.org/10.1891/2168-6653.28.3.126

Nosek, M. A., & Hughes, R. B. (2007). Psychosocial issues of women with physical disabilities. In A. E. Dell Orto & P. W. Power (Eds.), *The psychological and social impact of illness and disability* (5th ed., pp. 156–175). Springer Publishing Company.

Olkin, R. (1999). *What psychotherapists should know about disability.* Guilford Press.

Parker, R. M., Schaller, J., & Hansmann, S. (2003). Castastrophe, chaos, and complexity models and psychosocial adjustment to disability. *Rehabilitation Counseling Bulletin, 46*(4), 234–241. https://doi.org/10.1177/003435520304600404

Silver, R. L. (1982). *Coping with an undesirable life event: A study of early reactions to physical disability* (Unpublished doctoral dissertation), Northwestern University, Evanston, IL.

Vash, C. L., & Crewe, N. M. (2003). *Psychology of disability* (2nd ed., pp. 288–299). Springer Publishing Company.

Wright, B. A. (1983). *Physical disability: A psychosocial approach* (2nd ed.). Harper & Row.

CHAPTER 9

VULNERABILITIES, ABUSE, AND PSYCHOSOCIAL DISPARITIES OF WOMEN WITH DISABILITIES

DEBRA A. HARLEY AND CAROL E. JORDAN

LEARNING OBJECTIVES

After reading this chapter, you will be able to:

- Identify ways in which women with disabilities are vulnerable for IPV
- Describe the influence of intersectionality in the lives of women with disabilities
- Identify psychosocial disparites of women with disabilities
- Identify the importance of cultural competence to work with women victim-survivors of IPV
- Describe approaches for working with women with disabilities experiencing IPV

PRE-READING QUESTIONS

1. Why is it important to understand women with disabilities from an intersectional perspective?
2. What are the reasons why women with disabilities do not leave their abuser in IPV relationships?
3. In what ways are women with disabilities at risk for IPV?
4. What is the role of cultural competence in working with women with disabilities from different backgrounds?

Women are the direct victim-survivors of violence resulting in trauma and disability and often acquire disabilities because of battering and other forms of abuse. Vulnerabilities, abuse, and psychosocial disparities of women with disabilities warrant special attention because women with disabilities are abused at rates greater than women without disabilities and men with disabilities (United

States Department of Health and Human Services [HHS], 2020), are likely to experience a longer duration of abuse than women without physical disabilities (Breiding & Armour, 2015), experience disability-specific forms of abuse and vulnerabilities (Ledingham et al., 2022), and experience more profound negative health and mental health effects (Jordan, 2016). There are unequal power dynamics between women with disabilities and their perpetrator and/or care provider. Statistics suggest that women with disabilities have a 40% greater chance of intimate partner violence (IPV) than women without disabilities (American Psychological Association, n.d.). For the purpose of this chapter, IPV means various forms of abuse inflicted by one partner in an intimate relationship against the other partner (World Health Organization [WHO], 2021). The various forms include physical abuse, sexual abuse, psychological maltreatment, financial and other environmental controls, and stalking (Ricci, 2017). Additionally, for this chapter, victim-survivor means women who have been targeted by abuse. Using both the terms *victim* and *survivor* is more inclusive of the primary terms women often use to describe themselves. Mental health interventions for IPV should include risk assessment and safety planning, addressing legal issues, and strategic referral and service linkage tailored to meet the needs of the victim-survivor.

Women with disabilities are one of the largest and most marginalized populations in the United States (Nosek & Hughes, 2003). Women with physical, mental, and intellectual disabilities represent a population with high vulnerability for abuse and IPV, which often result in psychosocial disparities (Centers for Disease Control and Prevention [CDC], 2021a). Women with disabilities are two to three times more likely to experience IPV than nondisabled persons of the same gender identity, and 80% of women with disabilities are sexually assaulted at least once in their lifetime nationally (HSS, 2020). Furthermore, women of color (Black, Indigenous, People of Color [BIPOC]) with disabilities face unique issues related to the intersection of disability, diversity, and IPV (Jones & Thorpe, 2016; Lightfoot & Williams, 2009). Women with disabilities may also have increased vulnerability for abuse because of the combined cultural devaluation of women and persons with disabilities (Devkota et al., 2019). IPV is not a singular occurrence and does not exist as an isolated entity, and no two instances are identical (Vellidis, 2018). According to Redfern (2017), IPV is universal, and the difference is in how groups define abuse. In the United States IPV is recognized as a public health problem.

Vulnerability is associated with multiple factors, including the presence of a disability; need for personal assistance; social isolation; difficulty being believed about abuse; the woman's belief that abuse is the price to be paid for survival; the inability to escape due to lack of adaptive equipment or accessible buildings; learned understanding that abuse is normal; the perpetrator's belief that the woman is powerless to defend herself and, therefore, easy prey; and untreated depression of women with disabilities (Hague et al., 2011; Nosek et al., 2001a). The need for personal assistance and the difficulty in locating and retaining persons to provide that assistance make women with disabilities more tolerant of abusive behaviors (Nosek, 2002a, 2002b). The greater the number and extent of intersectional inequities (i.e., disability, gender, identity) a victim-survivor experiences, the more ability a perpetrator can control and coerce her, and the less likely she is to have access to help and safety (Tarrant et al., 2019). Too often the abuse experienced by women with disabilities may not be perceived as abuse because of the repeated exposure to mistreatment. In addition, nonphysical forms of IPV that typically occur earlier in a relationship may be less commonly identified as abusive by the victim/survivor (Minto et al., 2022). For example, a woman may not recognize that it is not supposed to hurt to have her hair combed. According to Powers and Oschwald (2005), women with disabilities who have been abused report greater difficulty in naming the abuse. The perpetrator may use subtle forms of abuse, such as name calling, to more overt forms such as physical abuse. See Exhibit 9.1 for examples of abusive tactics.

EXHIBIT 9.1. Examples of abusive tactics against women with disabilities

- Abandoning in a dangerous situation
- Removing or destroying mobility devices (e.g., wheelchair, scooter, walker)
- Disconnecting or hiding the telephone
- Denying access to prescribed medication
- Forcing someone to take medication against their will
- Forcing someone to lie in soiled clothing or bedding
- Preventing access to food
- Touching inappropriately while assisting with bathing or dressing
- Denying access to disability-related community resources
- Denying access to healthcare appointments
- Slapping, punching, biting, hitting, pushing, kicking, or dragging
- Physically attacking sexual parts of her body
- Denying access to money
- Calling her names or belittling
- Isolation, limiting her outside involvement
- Blaming the victim for the abuse
- Preventing or keeping her from getting a job

Women with disabilities who experience IPV face additional barriers of accessibility to IPV programs; failure of service providers to recognize abusive situations; limited training for police in the special needs of women with disabilities; and a host of other co-contributing factors, such as societal prejudices about disability and fear of otherness, lack of knowledge about disabilities, and isolation and segregation from the community, which may contribute to risk for abuse (Hughes et al., 2012). Women with disabilities are at a high risk of experiencing IPV because of social stereotypes that often serve to reduce their agency through infantilization, dehumanization, and isolation, making them vulnerable to various forms of violence, including institutional violence (Ortoleva & Lewis, 2012). Moreover, for women with disabilities, *ableism* (the belief that the abled body is preferred over the disabled body) creates misconceptions about IPV and places women with disabilities at greater risk for sexual assault (Nosek et al., 1997; Odette & Rajan, 2013).

In the United States, IPV is the leading cause of injury to women, more than auto accidents, muggings, and rapes combined; the costs of IPV alone exceed $5.8 billion per year, with $4.1 billion for direct medical and healthcare services; and every day more than three women are murdered by their significant other. About one in three women have been physically assaulted by an intimate partner in their lifetime and one in five experienced severe violence. The distinction for women with disabilities is that they are more likely to report more intense experiences of abuse, including the combination of multiple incidents, multiple perpetrators, and longer duration (Breiding & Armour, 2015). Similar rates of abuse are reported for lesbian, gay, bisexual, transgender, queer/questioning (LGBTQ) populations, with approximately one-third of women and men being victim-survivors of IPV (Brown & Herman, 2015). Among LGBTQ populations, bisexual women experience the highest level of psychological abuse, followed by lesbian women (Walters et al., 2013). Overall, over half of transgender individuals experience some form of IPV (James et al., 2016). It is important to recognize that cultural, institutional, and systemic factors make it more likely for LGBTQ persons to have a physical disability because of violence against them and a mental disability because of discrimination, closeted identity, and social isolation. For LGBTQ women with disabilities impacted by IPV, violence is not less dangerous or less serious because the partners are the same gender or gender identity (Safe Voices, 2021).

The purpose of this chapter is to identify issues of abuse and violence specific to women with disabilities and the influence of intersectionality in their lives. A general approach is presented on the topic with specific reference to various types of disabilities and group membership. Information is presented on (a) an overview of intersectionality, (b) barriers to seeking help, (c) women with disabilities and consequences of abuse and violence, including mental health outcomes, and (d) disparities in psychosocial outcomes. This chapter concludes with implications for working with women with disabilities to reduce disparities in their psychosocial adjustment and outcomes and discussion of the importance of cultural competence It is beyond the scope of this chapter to cover all types of disabilities; therefore, the focus is on disabilities in general, with some discussion of physical and mental disabilities. A glossary of terms is provided in Exhibit 9.2.

EXHIBIT 9.2. Glossary of terms

Control—means by which the perpetrator maintains dominance over the victim

Exploitation—taking advantage of a person to an extent that they are disempowered or unable to advocate for themselves

Intimidation—raising a hand or voice or using other looks, actions, or gestures to create fear

Isolation—denying the victim access to support systems

Privilege—making all the important decisions; providing care in a way to create dependence or vulnerability

Vulnerability—exposed to the possibility of being physically or emotionally attached or harmed

---

INTERSECTIONALITY

People are multifaceted in their social identities The term intersectionality was coined by Kimberlee Crenshaw (1989) and formed the framework for understanding oppression and the cumulative way in which the multiple forms of discrimination based on race, gender, identity, disability, sexual orientation, class, and other identities combine and overlap in the experiences of marginalized individuals or groups. Intersectionality moves away from defining people by a singular identity. Intersectionality explains that while women with disabilities share common oppressions, experiences of those oppressions are different as contextualized by other positionalities or identities. For example, a White lesbian with a disability may be privileged because of race and marginalized because of disability, gender, and sexual orientation. Another example of intersectionality is the case of Lynda (see Case Study 9.1). Lynda's case shows that as a BIPOC woman, her marginalization was further compounded by race, type of disability, poverty, parenthood, and systemic barriers.

CASE STUDY 9.1. THE CASE OF LYNDA

Lynda is a 32-year-old African American cisgender female. She has diagnoses of bipolar disorder and anxiety. She is married with three children. Her husband, William, was physically, emotionally, and sexually abusive. However, Lynda remained with him because she was financially dependent upon him while working on her college degree. When she decided to leave, she and her children faced financial hardship. She had to drop out of school, and her children went to live with her parents while Lynda was able to find housing in a shelter. Lynda was one of three BIPOC women in the shelter. Several White women residents in the shelter used racial slurs and insults toward BIPOC women. Although Lynda and the other two women registered complaints with the shelter director, nothing changed. Eventually, Lynda and the other two women were dismissed from the shelter when they engaged in a physical altercation with the White women. Lynda found herself experiencing even more hardship in her efforts to escape domestic violence and was further marginalized in what was supposed to be a safe space.

Discussion Questions

1. What cultural adjustments need to be made in the shelter?
2. How was Lynda further marginalized at the shelter?
3. What approach should be considered to address Lynda's intersectional oppressions?

Disability and gender (and other identities) are "interlocking categories of experiences that affect all aspects of human existence as they simultaneously structure people's lives" (Traustadottir, 2006, p. 81). Violence affects those with preexisting disadvantaged circumstances other than being a woman (Sullivan, 2018); however, being a woman decreases the chance of survival in an intimate partner relationship (Postmus et al., 2012). The presence of a disability increases the violence occurring and reduces the economic circumstances of the victim-survivor (Thiara et al., 2012). Individually and intersectionally, women with disabilities are adversely affected by structural inequalities. While inequalities are not new, understanding their sources, intersectionalities, and how they affect women with disabilities who are victim-survivors of IPV is important to recognizing the immediate and long-term consequences of victimization.

It is important that counselors and human service providers utilize an intersectional approach in service delivery to understand how women with disabilities are exposed to overlapping forms of discrimination and marginalization and how those intersections can lead to increased risk, severity, and frequency of experiencing multiple forms of violence (The Equity Institute, 2017). Utilizing an intersectional approach helps to reduce stereotypes and implicit bias when working with women with disabilities who are victim-survivors of IPV.

BARRIERS TO SEEKING HELP

Help-seeking involves both formal and informal sources. Help may be in the form of medical treatment, legal assistance, or psychological or mental health counseling. After experiencing IPV, various barriers to seeking help affect women in general. The first barrier to seeking help is the inability to admit that violence or abuse is taking place. Once a woman admits that she is a victim-survivor of IPV, she must then decide to act. That is, she must say something (tell someone) or do something (leave the abuser).

One of the greatest reasons women do not leave a domestic violence situation is fear, followed by a lack of resources, and fantasy that things will get better. The fear is well-founded, because the point at which a woman decides to leave an abusive relationship is when she is at an increased risk (i.e., of being killed). Fugate et al. (2005) identified barriers to include hassle, fear, concern for confidentiality, tangible loss, individual thresholds for the seriousness of the violence, a perceived requirement to end the relationship, and certain specific barriers. For minoritized identities, for example, LGBTQ and racial/ethnic groups, additional barriers include that reporting the traumatic experience will reflect negatively on their community, especially if the perpetrator also identifies with their community (Duke & Davidson, 2009); support systems ignoring or not knowing victim-survivors' needs because the institutions were not made with and for them; and a lack of explicitly inclusive systems (Ollen et al., 2017). For these victim-survivors of IPV who must navigate the effects of cumulative trauma, including discrimination, a noninclusive service system presents revictimization.

Women with disabilities face numerous barriers in decreasing their risk for abuse. Some of these barriers are related to seeking help and others to accessing IPV programs. In addition, women face various forms of cultural and IPV, as seen in the language, attitudes, and practices of people and in social constructs (Murthy et al., 2010). Other barriers to seeking help for abuse and violence include health problems, lack of mobility and/or transportation, schedule conflicts, fear of retribution, denial that the problem is real, alcohol and/or other drug abuse (both on the part of the perpetrator and their use as an emotional escape from the pain of abuse), and experiences with depression (Center on Research on Women with Disabilities [CROWD], 2002), being unaware of where to go, feeling embarrassed, feeling guilty about being a burden or feeling it was their fault, feeling that they could handle it themselves, beliefs about religious interpretation of scripture, and fear of not being believed (Milberger et al., 2003). In addition, women with disabilities realize that separation from the perpetrator does not mean cessation of abuse because the perpetrator continues to engage in various forms of emotional abuse (Jaffe, 2002).

Another area in which women with disabilities experience barriers to obtaining help is that of accessibility to IPV services (Milberger et al., 2003; Robinson et al., 2021). Many IPV shelters and services are not accessible for women with disabilities (Freer, 2022). In a survey of 2,703 IPV programs nationally (with a return rate of 22%) that deliver abuse-related services Nosek et al. (1997) found, on average, programs provided two services specific to women with disabilities, and 89% of programs provided fewer than five special services for these women. The most provided service available to women with disabilities was accessible shelter or referral to an accessible safe house/hotel room (83%). Other results from the study included that abuse programs provided individual counseling (80%), group counseling (73%), an interpreter for hearing-impaired women (47%), workshops/training on recognizing potentially violent situations (40%), safety plan information modified for use by women with disabilities (36%), and disability awareness training for program staff (35%). The service least likely to be offered was personal care attendant services (6%). Only 164 shelters indicated that they offer a woman with a disability their wheelchair-accessible emergency shelter, 23 said they would tell her they would call back when space becomes available, and 122 said they would suggest that she stay with a relative or friend. Other studies consistently identify the same types of barriers to accessibility in IPV services (e.g., Freer, 2022; Healey et al., 2013; Robinson et. al., 2021).

Additional architectural, attitudinal, and policy barriers to programs for women experiencing IPV include inability to meet needs for personal assistance with activities of daily living (ADL), inability of staff to communicate with deaf/hard-of-hearing women or those with speech impairments, lack of accessible transportation to the facility, insensitivity to LGBTQ inclusion, and incapacity to execute the tasks required to implement an escape plan (Nosek et al., 2001b). Effective service in shelters is highly dependent on having appropriately trained, qualified personnel who can address the multivariate needs of women with disabilities. Only 16% of programs in the Nosek et al. (1997) survey had a staff member who was specifically assigned to provide services to women with disabilities. These staff members, by training, included social workers (34%); peer counselors (22%); rehabilitation counselors (15%); psychologists (13%); and nurses, mental health specialists, legal and paralegal specialists, sign language interpreters, addiction specialists, or community volunteers (less than 5% each; Nosek et al., 1997).

Rems-Smario (2007) asserted that within the Deaf community there is a "double code of silence" related to IPV because services typically are not culturally sensitive or accessible to deaf survivors and because the Deaf community had misunderstood or minimized the problem. Research findings suggest "only a very small proportion of women with disabilities who are being abused, particularly those with physical or sensory disabilities, receive services from battered women's programs" (Nosek et al., 2004, p. 336). The disability group of women most likely to receive services from an IPV program was mental illness and the least likely were those with visual or hearing impairments (CROWD, 2002).

Healthcare and human services providers' negative attitudes is another barrier to women disclosing about abuse (Heron & Eisma, 2021). Heron and Eisma found women feared they would be judged or negatively evaluated. A lack of a positive relationship with their service providers was seen as a barrier. Lack of a positive relationship was considered to include not trusting the service provider, lack of continuity in the relationship, limited time with the service provider, and not expecting the service provider to be empathetic. If women perceived their service provider as having low capacity to help, this also prevented them from disclosing (Heron & Eisma, 2021). Furthermore, women did not disclose to healthcare providers about IPV because these women did not see healthcare services as an appropriate place to discuss abuse, as they perceived it was not a health issue to discuss with healthcare providers (Othman et al., 2014).

Too often women with disabilities must deal with a *credibility gap,* which refers to them being seen as unreliable narrators of their own experiences in the eyes of law enforcement, the judicial system, service providers, and support networks (Heron & Eisma, 2021). Broader cultural stereotypes about women include a lack of trust in women's self-report about what they are experiencing, resulting in a tendency to dismiss or psychologize complaints (GIVE, 2022). According to Martin et al. (2021), women with disabilities face different sociocultural (erroneous assumptions, negative attitudes, being ignored, being judged, violence, abuse, insult, impoliteness, and low health literacy), financial (poverty, unemployment, high transportation costs), and structural (lack of insurance coverage, inaccessible equipment and transportation facilities, lack of knowledge, lack of information, lack of transparency, and communicative problems) factors which impact their healthcare.

LGBTQ women with and without disabilities encounter the same help-seeking barriers as non-LGBTQ women, in addition to issues of homo/bi/transphobia and stigma in social service agencies and shelters, the inability of the authorities to understand that same-sex-couple IPV exists, the assumption that IPV is mutual in LGBTQ relationships, and insensitivity to and/or lack of awareness of the specific needs and issues of LGBTQ populations (Gluck, 2022; Parry & O'Neal, 2015). Individuals may not report IPV for fear that others will find out about their sexual orientation or gender identity, their abusive relationship, or both (Gluck, 2022). IPV occurs in LGBTQ populations at similar rates to the heterosexual population (Lorenzetti et al., 2015) and is more likely among lesbians than gay men (Leonard & Pitts, 2012). In addition, transgender women experience unique barriers to service not experienced by other sexual minorities. For example, trans women may not be considered female by service providers.

Research on the disparity in IPV in rural communities compared to urban areas is mixed. On one hand, studies reveal IPV in rural areas is higher compared to urban and suburban communities (Mantler et. al., 2020). In rural communities, IPV is more prevalent, injuries from IPV are more severe, homicides are three times as likely to involve IPV, and geographic isolation increases barriers to achieving safety (e.g., first responders will take longer to respond, lower likelihood others will witness or become aware of the violence, lack of transportation options; Peek-Asa et al., 2011; Strand & Storey, 2019). For rural women with disabilities, IPV problems are exacerbated by decreased access to resources, high and enduring levels of poverty, and high unemployment rates. In rural areas, less than half of violent crimes and just over half of serious crimes are reported to law enforcement (Morgan & Kena, 2018). In rural communities, victims tend to be well-acquainted with healthcare providers and law enforcement officers and, for that reason, they may be reluctant to report abuse. Other reasons for reluctance include fearing that their complaints will not be taken seriously, violation of confidentiality, and that they may incur more abuse (Rural Health Information Hub [RHIH], 2021). On the other hand, DuBois (2022) found that women living in rural isolation are at a lower risk of IPV victimization relative to women living in urban areas and small towns, who are most at risk of experiencing physical violence by an intimate partner.

Immigrant, refugee, and asylum-seeking women with and without disabilities face the same stressors and trauma of IPV as women born in the United States but must contend with additional barriers, including language and communication, cultural and traditional gender roles, immigration status and expired visa that may lead to fear and further isolation, fear of being deported, lack of awareness of their rights, and not knowing where to get help (Erez & Harper, 2018; Park et al., 2021). "Perpetrators of violence are aware, and leverage, that women with intersecting marginalization are less likely to receive helpful responses from their community or those agencies that are charged with their protection" (Tarrant et al., 2019, p. 21). These women face challenges that are twofold: (a) unfamiliarity with the legal system, and (b) the potential conflict between cultural background and new surroundings can make their victimization from abuse feel they cannot leave an abusive relationship or disclose their abuse to law enforcement (Salami et al., 2019). Immigrant women who are separated, divorced, and on visitor or temporary visas show the highest risk for IPV (Park et al., 2021). It is the intersection of these experiences, along with social, environmental, and political barriers for immigrant women that affects the experience of having a disability, and having a disability also alters the experience of migration (Pisoni, 2021).

Discussion of women with disabilities and IPV would not be complete without mention of a connection between COVID-19 and victimization. The COVID-19 pandemic created additional barriers to getting help after experiencing IPV. Although IPV was prevalent before the pandemic, public health restrictions put in place in response to the pandemic revealed an increase in IPV rates, leaving vulnerable women at increased risk and women vulnerable to injury. For women with disabilities, "the potential for physical dependence, higher levels of poverty, social isolation and perceived vulnerability by perpetrators contributed to a greater risk of violence and victimization" (Breiding & Armour, 2015, p. 455). Furthermore, a decrease in communication with counselors, social workers, medical doctors, and other service providers and a decrease in outside witnesses provided an increased opportunity for victimization within the home (Geiger, 2020). In their study on the intersection of IPV and brain injury (BI), Haag et al. (2022) referred to the impact of COVID-19 on IPV as the "shadow pandemic." Women in IPV situations are especially vulnerable to BI because more than 90% of physical IPV altercations focus on hits to the head, face, and neck and/or strangulation, and up to 75% of abused women have BI (Haag et al., 2019). BI occurs when strangulation restricts blood vessels and air passages, which turns into restriction of oxygen, not allowing oxygen to reach the brain and other parts of the body. Even if the victim survives the strangulation, she may eventually die due to complications of the strangulation, including blood clots, arterial complications, or respiratory issues. According to Brown (2019), BIs can be short- or long-term brain damage resulting in physical (headaches, sleep disturbance), sensory (vision and hearing distortions, sensitivity to light and sound), cognitive (executive function and memory), and mental health (depression, anxiety, mood fluctuations) symptoms. When untreated, BI can worsen over time and have permanent consequences. Haag et al. (2022) found increased experiences of violence and risk for violence for women because of survivors and perpetrators being confined at home without work, recreational, and social supports. COVID-19 proved to be "a very powerful tool of coercive control" for perpetrators (Haag et al., 2022, p. 46).

WOMEN WITH DISABILITIES AND CONSEQUENCES OF DOMESTIC AND INTIMATE PARTNER VIOLENCE

Women with intellectual disabilities tend to experience higher rates of victimization and poly-victimization throughout their lives (Codina et al., 2022). However, many of the issues and challenges of these women are unique, and they are often not addressed as a population requiring unique approaches and solutions, nor from an intersectional perspective. It is difficult to ascertain an accurate prevalence rate of violence against women with disabilities because early studies tended to use highly heterogeneous samples and mostly focused on people with cognitive or developmental disabilities (Nosek et al., 2004). Nevertheless, compared to women without a disability, women with disabilities are significantly more likely to report experiencing IPV, including rape, sexual violence other than rape, physical violence, stalking, psychological aggression, and control of reproductive sexual health (Breiding & Armour, 2015). In addition, women with disabilities are more likely to be victims of violence related to alcohol or drug use than men with disabilities and are at increased risk for developing substance use disorders as a direct result of IPV (Smith, 2021).

In a study of women with physical disabilities, 56% reported being abused. Of that group 87% reported physical abuse, 66% sexual abuse, 35% were refused help with a physical need, and 19% were prevented from using an assistive device they required. For women who had been abused, 74% reported ongoing victimization, and 55% reported multiple episodes of abuse in their adult lives (Milberger et al., 2003). In a survey of people with disabilities, Mandel (2005) found that 60% reported being forced to engage in unwanted sexual activity, and almost half never reported the assault. According to Ledingham et al. (2022), women with multiple disabilities experience the greatest prevalence and highest risk for abuse, and women with cognitive disabilities or multiple disabilities were significantly more likely to experience physical force during their first intercourse than nondisabled women. According to Boxall et al. (2021), although women with more severe long-term chronic illness and disability (CID) reported higher rates of IPV than women without disabilities before the start of the COVID-19 pandemic, during the pandemic the rates escalated, especially in the form of physical or sexual violence or coercive control in previously nonabusive relationships, physical or sexual violence or emotional abuse, harassment, and controlling behavior in relationships with a prior history of violence. Rates were higher for indigenous women, but the difference was not statistically significant (Boxall et al., 2021).

Physical Health Problems

One consequence of physical or sexual abuse is a wide range of health problems. These health problems consist of three categories: acute, chronic, and stress-related problems. *Acute health problems* include bruises, cuts, broken bones, vaginal trauma, and head injuries. *Chronic health problems* go beyond immediate injuries and are persistent, for example, chronic bowel syndrome, cognitive difficulties, and dizziness. *Stress-related health problems* manifest as physical symptoms such as chest pain, fatigue, sleep disturbance, headaches, eating disorders, and substance abuse. Chronic problems and stress-related problems are not mutually exclusive. Exposure to IPV can also exacerbate existing health problems such as hypertension, diabetes, epilepsy, migraine headaches, and arthritis (Logan et al., 2006).

Women with disabilities encounter adverse physical health consequences resulting from IPV, including backaches; headaches; skin disorders; maxillofacial injuries; pelvic pain; traumatic brain injuries; being raped with objects; broken bones; sexual health problems; unplanned pregnancies; sexually transmitted diseases; undiagnosed hearing, vision, and concentration problems and genitourinary problems in conjunction with emotional abuse; and threats of retaliation (Brown, 2019; Coker, 2007; Logan et al., 2006). In general, women who experience IPV are more likely to have chronic health conditions than women not exposed (Pico-Alfonso et al., 2006) and to suffer from more long-term health problems caused by IPV than men who sustain the same injuries (Alejo, 2014). Women victim-survivors of IPV with disabilities have pain or severe pain that impacts their daily functioning, and those with higher pain ratings report more difficulty participating in life roles (Ballan et al., 2021). Ballan et al. asserted that these findings underscore the need for trauma-sensitive approaches to pain management for IPV survivors with disabilities.

Vulnerabilities and Mental Health

Stressful life events, including abuse and victimization, are significant contributors to mental health disorders. The feeling that one has little or no control over a situation increases a sense of hopelessness, which leads to depression, anxiety, and other emotional and behavioral responses. Depression is more common in persons with physical disabilities than in the general population (Cree et al., 2020) and the most common symptom exhibited by women victim-survivors of IPV (Nathanson et al., 2012). Noh et al. (2016) found females having any disability presented higher levels of depression than their male counterparts. Women with a severe mental health–related disability are also more likely to be a victim of IPV compared to women without any mental health–related disability. This elevated risk is seen among women with depressive disorders, anxiety disorders, stress-related disorders, substance abuse, eating disorders, other addictive behaviors, obsessive-compulsive disorders, suicidal ideations, and especially posttraumatic stress disorder (PTSD; Ferrari et al., 2016; Trevillion et al., 2012).

Many women have experienced multiple forms of abuse throughout their lives, putting them at greater risk for a range of health and mental health consequences. For example, women are more likely to experience child sexual abuse, adult rape, and IPV than men, and the combination of childhood and adult victimization stressors may have more implications for mental health concerns than the kind of stressors men are more likely to experience (Gavranidou & Rosner, 2003). Although physical abuse tends to decrease with age, rates of emotional abuse appear to be constant over the life span. Among older adults, IPV is strongly correlated with physical and mental health problems, and the physical health of older victim-survivors may be more severely affected than younger victim-survivors (Knight & Hester, 2016). Women with physical disabilities report higher levels of stress than the general population (Hughes et al., 2005).

Severe abuse is associated with restricted coping skills and increased risk for anxiety and PTSD (Griffing et al., 2006). Although physical and psychological abuse often occur together, for some women the emotional abuse undermines their self-esteem, security, and self-confidence and is identified as a major reason for *suicide*. Trauma leads to a loss of agency (the feeling of overseeing your own life and having a say in what happens to you), causing the person's inner compass to shut down and depleting them of the ability to create something better (Women's Advocates, 2020). Women with disabilities who are victim-survivors of IPV are faced with internal barriers and issues of self-worth (Lundell et. al., 2018) as well as societal attitudes. Self-esteem in women with physical disabilities is more strongly influenced by social and environmental factors than by the fact of having a disability

(Nosek et al., 2001b). Nosek et al. (2004) identified internalized societal expectations to manifest in such factors as low self-esteem and self-worth, an external locus of control for decision-making, and being less competent. According to Domestic Violence (2022), "victims not only deal with their own demons that they are battling in their heads but also ones that society has placed in front of them as well after they have decided to leave their abusers". Vignette 9.1 provides a reflection of a victim/survivor of IPV about how her self-worth was diminished in an abusive relationship. Counseling with this survivor requires the counselor to first establish rapport before proceeding with focus on the woman's self-worth or the abuse.

VIGNETTE 9.1. THE CASE OF DIMINISHED SELF-WORTH

IPV does not happen all at once. It is a slow process. Little things happen, then more of them happen. At first you do not recognize that it is abuse. As time goes by you find yourself explaining it away. Next, it happens more often and with more intensity. You tell your family about it, and they do not believe he can do such things. You begin to question yourself about what is happening and believe that you cannot be worth much because no one else sees what you see. You start to believe that it is your fault. You begin to believe that your disability is harder on him than you. You rationalize that you deserve it because you stayed. As it happens more and more, you do not say or do anything because it will do no good. So, you stay, and you take it. You have taken it this long; you can endure anything.

The following is an example of how a counselor should proceed:

Client: I don't know why I am wasting your time with my problem. I have been able to handle it so far.

Counselor: Your time is so valuable. I am glad you took the time to come see me.

Client: I know you must think I am crazy for wanting to talk about this after all these years of doing nothing.

Counselor: I want you to think about how strong you are for doing this and how important you are.

Pico-Alfonso et al. (2006) found women exposed to IPV had a higher incidence and severity of depression and anxiety symptoms, PTSD, and thoughts of suicide than women without exposure. The symptoms of PTSD in women survivors of IPV may not be immediately visible. Symptoms can present as excuses, for example, the woman may say "I am just tired" or "I am having problems at work." This type of response is commonly associated with long-term verbal abuse. Verbal Abuse Journals (n.d.) emphasized that PTSD from domestic abuse can interfere with one's peace of mind even after leaving an abusive relationship. That is, after being in a continuous cycle of abuse, the survivor may not notice any difference between the symptoms of PTSD and her day-to-day stress (Mayo Clinic, n.d.). The case of Mary illustrates a survivor of IPV who has been in the cycle of abuse for years and does not realize her symptoms of PTSD or view herself as being in an abusive relationship (see Case Study 9.2). It is important to understand that IPV experiences do not always result in a psychological diagnosis; however, one's ability to maintain their mental health can be changed by experiencing abuse. Other ways in which a victim-survivor's mental well-being can be affected include difficulties with being productive at work, with caregiving, with establishing and engaging in healthy relationships, and with adapting to change and coping with adversity.

CASE STUDY 9.2: THE CASE OF MARY

Mary is a 53-year-old White lesbian. She has been in a committed relationship for 20 years. Mary acquired a spinal cord injury at age 40 because of an automobile accident resulting in paraplegia. She has been employed as a college professor for 18 years. Mary and her wife, Susan, married 5 years ago. Susan is a police officer. Both consider their relationship to be solid. Susan has never hit Mary but yells at her a lot and leaves her home alone until late into the night. The abuse increased since Mary's accident, in which Susan was the driver. Because of COVID-19 the two of them have spent more time together, with Mary working from home and Susan working on modified duties. During this time, Susan spends most of her time outside and interacts with Mary as little as possible. Susan now sleeps in a separate bed from Mary and does not turn on the intercom in her room, installed in case Mary needs something. During her last doctor's visit, Mary complained of headaches, not sleeping well, and feeling overwhelmed with work.

Discussion Questions

1. What are the implications related to sexual orientation?
2. How do you address issues related to the perpetrator?
3. What barriers exist for Mary in seeking help?

Women survivors of IPV may resort to self-injurious behavior or self-directed violence (e.g., cutting, suicide) as a coping strategy to regain control over their environment, to release tension, or to reduce overwhelming feelings (Temple et al., 2010). This type of affect regulation is described as providing relief in various ways, including distracting from emotional pain by replacing it with physical pain, providing a way of expressing or by allowing the individual to feel something in the face of dissociation and emotional numbing. It is short-term relief. "Self-harm is a response to psycho-socio-economic adversity and trauma" (Pickard, 2015, p. 81). Pickard distinguished self-harm from suicide, which is a desire for a permanent escape from suffering.

Intersection of Physical and Mental Health Disorders

Physical and mental health disorders are not necessarily mutually exclusive. Physical health problems can impact mental health, and mental health can influence the ways in which physical health problems are manifested; they are closely interwoven and interdependent (Sowers et al., 2009). The literature consistently confirms several key findings about a relationship between physical and mental health disorders: people with chronic physical conditions are at risk of developing poor mental health, physical problems can mask or resemble symptoms of depression, and people with serious mental health conditions are at high risk of experiencing chronic physical conditions (Doherty & Gaughran, 2014; Vaingankar et al., 2020). Ohrnberger et al. (2017) found significant direct and indirect effects of past mental health on present physical health and of past physical health on present mental health.

The intersection between physical and mental health in women who experience IPV manifests in short- and long-term consequences. Research reveals that IPV against women may be associated with mental health consequences that persist well into the life course (Ayre et al., 2016; Moulding et al., 2020). Moreover, "for women experiencing violence, mental health problems can overlap with trauma, making simple diagnoses and treatment difficult" (Australia's National Research Organization for Women's Safety [ANROWS], 2020, p. 4). Finally, Salter et al. (2020) emphasized that women who experience IPV can have ambivalence toward mental health labels because of the stigma of distressed women as hysterical, resulting in them being vulnerable to stigma and revictimization.

DISPARITIES IN OTHER PSYCHOSOCIAL OUTCOMES

There are two reciprocal views about disability and positionalities of gender and identity. One is that gender, gender identity, sexual orientation, and physical and mental disability are "dimensions that lead to health inequities primarily through the pathway of stigma and discrimination, leading to exclusion from accessing resources needed for well-being and health services through multiple pathways." The other is the dimensions of these positionalities "affect inequities constitutively, instrumentally through co-morbidities, and through stigma either directly or indirectly" (Nakkeeran & Nakkeeran, 2018, pp. 9–10). Nakkeeran and Nakkeeran articulated that the experience of stigma also forms the basis of identities and the difference between identities, which emerges as an important concept in the realities of disparities in health and psychosocial outcomes beyond measurable gaps. The premise of the argument of these authors is that because disability does not solely reside in the individual, one must recognize the mediation of social, economic, location, and other privileges or deprivileges in shaping and determining the degree of disability and vulnerability experienced by specific individuals. For women with disabilities who experience IPV, the social determinants of health and well-being and disability-specific stigmas (Nosek et al., 2001b) contribute to the structural mechanisms that constitute gendered disability-based disadvantage (Gartrell et al., 2018).

For women, sex (biology) and gender (social conditions) interact to determine women's disability and disease outcomes. Both sex and gender matter in health and have a wide influence on disability and CID (Buvinic et al., 2006). They influence etiology, diagnosis, progression, prevention, intervention, health outcomes of CID, and help-seeking behaviors and exposure to risk. The two differ in that sex is more prominent in etiology, onset, and progression of CID, and gender influences differential risks, severity of CID, access to and quality of care, and compliance with care. In addition, other social positions intersect with sex and gender and contribute to women's disproportionate CID (Buvinic et al.).

In general, women with disabilities, regardless of abuse and victimization status, fare more poorly in *physical function* and ADL across countries (Wheaton & Crimmins, 2016). On average, women with disabilities are more psychologically affected by inequitable workplace conditions compared to men with disabilities and women and men without disabilities because of exposure to more workplace stress, earning less, and being less likely to experience autonomous working conditions (Brown & Moloney, 2018). Women with disabilities also have a greater risk of psychosocial health problems than do men, have higher levels of isolation (Dembo et al., 2018; Nosek & Hughes, 2003), and are less likely to have spouses/partners (Meekosha, 2004). Women with disabilities have higher odds of severe distress following IPV compared to men or women without disabilities (Dembo et al., 2018).

For working women, IPV results in a total loss of millions of days of paid work each year. The financial impact of IPV of lifetime economic cost-associated medical services, lost productivity from paid work, criminal justice, and other costs is approximately $3.6 trillion, and the cost over a victim/survivor's lifetime is about $103,767 for women and $23,414 for men (CDC, 2021a). In addition, IPV can affect women's employment because of job interference tactics used by perpetrators. Perpetrators may exhibit job interference behaviors before, during, and after work, resulting in reduced job performance (i.e., absenteeism, tardiness, job leavings, and terminations). Swanberg and Logan (2005) found that even when women disclosed abuse to employers and job supports were offered, these led to short-term job retention, but fear and safety issues mitigated employers' attempts to retain workers.

Rothman et al. (2007) identified substantial ways in which *employment* is helpful to women experiencing IPV, including (a) improving their finances, (b) promoting physical safety, (c) increasing self-esteem, (d) improving social connectedness, (e) providing mental respite, and (f) providing motivation or a purpose in life. Women with disabilities are more likely to be unemployed and, accordingly, women victim-survivors of IPV are more likely than nonvictims to be unemployed, report lower personal income, and rely on public assistance (Postmus et al., 2010).

Challenges faced by *BIPOC women* differ from those of White women experiencing IPV. BIPOC women face racism, discrimination, and stereotypes that shape their experience and response to IPV. For example, BIPOC women are often more afraid of what will happen if they report abuse than they are of the violence they are enduring. In addition, while Black women experience IPV at exceedingly high rates (Lacey et al., 2016), they also are disproportionately more likely to be criminalized by the judicial system when seeking help (e.g., arrested when trying to defend themselves against abuse; Henderson, 2015). Black women also are disproportionately impacted by *lethal IPV*, at nearly three times the rate of White women (Petrosky et al., 2017). Moreover, residual effects of IPV disproportionately affect the long-term health of BIPOC women.

LGBTQ women experience IPV at significantly higher rates than heterosexual women (CDC, 2013). Although sexual orientation and gender identity data collection has increased in population-based health survey, administrative datasets (e.g., healthcare, social services, coroner and medical examiner offices, law enforcement) do not meet the needs of scaled public health interventions to effectively record and curb IPV among sexual and gender minority communities (Blosnich, 2022).

Disparities in *law enforcement* treatment of domestic violence cases show that while police officers have broad discretionary powers when investigating crime, officers use added discretion in IPV cases. That is, officers can be more or less lenient when making arrests or reports than with other crimes. In instances of IPV involving women with disabilities, police are less likely to respond (77%) than they are to reported violence against persons without disabilities (90%; Harrell & Rand, 2010). For women with disabilities who experience IPV in their interaction with law enforcement, "justice can be impacted at the intersection of mental health and violence, because the criminal justice system is not designed to accommodate trauma" (ANROWS, 2020, p. 7).

IMPLICATIONS FOR WORKING WITH WOMEN OF VULNERABILITY AND ABUSE

In 1994, Congress passed the Violence Against Women Act (VAWA), which directed the National Research Council to develop a research agenda aimed at broadening the understanding of the scope and dynamics of domestic violence and rape (Jordan, 2009). VAWA has since been renewed and strengthened three times, in 2000, 2005, and 2013, and most recently, the 2022 reauthorization of VAWA strengthens this landmark law by including reauthorization of current VAWA grant programs to increasing services for underserved and marginalized communities (The White House, 2022). These requirements provide increased protection and courses of action for women victimized by IPV, with a specific focus on marginalized communities (e.g., women with disabilities, BIPOC women, and LGBTQ women).

Counselors working with women with disabilities in most settings will encounter clients impacted by IPV, and are more likely to encounter women at the survivor stage rather than those still in an abusive situation (Bray, 2014). It is important to understand that IPV of women with physical disabilities is a problem largely unrecognized by rehabilitation service providers (Powers et al., 2002; Young et al., 1997) and is addressed to only a limited extent in the rehabilitation counseling literature. Although women with disabilities are more likely to be targets of IPV, they are less likely to receive assistance or services (Nosek, 2002a, 2002b; Nosek et al., 2006).

One of the reasons that IPV against women with disabilities too often goes unidentified and unaddressed is the limited understanding of the nature of gendered disability violence (Frohmader et al., 2015). Because rehabilitation professionals have been the primary service providers for people with disabilities, Siu (2008) conducted a cross-sectional survey of rehabilitation professionals to determine their knowledge of, self-assessment concerning, and opinions about helping female consumers with abuse issues. Siu (2008) found gender to be statistically significant on subscale scores on knowledge and self-assessments and experience was not significant, and certified rehabilitation counselor (CRC) status was statically significant. An examination of rehabilitation counseling master's students' beliefs and attitudes about IPV toward women found African American students and students ages 25 to 30 scored lower in IPV knowledge, and participants who indicated having training in IPV and those who had a previous history of IPV had a higher level of competency than those with no training in or no previous experience with IPV (Davis, 2013). It is critical that counselors recognize the psychosocial disparities in vulnerability and abuse when working with women with disabilities, to be mindful of intersectionalities, and to do so through the lens of cultural competence. Another key consideration in working with women with disabilities who are survivors of IPV is recognition that although these women encounter difficulties in responding to abuse, they challenged assumptions about passivity, and this resistance helped them navigate IPV (Jordan, 2022).

Resilience of Women Survivors of Domestic Violence/Intimate Partner Violence

Resilience has been found to be an important component in positive mental health and psychosocial outcomes among victim-survivors of IPV. For some women, social and spiritual support were instrumental in recovery, growth, and resilience in the aftermath of IPV (Anderson et al., 2012). Other trajectories of resilience of women victim-survivors of IPV include the strength of maternal love when their children became victims of violence, interrupting the cycle of violence and making resilience possible (Trigueiro et al., 2014); utilization of community resources; prioritizing their role as a mother; reconstructing their own identity through the assumption of new roles (Crawford & Liebling, 2009); and characteristics of their cultural background. Cultural factors can positively influence coping with the impact of trauma, but victim-survivors may also be ostracized from their community because of the cultural meaning or perception of trauma (Substance Abuse and Mental Health Services Administration [SAMHSA], 2014a). Strategies to promote resilience include (a) social support to help buffer an individual's stress response (The Trevor Project, 2019), (b) returning to a sense of normalcy to help create a sense of structure and purpose after experiencing trauma, and (c) creating meaningful reasons for why the event may have occurred and how to create some positive take-aways from the experience to help facilitate recovery (Falbo-Woodson & Madra, 2018).

Counseling Approaches

Counseling intervention and support for women with disabilities experiencing or having experienced IPV can be critical in promoting coping and mediating potential long-term impacts (Gormley et al., 2022). The goal of counseling or therapy for women who are victim-survivors of IPV is to improve coping skills, develop new ways of working through problems, enhance self-confidence and empowerment, and strengthen resilience and resourcefulness (Women's Advocates, 2020). Therefore, empowerment becomes essential in working with women who are IPV victim-survivors. Interventions require a multiphase approach and a combination of interventions based on the needs of the individual.

Women victim-survivors of IPV usually employ emotion-oriented strategies to cope with violence or its outcome, and they mostly do not have problem-solving strategies (Waldrop & Resick, 2004). Given that individuals possess different coping styles, coping styles are associated with all kinds of violence, and the rate of resilience is associated with all kinds of violence (Fakari et al., 2022), the authors of this chapter selected several highly effective evidence-based approaches to counseling victim-survivors of IPV to present, including trauma-informed care (TIC), cognitive behavioral therapy (CBT; Bisson et al., 2019; SAMHSA, 2014a; Sullivan et al., 2013), person-centered counseling (PCT), and feminist therapy (FT). In the application of intervention with women with disabilities who experience IPV, one should understand the different types of traumas and which type is experienced by the individual, as well as be mindful that an individual may experience multiple types of traumas. Typically, women who have experienced one type of IPV often experience other types of gender-based violence in their lifetime (e.g., child sexual abuse; Cox, 2016). In addition, women who experience IPV usually experience repeated violence (Webster et al., 2018). Exposure to multiple repeated forms of interpersonal victimization, along with the resulting traumatic health problems and psychosocial challenges, is called *complex trauma* (Salter et al., 2020). The reader is reminded that it is best to explore other forms of counseling approaches as well and to be cognizant of the relationship between psychosocial, gender, and cultural aspects of disability.

Trauma-Informed Care

Trauma-informed care is an approach that assumes an individual is likely to have a history of trauma, recognizes the presence of trauma symptoms, and acknowledges the role trauma may play in an individual's life. The key to TIC is to promote healing and avoid retraumatization. The focus is on the whole person. The application of TIC involves a paradigm shift from asking "what is wrong with this person" to "what has happened to this person" (Harris & Fallot, 2001). There are *five principles of TIC*. The first involves ensuring that a victim-survivor has physical and emotional *safety*. Second, *trustworthiness* is demonstrated through establishment of and maintaining in practice interpersonal boundaries and clarity of what is expected regarding tasks. Third, the victim-survivor is afforded *choice* and control over their intervention experience. Fourth, *collaboration,* which goes together with choice, means the victim-survivor can make decisions and share in the power about her recovery. Finally, *empowerment* involves skill building of the victim-survivor. In practice, the survivor is validated and affirmed in each interaction with the counselor (Harris & Fallot, 2001). SAMHSA (2014b) has also identified these principles of a trauma-informed approach, with the addition of cultural, historical, and gender issues. An emphasis on cultural, historical, and gender issues is incorporated to make sure cultural stereotypes and biases (based on race, ethnicity, sexual orientation, gender identity, etc.) are not barriers to services and victim-survivors have access to gender-responsive interventions, utilization of healing values of traditional cultural connections, and historical trauma is recognized and addressed in protocols and process that are responsive to the cultural and identity needs of victim-survivors (SAMHSA, 2014b).

The application of TIC is advocated for across systems of care when working with women victim-survivors of IPV (Anyikwa, 2016; Taft et al., 2016; Wilson et al., 2015) and persons with disability (Williamson & Qureshi, 2015). TIC has been found to be effective in working with women victim-survivors of IPV and abuse. In a study to address TIC for women with mental health problems who experienced IPV Hegarty et al. (2018) demonstrated the need for a holistic service model for addressing complex needs of women in tandem with other structural oppression and marginalization. TIC mindfulness-based stress reduction was effective in reducing posttraumatic stress disorder (PTSD) symptoms, depressive symptoms, and attachment patterns with female survivors of IPV

(Kelly, 2015; Kelly & Garland, 2016). Gatz et al. (2007) found TIC effective in treating women with co-occurring disorders and histories of trauma. Trauma-informed messages (TIM) were used with heterosexual women who experienced IPV and who had adverse childhood experiences, and TIM predicted greater IPV termination attitudes, including leaving intention, trauma knowledge, and safety-related empowerment aspects. The effectiveness persisted among those with borderline personality disorder symptoms and unhealthy attachment patterns who naturally expressed impaired social information processing. However, TIM was less pronounced among women who scored higher on the trauma-driven traits (Chansiri, 2021). For many women victim-survivors of IPV, the intersection of trauma with the need for safe, stable, sustainable, and long-term housing is a concern. Ward-Lasher et al. (2017) implemented TIC using a case study approach in a housing program for victim-survivors of IPV and found most clients in the program retained housing up to three months after services ended and increased their safety and knowledge of IPV.

Cognitive Behavioral Therapy

CBT is designed to change thinking patterns. It has been used with women survivors of IPV to understand how they negatively appraise the trauma to gain insight into their symptoms. Ehlers and Clark (2000) found using CBT to modify cognitive appraisals and to address maladaptive coping strategies such as manipulation reduced PTSD symptoms and increased IPV survivors' ability to process information successfully, which in turn, enhanced the formation of a healthy belief about the self and the future. Johnson and Zlotnick (2009) used CBT with women living in domestic violence shelters by targeting their sense of control, power, safety, self-esteem, and intimacy to decrease severity of PTSD and depression symptoms, while increasing interpersonal relationships. Muthami (2017) found tailored CBT to have both short- and long-term impact on the lives of women in Kenya exposed to IPV and psychological disorders. However, these women needed a minimum of 14 to 16 sessions, as well as support systems that were responsive to restructuring strategies of alleviating the negative impacts of IPV. Women experiencing IPV who received CBT showed significant differences in posttest stage in mental health score and its dimensions in those participating in interventions programs compared to women in the control group. In addition, the women had significant differences in the posttest stage in the mindfulness score compared to the other group (Sabzevari et al., 2022). Similar results were found using CBT for women in domestic violence situations in Brazil with symptoms of anxiety, depression, and PTSD, showing a significant reduction in anxiety, depression, and stress symptoms, and life satisfaction levels increased significantly (Habigzang et al., 2018).

Cognitive Trauma Therapy for Battered Women (CTT-BW) was developed for women with PTSD and IPV who are no longer in abusive relationships. However, CTT-BW has not been evaluated with women still in abusive relationships. CTT-BW uses psychoeducation, CBT techniques, and modules specific to IPV (trauma-related guilt, other trauma histories, managing ongoing contact with abusive ex-partner, and risk for revictimization; Beck et al., 2016).

Person-Centered Therapy

PCT, or client-centered therapy, uses a nonauthoritative approach that allows clients to take more of a lead in counseling, and in the process, they discover their own solutions. PCT permits the survivor of IPV to regain power and control over her life by making independent decisions (Ivory Research, 2019). For survivors of IPV, PCT offers movement toward *self-actualization* or *personhood* as she learns to trust her own perceptions and feelings. In a study inquiring about the role of PCT in empowering women of IPV, Houston (2019) suggests PCT promotes this view of self-actualization from an intersectional perspective and mostly succeeds in empowering women to take control of their lives and to gain insight and self-awareness.

Feminist Therapy

Feminist scholars indicate that women tend to report greater depressive symptomology than men because this is a culturally normative and socially acceptable way for women to express dissatisfaction and unhappiness with social and relational contexts. Thus, depressive symptoms are considered useful for identifying cognitive vulnerabilities associated with social inequities and IPV for women (Ussher, 2010). At the core of feminism is political, social, and cultural intersections of women's lives informed by patriarchy and social norms (Lengermann & Niebrugge (2010). FT as a self-forgiveness framework for counselors is useful in helping victim-survivors of IPV forgive themselves for the harm they have experienced. The approach is to help them resolve the blame, guilt, and shame commonly associated with IPV and abuse (Turnage et al., 2003). Smailes (2004) asserts PCT's commitment to the client's internal frame of reference is effective in women victim-survivors' of IPV realizing their full potential because it yields an environment in which they can experience themselves and their world. PCT works well with feminist therapy because both honor the woman's individual reality and her understanding of her world socially and politically. The strength of combining PCT and FT for victim-survivors of IPV lies in being able to locate them within the political arena (Smailes, 2004).

Other therapies proved effective with survivors of IPV include narrative therapy because of the techniques it utilizes to empower these women and reshape their lives (Reyes-Foster, n.d.) and Helping Overcome PTSD through Empowerment (HOPE; Iverson, 2020). Iverson stresses that while there is no universal approach to address IPV, CBT and HOPE psychotherapies have demonstrated efficacy specifically for women victims/survivors.

CULTURAL COMPETENCY

Unfortunately, implicit bias is embedded in the counseling and helping professions by those who enter them. This unchecked implicit bias creates more trauma for clients. When service providers do not see the "whole" person, including disability, race, gender, gender identity, and sexuality, services may not be culturally appropriate, inclusive, and identity-sensitive. Although IPV has definitions that are universal, cultural beliefs also inform perceptions and definitions of abuse. Fernandez (2006) encourages culturally viable options for women who are operating within diverse cultural frameworks and experiencing IPV that is sensitive to and inclusive of a range of IPV across cultures and enhances communication among victim-survivors. Cultural competence is more than simply understanding cultural practices or hiring a person of the same culture to provide services, but is about understanding how culture experienced by the individual influences what they do, think, and understand (Lee et al., 2002). Cultural responsiveness in IPV services requires an understanding of how culture shapes (a) an individual's experience of violence, (b) whether perpetrators accept responsibility, (c) whether services are equally accessible to all, and (d) counselors' and service providers' own responses within the culture of the systems and organizations in which they work (Future Without Violence, 2016). For example, Case Study 9.3 demonstrates concerns of a victim-survivor of IPV from a cultural perspective in which Li Chow is seeking help for her husband because she is not interested in separating her family. According to Bent-Goodley (2007), "having a clear understanding of the individual's experiences and unique circumstances is needed to fully engage in assessment and planning" (p. 93). Codes of ethics for counseling and human services professions specify that cultural competence speaks to providing services that are ethical, competent, and effective. Because counselors and human services professionals hold a position of trust within society that affords them certain privileges that are not given to members of the public at large, they are expected to adhere to ethical principles, cultural competence, and social responsibility (Harley et al., 2021).

CASE STUDY 9.3: THE CASE OF LI CHOW

Li is a 37-year-old female who immigrated to the United States from South Korea. She has been married for 12 years and has three children, ages 10, 7, and 5. Li worked as a nurse's aide for eight years but stopped working when she injured her back. She has not been able to do any substantial physical labor. The loss of her job reduced the family's income. She helps her husband in their takeout restaurant. She and her husband argue a lot, and he hits her often. During one of their fights, a neighbor called the police. Upon arrival they observed Li had a black eye and swollen lip. Her husband was arrested, and a social worker was assigned to her case. Li has been running the restaurant along with two of her friends and oldest son. Li explained to the social worker that her husband is not "mean," and she wants her to help him so he can come back to work and take care of the family because that is what he needs to do.

Discussion Questions

1. What is Li's perception of what is going on?
2. What has Li identified as her goals?
3. What are the cultural issues to be addressed?

CONCLUSION

The prevalence and rates of lifetime IPV are high among women with disabilities and have lifelong and debilitating effects compared to women without disabilities. Women with disabilities experience IPV differently and intersectionally. Acts of IPV against women with disabilities often go unreported, which makes it difficult to document and respond to the true scope of this abuse and victimization. Major concerns in addressing IPV against women with disabilities are the barriers to treatment, public perception, lack of self-awareness of abuse (not seeing themselves as such), lack of sufficient training among service providers and law enforcement officers, and risk of continuous abuse in some form even after leaving the abusive situation. Frequently barriers to treatment and services create a revictimization of women with disabilities.

In addition, cultural, religious, and geographic issues tend to further complicate access to help for women who experience IPV, which is exacerbated for women with disabilities. Clearly, IPV against women with disabilities is a crisis with far-reaching health impacts, requiring substantially more medical treatment, mental health counseling, and psychosocial adjustment than nonvictimized women. An intersectional approach allows for a more holistic understanding of women with disabilities who experience IPV through addressing the complexities of life, especially regarding type of disability, race, sexual orientation, oppressed and marginalized identity, poverty, geographic influence, and issues of accessibility to resources and services.

CLASS ACTIVITIES

1. For many women with disabilities, the only immediate resource they may have to access when experiencing IPV is a domestic violence crisis hotline. Research the purpose of such a hotline and volunteer to work at a crisis hotline. Write a reflection paper in which you discuss your observations and emotions during this process. Conclude with what you see as your role as a future practitioner to address IPV among women with disabilities.

2. Because of the sensitive nature of IPV, women are hesitant to participate in interviews and share their experience. Contact and interview a therapist or social worker who works with women who experience IPV. Include questions such as: (a) Why did you want to work with women who are abused? (b) What type of training did you have to get? (c) What has been the most devastating situation you have encountered working with these women? (d) What type of distinguishing issues are presented by women who (1) have disabilities, (2) are LGBT, (3) are women of color, and so forth? (e) How do you approach intersectionality? (f) How do you disconnect from the traumatic experiences of these women and not become emotionally consumed? (g) What advice do you give to someone planning to work with this population? These are only some example questions. Be sure to develop a list of your own questions.

3. For women experiencing or who have experienced IPV, one of the most important things to do is to develop strategies for safety and survival. Develop a safety plan for a woman who is still experiencing violence. Be sure to identify her disability(ies), functional limitations, and barriers to accessing services.

4. Challenge beliefs and feelings about LGBTQ women and domestic violence through self-examination using role-play through which students explore their feelings, beliefs, perceptions, and attitudes about LGBTQ women's sexuality, identity, roles, and orientation. Encourage students to use an intersectional perspective. Role-play occurs in the context of a counseling session. One student plays the role of the counselor/therapist, and the other student plays the role of a lesbian, bisexual, or trans woman with a disability (select one). Roles can then be reversed. Other students are to observe the interaction and at the end of the role-play provide feedback about the interaction and recommendations of how things about the interaction can be changed. The class can be divided to do several role-play situations at one time.

KEY REFERENCES

Only key references appear in the print edition. The full references appear in the digital product on Springer Publishing Connect™: https://connect.springerpub.com/content/book/978-0-8261-5111-7/part/partII/chapter/ch09

Breiding, M. J., & Armour, B. S. (2015). The association between disability and intimate partner violence in the United States. *Annals of Epidemiology, 25*(6), 455–457. https://doi.org/10.1016/j.annepidem.2015.03.017

Fugate, M., Landis, L., Riordan, K., Naureckas, S., & Engel, B. (2005). Barriers to domestic violence help seeking: Implications for intervention. *Violence Against Women, 11*(3), 290–310. https://doi.org/10.1177/1077801204271959

Hague, G., Thiara, R., & Mullender, A. (2011). Disabled women, domestic violence and social care: The risk of isolation, vulnerability, and neglect. *British Journal of Social Work, 41*(1), 148–165. https://doi.org/10.1093/bjsw/bcq057

Heron, R. L., & Eisma, M. C. (2021). Barriers and facilitators of disclosing domestic violence to healthcare service: A systematic review of qualitative research. *Health and Social Care, 29*(3), 612–630. https://doi .org/10.1111/hsc.13282

Ledingham, E., Wright, G. W., & Mitra, M. (2022). Sexual violence against women with disabilities: Experiences with force and lifetime risk. *American Journal of Preventive Medicine, 62*(6), 895–902. https:// doi.org/10/1016/j.amepre.2021.12.015

Lundell, W. I., Eulau, L., Bjarneby, F., & Westerbotn, M. (2018). Women's experiences with healthcare professionals after suffering from gender-based violence: An interview study. *Journal of Clinical Nursing, 27*(5/5), 949–957. https://doi.org/10.1111/jocn.14046

Nosek, M. A., Hughes, R. B., Taylor, H. B., & Taylor, P. (2006). Disability, psychosocial, and demographic characteristics of abused women with physical disabilities. *Violence Against Women, 12*(9), 838–850. https://doi.org/10.1177/1077801206192671.

Pico-Alfonso, M. A., Garcia-Linares, M. I., Celda0Navarro, N., Blasko-Ros, C., Echeburua, E., & Martinez, M. (2006). The impact of physical, psychological, and sexual intimate male partner violence on women's mental health: Depressive symptoms, posttraumatic stress disorder, state anxiety, and suicide. *Journal of Women's Health, 15*, 599–611. https://doi.org/10.1089/jwh.2006.15.599

Powers, L. E., Curry, M. A., Oschwald, M., Maley, S., Saxton, M., & Eckel, K. (2002). Barriers and strategies in addressing abuse: A survey of disabled women's experiences. *Journal of Rehabilitation, 68*(1), 4–13.

Powers, L. E., & Oschwald, M. (2005). *Violence and abuse against people with disabilities: Experiences, barriers, and prevention strategies.* Center on Self-Determination.

Salter, M., Conroy, E., Dragiewicz, M., Burke, J., Ussher, J., Middleton, W., Vilenica, S., Martin Monzon, B., & Noack-Lundberg, K. (2020). *"A deep wound under my heart": Construction of complex trauma and implications for women's wellbeing and safety from violence.* Research Report, 12/2020. ANROWS.

CHAPTER 10

SEXUALITY AND DISABILITY

NOREEN M. GRAF AND RORY L. GLOVER

LEARNING OBJECTIVES

After reading this chapter, you will be able to:

- Identify and recognize the unique terms associated with sexuality, gender identity, and sexual orientation
- Identify and recognize the sexual stigmatization and discrimination associated with being a person with a disability
- Analyze specific impacts of disability on sexuality based on the type of disability, severity of disability, and the type of intimate relationship
- Identify the frequency, dynamics, and contributing factors of sexual abuse against women with disabilities
- Recognize the trends and legislation relevant to sexuality and disability

PRE-READING QUESTIONS

1. What are the misconceptions and myths about persons with disabilities in relation to their sexuality?
2. Differentiate some of the sexuality issues faced by persons with various types of disabilities (cognitive, learning, physical, psychiatric, and chronic illness)?
3. Describe your beliefs about people with disabilities becoming parents? Do your beliefs about parenting change based on the type of disability such as developmental, mental health, physical, or sensory impairments?

Sexuality in relation to disability has been neglected by service providers, educators, and researchers, despite consensus that sexuality has a direct impact on consumers' quality of life and social adjustment (McCray et al. 2022). In their review of the literature, Kazukauskas and Lam (2010) identified the reasons for this neglect: inadequate supports, time constraints, no guiding policies in facilities, lack of training, negative attitudes, lack of knowledge, and discomfort on the part of counselors. Additionally, they noted areas of discomfort included addressing topics such as bowel and bladder function, body image, sexual acts and behaviors, sexual preference, and reproductive function and choice.

In a systematic review of healthcare professionals' knowledge, attitudes, and behaviors, most healthcare professionals did not include assessment of sexuality. They had limited knowledge and confidence in addressing sexuality and expressed discomfort at raising issues of sexuality with consumers who had chronic illnesses or disabilities (McGrath et al., 2021). Similarly, in an examination of organizational supports for intimate relationships, only half of the organizations supported participants' rights to pursue and maintain relationships and less than half addressed barriers toward relationships (Friedman, 2019). In a recent study of 27 rehabilitation counselor educators, McCray et al. (2022) found levels of comfort were self-reported as high and attitudes toward sexuality were positive, but they also indicated lower levels of specific knowledge regarding sexuality and people with disabilities (PWDs).

Kazukauskas and Lam (2010) contend that rehabilitation counselors may be the only professionals who remain with consumers throughout the process of rehabilitation and are ethically committed to be competent and knowledgeable about issues of sexuality so that consumers can become as fully integrated and independent as possible. Based on their study of 199 certified rehabilitation counselors related to knowledge, attitude, and comfort in addressing the sexuality and disability issues of consumers, the authors recommended enhancing training and education.

This chapter focuses on (a) sexuality and related components; (b) disability and intimate relationships; (c) disability type and related sexual issues; (d) sexual orientation, sexual functioning, procreation, and parenting; (e) sex education, sex therapy, and sexual surrogates; and (f) sexual abuse.

SEXUALITY AND RELATED COMPONENTS

Defining Sexuality

Defining sexuality is complex because it involves all the factors that affect how individuals view themselves and behave in relation to their gender and gender identity. They are influenced by their upbringing, the culture they associate themselves with, and society at large. The World Health Organization (WHO) states, "The definition of sexuality is complex: it includes gender roles and sexual orientation and is influenced by the interaction of biological, psychological, cognitive, social, political, cultural, ethical, legal, historical, religious and spiritual factors" (World Health Organization, 2010a, p. 4). The WHO (2006) report also stated that "sexual health requires a positive and respectful approach to sexuality and sexual relationships, as well as the possibility of having pleasurable and safe sexual experiences, free of coercion, discrimination and violence" (p. 5). Further, the WHO defines attainment and maintenance of sexual health as necessitating "the sexual rights of all persons must be respected, protected, and fulfilled" (p. 5).

Daily (1984) views sexuality from a psychological, emotional, and functional perspective and describes sexuality as having five components: identity, intimacy, sensuality, sexualization, and reproductive aspects. *Identity* is the continual process of discovery of who we are in relation to our sexuality; *intimacy* refers to emotional closeness with others; *sensuality* is the experience of our body through our five senses; *sexualization* is the use of the body for the benefits of control, manipulation, and influencing others; and finally, *reproductive aspects* involve the functions of conceiving and child-rearing.

The following definitions are offered to clarify our understanding of terms related to human sexuality:

- Sexual orientation is considered a piece of one's identity that involves attraction to others as well as the resulting behaviors and associations. Attraction to others may include attraction to either men or women, to those who are both/neither, or persons with various gender identities. Terms associated with gender identity include but are not limited to heterosexual, lesbian, gay, and bisexual as well as asexual, pansexual, and queer.

- Gender identity: This term is used to define a person's internal connection to being male or female. It can also refer to alternate identities that do not conform to gender binary distinctions such as gender neutral, gender nonconforming, or gender queer. Gender identity does not necessary correspond to one's at-birth sexual assignment.

- Cisgender: This term is used to denote correspondence with sexual identity and at-birth sexual assignment.

- Transgender: This term encompasses a wide range of people whose gender identity does not conform to traditional associations with at-birth sexual assignment.

- Genderqueer: This term describes person who do not align their gender identity with traditional binary distinctions and may see overlap in gender dichotomies. (American Psychological Association, n.d)

A recent focus on adaptation of pronouns to convey gender identity more accurately has emerged with a focus on gender pronouns. In addition to familiar pronouns such as he and she, pronouns such as "they," "ze," and "hir" are being used to define identities that do not conform to traditional sexual identity norms. This development of language is an outgrowth of lesbian, gay, bisexual, transgender, queer and questioning (LGBTQ) communities and is a push toward awareness and inclusion of individuals of various sexual identities. Asking a person how they would like to be addressed or what pronouns they prefer is both a courtesy and, in some agencies, a requirement.

It is important to understand that components that contribute to sexuality are integrally connected and influenced by society and culture and by the rules set up to govern sexual behaviors, including the selection of a socially acceptable mate. Even though society seems to be allowing for greater flexibility regarding sexuality, it is more aptly described as increased tolerance for those who deviate from the expected norm. Persons who choose same-sex relationships are now considered somewhat socially acceptable. Thirty-two countries allow and recognize same-sex marriages and, since 2015, all 50 U.S. states allow for same-sex marriage (World Population Review, 2022). Hard-fought legal sanctions against discrimination based on race or ethnicity have created tolerance for marriages between persons of differing cultures, but tolerance of sexual relationships and sexual expression for persons with disabilities is yet to be achieved. Even within the counseling profession, sexual education related to clients is by and large focused on pathology and dysfunction rather than health (Zeglin et al., 2019).

Sexual Stigmatization

Despite efforts at inclusion and education, sexual stigmatization of persons with disabilities continues. Healthcare providers, direct care providers, and family members persist in their beliefs that PWDs are asexual, cannot provide informed consent for sexual activities, cannot or should not bring a pregnancy to term, and cannot be good parents. Despite this, an increasing number of women with disabilities are having children. With the gradual recognition that people with disabilities have the right to appropriate sexual expression and reproductive healthcare, social service providers and healthcare workers are beginning to inform and support their consumers with disabilities (Long-Bellil, 2022). Progress in this arena is essential. Horner-Johnson et al. (2019) stated that the birth rate for women with disabilities is now comparable to that of women without disabilities.

Nearly 20 years ago, Vash and Crewe (2004) discussed the historical sexual stigmatization of PWDs as originating from biological and social sanctions that attempted to eliminate what was viewed as a "defective gene pool" because survival was based on physical abilities. As society has progressed, survival is no longer contingent on physical ability. Vash and Crewe (2004, p. 85) point to a lessening of "the rejection of disabled mates." This is a far cry from "acceptance," which is apparent to those PWDs seeking mates and may profoundly affect self-esteem, since finding a mate is often regarded as symbolic of one's desirability and worth.

Many of the sexual myths associated with PWDs and delineated by Olkin in 1999 remain a source of misinformation and stigmatization. Olkin noted that much of society views PWDs as lacking sex drive, incapable of sexual performance, and lacking both the social skills and appropriate judgment to be sexually appropriate. Persons without disabilities (PWODs) who partner with PWDs are frequently viewed as either deviant or desperate. Morris (1993) discussed myths from an insider perspective related to the sexuality of women with disabilities (WWDs), which negatively affect the behavior of individuals in society and the willingness to engage in romantic and intimate relationships with PWDs:

That we are naïve and lead sheltered lives

That we are asexual or at best sexually inadequate

That we cannot ovulate, menstruate, conceive, or give birth, or have orgasms,

That if we are not married or in a long-term relationship it is because no one wants us and not through our personal choice to remain single or live alone

That our only true scale of merit and success is to judge ourselves by the standard of their world

That we are sweet, deprived little souls who need to be compensated with treats, presents, and praise. (Morris, 1993, p. 16)

The impact of rigid social role expectations on PWDs has been profound. As early as the 1980s the rehabilitation literature discussed the psychosocial issues related to the stigmatization of WWDs as asexual and dependent. When women are viewed as unable to meet their obligations to have children or nurture children and when they are viewed as unable to be employed, society views them as both roleless and sexless (Buonocore Porter, 2018; Danek, 1992; Thurer, 1991).

Social Construction of Gender Identity and Body Image

Clearly, PWDs are deprived of sexual equality despite social advances. In order to further understand this disparity, it is necessary to examine the social construction of gender identity and body image. While gender usually refers to the biological makeup of a person, there is also a strong social component that contributes to how we define sex differences. Our gender expectations, roles, and interactions are also determined by the social distribution of sex-based power and resources. In a gender-stratified society, it is therefore important that gender be clearly defined. Today, what men do is still more highly valued, and a lack of clarity about gender contributes to evaluation confusion and challenges the sense of security offered through dichotomous thinking and rules (Lorber, 2018).

Gender-based roles influence how individuals think and feel about themselves and others as males and females. For example, in a traditional North American household, women are expected to have greater responsibility tending to the household and the children, and men are expected to take on greater responsibility in providing financial support for the family. These roles reinforce the woman as a psychological/emotional caretaker and the man as a physical/financial caretaker. If a woman is physically, psychologically, sensually, or developmentally impaired, how will she clean the house? How will she bathe the children? Will she be able to engage in sexual activity with her husband? If a man is impaired, how will he make money to pay the bills? How will he be able to manage house repairs?

While these questions are still relevant today, it is clear that the lines that define the traditional role distribution have become increasingly blurred. It is frequently necessary for both partners to have full-time jobs to support the family, parenting roles and responsibilities are shifting, and there is an increase in single-parent households. Even so, traditional roles and attitudes appear resistant to change because they are deeply ingrained in today's social structure. Questions about being able to meet traditional roles and responsibilities continue to contribute to the reluctance to consider PWDs as intimate and sexual partners and to recognize and normalize the sexual needs and desires of PWDs.

Sedikides et al. (1994) examined gender differences in relation to romantic relationships. In a study of the costs and benefits of romantic relationships, the authors noted that for both males and females, the most important benefits were described as companionship, feeling loved and loving, and happiness. However, females viewed intimacy, self-growth and understanding, and increased self-esteem as more beneficial, and males viewed sexual gratification as more beneficial. Females viewed a loss of identity and innocence as a greater cost, and males viewed monetary loss as more consequential. In other words, females continued to believe they would be emotional caretakers at the risk of losing their identity, and males continued to believe that they were less intimate and more responsible financially. Similarly, when investigating desired changes by couples in relationships, Heyman et al. (2009) found women desired increases in their male partner's compassionate and emotional behaviors, parenting, and instrumental support, while men desired increases in sex. For males, this may be due to satisfaction with other areas in the relationship rather than an indication of disinterest or lack of valuing emotional and supportive properties.

Impact of Gender-Based Values and Social Roles on People With Disabilities

In our society, even our values tend to have either a masculine or feminine orientation, which leads to cultural bias and underrepresentation of women in male-dominated professions (Cheryan & Markus, 2020). For example, assertiveness is associated with males and compassion with females. Interestingly, many of the values that guide rehabilitation professionals are masculine based rather than feminine based. Independence is viewed as a masculine-oriented goal, whereas interdependence and the importance of relationships tends to be seen as a feminine orientation. Yet most rehabilitation counselors are quick to vocalize the importance of the greatest amount of independence possible as the ultimate outcome goal. This lack of taking gender identities into account can pose difficulties for consumers who have a strong "female" orientation. While *interdependence* is still not a focus of rehabilitation, some agencies write and follow policies that reflect as much independence *as desired* by the consumer. In New York, the Vocational and Educational Services for Individuals with Disabilities (VESID) website lists: "One major goal of the vocational rehabilitation process is to foster the greatest degree of independence and responsibility, as desired by an individual" (VESID, 2017, para. 3). While still not an acknowledgment of a feminine perspective as equally viable, it leaves open the possibility of accommodating potential gender differences.

Early on, Burns (1993) and Scotti et al. (1991) noted that in terms of sexuality, treatment discrepancies are apparent. For example, when male consumers exhibit inappropriate behaviors, they are more likely to be viewed as behaving "badly." Similar inappropriate behaviors from female consumers will be considered "psychological problems." Women are more likely to be punished or medicated for equivalent sexual behaviors that may be ignored or rationalized when exhibited by male clients. In a qualitative study of staff who provided services for persons with intellectual disabilities, unfavorable attitudes toward sexuality were found to correlate with traditional gender stereotypes. Women were perceived as sexually innocent and men as sexually motivated. Negative social stereotypes were reflected that denied positivity of sexual expression. Further, staff expressed anxiety and a lack of awareness around the topic of sexual expression and disinterest in proactive support for client rights of sexual expression (R. Young et al., 2012). Clearly, much needs to be done to create equality in treatment that gives consideration to issues of gender in terms of values, expectations, desires of consumers, and consumer rights.

Self-Esteem and Body Image

The effect of social messages about sexual roles and expectations is profound. Messages from society, treatment professionals, caretakers, and the portrayal of sexuality by the media have had great impact on how PWDs feel about their bodies and themselves. The fact that beauty is socially dictated is historically evident. From the painting of Rubin, when larger sizes were an indication of beauty and prosperity, to the fashion photography of the present, where there have been bans against using severely underweight models in advertisements, there is always a clear message from society regarding physical beauty and sexual desirability.

Today the average person in the United States is exposed to between 4,000 and 10,000 advertisements a day (Pyle et al., 2022). Billions of dollars are spent on making the body fit into whatever socially constructed image of beauty is currently accepted. People subject themselves to endless diets. They have surgeries to alter the face; to add and subtract from breasts, hips, and stomach size and shape; and recently, surgeries to increase height that involves cutting and lengthening of leg bones. People have injections to reduce lines on the face, have hair transplants, and spend billions of dollars on products that claim to make them appear younger. All this is for the sake of conforming to socially imposed standards that people hope will render them attractive to others and therefore more desirable and ultimately more lovable. What is the message in all this to persons with physical deformities, with losses of limbs or other body parts, and for those who need mobility aids?

In a study of sexual identity, body image, and life satisfaction among 134 women with and without physical disabilities, Moin et al., (2009) noted similar sexual desires and needs but differences in lower levels of body image, sexual self-esteem, and sexual and life satisfaction for WWDs when compared with women without disabilities (WWODs). These differences were even more apparent in younger women. The study also found that about one-third of the WWDs did report sexual satisfaction and that sexual satisfaction was also found to be strongly correlated with life satisfaction.

When physical appearance is altered as a result of disability, the body falls further away from the expectations of society and body image, and the attitude one has toward the physical self may decline and affect self-esteem. A low self-esteem affects a person's willingness and confidence to engage in social activities and to engage in relationships with others. Lack of socialization can further contribute to a person's isolation, lower quality of life, and lack of self-confidence to the point that the possibility of rejection appears so great that it may no longer seem worth the risk. Persons with physical anomalies may fear that others will laugh at them, reject them, or come to think of them as deviant. Even more than the body, the face plays an important role in a person's self-image and self-identity and is distinctly different from that of the rest of the body.

Callahan (2004) theorized that each body part holds a symbolic meaning as well as functional use; arms symbolize strength, hands symbolize creativity and the ability to provide, legs represent speed and vitality, and reproductive organs indicate pleasure, intimacy, and procreation. In her examination of facial disfigurement (one's self-presentation to others) in persons with head and neck cancer, Callahan described the "profound psychological trauma" (Callahan, 2004, p. 73) that can occur in terms of one's body integrity and sense of self. Similarly, 70 years ago, in reviewing psychosocial problems associated with facial deformities, MacGregor concluded that coupled with the adjustment problems of the person and societal negative attitudes, prejudice, and discrimination: "Wherever plastic surgery can correct or improve the facial injury or congenital malformation, it should be undertaken as early as possible in order to avoid not only the obvious disadvantages, but to prevent deep psychological wounds which may be incurred but not so easily eliminated" (MacGregor, 1951, p. 638).

In brief, accepting and loving one's body as it is in a society that does not endorse or support such a notion is challenging. A number of practices can assist in increasing body image, but much of it relies more on changing one's thinking more so than one's body, refusing to accept the media-portrayed image of the beautiful man or woman, and giving up the practice of comparing oneself with those photo-altered images of often-emaciated women or muscle-bound men. Yuen and Hanson (2002) concluded that physical activity could increase body image for persons with acquired mobility impairments. In their study, persons who were physically active evaluated both their physical appearance and their health as more positive; they showed more concern about their physical fitness and were more satisfied with their bodies than those with mobility impairment who were not active. A number of studies also suggest that attention to making oneself as attractive as possible has positive effects on self-image and physical appearance for PWDs (Kammerer-Quayle, 2002).

A controversy over cosmetic surgery for children with Down syndrome (DS) brought to light the ethical dilemmas involved in such a practice when in 2008 the parents of a child with DS subjected the 5-year-old to a number of surgeries on the tongue, eyes, and ears to correct the facial indicators of DS. As parents, they sought to eliminate the future stigmatization their child would face, but a number of bioethicists argued that it was an unnecessary and elective surgery that should have waited for the child to reach the age of consent (Fox News, 2008). Adult protective services have also expressed concerns related to a growing increase in cosmetic surgery for persons with intellectual disabilities (Cambridge, 2002), and a number of cases have come before hospital ethics boards weighing the value of enhancement and restorative procedures in adults and children (Opel & Wilfond, 2009). A 2019 study of parents of children with DS found favorable attitudes toward surgeries that they viewed could decrease stigmatization and parental anxiety (Michael & Jarrett, 2019). The National Down Syndrome Society (NDSS, 2011), which previously acknowledged cosmetic surgery for children with DS as a personal choice of parents, no longer includes any relevant materials on the topic outside of medically beneficial and necessary surgeries (NDSS, 2022). They offer no position, education, support, or guidance for parents or consumers considering the option of cosmetic surgery.

For rehabilitation counselors, simply ignoring the importance of physical appearance or waiting for adjustment to occur is not appropriate, because appearance is clearly tied to how people feel about themselves and interact with others. Kleve et al. (2002) demonstrated the importance of social supports and interactions in positive adjustment to disfigurement. However, interaction may depend on self-esteem, and self-esteem may be tied to body image. Thus, attention to physical appearance may need to move beyond basic hygiene concerns to application of cosmetics and, in some cases, cosmetic surgery. These considerations have historically been extended to PWDs only on a limited basis, such as for those with facial burns. However, a person's level of adjustment to having an apparent physical difference also needs to be taken into consideration because those with poor adjustment may demonstrate feelings of depression, social avoidance and anxiety, fear of being evaluated negatively by others, and shame. Demographic variables, including age and sex, can also influence adjustment to physical differences. Overall, women reporting more difficulty than men with visible physical differences and late adolescents and young adults also typically have greater concern for visible differences. Even hidden physical differences can interfere with adjustment because if the physical differences are typically concealed, distress may also be high due to fear of others finding out, suggesting that the secrecy and anticipated discovery by others can also increase distress (Moss & Rosser, 2008).

For people paying attention, the slow but deliberate civil rights movement has been making gains beyond demanding civil rights to a place of disability pride where disability is viewed as valuable, enriching, and positive. In a study of 710 PWDs, disability pride was able to mediate the association between stigma and negative self-esteem, thereby providing some ego protection (Bogart et al., 2018).

DISABILITY AND INTIMATE RELATIONSHIPS

Partnering Desires and People With Disabilities

In 1943, Abraham Maslow identified basic human needs as love, affection, and belonging that encompass both the need to love and the need to feel loved in order to overcome loneliness and feelings of alienation. While recognizing the need for love, Vash and Crewe (2004) discussed pairing as a part of a preprogrammed biological drive that is reinforced, if not required, by society. The state of being without a partner is viewed by society as an indication of one's inferior status, bringing humiliation and disgrace to the individual. The proof of one's worth often comes with the acquisition of a partner. Clearly, much of today's values are embedded in past survival needs that are no longer relevant; a time when a lack of medical sophistication led to numerous infant deaths and death of mothers during childbirth. Because successful procreation was far more contingent upon physical makeup, PWDs were generally excluded from consideration as life partners and dismissed as sexually responsive or desirable. Changes in survival rates and medical advances appear to have little effect on some attitudes, as persons who do become partners of PWDs are frequently seen as being less intelligent, and less sociable, than partners of PWODs (Goldstein & Johnson, 1997).

PWDs are not excluded from experiencing partnering desires or, unfortunately, from the messages imposed by society. They look to attract partners for reasons of love, intimacy, and security, yet it is difficult to see role models with disabilities represented as sexually and physically attractive. For some PWDs, values of physical beauty will become less meaningful to the fulfillment of their lives, yet the importance of relationships and pairing will not necessarily diminish (Wright, 1960). Vash and Crewe (2004) note that, like PWODs, not all PWDs will be interested in pairing or having children, but for most people partnering is a strong urge. Not only will they need to deal with the devices that indicate disability, such as wheelchairs, canes, and so on, which may cause people to reject them, but they will also need to overcome the negative or dismissive attitudes of others. Numerous recent podcasts run by PWDs, such as the Accessible Stall, have begun to candidly address issues of accessibility and sexuality and disability (https://www.theaccessiblestall.com).

In a recent study of 1,443 individuals without disabilities regarding intimate relationships that examined friendships and romantic relationships, Friedman (2018) stated, "In addition to the general benefits provided by intimate relationships, such as lover, comradery, and closeness, intimate relationships are especially fruitful for adults with disabilities as they can help them deal with ableist attitudes and promote a sense of disability community and pride, and support them as they navigate the service system" (p. 16).

Attitudes of Persons Without Disabilities

Perhaps the greatest barrier to partnering is the attitudes of PWODs. Several researchers have studied how attractive PWODs will find PWDs (Man et al., 2006; Marini et al., 2011; Miller et al., 2009). Rojahn et al. (2008) found that college students reported similar romantic attractiveness to people with and without disabilities but noted a clear preference shown for physical health, suggesting a disconnection between the explicit ratings and implicit attitudes. A number of researchers have also investigated attitudes toward having relationships with PWDs (Howland & Rintala, 2001; Kreuter, 2000; Snead & Davis, 2002; Wada et al., 2004). Wong et al. (2004) concluded that the type and severity of the disability are major determinants in the choice to become involved with a PWD. Miller et al. (2009) found that college students were willing to have friendships and acquaintanceships with PWDs and also willing to date PWDs; however, they were least willing to marry or have a partnership with PWDs, especially with those having a severe disability. Additionally, PWODs were more willing to become involved with persons with physical disabilities and least willing to engage with persons with psychological disabilities.

The Impact of Type of Disability

Antonak (1981) noted a hierarchy of stigma attached to disability; those with physical disabilities receive the least social stigma, and those with psychiatric disabilities receive the greatest stigma. Gordon et al. (2004) assessed attitudes regarding friendship and marital relationships with PWDs and concluded that the majority of students were more willing to be friends with persons with medical, physical, and sensory impairments but were less inclined to want friendships with persons with mental retardation and psychiatric illness; only 13% stated that they would marry someone with a psychiatric illness and 4% with mental retardation. In their study, Miller et al. (2009) found that college students were the least willing to marry or have a partnership with persons with cognitive or psychiatric disabilities. In a study of attitudes toward disability that looked at physical versus psychiatric disability, involvement in a sexual relationship was associated with more negative attitudes when the person had a psychiatric disability (Hasson-Ohayon et al., 2014).

The Impact of Severity of Disability

Taleporos and McCabe (2003) found that people who reported greater severity of disabilities as measured by level of independent functioning were less likely to have partners or to be married than those with less severe disabilities. Individuals with the most severe disabilities were also less likely to have partners and were less likely to be married than persons with less severe or no disabilities. Similarly, Miller et al. (2009) determined that the more severe the disability, the less willing PWODs were to engage in a relationship. While this finding is expected and distressing, they also found that the personal attributes of intelligence, kindness, and humor in PWDs were the most likely to overcome intimacy reluctance on the part of PWODs by increasing their reported willingness to enter into more intimate relationships with PWDs.

While not often seen in the rehabilitation literature, Vash and Crewe (2004, p. 97) noted that some persons are sexually attracted to amputees. While they term this as "unwholesome turns," they also note that there is some discussion regarding if such an attraction "empowers or exploits people with disabilities" (Vash & Crewe, 2004, p. 98). The notion of rejecting society's repulsion of a stump is powerful. Terming such an attraction as "sick" plays into the ever-present insistence that beauty is regulated by society. If, however, there is coercion, manipulation, or force used in the satisfaction of one person's desires, the health of the fantasy is a moot point because abuse is in place. In a 1998-documentary titled *My One-Legged Dream Lover*, Kath Duncan explores amputee fetishism (Duncan & Goggin, 2002) as having a limited number of researchers (Dixon, 1983; Kafer, 2000). The website ASCOT-World (www.ascotworld.com) is a disability and amputee support group and social club that contains a matchmaking online service that welcomes devotees (the term used for nondisabled persons who are attracted to persons with amputations).

The Impact of Types of Relationships

For a number of reasons, PWDs often have more difficulty forming friendships and finding partners for romantic relationships than PWODs (De Loach, 1994; Goldstein & Johnson, 1997; Howland & Rintala, 2001; Rintala et al., 1997). One reason revolves around the process of obtaining a mate, which generally progresses from an acquaintance relationship to friendship, courtship, romance, and finally to a long-term commitment. While most people seem willing to acknowledge and interact with PWDs on an acquaintance level, some studies have shown that many people are less willing to progress to dating and marriage.

A few studies have examined the attitudes of PWODs in relation to engaging in intimate relationships with PWDs. These studies have concluded that PWDs may have difficulty making friends, forming romantic relationships, and finding partners. For the most part, these studies are discouraging in that PWODs express a willingness to have casual relationships but are less willing to date or marry

PWDs (Miller et al., 2009). A recent large-scale study (n = 2208) surveying young adults in Australia and Hong Kong showed "considerable resistance towards dating PWD. . . .Male participants generally expressed less willingness than female participants towards dating PWD . . ." (Ip et al., 2022, p. 240).

In a survey of 1,013 students, Hergenrather and Rhodes (2007) found that females held more positive attitudes toward dating and marrying PWDs than did males. Measuring attitudes is important; however, attitudes do not necessarily translate into action. Despite more reported positive attitudes among females without disabilities, males with disabilities reported that WWODs were only interested in friendships. Likewise, WWDs believed that men made judgments not to date them based on devices such as wheelchairs and prosthetic devices.

Fear and discomfort may also play a role in persons' decisions related to intimacy with PWDs. Milligan and Neufeldt (1998) found that women were more willing to date men with spinal cord injury (SCI) if they had previously been in relationships with PWDs, suggesting that initial discomfort may be overcome with exposure. Another important factor in this study was the level of independence and adjustment of the male as being relevant to female willingness to consider partnering; those perceived as more adjusted were more desirable partners. Thus, not only does the PWOD need to work through discomfort and uncertainty but the PWD is more desirable if viewed as adjusted and more self-sufficient. In this study, other concerns of females about dating persons with SCI were reported as care giving, health concerns, restriction of activities and physical limitations, financial issues, and sexuality/conception issues.

Similarly, in a study examining the attitudes of 395 college students, Marini et al. (2011) found that 66% of students surveyed indicated that they would not have a problem dating someone in a wheelchair after having seen a photograph and reading a brief bio of the individual. Of the 33% who indicated that they would not be willing to become intimately involved with people in wheelchairs, the top-rated reasons included the perception of caretaking as being too much work, feeling awkward in not knowing what to say or how to treat them, believing the person would be sick too often, and believing that the PWDs could not be sexually satisfying. Those students who had had a previous close relationship with someone with a disability, however, were more likely to be open to having a more intimate relationship. The authors concluded that students with a past close disability relationship could separate societal myth and misconceptions regarding wheelchair users.

For many people, a committed and loving marriage is the ultimate goal. The ability of a relationship to withstand challenges will depend on the particular strengths of the couple both individually and as a pair. Couples who enter a relationship where disability is already a factor do so with at least some anticipation of the potential challenges they will face. However, when disability occurs after the establishment of a relationship, greater difficulties have statistically been supported, and divorce is more likely to occur (DeVivo & Richards, 1996). In a study examining divorce among PWDs, the onset of disability increased the likelihood of divorce if the PWD was the wife. Divorce rates did not increase if the PWD was the husband (Karraker & Latham, 2015).

Kreuter (2000) examined the relationships of 49 persons with SCI and concluded that those who were injured before the marriage had more stable marriages than those injured after marriage. Similarly, sexual satisfaction was reported as greater among couples where the marriage is postdisability (Crewe & Krause, 1988). In predisability marriage, when one partner became the caregiver of the other, there was a negative impact on the relationship, and when the partner with the disability was female, there was a greater, likelihood of divorce. Overall, divorce statistics for PWDs are high, and there is a lower rate of marriage among this population (DeVivo et al., 1995; Urey & Henggeler, 1987). DeVivo et al. (1995) examined over 600 recorded marriages among persons with SCI and found almost twice as many divorces as would be expected among nondisabled persons of the same age and gender. More recently, between 2009 and 2018, over a million PWDs were divorced. This was nearly twice as many as those who were married during those years. Comparatively, only a third of the people who were married without disabilities were divorced during this time frame (Kim, 2021). Unfortunately, these figures did not track the onset of the disability as occurring before or after marriage for those getting divorced.

DISABILITY TYPE AND SEXUAL ISSUES AND CONCERNS

Sexuality and Physical Disabilities

In a study to examine sexuality and quality of life, McCabe et al. (2000) reported that persons with congenital physical disabilities had low levels of sexual experience and knowledge and had negative feelings related to sexuality, but they had high sexual needs and desired to increase their sexual knowledge. In terms of sexual experiences, 12% had never romantically kissed or hugged anyone, nearly 30% had never held someone while naked, almost 40% had never engaged in sexual intercourse, and 60% were not currently having intercourse in a relationship. Their study determined that while sexuality was associated with quality of life, it was not associated with life satisfaction, making the point that, at least for their sample, sexuality and sexual experiences add an important and desired dimension to life but are not necessary for achieving satisfaction in life.

Shakespeare (2000) noted the social and financial difficulties related to establishing a sexual relationship as follows:

> It also helps to have someone to have sex with. Most people meet potential partners at college, at work, or in social spaces. Unfortunately, disabled people often don't get to go to college, or to work, or achieve access to public spaces because of physical and social barriers. Being sexual costs money. You need to buy clothes, to feel good about, and go places to feel good in. If you are poor, as 50% of disabled Americans are, then it is correspondingly harder to be sexual. More than money, being sexual demands self-esteem. It demands confidence, and the ability to communicate. (Shakespeare, 2000, p. 161)

Taleporos et al. (2002) point to the positive connection between sexuality variables and psychological well-being. In a study of 748 PWDs and 448 PWODs, they found that persons with higher self-esteem were more likely to be sexually satisfied and feel good about their bodies and their sexuality. However, because WWDs are frequently viewed as asexual (Di Giulio, 2003), little attention has been paid to their sexual functioning, creating barriers to sexual fulfillment faced by women. Stinson et al. (2002) found that due to negative stereotypes, women with developmental disabilities lacked access to gynecological healthcare, were given limited choices regarding reproductive issues, and had a lack of sex education. In addition, several social, psychological, and physical barriers prevent women from sexual expression and functioning (Christian et al., 2001; Westgren & Levi, 1999). In a qualitative study of adults with physical disabilities, Kattari (2014) found there was a lack of confidence among participants to bring up disability in sexual negotiations. Participants' previous attempts to discuss needs associated with their disability had resulted in their partners shutting down, being unsupportive, or exhibiting behaviors that hurt their feelings. Even participants who described their partners as open and validating around sexual topics struggled with self-esteem and lacked confidence to ask for their wants and needs to be met.

Vash and Crewe (2004) point to a number of physical issues related to sexual activity, including the effects of paralysis, pain, amputations, neurological impairments, and bowel and bladder dysfunction upon the ability to experience erotic sensation. In a study of 504 WWDs and 442 WWODs to compare sexual experiences, Nosek et al. (1997) reported that women with physical disabilities did not differ from WWODs in sexual desire, but they did find significantly lower levels of sexual activity, satisfaction, and response. The level of sexual activity among WWDs was predicted by living with a significantly positive attitude. Women who had a more positive self-image and viewed themselves as approachable reported higher sexual activity. Interestingly, the severity of their disability was not a factor in the level of sexual activity. Factors related to positive sexual response included having a positive attitude toward using assistive devices, higher income level, and less stereotypical concern. Greater sexual satisfaction was predicted by sexual activity and a more positive attitude about assistive devices.

Problems related to sexual functioning after SCI are reported as arousal, frequency of sexual activity, initiation, and enjoyment (Klebine, 2007; Kreuter et al., 1994). Two interesting qualitative studies conducted by Whipple et al. (1996) and Richards et al. (1997) reported that women with SCI initially dissociate themselves from their sexuality, believing that they can no longer experience sexual pleasure. Over time they may become ready to reintegrate sexuality into their lives. Men with SCI are more likely to report limited opportunity for sexual expression and are often unsatisfied with their sexual lives.

In a study to examine issues that negatively impact sexuality for men with SCI, Sakellarious (2006) identified the topics of *dependency, spread, body beautiful, social disapproval, personal assistance,* and *impairment* as barriers. Participants revealed that the frustration that comes from societal views of independence is more closely related to body performance rather than self-direction. Participants stated that others were more likely to see the wheelchair than the person in it. Like women, participants believed that they were being held to a standard of the socially prescribed beautiful body, which they could not attain, leading to "aesthetic anxiety." Practically, the need for a personal assistant was also noted as a barrier to sexual expression because privacy was limited in that attendants needed to undress, empty the bladder, and position the individual for them to participate in sexual activity. Physical impairment of bodily sensation also was noted as a barrier for some, as were financial resources and environmental barriers that limited accessibility.

Sexual Concerns and Learning Disability

Concerns related to the sexual function of persons with developmental disabilities differ greatly from those related to people with physical challenges and are frequently based on the capacity of the person to understand sexual functioning in terms of consequences and the rights of others. Szollos and McCabe (1995) noted that persons with intellectual disabilities frequently have misinformation related to sexual functioning. Staff members who care for persons with learning disabilities frequently experience discomfort with the sexual expression of such individuals. Double standards are commonplace in the beliefs related to sexuality and persons with learning disabilities. One study, for example, found that even persons opposed to abortion on moral grounds believe that it should be made available if the woman has a learning disability. Staff members were also found to frequently rely on personal judgments rather than facility policies when they felt a need to address sexual behaviors by residents. Many times this led to the cessation of normal sexual expression and interaction. At other times, staff members tolerated inappropriate behaviors or sexual harassment rather than deal appropriately with these behaviors (Parkes, 2006).

There are also concerns related to the sexual abuse of others that appears to occur with greater frequency among this population than the general population (Brown & Stein, 1997). In a study of mild and moderate learning disabilities to investigate how women experience their sexual lives, McCarthy (1998) reported that these women commonly find themselves engaged in sexual activity that is not to their liking and not of their choice and point to a lack of preparation of social service providers on how to deal with behaviors and events related to sexual abuse by and to people with developmental impairments (Brown & Turk, 1992; Brown et al., 1994).

Men with learning disabilities may present caregivers with a number of challenging behaviors, including the use of pornographic material, cross-dressing, prostitution, and pedophile tendencies. When looking at the sexual encounters of men and women with learning disabilities, it is interesting to note that women without learning disabilities do not engage in sexual contact with learning-disabled men, but men without disabilities do engage in sexual activity with both men and women with learning disabilities. Pornography is often gained through those sexual encounters and intended to create sexual vulnerability. Cross-dressing is problematic when theft of women's clothing takes place, when embarrassment or ridicule results, or when it results in abuse of the PWDs. Prostitution also renders men, like WWDs, vulnerable to sexual assault, sexually transmitted diseases, and exploitation. Men with disabilities may be offered goods and money for sex in public parks and toilets. Whereas WWDs tend to be at greater exploitation risk in treatment facilities, men are at greater risk in public areas. This type of exposure may lead to sadomasochistic sexual activities that can be adopted by the PWDs and then perpetrated on others. Finally, there is concern that men with learning disabilities may have pedophile tendencies. Generally, while this may be an accurate representation of some males with developmental disabilities, behaviors that indicate sexual interest in children seem to indicate developmental immaturity; identifying with and relating to children may be due to the neglect of their sexuality (Cambridge & Mellan, 2000).

Sexuality and Cognitive Disabilities

Cognitive impairments, such as those that occur as a result of a cerebrovascular accident (stroke) or a traumatic brain injury (TBI), can include physical impairments but typically include behavioral, emotional, and intellectual problems. According to the Centers for Disease Control and Prevention, there are about 1.5 million TBIs per year, and most occur in young males, with 85% occurring before the age of 25. Sexual dysfunction following brain injury is common and may include impotence, lack of ability to ejaculate, premature ejaculation, loss of sensation, diminished sexual libido, body image and sexual identity problems, decreased self-esteem, disturbing exhibitionist behaviors, sexual preoccupation, and masturbation (Ducharme, n.d.; Ducharme & Gill, 1990; O'Carroll et al., 1991).

Because the ability to regulate behaviors is diminished in persons with head injury, other behaviors may also emerge that are detrimental to satisfying sexual experiences. For example, persons with head injuries may be distracted during sexual activity, may talk incessantly or aimlessly, or may experience fatigue and confusion. Emotionally, persons with TBI may be lacking in emotional connection or sensitivity toward their partners and may exhibit self-centered behaviors, showing little regard for their partners' needs or desires. Treatment for sexual and other behavioral problems includes medications and behavioral therapy (Ducharme, n.d.).

Sexual Concerns and Psychiatric Illness

Intimate relationships among persons with serious mental illness (SMI) also differ from people in the general population in that there is generally less intimacy and less commitment in these relationships. They tend to have sex sooner and the relationships are for a shorter term. They are also more likely to have concurrent sexual relationships and report being less sexually satisfied in their sexual encounters (Perry & Wright, 2006). According to a review by Matevosyan (2009), "Women with SMI have more lifetime sex partners, low contraceptive usage, higher rates of unwanted pregnancies, and are at high risk for sexually transmitted infections" (p. 109). Of all the types of disability, psychiatric disabilities are the most stigmatized, and that contributes, along with lower income and fewer social opportunities, to these persons pairing with other persons who are also less socially accepted. According to Perry and White (2006),

> People with serious mental illness are often forced to try to meet their sexual needs or forge a relationship with other "social undesirables." In short, they seem to take what they can get in terms of where, when, and with whom to have sex. This not only results in relationships that are less satisfying, less intimate, and much shorter lived, but also increases HIV risk by concentrating sexual activity within high-risk populations like IV drug users, sex workers, and others with serious mental illness. (Perry & Wright, 2006, p. 180)

In general, people with mental illness do not use safe sex practices, report lack of satisfaction with their sexual and social lives, and lack a sense of intimacy in relationships. Consumers who live in residential care settings also lack privacy. A number of barriers exist to fulfilling sexual activity in residential settings, including policies that require shared rooms, no sexual activity, frequent histories of sexual abuse, social stigmatization, low self-esteem, medications that interfere with desire and function, intrusive symptoms, social skill deficits, and a lack of support and education related to sexual expression and activity (Cook, 2000).

In an overview of sexuality and psychiatric disabilities, Knoepfler discusses differences in sexual functioning, noting that persons with depression are likely to show little sexual desire, as opposed to persons with manic disorders who may exhibit rapid transitions in desire and rapid escalation. Knoepfler states that persons with personality disorders are varied but "tend to act in impulsive ways disregarding consequences" (Knoepfler, 1991, p. 214) and that persons with schizophrenia, who experience an inability to distinguish between fantasy and reality, may imagine or engage in bizarre sexual behaviors (Knoepfler, 1991). As there are different types of schizophrenia, this characterization is likely true for only a small portion of individuals with the disorder; however, one contribution of this work is that it makes clear that it is important to consider the effects of specific diagnoses on sexuality to avoid the trap of stereotyping individuals in terms of sexual needs, desires, and behaviors.

In a study specific to understanding sexuality among persons with schizophrenia, Volman and Landeen (2007) studied five women and five men with schizophrenia. They found that participants did form and maintain intimate relationships. They viewed their sexuality as one of the factors that made them the same as persons without mental illness. They considered their sexuality as part of their well-being and essential in their lives. Sexuality was viewed as physical and emotional and more meaningful when sex was within the context of an intimate relationship. However, all the participants felt that the symptoms of their illnesses and effects of the medications had a strong impact on their sexuality and compromised their view of themselves, sexual functioning, and ability to have intimate relationships. They noted problems with hearing voices, weight gain, difficulty with achieving orgasm, and decline in libido. Participants also discussed the effects of social stigma that resulted in being judged and rejected, delaying the age of sexual knowledge and experience until much later in life. Finally, strategies that helped participants were identified as using counseling, medical compliance, positive self-talk, and engaging in a healthy lifestyle. However, talking about sex was identified as causing shame and embarrassment, often leading to not bringing up important concerns with clinicians.

Sexual Concerns and Chronic Health Conditions

For persons with chronic health conditions, physical limitations and pain as well as emotional state may affect sexuality. Persons need to be able to communicate changes in sexuality, including interest, a need for different types of sexual stimulation, and altered positioning and activities. Body pain may have a direct influence on sexual activity and persons may need to make adjustments, such as interrupting sexual activity multiple times to deal with pain or wait for it to subside. This may lead to avoidance of sex with a partner and feelings of grief over the loss and fear of impotency. Partners may feel unloved, angry, and resentful. They may also feel guilty for diminished empathy and causing pain to their partners. Pain management, sexual preferences, and alternatives that consider religious, cultural, and personal beliefs may be assistive, along with couples' therapy (Claiborne & Rizzo, 2006). In a study to examine the impact of gynecological cancer on marriage and levels of loneliness, Kömürcü et al. (2015) found nearly 80% of the patients reported their sexual lives changed and almost half the patients stated they felt lonely. Approximately 60% felt their husbands were less supportive and half believed they were in need of psychological support.

Other chronic health conditions are HIV and AIDS. For this population, most of the literature focuses on the prevention of infecting others through abstinence or the use of condoms. In a study of over 2,000 men who had sex with men, 40% were found to engage in unprotected anal sex with a person of unknown HIV status (Golden et al., 2004). While much of the sexuality literature for persons with other disabilities focuses on assisting persons to engage in healthy sexual behaviors, little is written for persons who are HIV positive. Not only do they need to focus on not infecting others but also they must protect themselves from acquiring new strains of the virus or other sexually transmitted diseases (STDs), placing them at greater health risk. In addition, persons who are HIV positive will have concerns related to telling partners, anger if they believe their partners transmitted the disease to them, and fear or guilt if they have transmitted the disease to their partners (HIV InSite, 2005). For women who are HIV positive and become pregnant, the risk of the child contracting HIV is about 25% if precautions are taken and considerably less with appropriate use of medication. Because vaginal delivery and breastfeeding increase the risk of contraction, these are avoided for HIV-positive women. Couples who wish to have biological children risk infection of one another (if one partner is not seropositive) and the child. The risk may be reduced by minimizing the number of unprotected sexual interactions through only engaging in unprotected sex at the point of ovulation. Another method is to use intrauterine insemination after washing the sperm free of HIV (Gilling-Smith, 2000).

SEXUAL ORIENTATION, SEXUAL FUNCTIONING, PROCREATION, AND PARENTING

Sexual Orientation and People With Disabilities

Kline (1991) referred to sexual orientation as encompassing heterosexual, bisexual, and homosexual relations. There are also numerous persons who do not engage in sexual activity who are referred to as nonsexual and persons who have a lack of any sexual orientation referred to as asexual. Kline also distinguishes sexual orientation from gender identity that includes a psychological self-connection to a gender, to both genders, or to neither. *Transgendered* refers to persons who identify with the opposite gender. *Transsexuals* have received sexual reassignment procedures to physically change their biological identity, and *transvestites* utilize clothing and makeup to identify with the opposite gender.

In 2021, the U.S. Census Bureau collected data for the first time on sexual orientation within households in the Household Pulse Survey, finding that approximately 8% of adults identified as gay, lesbian, bisexual, or transgender. Another 2% identified as "other," which may include asexual or pansexual (gender-blind) identification (U.S. Census Bureau, 2021). Nosek et al. (1997) examined sexual orientation of women with physical disabilities and found that 87% of the women with SCI were attracted to men, 4% were attracted to women, 7% to both men and women, and 2% were not attracted to either gender. McCabe et al. (2000) found that 16% of their sample of PWDs reported at least one same-sex experience and about 5% reported frequent same-sex activity.

Studies related to the cumulative effect of belonging to more than one stigmatized minority status are scant, but it can be assumed that negotiating living with a combination of racial minority status, disability, and gender identity issues might enhance marginalization. Persons with disabilities who identify as LGBTQ may struggle with numerous stigmatized identities and face discrimination, bullying, and rejection from the able-bodied and disability communities and heterosexual and LGBTQ communities (Santinele-Martino, 2017). Rembis (2010) examined persons who were disabled and identified as lesbian and noted acceptance resistance from both the lesbian and the disability communities. In their review of the literature related to the challenges of lesbians with disabilities, Vaughn et al. (2015) noted *concealing* disability and sexual orientation and *controlling* who is told about invisible disability and sexual orientation are implemented to manage stigma. "Because of the stigma experienced as a person with a disability and as a lesbian, many women try to hide their sexual identity until they feel safe enough to disclose and if at all possible, they hide their disability identity for as long as possible to avoid being ostracized" (p. 53).

Sexual Functioning

Overall, sexual functioning is important to PWDs, but sexual dysfunction is far more prevalent. In a study of 681 persons with SCI, return to sexual functioning was listed as the top personal priority for persons with paraplegia. It was the second priority for persons with tetraplegia, with only the desire for recovery of arm or hand function superseding sexual recovery desire (Anderson, 2004). For women with SCI, Jackson and Wadley (1999) found an overall substantial decrease in sexual activity following injury. However, over time, participation increased from 49% 1 year after injury to 76% after 10 years.

Sexual dysfunction among couples in the general population is about 13% compared with 40% of persons with chronic diseases and 73% for persons with multiple sclerosis (MS; Zorzon et al., 1999). Sexual functioning for most WWDs is generally not physiologically impaired, but depending on the type and extent of the disability, a number of concerns may need attention. For women with injury in the spinal cord, sexual dysfunction is most often related to a lack of desire to engage in sexual activity and may be more of an emotional and psychological problem than a physiological one. Initial concerns may be related to sexual satisfaction, exploration, and arousal. Individuals and couples may or may not need to try different methods for achieving sexual pleasures. Sexual arousal is both an emotional and physical response that may occur through any of the senses. Arousal can be achieved through the stimulation of any body part, including not only the clitoris and vagina but also breasts, mouth, ears, and feet. A willingness to explore options and discuss body pleasure and sensations will be mutually beneficial.

A number of physiological issues are also of concern for women with SCI, including bladder management, bowel management, autonomic dysreflexia (AD), and spastic hypertonia. Bladder and bowel accidents can be minimized or avoided through management of food and fluid intake and establishing a consistent routine for emptying the bladder and bowel. For women with catheterization, the bladder can be emptied prior to sexual activity. Depending on the type of catheter, the catheter can be removed or partially removed, and the tubing may be fastened down with tape to avoid kinking or accidental removal. AD is a life-threatening condition that may be of concern for individuals with SCI. While laboratory studies have not shown AD to be induced by sexual activity, an onset of multiple symptoms (rise in blood pressure, irregular heartbeat, fever, face flushing, chills, headaches, blurred vision, nasal congestion, and sweating) would require ceasing sexual activity and seeking medical assistance or advice (Spinal Cord Injury Information Network, 2007).

Males with SCI experience both emotional and physiological changes associated with their sexuality and sexual performance. In the general population, men experience psychogenic erection due to psychological arousal (sexual thoughts or visual or auditory stimuli) and reflex erections due to physical contact. For men with SCI, depending on the level and completeness of injury, impairment may occur to one or both of these functions. Men with low-level injuries may retain psychogenic arousal, but higher-level injuries will result in impairment of this function. However, most men with SCI can achieve reflex erections (unless the S2–S4 nerve pathways are damaged). Also, erectile dysfunction (ED) is not uncommon among men with SCI in that they may not be able to sustain an erection that is sufficient to meet couples' desires. ED can be treated through medication or a variety of alternative treatments. Oral medication consists of phosphodiesterase inhibitors, such as sildenafil (Viagra) or tadalafil (Cialis), that increase blood flow into the penis. Risks of engaging in sex can include priapism (prolonged erection) that can be very painful because the blood fails to drain from the penis and can lead to permanent damage to the ability to have erections, and any onset of symptoms must be medically attended to immediately. Alternative treatments include injections directly into the side of the penis that produce erections that last several hours, placement of a pellet into the urethra (medicated urethral system erection [MUSE]), and the use of a hand- or battery-operated cylinder vacuum pump that pulls blood into the penis that is then constricted with a band (Spinal Cord Injury Information Network, 2007). A number of sex and masturbation products are available through Disabilities-R-Us (http://disabilities-r-us.com), a support and resource website created by PWDs. Another type of assistive treatment involves surgical implantation of a penile prosthesis of variable firmnesses or inflatable devices.

Similar physiological concerns (altered libido, bladder and bowel dysfunction, and spasticity) are present for persons with MS that has an onset between 20 and 40 years of age and is twice as common in women as in men (van den Noort & Holland, 1999). For women, decreased vaginal lubrication, impaired ability to masturbate, genital numbness, fatigue, depression, and decreased self-esteem are also of concern (Foley & Sanders, 1997); physical symptoms may be reduced through the use of vibrators, lubricants, and medication to reduce nerve pain. Christopherson et al. (2006) reported that educational materials are also beneficial in diminishing sexual difficulties for partners but recommend additional counseling for relaxation and positioning as well as dealing with pain and depression. For all persons with neurological impairments, body mapping may be a useful technique because it involves discovery and mapping of the body parts that receive sensory pleasure, those that involve discomfort, and those that are neutral. This mapping identifies body areas that experience arousal and those that need to be avoided or protected (Matthews, 2009).

Fertility

Fertility issues for men deal primarily with issues of achieving ejaculation and collecting healthy sperm. Because the quality of sperm generally declines following SCI, the collection of sperm within a week of the injury may prove important for men who wish to father biological children. After that time sperm quality may not be sufficient for the production of children. Additionally, most men with SCI are unable to reach ejaculation, and the collection of sperm may need to be assisted through the use of penile vibratory stimulation (PVS), which utilizes a vibrator designed to provoke ejaculation. Semen is collected and processed in a medical setting to reduce the risk of AD. Other methods of collecting semen include electroejaculation, which applies electrical stimulation through the anus and induces the release of semen; prostrate massage, which applies pressure and massage to the prostate gland; and surgical removal of sperm, which is both costly and the least effective method of viable sperm collection (Brackett et al., 2010).

For women with SCI, menstruation may cease at the onset of injury, but for the majority of women it resumes within 6 months. Becoming pregnant and giving birth are generally not impaired, and birth control is resumed for women who are sexually active. Jackson and Wadley (1999) found that sexually active women with SCI showed a decrease in the use of birth control pills and an increase in elected sterilization and condom use.

Reproductive Choice

"Reproductive health implies that people are able to have a responsible, satisfying, and safe sex life and that they have the capability to have children and the freedom to decide if, when, and how often to do so" (WHO, 2010b, para. 2). Public controversy over the right of some persons with disabilities to marry stems largely from concerns related to the upbringing of children that may result from that union. Influenced by the eugenics movement in the early 1900s, tens of thousands of persons with cognitive disabilities were institutionalized and prohibited from sexual relations until, in the 1920s, the cost of segregating and overseeing such large numbers became prohibitive, and sterilization was implemented as a means of ultimately extracting "feeble-mindedness" from society (Block, 2000). In order to control reproduction among persons with disabilities, nearly 30 U.S. states passed laws that permitted involuntary sterilization of people with disabilities (Silver, 2004), resulting in the forced and indiscriminate sterilization of approximately 60,000 PWDs, in particular adolescents who reached the age of sexual maturation (Reilly, 1991).

Sterilization has become more restrictive and regulated by federal rules and state laws. Consideration is also given to several ethical issues and revolves around the rights of the individual to be sexually active, to be expressive, and to procreate that are weighed against the rights of the unborn child to receive adequate care (American Academy of Pediatrics, 1999). Although sterilization is still used as a parenting deterrent, fewer physicians are willing to conduct sterilization without a court mandate (Block, 2000). However, forced sterilization is allowed in most states, and laws permitting forced sterilization are present in 31 states and Washington, DC (National Women's Law Center, 2022).

Parenting

Historically, the right to reproduce and become a parent has been violated for PWDs. Systematic and persistent discrimination of parents with disabilities in family law, child welfare, and adoption and foster systems is well established (Callow et al., 2011). For PWDs, creating families has not kept pace with progress in other arenas of disability rights and community participation. Parents with disabilities have more difficulty adopting children, gaining access to reproductive health care, and are more likely to lose child custody in the case of a divorce (Powell, 2014). Accessible services within the child welfare system have also been identified as barriers to parents with disabilities maintaining their parental rights. (Albert & Powell, 2021; Powell & Parish, 2017). Indeed, parenting has been deemed the last frontier in disability rights (Kirshbaum, 2002; Kirshbaum & Olkin, 2002). In her article, O'Toole (2002) states that although little research has explored parenting and PWDs, many WWDs are successful parents despite societal barriers and a lack of sex education, expectations of celibacy, social views of PWDs as undesirable partners, sterilization, high rates of divorce at disability onset for married women, and removal of child custody from WWDs.

Termination of parental rights and child welfare system involvement are higher for PWDs, particularly intellectual and psychiatric disabilities (e.g., DeZelar & Lightfoot, 2018; Kaplan et al., 2019; LaLiberte et al., 2017; Lightfoot & DeZelar, 2016). According to Powell (2014) "Parents with disabilities are the only distinct community of Americans who must struggle to retain – or even gain in some situations – custody of their children" (p. 15). The rate of child removal from parents with psychiatric disabilities is as high as 70% to 80%. Removal rates for parents with intellectual disabilities is between 40% and 80%, and the removal rate for those parents with physical disabilities is 13%. Parents with disabilities, especially in cases where the other parent does not have a disability, are commonly denied visitation and custodial rights (Breeden et al., 2008; Economou, 2016; Lanci, 2018; Powell, 2019).

The 2012 National Council on Disability (NCD, 2021) issued a groundbreaking policy study that displayed the pervasive discrimination faced by parents with disabilities in the court systems in a call to reform state and federal legislation. At the time, in every state, disability was a consideration in family and child dependency court, and two-thirds of states allowed parents to be deemed unfit based solely on the basis of the parent's disability and could terminate parental rights. In several states, physical disability is allowed to be the sole grounds for terminating parental rights even without evidence of abuse or neglect. While some states have amended or adopted such prejudicial legislation, many state laws remain unchanged. Advocacy and legislative reform of bias laws remain a urgent need for the rights of parents with disabilities in creating and maintaining families (NCD, 2012).

Societal concerns for parenting by PWDs are based on physical ability and cognitive capacity concerns. The decision to become a parent for a person who has a physical impairment and limitations was examined by McNary (1999). Her interviews revealed that the parenting decision was influenced by a number of concerns related to physical considerations, such as having the stamina and energy to raise children and the emotional and financial effect of their disability on their children. Physically, they wondered about their ability to perform childcare tasks, particularly if they ". . . ended up in a wheelchair" (McNary, 1999, p. 99). They also worried about the safety of their children and their ability to sufficiently respond when necessary. Despite these concerns, participants revealed significant determination and belief in their ability to manage; as one participant stated, "I can conquer it. . . . I'm not going to let it stop me from doing something that I have wanted all my life" (McNary, 1999, p. 98).

In the United States, approximately 10% of parents have disabilities. These 4.1 million parents make up 6.2% of parents with children under the age of 18. Among parents with disabilities, 2.8% are mobility impaired, 2.3% cognitively impaired, 2.3% have a daily activity limitation, 1.4% have a hearing impairment, and 1.2% have a visual impairment. Due to scant research on the prevalence and classification of parents with disabilities, the number of parents with disabilities is likely significantly underestimated (NCD, 2012).

In a study to examine the outcomes of children raised by mothers who had intellectual impairment, Powell and Parish (2017) noted the children had poor cognitive and behavioral outcomes when compared to children whose mothers were not intellectually impaired. However, "families headed by mothers with intellectual impairments experienced multiple hardships related to socioeconomic factors, limited social supports and poor self-reported health" (p. 50). The authors conclude effective policies and programs needed to be implemented to support child development as well as assist with financial impediments.

A number of changes have taken place that give recognition to the idea that parenting problems for PWDS are more likely related to lack of services and supports, low income, and knowledge deficits than to the abilities of PWDs to raise a child who is physically, intellectually, and emotionally healthy.

Growing research shows beneficial outcomes for parents with disabilities who receive parental skills training. Wade et al. concluded that "home-based behavioral parent training leads to successful learning of parenting skills among parents with intellectual disability" (2008, p. 362). A randomized control study of 85 parents with mild intellectual disabilities in the Netherlands found that video feedback intervention of parental sensitivity and responsiveness reduced parental stress (Hodes et al. 2017). Self-determination practices and parental interventions also benefit parents with intellectual disabilities (Knowles et al., 2017). Contextual and skills-based interventions for parents with disabilities can provide support to this community, which has historically been lacking in support in the broader community.

Legislative changes related to disability and parenting have included the removal of discriminatory language from legal proceedings related to child custody, parent rights, adoption, and divorce (Callow et al., 2008). However, discriminatory legislation toward parents with disabilities continues to be a significant barrier to disability rights. Three identified barriers in protecting parents with disabilities have been labeled as (a) legislators' pejorative attitudes toward parents with disabilities, (b) external opposition, and (c) legislative barriers (Albert et al., 2022). Several websites provide resources, support, and advocacy information are now available to provide parents with disabilities with support and information, such as the National Research Center for Parents with Disabilities. The International Association for the Scientific Study of Intellectual and Developmental Disabilities (IASSIDD), Special Interest Research Group (SIRG) on Parents and Parenting with Intellectual Disabilities promotes research, support, and networking for parents with intellectual disabilities.

SEX EDUCATION, SEX THERAPY, SEXUAL SURROGATES, AND SELECTIVE ABORTION

Sex education is not a one-time event that occurs in the early schooling years, but rather a continued process of learning about physical, emotional, and psychological sexual interactions and functions. When changes to the body and psyche occur due to disability, aging, or other significant events, there is frequently a need for additional learning related to sexuality issues. Unfortunately, sex is an uncomfortable topic for many people, including health professionals and caregivers. Health providers may assume counselors are addressing the topic, and counselors believe these needs are being addressed by health workers.

Although sex education is a part of the curriculum in many schools, children and adolescents with disabilities are sometimes excluded (Barnard-Brak et al., 2014). This is problematic in that they also receive less information about sex and sexuality from peers and family (Schmidt et al., 2020; Wilson & Frawley, 2016). A lack of information leaves them vulnerable to sexually transmitted infections and unintended pregnancy and sexual abuse (Barnard-Brak et al., 2014; Streur et al., 2020; Treacy et al., 2018). Among cancer patients, only between 17% and 23% reported that sexuality concerns were addressed. However, 67% of men and 39% of women felt it was important to discuss sexuality. They wanted to be asked about their sex lives and wished for information on body image, libido, fertility, and general well-being (Southard & Keller, 2009).

Lack of knowledge about sexuality and sex has been reported about a number of disabilities and is reflective of the need for more sex education. Little sexual knowledge has been reported for persons with physical and intellectual disabilities (McCabe, 1999). In a qualitative study to examine sex education among youth with physical disabilities, East and Orchard (2014) found a "tendency for parents, educators and health professionals to place the responsibility of delivering sex education to young people with physical disabilities on someone else who they believe to be more appropriately qualified to handle these types of situations" (p. 335). This resulted in adolescents lacking in a comprehensive understanding regarding their sexual capacities and as well as insufficient information to make informed decisions about intimate relationships and sexual health. Simlarly, Sawin et al. (2002) found 29% of teenagers with spina bifida reported no one had ever discussed sex with them.

For persons with intellectual disabilities, there are a number of concerns related to education. One fear is that talking about sexual issues will encourage inappropriate sexual behaviors. This has led parents and schools to avoid conversations related to sex. Another issue centers around the feelings of the person; it is anticipated that talk about sexual issues will lead to distress or embarrassment, that it may be intrusive, or that some PWDs may not be able to give consent, or there is not sufficient benefit for the PWD (Bryen, 2016; Stein & Dillenburger, 2017). Even researchers hesitate to conduct research to examine sexuality because they fear they may cause some type of emotional damage (McCarthy, 1998) or that they may be accused of sexual abuse by the participant (Brown & Thompson, 1997). In their study to examine college students' with learning disabilities reactions to sexuality research, Thomas and Kroese (2005) found that while a few participants were embarrassed, the majority of participants showed no embarrassment or distress, and no inappropriate behaviors were apparent. In fact, several students reported positive affects related to having the opportunity to talk about sex.

Probably one of the most controversial topics for PWDs is the use of sex therapy, sex coaches, and sex surrogates. Sex therapy is generally a short-term psychotherapy that centers around issues of sexual intimacy, feelings, and functioning provided by licensed therapists who may be certified through the American Association of Sexuality Educators, Counselors, and Therapists (ASSECT). PWDs might receive sex therapy for a number of issues related to sexual desire, arousal, functioning (anorgasmia, premature ejaculation, and dyspareunia), or intimacy problems associated with disability (Mayo Clinic, 2010).

From the standpoint that sexuality and sexual expression are human rights, Shapiro (2002) argues that sexual surrogacy is an appropriate means of sexual gratification for PWDs and an opportunity not only to be sexual but also to reclaim their bodies.

> Simply put, sexual surrogacy is not prostitution nor is it simply gratification in its most vulgar meaning. Sexual surrogacy is a therapeutic process which attempts to have the patient begin a dialogue with their own body in a meaningful way, transcend simple gratification. (Shapiro, 2002, New Thinking and Approaches, para. 1)

Shapiro further believes that surrogacy should be government supported as a "therapeutic mechanism in the on-going rehabilitation of persons with disabilities" (Shapiro, 2002, Introduction Section, para. 5).

In a brief description on Disaboom (www.disaboom.com), an information website for persons with disabilities, Fulbright (n.d.) lists the advantages of working with a sexual surrogate as overcoming a sexual disorder, gaining self-confidence, and developing skills and attitudes for healthy sexual functioning and well-being. According to the International Professional Surrogates Association (IPSA, n.d.-a):

> In this therapy, a client, a therapist and a surrogate partner form a three-person therapeutic team. The surrogate participates with the client in structured and unstructured experiences that are designed to build client self-awareness and skills in the areas of physical and emotional intimacy. These therapeutic experiences include partner work in relaxation, effective communication, sensual and sexual touching, and social skills training. Each program is designed to increase the client's knowledge, skills, and comfort. As the days pass, clients find themselves becoming more relaxed, more open to feelings, and more comfortable with physical and emotional intimacy. The involvement of the team therapist, a licensed and/or certified professional with an advanced degree, is a cornerstone of this therapy process. (para. 1)

A number of disadvantages exist, including access outside of the states of Florida, California, New York, and Pennsylvania. Due to legal and ethical concerns, many surrogates keep their practice secret. Also, sex workers may falsely present themselves as surrogates (Fulbright, n.d.). The cost of this service is prohibitive for many PWDs. While individual session cost is said to mimic local therapist charges, the cost of intensive therapy for 1 or 2 weeks would range from $4,000 to $8,000 (IPSA, n.d.-b).

A final topic of controversy regarding disability and sexuality has to do with genetic testing, therapeutic abortion, and embryonic selection. In 1996, Glover and Glover explored the legal and ethical issues of postviability abortions for fetuses who were found to have DS. They concluded, "Although viability is a strong legal and moral consideration for a presumably healthy fetus, it does not appear to be so for a fetus who has Down syndrome. Such inconsistencies strongly test ethical principles because society has chosen to erect a legal double standard of unequal treatment that is fundamentally discriminatory and constitutionally impermissible" (p. 213). A decade later, Adrianne Asch (2003) wrote, "Is it possible for the same society to espouse the goals of including people with disabilities as fully equal and participating members and simultaneously promoting the use of embryo selection and selective abortion to prevent the births of those who would live with disabilities?" (p. 315).

Both preimplantation and prenatal screening can allow prospective parents to decide which embryo to bring to term. Research suggests 60% to 90% of positive screens for DS result in abortion of the fetus (Natoli et al. 2012). Similarly, embryos that are determined to carry a deficient genetic makeup are discarded routinely. While there is heated controversy surrounding trait-based selection (gender, eye color, etc.), selecting against disability is generally accepted. Those who oppose argue:

- Selection against disability suggests persons with disabilities are unworthy of being born.
- Encourages intolerance of human variation.
- Selective termination is based on misinformation and myths about the experience of living with a disability.
- Selective termination is based on a single trait and does not take into account the whole of a human being. (Ouellette, 2015)

At the opposite end of the spectrum is the practice of selection for disability. If selective termination against disability carries ethical concern, what of those individuals who seek a child with a disability? Philosopher Melissa Seymour Fahmy (2011) examines the ethics of Deaf parents using preimplantation genetic diagnosis to select for deaf children. While most persons consider deafness a disability, in the Deaf culture, it is not viewed as a negative attribute. Fahmy considers the central questions of harm to the child, the child's right to an open future, the introduction of avoidable suffering and/or limited opportunity, and parental and civic responsibility. She concludes, "The lesson to be learned from the deaf case is that we need norms that govern not just the use of reproductive technology, but procreation and procreative decision-making in all of its various forms" (p. 1467).

SEXUAL ABUSE OF PERSONS WITH DISABILITIES

Frequency of Sexual Abuse

A limited number of studies have attempted to estimate the prevalence of abuse against PWDs. In a recent study of 187 college students with disabilities examining sexual victimization, Holloway et al. (2022) used an online survey and determined 71% of the sample reported one or more incidences of lifetime sexual assault and/or rape, and 51% indicated sexual victimization since their attendance at the university. Lund and Vaughn-Jensen (2012) conducted a meta-analysis of victimization studies of PWDs and determined children with disabilities are 2.9 times more likely to be sexually abused than children without disabilities. Similarly in a study of approximately 9,000 women and 7,000 men, women with disabilities were at greater risk of rape, and men with disabilities were at greater risk of being forced to penetrate a perpetrator. (Basile et al., 2016). Similarly, a recent meta-analysis revealed PWDs are twice as likely to be sexually victimized during their lifetimes when compared to PWODs. The highest victimization rates were found for persons who are blind (Mailhot Amborski, et al., 2022).

Children with mental health and intellectual disabilities are at even greater risk and are 4.6 times more likely to be sexually abused as children without disabilities. According to Smith and Harrell (2013):

> *...sexual abuse of children with disabilities has not garnered the attention of policymakers, practitioners, advocates, or community members. These children are also less likely to receive victim services and supports that are more readily available to other victims because of a variety of factors including barriers to reporting and a lack of responses tailored to meet their unique needs. Without receiving support, these children suffer serious long-term aftereffects, including post-traumatic stress disorder, anxiety, and depression, as well as an increased risk of victimization in adulthood.* (p. 102)

Sobsey (1994) estimated that WWDs are raped at least one and a half times more often than women in the general population. WWDs, like WWODs, are most frequently assaulted by a familiar person, in a familiar place, such as at home or at work (Andrews & Veronen, 1993). In reviewing the prevalence of abuse, it is apparent that the less likely a person is to defend oneself, either physically or psychologically, the greater is the chance of being abused. The less credible they are considered, such as those with cognitive or physiological impairments, the more they are likely to be abused and the less likely they are to prosecute. Several studies have found that prosecution of cases of sexual abuse for victims with cognitive impairment is only between 5% and 9% (Brown et al., 1995; Mansell, 1995).

Among persons with developmental disabilities, sexual abuse is particularly high. Civjan (2000) found a rate of sexual abuse among women with developmental disabilities of 83%, and Wilson and Brewer (1992) found that women with developmental disabilities were 10.7 times more likely to have been sexually assaulted than WWODs. Brown et al. (1995) noted that victims ranged from profoundly to mildly disabled but that most (61%) fell into the severe-to-moderate (IQ 21–50) categories. Interestingly, among this disability group, males and females were equally likely to be abused, but almost all of the perpetrators were male and known to the victim. Several studies have noted that only 2% to 3% of perpetrations are committed by persons unknown to victims with mental retardation (Brown et al., 1995; Furey, 1994); 53% of identified perpetrators of sexual abuse against persons with developmental disabilities were other consumers, and 20% of perpetrators were identified as staff/volunteers (Brown et al., 1995).

Institutionalization also increases the risk of abuse. Sobsey and Mansell (1990) found that the risk of sexual abuse among persons living in institutional settings was two to four times higher than for those living in the community. Perpetrators who are staff members may use threats or bribes (Andrews & Veronen, 1993) or may sexually victimize persons while they are unconscious, medicated, or restrained (Musick, 1984), and the risk of exposure to multiple offenders is increased by high turnover rates due to low wages and minimal employee screening.

Persons who have sensory impairments are also sexually abused at high rates. Welbourne et al. (1983) reported that among women who were blind from birth, 50% had been sexually abused. However, studies of persons with sensory impairment are scarce and tend to be limited to clinical populations that are not generalizable to the general population. Another study found that the overwhelming majority of deaf children and adolescents admitted to a psychiatric facility had histories of sexual abuse (Willis & Vernon, 2002).

The rate of sexual abuse of women with physical disabilities is similar to that of women without disabilities (Young et.al, 1997), but Nosek et al. (2001) concluded that these abusive relationships tend to continue for longer durations. Unlike other disabilities, much of the research conducted with women with substance abuse disabilities examines abuse that occurred prior to the onset of the disability. Abusive histories have been found to be prevalent among the majority of women in treatment for chemical dependency (Glover et al., 1996; Wadsworth et al., 1995) and believed by many researchers to be a contribution to the onset of chemical dependence.

The Dynamics of Abuse Against Women With Disabilities

Sexual abuse is motivated by a need for feeling of power and control, and it is frequently maintained by manipulation, coercion, and threats. Most perpetrators share similar characteristics, including a need for immediate gratification, poor impulse control, and anger. Girls with disabilities may be particularly vulnerable to abuse because they are frequently unwelcome in social activities and have less exposure to social interaction. When they reach dating age, they may have confusion associated with their own needs and desires. Their desire to feel like "normal women" may lead to relationships that make them more susceptible to abuse. They may come to believe that their choices are limited to celibacy or sexually violent relationships and that they should be grateful for any sexual attention (Womendez & Schneiderman, 1991). Cattalini (1993) noted additional factors that may increase vulnerability to abuse as physical and emotional isolation from others, feelings of powerlessness, low resistance to bribery and coercion, sexual repression, little understanding of abuse, and poor self-protection skills. In a qualitative study of 72 women with physical and cognitive disabilities, Saxton et al. (2001) identified difficulties with personal boundaries, imbalances of power, and a sense of loyalty and obligation to service providers as interfering with the willingness to end or report the abuse, particularly if the perpetrator was a family member.

It is also important to note especially for women that the disability may have been caused by abuse. Over 2 million women are seriously assaulted by their male partners every year (Coble et al., 1992). Sobsey (1994) estimated that violence was a contributing factor to the cause of 10% to 25% of development disabilities. For women with violence-induced disability, it is important to consider who caused the disability and whether the perpetrator is now a caretaker (CALCASA, 2001).

Contributing Factors to Sexual Abuse

The sexual abuse of PWDs must be viewed within the framework of societal attitudes and structure. Historically, WWDs have been sexually regulated by society through forced sterilization, forced contraception, and forced pregnancy termination, and some physicians continue to recommend sterilization for WWDs but rarely suggest the same for males with similar disabilities (Beck-Massey, 1999).

The societal view that WWDs are asexual and roleless has further served to devalue and dehumanize WWDs, making it easier for caregivers and perpetrators to excuse abusive behaviors with the rationalization that WWDs do not understand perpetrated sexual acts as negative or even that they are helping their victim in some way. Additional stereotypical assumptions and stereotypes that contribute to the vulnerability of WWDs were outlined by Chenoweth (1993) as promiscuity, unattractive and grateful for attention, childlike, compliant, maternally inept, and insensitive to sexual trauma. These perceptions have led to a lack of sexual education, learned passivity, low reporting, exposure to multiple people without preventative measures, and low help-seeking.

The view that WWDs are asexual has also contributed to making WWDs with disabilities vulnerable because little to no attention is given to training women to recognizing potentially abusive situations, self-defense, or reporting abuse. Nosek (1996) found that vulnerability to abuse was increased through architectural barriers, inappropriate mobility aids, and exposure to medical and institutional settings because these limited the ability of PWDs to escape. Unfortunately, even exposure to disability services has been found to increase sexual abuse. Sobsey and Doe (1991) found that 44% of their sample of 162 PWDs who were sexually abused had perpetrators who gained access to them by way of disability services, including paid service providers, psychiatrists, and residential staff. They estimated that exposure to the disability service system increased the risk of sexual victimization by 78%.

In a review of the literature, Andrews and Veronen (1993) identified eight areas that contribute to greater vulnerability to abuse for WWDs, including (a) dependency on others for care, (b) perceptions of powerlessness, (c) lower risk of perpetrator discovery, (d) lower believability, (e) lack of appropriate and comprehensive sexual education for PWDs, (f) social isolation, (g) physical helplessness, and (h) mainstreaming without consideration for self-protection. They also concluded that sexual involvement with personal attendants was not uncommon. Other contributing factors to sexual vulnerability include the imbalance of power, difficulties in recognizing and reporting abuse, and the dynamics involved in using relatives and friends to provide services (Saxton et al., 2001).

When PWDs are abused, crisis intervention may include having an escape plan in place, a temporary stay at a confidential women's shelter, and making permanent plans to separate from the abuser (Nosek et al., 1997). Unfortunately, services such as those within the justice systems, women's shelters, and medical services can present barriers that inhibit access and participation. Barriers to acquiring assistance after violence is identified by the Center for Research on Women with Disabilities (CROWD) from WWD reports as including (a) they were not believed, (b) they were discriminated against, (c) transportation was not available, (d) referrals were inappropriate, and (e) services were inaccessible. Many existing programs and shelters frequently do not include alternative formats such as Braille, do not provide attendant care, and are not fully accessible.

Legislation and Trends

Originally enacted in 1994, the Violence Against Women Act (VAWA) was reauthorized in 1998 and in 2000 with new language that specifically includes WWDs, allocating millions of dollars for research and programming to enhance protection, strengthen education, and end violence and abuse (Whatley, 2000). It was again reauthorized in 2022 through fiscal year 2027 for "programs and activities under the Violence Against Women Act that seek to prevent and respond to domestic violence, sexual assault, dating violence, and stalking. The bill also authorizes new programs, makes changes to federal criminal laws, and establishes new protections to promote housing stability and economic security for victims . . ." (Congress.Gov, 2022, para. 1).

Included in the office funding stream are grant competitions related specifically to WWDs. In 1998, the Crime Victims with Disabilities Awareness Act was passed, which mandates that disability status needed to include information gathered from crime victims. Accurate data on the prevalence of crime and violence perpetrated against WWDs would strengthen calls for more services and supports.

For PWDs, current legislation issues related to sexuality are related to marriage penalties, child custody, and childcare. For PWDs, the decision to marry and cohabitate may be a costly one that they simply cannot afford because funding decisions are based on combined income. Marrying can cause Social Security benefits to be reduced or lost, and couples are at risk for losing Medicaid and personal assistant benefits. Couples who cannot afford to lose these benefits are put in the position of living together in secret, which will impact employer health benefit coverage (Fiduccia, 2000).

Issues of child rearing can be complicated by regulations related to personal assistance services. Only a few states include childcare as an activity of daily living, and that has profound implications for child care when there are functions related to children that cannot be provided by a parent with a disability. Many states prohibit personal assistants from providing childcare activities, which has implications for both childcare and child custody should the couple divorce (Fiduccia, 2000).

Finally, little attention has been paid to providing persons with physical impairment alternative self-defense strategies. Training has emerged in self-defense from the seated position while in a wheelchair and self-defense utilizing the wheelchair and mobility aids as weapons against would-be perpetrators. In addition, specific weapons training is also emerging for PWDs that takes into account the strength and mobility of PWDs (Madorsky, 1990; McNab, 2003). These trainings are available to PWDs through associations such as the International Disabled Self-Defense Association (www .nchpad.org/Directories/Organizations/2687/International~Disabled~Self-Defense~Association), and the National Rifle Association now lists adaptive shooting programs and resources on its website, stating:

> *The NRA Adaptive Shooting Program would like to showcase businesses offering gear, services, and training for people with disabilities while also providing a useful resource for the adaptive community. This project acknowledges the effort required to reimagine the traditional, open doors, and make the outdoors accessible.* (NRA Explore, 2022, para. 1)

CONCLUSION

Issues related to sex and sexuality for PWDs incorporate a number of important topics that can affect how PWDs view themselves and live their lives. This chapter discussed the social construction of gender identity and body image and the role that social construction plays in the sexual stigmatization and abuse of PWDs. Societal attitudes additionally play a role in self-esteem and body image for PWDs and affect their intimate partnering choices. Additionally, PWDs have a number of issues and concerns that are specific to the type and severity of their disability and may impact their sexual functioning, reproductive choices, and feeling about parenting.

CLASS ACTIVITIES

1. Ask students if any of them have held misconceptions about people with disabilities or believed any of the myths described in this chapter and if they are willing to share their thoughts before and after the reading the chapter.

2. Discuss the reasons that sexuality in relation to disability has largely been neglected and ignored by researchers, health professionals, and treatment providers.

3. Discuss the legal and ethical implications of controversial topics such as selective abortion based on disability, sexual surrogates for people with disabilities, forced sterilization of persons with disabilities, and cosmetic surgery for children with Down syndrome.

KEY REFERENCES

Only key references appear in the print edition. The full references appear in the digital product on Springer Publishing Connect™: https://connect.springerpub.com/content/book/978-0-8261-5111-7/part/partII/chapter/ch10

Albert, S. M., & Powell, R. M. (2021). Supporting disabled parents and their families: Perspectives and recommendations from parents, attorneys, and child welfare professionals. *Journal of Public Child Welfare*, *15*(5), 529–529. https://doi.org/10.1080/15548732.2020.1751771

Friedman, C. (2019). Intimate relationships of people with disabilities. *Inclusion*, *7*(1), 41–56. https://doi.org/10.1352/2326-6988-7.1.41

Hasson-Ohayon, I., Hertz, I., Vilchinsky, N., & Kravetz, S. (2014). Attitudes toward the sexuality of persons with physical versus psychiatric disabilities. *Rehabilitation Psychology*, *59*(2), 236–241. https://doi.org/10.1037/a0035916

Miller, E., Chen, R., Glover-Graf, N. M., & Kranz, P. (2009). Willingness to engage in personal relationships with persons with disabilities. *Rehabilitation Counseling Bulletin, 20,* 1–14. https://doi .org/10.1177/0034355209332719

Nosek, M. A., Foley, C. C., Hughes, R. B., & Howland, C. A. (2001). Vulnerabilities for abuse among women with disabilities. *Sexuality and Disability, 19,* 177–189. https://doi.org/10.1023/A:1013152530758

Vash, C. L., & Crewe, N. M. (2004). *The psychology of disability.* Springer Publishing Company.

CHAPTER 11

ABLEIST MICROAGGRESSIONS

DENIZ AYDEMIR-DÖKE

LEARNING OBJECTIVES

After reading this chapter, you will be able to:

- Define and identify different types of microaggressions and the different ways they are expressed
- Understand microaggressions and their relationship with ableism
- Identify the different domains of ableist microaggressions and how disabled people are impacted
- Understand the impact of microaggressions that occur in the counseling setting and how to intervene
- Explore different ways of responding to microaggressions

PRE-READING QUESTIONS

1. What are microaggressions? How are they different than overt discrimination? How are they similar?
2. Why do you think disability microaggressions might not be as obvious to nondisabled people as those stemming from other kinds of biases?
3. How might you interrupt a microaggression if you were to witness one?

"Ever since I started to go out on my own, I have had people not respect my personal space. I've always been grabbed. Any part of my body is up for being grabbed, stroked, pushed, pulled, and that includes my cane, mobility, or guide dog. Her body, her harness, and leash, whatever people can lay their hands on, they will grab it and tried to pull me around. I thought when the pandemic hit that would lessen, but that has not been the case at all. I am still grabbed. I am still yelled in the face. And when I asked people to stop, they always have an excuse like, 'Oh, I am trying to help.' Well, we still of social distance, and they just get very defensive. So, the sort of grabbing and being pulled around has not lessened at all, which [has] made going out very scary for me."

—A blind participant for a focus group study (Aydemir-Döke & Spencer, 2023)

DEFINITION OF MICROAGGRESSIONS

Microaggressions are the brief and usually unintentional daily slights and insults targeting oppressed identities such as race, disability, sexual orientation, and gender that communicate hostile, derogatory, or negative messages (Sue et al., 2007). Microaggressions give messages to the targets on inclusion/exclusion, inferiority/superiority, desirability/undesirability, and normality/abnormality. Targets may include racial minorities, people with disabilities, affectional and gender minorities, and women, who are on the margins of the social consciousness and desirability (Sue, 2010a). Those marginalized groups are disadvantaged in social, cultural, political, and economic systems; they are assigned to low status in society and have a negative image for the general public. Marginalization of those groups causes oppression where those groups experience systematic exclusion and injustice (Sue, 2010a).

After the civil rights movement, which highlighted the harmful effects of systemic marginalization, oppressive worldviews evolved into a more subtle way of expression (Sue, 2010a, 2010b). For example, racism evolved from overt expressions to covert, more implicit forms, which were defined as *aversive racism* (Gaertner & Dovidio, 2005). Aversive racists are the White people who genuinely support egalitarian values but also hold negative beliefs about Black and other racial minorities. Those people are uncomfortable around racial minorities and keep their interactions with minorities to a minimum. When they are engaging with racial minorities, they are preoccupied with wrongdoing. However, they express their negative beliefs in subtle and indirect ways (Gaertner & Dovidio 2005). Sue (2010a, 2010b) explained that microaggressions are conceptually close to aversive racism.

In the microaggression research, the focus can be on any minority group that has been oppressed and has been targeted with those unconscious insults because of overt racism, sexism, heterosexism, ableism, and so on. In the rest of this chapter, we will focus on microaggressions that are a direct result of ableism and experienced by disabled people.

WAYS OF EXPRESSING MICROAGGRESSIONS

Microaggressions can happen in different forms, including verbal, behavioral, and environmental (Sue et al., 2007). The common feature is that through words, actions, or environmental cues individuals are expressing their implicit bias related to disability by conveying views that disabled people are less valuable, less desirable, and outside of the "norm" as compared to nondisabled people. Examples of verbal microaggressions toward a disabled person may be: "I think you are faking it" or "How can a blind person find her way in this campus? Even I am losing my way all the time." An example of a behavioral microaggression would be avoiding eye contact with a disabled person or making gestures of disgust. Another way of expressing microaggressions is environmental. The most basic example of this is inaccessibility to the built environment such as not having ramps or accessible bathrooms. Here, even having an accessible entrance to a building that is different than the main entrance can be considered an environmental microaggression.

TYPES OF MICROAGGRESSIONS

Sue defined three different types of microaggressions, differentiated according to conscious awareness of the perpetrator and type of impact. The first one, *micro-assault*, involves a conscious awareness by the perpetrator and, as such, represents an explicit behavioral or verbal act such as name-calling, teasing, or bullying that aims to hurt the targeted person. An example of this type of microaggression can be pushing a person who is using crutches to walk. Micro-assault is the most obvious form of microaggression. The only thing that makes it different from the general understanding of bullying or bigotry is that the person is targeted specifically because of their marginalized identity. The second form, *micro-insult* is often unconscious to the perpetrator. Micro-insults are interpersonal interactions or environmental cues demeaning to the marginalized identity. These comments communicate messages that express insults, rudeness, and slights about the identity of the targeted person but may also be presented in the form of a compliment. An example of this type of microaggression can be a comment such as "I cannot believe that you are so successful in spite of your disability; you are such an inspiration." The message portrayed through this statement is that if a disabled person is successful, they must be an exception. The last form, *micro-invalidation*, occurs through interpersonal and environmental cues where the perpetrator unconsciously denies the reality of the marginalized person (Sue, 2010a; Sue et al., 2007). An example of ableist micro-invalidation is someone saying, "No one is perfect, everybody has some kind of disability." This kind of microaggression is harmful because it diminishes the experience of disabled people.

IMPACT OF MICROAGGRESSIONS

Sue et al. (2007) identified four psychological dilemmas in the experience of microaggression, where the target must reflect on their interpretation and wonder whether the incident has to do with their identity (i.e., disability status, race, gender) and consider whether the perpetrator intended to harm or whether the harm was unintentional. A nondisabled person would not have the same kinds of questions in a similar experience and thus would not face the same dilemmas. The first psychological dilemma experienced as a result of a microaggression is described as the clash of realities. Here, the reality of a person from a minority group(s) might be significantly different from a person from a privileged group(s) who holds the power and means to determine the reality via education, mass media, and social institutions (Sue, 2010a). As Sue (2010a) states, the group holding the power determines the reality and imposes it on the others, including the oppressed groups. When a clash of realities happens, the reality of the oppressed would not be held as valid because it conflicts with the reality imposed by the privileged group or individual. In such instances, the perpetrator of the microaggressions would accuse the target of being inaccurate, oversensitive, or paranoid (Sue, 2010a).

The second dilemma is the invisibility of unintentional expressions of bias. Because of the unconscious, implicit nature of the microaggressions, the perpetrators do not recognize what they did is biased (Sue et al., 2007). Perpetrators can find alternative reasoning for their behaviors and deny their implicit biases (Sue et al., 2007). Here, two mechanisms are working together for the perpetrator: first, the lack of awareness of the prejudices and unintentional discriminatory behaviors, and second, the need to maintain a self-image as an unbiased and good person (Sue, 2010a). In such cases, people are not aware of the biased attitude that they hold and perpetrate unintentionally and stick to a self-image that is inherently good. It is then challenging for the target of the microaggression to make the invisible visible and confront the perpetrator with the harmful message and impact of the microaggression (Sue, 2010a). This is a common situation for disabled people. If they address the microaggression, they can be accused of not having gratitude for the help that others are providing for them or insulting a person who sees themselves as trying to help.

The third dilemma is the perceived minimal harm of microaggressions (Sue, 2010a; Sue et al., 2007). This dilemma refers to the idea that people often accuse the recipient of the microaggressions of making a mountain out of a molehill. Although microaggressions are slight, the impact of those slight experiences is significant because they are happening daily and accumulating over time (Sue, 2010a). Cumulative effects of repeated microaggressions include feelings of self-doubt, frustration, and alienation (Sue et al., 2007) and can impact mental health (Conover et al., 2021). The last dilemma is the catch-22 of responding to microaggressions. Microaggressions place the recipient in a difficult position. The recipient has to figure out the motivation behind the microaggression and decide when and how to respond, which can be challenging (Sue, 2010a). The unconscious, ambiguous, and unintentional nature of the microaggressions makes the recipient skeptical about his or her own experience (Sue, 2010a; Sue et al., 2007). Individuals may questions themselves in the moment or experience conflict about their interpretation of the comment or behavior. Oftentimes, if the person does not address it, they can feel a loss of self-integrity. Alternatively, addressing a microaggression can cause other problems (Sue, 2010a; Sue et al., 2007). Disabled people who point out microaggressions when they happen may become the target of resentment, frustration, or anger, and the responsibility of repeatedly pointing out microaggressions can be exhausting.

MACROAGGRESSIONS: A RELATED BUT DISTINCT CONCEPT

In their work, Sue et al. (2020) clearly differentiate between micro- and macroaggressions. As we already covered, microaggressions are interpersonal or environmental insults and slights targeting oppressed identities. Micro versus macro differentiation is not about the significance of the event, but rather the scope. The term *micro* indicates the daily happening of slights and insults. The term *macro* indicates overt and system-wide offenses and abuses directed at minoritized individuals. Thus, macroaggressions are the perpetuation of the bias toward oppressed identities in the philosophy, programs, policies, practices, and structures of governmental and social institutions like legal, education, and healthcare systems, as well as business and industry (Sue et al., 2019). So, the perpetrator is not an individual, but rather an institution, community, or society. Another difference between micro- and macroaggressions is the target. While microaggressions are targeting an individual, macroaggressions are targeting an entire group. Lastly, correcting a microaggression is about fixing an individual's bigotry, whereas for a macroaggression to be fixed, the change needs to happen at the policy level (Sue et al., 2020). Sue et al. (2019) explained the relationship between racist micro- and macroaggressions as "racial macroaggressions represent an overarching umbrella that validates, supports, and enforces the manifestation of individual acts of racial microaggressions" (p. 132). Thus, we can assume this definition would apply to micro- and macroaggressions based on other -isms like ableism, sexism, heterosexism, and classism.

ABLEIST MICROAGGRESSIONS

The origins of disability microaggressions are in the worldview of dis-ableism or ableism (Keller & Galgay, 2010). Ableism is the worldview that assumes disability is inherently negative and that any form of impairment should be cured or minimized at the least (Campbell, 2009). Thus, ableism is a system of beliefs, practices, and processes of defining a standard of the perfect human body and self, where having a disability becomes a diminished way of being (Campbell, 2009). As racism has evolved from coercive to aversive, explicit forms of ableist discrimination have evolved to more implicit ones since the passage of the Americans with Disabilities Act (ADA; Keller & Galgay, 2010; Palombi, 2013). Friedman (2018, 2019) conceptualized ableism using the framework for racism and found out that a majority of people can be categorized as aversive ableists, those indicating that they do not have any preference for disabled or nondisabled at the explicit level and prefer nondisabled over disabled at the implicit level. Research indicates that people who identify as males, have no disabilities, are less educated, and do not have contact with a person with a disability hold more implicit prejudice toward disabled people (Harder et al., 2019). Harder et al. (2019) also found that while explicit prejudice toward people with disabilities is decreasing over time, implicit prejudice is increasing. Thus, people with disabilities are one particular group of marginalized people who have been the target of microaggressions (Aydemir-Döke & Herbert, 2021; Calder-Dawe et al., 2020; Conover & Israel, 2018; Conover et al., 2017; Kattari, 2019; Kattari, 2020; Kattari et al., 2018; Keller & Galgay, 2010; Lee et al., 2019; Lett et al., 2020; Olkin et al., 2019).

DOMAINS OF ABLEIST MICROAGGRESSIONS

Keller and Galgay (2010) conducted the first study on ableist microaggressions in which they defined nine main ableist microaggression domains. Those are denial of privacy, helplessness, secondary gain, infantilization, patronization, second-class citizenship, denial of identity, spread effect, and de-sexualization. It is possible that a given microaggression may not fit any of those domains or can fit in multiple domains. Please note that these domains do not encompass all of the ableist microaggression experiences, but we present them, as they are helpful to provide a general framework for understanding these experiences.

In *denial of identity*, the perpetrator disregards any significant identity of the person except for the disability. In denial of identity, any quality of the disabled person such as skills, expertise, or membership of the person is overridden by disability, and the person is reduced to their disability. The basic message of this microaggression is that the only thing that I can recognize about you is your disability. A simple example of this is a comment like, "I cannot believe you are a professor." Not recognizing that disabled people with the same disability type have different and unique skills and capabilities can also be included in the denial of identity, for example, assuming that all autistic people are gifted musicians.

Denial of disability-related experience is the next form of ableist microaggression (Keller & Galgay, 2010). In these microaggressions, perpetrators deny or minimize the negative or unfair experience of the disabled person. The target can be accused of being too sensitive or critical. Another theme under this domain is asking for documentation to prove the disability. This can happen to those with both visible and invisible disabilities. The main message is: "What you are experiencing is not real and I don't believe you." A real-life example of this happened to me during a job interview. The high-ranking administrator said, "I was talking about you with my wife last night, and I told her 'Not everybody can do everything, like we all are disabled.'" Another common example for this domain is "Hey, you can walk! How come you are parking in the reserved disability space?" or "Isn't it nice to have extra time for all of your exams? You should see my GPA if I also had that!"

The next form of ableist microaggression is the *denial of privacy* (Keller & Galgay, 2010). Here, perpetrators ask for disability information in explicit or implicit ways in situations where the request is inappropriate and violating and would never be asked of a nondisabled person. The disabled person is forced to identify themselves, talk about their disability, or be expected to be the disability ambassador to educate people and answer other private questions. They sometimes are even expected to ease the discomfort of the perpetrator. For example, a stranger sitting next to you at the bus stop asks, "Isn't it difficult to live like this?," "Did you have an accident?," or "Is there a cure for this?" People even ask very private questions like "Can you have sex?" Denial of privacy also can happen in the form of touching the body of the disabled person or touching their assistive technology, mobility devices, or support animals without permission. The message communicated to the disabled person is that nothing about you can be private. "I am often touched, patted, grabbed or pulled by random strangers who seem to have no idea that their behavior is inappropriate . . . treating me like an animal or a piece of luggage" (Nario-Redmond et al., 2019, p. 17).

Expectation of helplessness is another form of microaggression that disabled people are experiencing (Keller & Galgay, 2010). A person with a disability is usually assumed to need help, and that assumption reflects the low expectation that people have of them. Another assumption of helplessness is that the disability is a catastrophic experience and there is no way to have a fulfilling life for a disabled person. The main message is that it is not worth living a life with a disability. Receiving those messages daily is very degrading for people with disabilities (Keller & Galgay, 2010). I can share a personal experience dealing with this. I was crossing the road with my cane in my right hand and my infant's car seat in my left hand. My dad and my two young sons were also with me but they were not going to come with me yet. My dad ran after me, so I told him to stay with the boys under the shade. He said, "How are you going to cross the road?" and I replied, "Like I always do!"

The next form of microaggression is *secondary gain* (Keller & Galgay, 2010). In this microaggression, perpetrators interact with the disabled person with a concealed agenda of having a gain, like recognition for their good deeds. Another way of this microaggression is comparing oneself to a disabled person and feeling grateful for not having a disability. An example is "I have had people tell me that if they ever become as ill and disabled as I am, they would probably kill themselves, and kudos to me for not killing myself." (Nario-Redmond et al., 2019, p. 17). Secondary gain can also be observed in charity campaigns. Like running a campaign to provoke a pity response so that the campaign can collect more donations. Although outdated, telethons were a good example of this (Longmore, 2015).

Spread effect (Keller & Galgay, 2010) happens when perpetrators overgeneralize impairment in one aspect to other aspects of the person with a disability. This overgeneralization often occurs in a negative direction that diminishes the capabilities of the person with a disability and is an expression of the assumption that disabled people are generally incapable. Talking loudly to a blind person is a generic example of this, reflecting the idea that a person who cannot see also cannot hear. Overgeneralization of the capacity of the person with a disability can happen in a positive way, which is the cause of positive stereotypes, such as the ideas that blind people can memorize everything or autistic people have extreme talents in a particular area.

Patronization is another form of ableist microaggressions (Keller & Galgay, 2010). Under this domain, we can see false admiration, namely the appraisal of people with disabilities for almost anything that they are doing. This microaggression is very close to the concept of "inspiration porn." For example, congratulating a person in a wheelchair for "getting out of the house." One individual explained their experience with being labeled inspiring for engaging in an everyday activity:

> I have probably been told I am inspirational on at least a weekly basis. In one memorable instance, a creepy guy at the gym came up and told me that I inspired him to go exercise. He explained that he has some kind of knee discomfort and often feels unmotivated to go to the gym, but then when he remembers seeing me at the gym, it gives him the push he needs to get up and go. (Nario-Redmond et al., 2019, p. 18)

Infantilization is the microaggression where a disabled adult is treated like a child. Sentimentally talking to a disabled person, calling them inappropriately "sugar" or "hun," not using appropriate pronouns, and talking to the person accompanying them instead of the disabled person are among the examples. This microaggression can result in significant consequences to autonomy if individuals are blocked or prevented from making their own decisions or receiving information they will need to make important choices. I have a personal example for this one as well. At the university where I worked, the department that I worked in was having a table at an event during disability awareness month to introduce students to the Rehabilitation and Human Services Program. I had my cane with me and was visibly pregnant. I was sitting with the other hosts from our same program on the same side of the table. My coworkers that were with me were White women with no visible disabilities. I was writing the students' names with braille who were visiting the table. A male student asked, "Is she a student?" I did not realize that I was the "she" that he was asking about. My coworker responded, "No, Dr. Aydemir-Döke is a professor in our program." The student then asks, "How does she write these?" Knowing that the question was meant for me, I started to address the student, and I answered his questions. He could not accept promoting me from being "she" to being "professor" and perhaps did not believe that I was capable of addressing his questions.

Second-class citizenship is the next form of ableist microaggressions. In this domain, the disabled person can be ignored or avoided, or it can be a more structural or systemic level. Thus, the rights of the person with a disability are perceived as unreasonable, unjustified, and bothersome by the perpetrators (Keller & Galgay, 2010). Environmental microaggressions, such as structures or applications that do not allow equal access or allow just a separate access to disabled people is an example of this, for example, selecting a nonaccessible restaurant for a dinner with friends without recognizing that it means a friend who is a wheelchair user will not be able to go. Other common examples can be found in the area of disability accommodations, for example, asking if someone "really needs" the accommodation they requested or asking a disabled person to accept a lower form of access because providing full access would be inconvenient or costly. Avoiding eye contact with a disabled person is another common way for second-class citizenship ableist microaggressions to surface.

The last domain of ableist microaggressions proposed by Keller and Galgay (2010) is *de-sexualization*. In this domain, sexuality and the sexual or gender identity of a person with a disability are ignored. The message delivered is that a person with a disability should not seek sexuality or sexual partners, cannot be in romantic relationships, and are not desired as a sexual partner, at least by nondisabled people. Thus, in this domain, people with disabilities are seen as incapable of participating in sexual activities or even having sexual desires (Keller & Galgay, 2010). Robb (2015) provides an example of this domain of microaggressions. "I had a guy flirting with me, well we were flirting, and then he goes, 'You know, you'd be really hot if you weren't a cripple.' That was actually one of the first times that I realized that people did not see me, they saw the bike. Like they didn't see me as a person, they saw a person on a bike. Like, I can't be attractive unless I'm not on it. That's really painful because it's college. I want to have a relationship, like a normal relationship with somebody." (Robb, 2015, p. 116).

RESEARCH ON ABLEIST MICROAGGRESSIONS

The research on ableist microaggressions is still limited compared to the number of studies conducted on the topic with individuals of other marginalized identities. Available studies indicated that disabled women and those with visible disabilities were reported to be bothered more by ableist microaggressions (Aydemir-Döke & Herbert, 2021). Exposure to ableist microaggressions is correlated to negative outcomes such as depression and anxiety (Andreou et al., 2021; Conover & Israel, 2018; Kattari, 2020), reduced levels of self-esteem and life satisfaction (Andreou et al., 2021), lower academic self-concept (Lett et al., 2020), and work-related stress (Lee et al., 2019). A study showed that the more ableist microaggressions the disabled people reported experiencing, the more accurately they can identify an ableist microaggression vignette. Additionally, they are not likely to misidentify a neutral vignette as ableist (Conover et al., 2021). Experiencing ableist microaggressions causes feelings such as being stigmatized, shame, and frustration (Kattari et al., 2018). Both disabled and nondisabled people find ableist microaggressions insulting, hurtful, disrespectful, and annoying (Conover et al., 2021). Ableist microaggressions committed by family members were interpreted as more harmful compared to medical providers or friends (Conover et al., 2021). The closeness of relationship with the perpetrator of the microaggression influences the emotional consequences of the experience.

Disabled people with intersectional identities might be more vulnerable to the cumulative impact of intersectional microaggressions (Aydemir-Döke & Herbert 2021), yet there are very few studies focusing on intersectional microaggressions that disabled people with other marginalized identities are experiencing (Conover & Israel, 2018; Miller & Smith, 2021; Olkin et al., 2019). In the qualitative study by Miller and Smith (2021), disabled LGBTQ participants reported almost three times more ableist microaggressions than LGBTQ microaggressions, which might suggest that disability, particularly visible disability, might be a more salient marginalized identity. This may be because it might be possible to pass as heterosexual/cisgender but it may not be possible to pass as nondisabled when you have a visible disability. Conover and Israel (2018) found that disabled people who are also sexual minorities are experiencing ableist microaggressions in the sexual minority community and homonegative microaggressions in the disability community. Experiencing ableist microaggressions in the sexual minority community is linked to lower social support satisfaction within this community, yet the researchers did not observe the same pattern for the homonegative microaggressions experienced within the disability community. Thus, when working with sexual and gender minority clients with disabilities, counselors should pay specific attention to the double marginalization that this group is experiencing and plan interventions to empower their clients against the combined impact of ableism, heterosexism, and sexism. Also, there is a clear need to integrate the intersectional understanding within those minority communities so that they would not marginalize their own people.

ABLEIST MICROAGGRESSIONS AS IT APPLIES TO COUNSELORS: CAN COUNSELORS BE ABLEIST?

Those in the helping profession, by nature of their socialization, have been exposed to -isms such as racism, ableism, sexism, and heterosexism. Thus, counselors are not immune to perpetrating similar kinds of unintended, yet harmful messages. To the contrary, the literature indicates that counselors commit microaggressions in both individual and group counseling settings (Constantine, 2007; Davis et al., 2016; Kivlighan III et al., 2021; Miles et al., 2021; Morris et al., 2020; Owen et al., 2010; Owen et al., 2011; Owen et al., 2014; Shelton & Delgado-Romero, 2013). Owen et al. (2018) ran an experimental study where they found that only 50% of the counselors watching the counseling vignettes with three racist microaggressions were able to identify at least one microaggression and only 25% were able to identify two or three microaggressions. Thus, at least half of the counselors watching the vignettes with microaggressive instances were able to identify none of them. Being able to identify a microaggression is the first step in addressing it. Specifically, counselors' microaggressive behaviors have a detrimental impact on the therapeutic alliance, client satisfaction with counseling services, and perceived improvement due to the services received (Constantine, 2007; Davis et al., 2016; Morris et al., 2020; Owen et al., 2011). Further, counselor incompetence leads to clients expressing anger, frustration, powerlessness, and rejection (Constantine, 2007; Shelton & Delgado-Romero, 2013). Experiencing microaggressions in counseling relationships reduces the likelihood of seeking help and was linked to client dropout (Shelton & Delgado-Romero, 2013).

When examined specific to the counseling of disabled clients, research suggests that counselors in training do not receive adequate training on disability counseling competencies and do not feel confident working with this specific minority group. In a study conducted by Hunt et al. (2006) disabled lesbians indicated that their therapists were not competent to work with their intersectional identities, they did not receive satisfactory services, and they even experienced bias and discrimination in the therapy. One might assume that among the helping professionals, rehabilitation counselors would not commit ableist microaggressions given that they receive extensive training on serving this specific population, yet the opposite has been demonstrated. In a qualitative study on premature termination of vocational counseling, participants reported experiencing relationship problems with their counselors (Rigles et al., 2011). Clients reported that their counselors were inclined to undermine their experiences associated with disability (denial of disability), did not believe in their potential (helplessness/patronization), and/or treated them like children (infantilization).

Overall, despite the expectation, counselors do commit microaggressions, which in turn negatively impact the client–counselor relationship and counseling outcomes. Despite a thorough search, I was not able to find a study examining the occurrence or impact of ableist microaggressions within the counseling relationship, but there is some indirect evidence that disabled people are experiencing ableist microaggressions both in mental health and rehabilitation counseling settings (Hunt et al., 2006; Rigles et al., 2011). Since counselors can commit microaggressions, what should we do to prevent it or intervene if it happens?

INTERVENTIONS FOR ABLEIST MICROAGGRESSIONS COMMITTED BY COUNSELORS

Microaggressions might emerge in a counseling setting in different ways. Counselors themselves might commit them, or clients may want to discuss their experiences in their day-to-day life. Microaggressions happening in the counseling setting cause ruptures in the therapeutic process, and research indicates that addressing microaggressions committed by the counselors themselves is linked to better outcomes (Owen et al., 2014; Yeo & Torres-Harding, 2021). Having a collaborative approach with your clients and showing openness, empathy, and flexibility with the client are reported as some of the ways that a counselor can engage with their client upon perpetrating a microaggression (Yeo & Torres-Harding, 2021).

Recently, counselors started to adopt the cultural orientation as opposed to the cultural competency approach to work with clients who are culturally different than the counselor (Hook et al., 2017; Mosher et al., 2017; Zhu et al., 2021). Cultural orientation has three basic components: cultural humility, attending to and eliciting cultural opportunities, and cultural comfort (Hook et al., 2017). For the purpose of this discussion, I will focus on humility.

Humility refers to the process, values, and interactions between the counselor and client (Hook et al., 2017). Having cultural humility means that, as the counselor, you recognize that you are limited in terms of having a complete understanding of the cultural background and experiences of your client (Hook et al., 2017). Thus, you do not assume that you are the expert of your client's life. This is particularly meaningful for disabled people because they have been in a subordinate position where they have been viewed by experts as someone who needs to be fixed (Olkin, 2007). Acknowledging that your client is the expert of their life and you are just someone who is trying to help is a good starting point. With this approach, you might avoid stereotypical thinking about a given impairment and what one can or cannot do with that impairment. This approach would eventually help you to avoid committing microaggressions and would also empower your client. This does not mean that you should not educate yourself about impairment and possible functional limitations with that impairment. You simply need to recognize that each of your clients is unique with their limitations, capabilities, and intersecting identities. For example, as a person who never had special education help and never attended schools for the blind, I was limited in my reading of braille. However, I can use a screen reader very well. So, someone counseling me would need to know what braille is and what a screen reader is and still keep in mind that some Blind people may not use either of these methods to access information. For example, some might be able to read large print. Therefore, it is best to ask individuals their preferred format if you are giving an informed consent form or any other material.

Cultural humility has two dimensions: *intrapersonal,* where the counselor uses self-exploration and reflection about their own biases as well as being able to self-criticize themselves, and *interpersonal,* where the counselor is oriented to the client's cultural background (Hook et al., 2017; Mosher et al., 2017). Supervision or individual counseling can be used to support growth on the interpersonal dimension (Mosher et al., 2017). Counselors can also self-examine their reactions to their encounters with disabled people by reflecting on questions like: What do I feel: discomfort, pity, admiration?

What are my unregulated thoughts? What does my body feel like, for example, is my heart rate increased? What are my external behaviors, like staring, not forming eye contact, or smiling? Are these reactions different from my other encounters with disabled or nondisabled people? If yes, why, and what is different with that person? For example, are you feeling more comfortable around wheelchair users than blind people?

Hook et al. (2017) gave a detailed recommendation for counselors to repair possible ruptures that may have occurred in the counseling relationship. To be able to repair something, first, you need to know that it is broken. To do this you need to expose yourself to the microaggression literature, as you are doing now by reading this chapter. Also, as the counselor, you need to be able to sense that something has changed. For instance, take notice of cues from the client, such as a decrease in engagement. After noticing what had happened, the most important thing to do is own what you have done and attend to the other person's emotions. Microaggressions, by their very nature, are ambiguous and unintentional. It is important to recognize that as the perpetrator, defensiveness is a common reaction (Hook et al., 2017). Avoid clarifying, justifying, or defending your behavior, and don't expect your client to ease your feelings. The client is in that session with the opposite expectations. You are there to help them (Hook et al., 2017). It is critical to create a safe environment where your clients can disclose what happened. Getting client feedback is another thing you might do. You can informally assess the therapeutic relationship and check in with your client regularly. See Hook et al. (2017) for specific strategies that you might utilize during a session.

Hook et al. (2017) also gives a seven-step action plan where counselors: (a) check in with themselves and examine their emotions; (b) consider the client's perspective and try to understand their feelings; (c) examine their motivation, how would addressing the microaggression help you and your client; (d) consulting and/or getting supervision on the issue; (e) owning and addressing it during the session; (f) asking the client's perspective and feelings; and (g) apologizing where you would own your behavior and take responsibility. The apology should be beyond saying "I am sorry" and should have the following ingredients: starting the apology by naming what you are apologizing for, taking responsibility for your behavior, expressing your emotions, attending to your client's emotions, and making a commitment for future behavior (Hook et al., 2017).

The recommendations provided would work both in the individual and group counseling settings where the counselor is the perpetrator. However, things get more complicated in group counseling settings where another group member is perpetrating the microaggression (Kivlighan III et al., 2021; Miles et al., 2021). In group settings, it is recommended to build a group multicultural orientation in the preparation stage. By building a group multicultural orientation through setting norms and modeling, the members would be empowered to intervene in the case of a microaggression. This can be implemented right in the first session where members can be encouraged to talk about their different identities and how it feels to be around people having those different types of identities (Miles et al., 2021). Also having a metacommunication about addressing difficult dialogs, including microaggressions, in the early stages of the group and setting norms on how to process such instances is another recommendation (Miles et al., 2021). Miles et al. (2021) also suggested that group counselors can make use of the strategies that are proposed for bystanders and targets alike, which is the next topic.

COUNSELOR RECOMMENDATIONS FOR ASSISTING CLIENTS IMPACTED BY ABLEIST MICROAGGRESSIONS

The daily experience of ableism is likely to emerge as a topic that clients would bring to the counseling setting. Counselors, regardless of their specialty, have to be knowledgeable about ableist microaggressions and should be able to process them effectively with their clients (Aydemir-Döke & Herbert, 2021;

Conover et al., 2021). Scales such as the Ableist Microaggression Impact Questionnaire (Aydemir-Döke & Herbert, 2021) can be used to explore the experiences of disabled clients.

The most salient activities that counselors can do to support clients include validating the microaggression experience, processing the implied meaning of the microaggression, and identifying its impact on the client. Other approaches include helping the client not internalize those frequent messages, educating them about the social model of disability, and attributing the experience of microaggression as external to the person, to the stigma and discrimination. However, Olkin (2017) warned that focusing on microaggressions can create a heightened awareness of the hassles one has to go through on a daily basis and can cause a dysphoric and angry effect. However, counselors can warn their clients about possible negative emotions that one can experience by focusing on ableist microaggressions and how to channel those emotions (such as *righteous anger*). Counselors can help individuals understand that this negative emotional response would probably be a short-term change, and clients can also benefit from naming their experiences and figuring out where those feelings are coming from (Olkin, 2017).

A counselor can teach their clients micro-intervention strategies and can even role-play their reaction for the next event or can support them by advocating on their behalf. Before deciding on any action, possible consequences, such as importance of the micro-intervention, retaliation, or rejection, should be thoroughly discussed with the client. Counselors can also help their clients to choose the battles that they want to fight. Olkin (2017, p. 143) recommends addressing the following questions: "(a) Is this important to me in my daily life and functioning? (b) Is there a possible solution? (c) What are the consequences to me if nothing changes? (d) Is there anyone who might help me with this issue? (e) How likely am I to be successful?" If clients choose not to intervene, focusing on the well-being of the person, and teaching clients self-care techniques like mindfulness can be another thing that a counselor can do.

BYSTANDER INTERVENTIONS FOR ABLEIST MICROAGGRESSIONS

You might be the target of microaggression or be an ally or a bystander. In those roles, there are strategies that you can use to intervene (Sue et al., 2019; Sue et al., 2020). Sue et al. defined micro-interventions as "antibias actions used by targets, parents/significant others, allies and well-intentioned bystanders to counteract, challenge, diminish, or neutralize the individual (microaggressions) and institutional/societal (macroaggressions) expressions of prejudice, bigotry, and discrimination" (2019, p. 42). Sue et al. (2020) categorized the intervention strategies based on the strategic goals. Although their work is about racist microaggressions, I will adopt their recommendations for ableist microaggressions.

GOAL 1: MAKING THE INVISIBLE VISIBLE

Since micro-assaults are obvious bigotry, there is no need to question their meaning or intention. Micro-insults and micro-invalidations are more ambiguous in nature; thus, those experiences are more prone to remaining invisible (Sue et al., 2007).

Developing Perspicacity

Developing perspicacity, defined as being able to infer underlining meaning, or the ability to read between the lines, is an important part of identifying and addressing microaggressions. This ability means the intervening actors can accurately identify biased statements, actions, or discriminatory practices. This is the prerequisite for all of the other responses. For targets, perspicacity would diminish the self-doubts about their experience (Sue et al., 2020). As ableism is not recognized as much as other -isms, and sometimes the humiliating treatment of disabled people can be done in a compassionate, assumingly innocent way (like over-helping), learning about ableism and ableist messages is critical to help develop perspicacity. The best ways to learn include reading and watching disabled authors and artists and also learning about the disability history and culture. Likewise, interacting with disabled people will definitely help. But be mindful in those interactions and monitor your emotions, cognitions, and behaviors as has been recommended in the section earlier.

Naming the Micro-Insult

The second strategy identified by Sue and colleagues (Sue et al., 2019; Sue et al., 2020) is disempowering the innuendo by naming it. Naming what has happened demystifies, deconstructs, and makes the invisible visible (Sue et al., 2020). It also reassures the target that they are not making things up and validates their experience. Naming it can be used by bystanders and targets. This can be as simple as saying, "It is a stereotype" and "What you have just done was not okay." For example, if someone kneeled down to pet a guide dog of a blind person, you might let them know this behavior is inappropriate by saying, "She is working and you should never pet service animals."

Undermining Metacommunication

Undermining metacommunication is the next tactic. According to Sue et al. (2020), although simple, this tactic serves several purposes like recognizing a conscious compliment of the perpetrator, lowering defensiveness for the follow-up, undermining the unspoken assumption of microaggression, and creating the possibility for future awareness of false assumptions. An example exchange could be if someone tells a disabled person: "You are amazing. You have such a positive outlook," they can respond, "Thanks, I have a very nice job and a loving family." This addresses the incorrect assumption that a disabled person cannot have reasons to be happy.

Challenging the Stereotype

Challenging the stereotype is the fourth micro-intervention (Sue et al., 2020). Here metacommunication by the micro-aggressor is being addressed, exposed, and challenged. Unlike the tactics earlier, this is more confrontational and can induce defensive, negative, and antagonist reactions. The advocate must decide if they would like to engage in a longer conversation or cut it there (Sue et al., 2020). An example exchange could be a waiter asking, "What would she like to eat?" and the companion answering, "Why don't you ask her? I do not speak for her."

Broadening the Trait

The next approach is to broaden the ascribed trait to a universal human behavior (Sue et al., 2019; Sue et al., 2020). Stereotyping a group might mean that selectively some common attributes are exclusively attributed to marginalized groups (Sue et al., 2020). You are generalizing the stereotype to a broader group. This is good for sentences starting with "Those people are…" A response to broadening the ascribed stereotypic trait can be presenting information that challenges the perpetrator's thinking and providing alternative perspectives.

Asking for Clarification

Asking for clarification for a statement or an action is another micro-intervention to make the invisible visible. Asking for clarification would require the perpetrator to elaborate on what they have done or said and potentially can lead them to recognize their bias. This is a more confrontational method where "the intent of these questions is to (a) force the perpetrator to stop and consider what they just said or did, (b) communicate your disagreement or disapproval, and (c) encourage a further exploration of the belief or attitude of the person" (Sue et al., 2020, p. 123). Some general questions presented in Sue et al. (2020, p. 123) are: "What exactly do you mean?," "Come again. Did I hear you correctly?," "Do you realize what you just said?," and "I can't believe you just said that. Tell me what you mean."

An example of this specific to an ableist microaggression could be that after learning that the student with learning disabilities had the highest score on an exam, another student might say, "If I also had that much time, I would get all A's for all of my classes." The response could be, "What do you mean? Can you clarify?" Another example dealing with a common ableist microaggression could be a person saying to a disabled person, "You don't look disabled." They might ask, "What is wrong with being disabled?"

Making the Metacommunication Explicit

The next tactic is making the metacommunication explicit via rephrasing or restating it (Sue et al., 2020). Metacommunication refers to covert messages that are conveyed subtly and may modify the meaning of the primary communications. This tactic is done with a questioning tone or by checking with the perpetrator to clarify their meaning. An example can be at a managerial meeting where several senior managers are discussing promotions and an ally states, "So you are not going to promote Caleb to be a store manager just because you think customers would be uncomfortable to see a wheelchair user?" or "You think Mike is less intelligent just because he cannot talk fluently?" This, again, is a more confrontational strategy with the possibility of evoking a defensive reaction. This strategy aims to make the perpetrator face the meaning of their words (Sue et al., 2020).

Engaging the Perpetrator

Reversing, redirecting, or mimicking the statements or actions of the offender as if it was meant for the perpetrator is another tool in the micro-intervention toolbox (Sue et al., 2020). This might be a humorous and sarcastic way of engaging a perpetrator by making them the target of the offense. An example of an exchange might be the perpetrator saying, "You are pretty for a blind woman" and the blind person responding, "Thanks. You are also pretty for a sighted woman."

Another tactic that I use as a blind person in my interactions is dry humor. I cannot do it all the time, however, because it requires a state of mind of creativity, not stress or frustration. This can be a good strategy for repeated offenses because usually, you can think of a response to a behavior after the fact. Here is my favorite personal example. I was pregnant, and you need to give a urine sample periodically when you are pregnant. During one of my visits with the OB/GYN, the nurse asked my husband if I can pee in a cup. She had asked my husband this on previous occasions. Previously, my response had been that I would be okay. But this time, I responded with, "I am potty-trained. No worries." As I was laughing at the time, it did not create tension. This was not very educational, but rather a little punitive, but it was a relief on my end at least. Here is another example that I heard from a Turkish friend. When a person said to them, "You people are doing nothing and living on disability income.

Isn't it nice? You don't have to work." My friend responded, "I wish God would give you the same so that you also can enjoy the disability income."

GOAL 2: EDUCATE PERPETRATORS AND STAKEHOLDERS

The main aim of micro-interventions is to bring about change by engaging the perpetrators so that they can realize that what they have done was offensive, that they can identify the underlying assumption of their behavior, and that they are aware of the perspective of the target (Sue et al., 2020).

Focus on Impact, Not Intention

A primary approach to addressing microaggression is to challenge the person to focus on the impact instead of the intention. The reason this is important is because the first reaction (and often defensiveness) of the perpetrator is to state their intention and avoid recognizing the harm. The aim of this tactic is that it "(a) avoids an accusation of bias, thereby lowering defensiveness, (b) allows the discussion to center on the interpersonal transaction, rather than arguing over intent, (c) encourages empathic understanding of why the impact was poorly received, and (d) hopefully, results in an educational dialogue that has a lasting impact" (Sue et al., 2020, p. 138). An example can be stated "I know you like to help but you not letting me do the things I am capable of is frustrating. I will ask for help if I need it." Another example that a bystander might say is, "I know you like to help her but you should not touch her without her permission. This is violating her privacy." If a perpetrator continues to emphasize their intention, it might help to recognize their meaning and ask them to also recognize their impact.

Contradicting Stereotypes Through Personalization

Contradicting the group-based stereotype with opposing evidence by personalizing it to specific individuals is another approach to addressing microaggressions (Sue et al., 2020). Stereotypes are applied to groups as if every member shares the same traits. Here, you are providing personalized opposing evidence. Asking about whom the person is talking can challenge the group stereotype. An example of an exchange could be where a person states, "Those mental people are all dangerous" and a response could be, "My cousin has schizophrenia and he is working as a science teacher, and he never hurts anyone." I personally think this strategy may not work well against ableism, sometimes even the people very close to a disabled person can be ableist and say ableist things. In those situations, they are assimilating the positive example from the rest of the group and see that example as an outlier.

Appealing to Values and Principles

Appealing to the offender's values and principles is another approach, where you point out the discrepancy between their statement or behaviors and how they view themselves (Sue et al., 2020). Microaggressors often hold egalitarian liberal values on the explicit level and are not aware of their implicit bias, so appealing to their conscious values while indirectly pointing out the discrepancy with their behavior might create a realization (Sue et al., 2020). An example statement is, "I know you like to be fair and would like to provide a nice work environment for all, but when Jon asked if he can have a special chair so that he can sit without pain, you refused his request. Would you like to reconsider this?"

Pointing Out Commonalities

Pointing out commonalities is the next method recommended by Sue et al. (2020). In this strategy, you are pointing out something that the perpetrator and the target have in common. For example, when a friend does not invite your disabled friend to a party, you might respond with, "You think hanging out with Julie would not be fun and did not invite her, but she is one of the most fun people that you can ever meet. Did you know that she also is a professional swimmer just like you?"

Promote Empathy

In promoting empathy, the aim is to promote compassion (Sue et al., 2020). But, as I have already indicated, some of the ableist microaggressions are based on feelings of compassion, so if you are trying to promote empathy for disabled people, avoid passing over the line toward pity. Here you should take the minority or social model of disability and focus on the oppression and the discrimination that disabled people are experiencing instead of their impairments or functional limitations. An example of something that you might say is, "You are complaining about finding a restaurant with an accessible entrance and restroom for the Christmas get-together, even finding an accessible place to eat is this difficult. Think about all the other things. So, we may not go to the steakhouse that you like to always go to, but how about this Thai restaurant? They also have an accessible parking lot."

Emphasizing How the Perpetrator Would Benefit

Emphasizing how the perpetrator would benefit is an approach that emphasizes personal growth and development by increasing your understanding of diversity and seeking out exposure to different people (Sue et al., 2020). If you observe a person committing microaggressions, particularly if it is a pattern, you might bring it to their attention and suggest a way to pursue personal development work. Something that you might say to a perpetrator is, "You said you feel uncomfortable about volunteering at the group home, but I think this experience will enrich your clinical skills and you will learn a lot about people with severe mental illness and will realize they are not different than you or me."

GOAL 3: DISARM MICROAGGRESSIONS

Sue et al. (2020) proposed several tactics to disarm microaggressions. These include strategies to identify microaggressions when they are happening and respond by challenging, redirecting, disagreeing, or simply asking the person to stop because you find their words or actions offensive. For example, you observe a person bullying a classmate with a developmental disability and they are using derogatory words. As a bystander or ally, you can stop the offender by saying "That's not actually funny. Stop bothering him." Such an intervention "(a) stops the demeaning comments, (b) expresses personal disapproval, (c) briefly indicates their 'hurtfulness' or impact, and (d) redirects it to the problem at hand" (Sue et al., 2020, p. 156). By expressing the disagreement, you stop the false consensus about the marginalized group.

Another approach is to state your values and set boundaries (Sue et al., 2020). This method is most effective when directed at a person with whom you have at least some relationship. A statement such as, "You know that treating disabled people with the same respect that I would treat other people is very important for me. Can you please stop making those comments?" Another way to disarm micro-aggressions is just to express disagreement (Sue et al., 2020). Some example statements by Sue et al. (2020, p. 157) are: "That's not how I view the situation." "I don't agree with what you just said (or did)." "That doesn't sound right to me." and "I don't think that's true at all." Another method is to describe what is happening and confront the perpetrator with your observations. For example, "Each time we come across your neighbor with cerebral palsy, I noticed your smile turns into an expression of pity, and you are not even responding to his efforts to chat, I do not think this is a good way to engage with anyone." You might also use nonverbal communication to express your disapproval, by frowning, shaking your head, or removing yourself from the infraction (Sue et al., 2020). Finally, reminding the perpetrator of the rules such as organizational values and code of conduct or policies regarding diversity is the last micro-intervention tactic that is proposed by Sue et al. (2020).

GOAL 4: SEEKING EXTERNAL SUPPORT/VALIDATION

Dealing with ableism daily can be very draining. Because of the widespread ableism in contemporary society, a person may have very few, if any, spaces where they do not experience ableist microaggressions. Strangers, acquaintances, friends, and even family members can be perpetrators of ableist microaggressions. A protective strategy is to seek external support and validation. Sue et al. (2020) recommend some avenues for external support, including reporting incidents to leadership and giving them the opportunity to help and seeking formal or informal supports through counseling or community supports.

If the ableist microaggressions that you are observing or experiencing are happening at an organization like a school, a restaurant, or a workplace, you might consider reporting them to leadership or management (Sue et al., 2020). Leveraging the support of leadership can be a more effective way to stop microaggressions from happening, and the target can receive support. Reporting the incident is a more formal way of getting external support; however, it may not be safe to do so. In that case, keeping an officially dated record would help later on if the target wanted to later proceed and take action.

Sue suggests receiving counseling or psychotherapy to get validation and external support if you are experiencing microaggressions (Sue et al., 2020). Seeking spiritual, religious, and community support is another way to cope (Sue et al., 2020). Being in these inclusive settings can provide a sense of validation. In these spaces, you can build long-lasting relationships with the people who have commonalities with you. These spaces might provide opportunities for activism and organizing. Also in these spaces, you can learn about healing tools like praying and meditation. Community organizations can provide resources such as referrals for social services and economic and legal support (Sue et al., 2020). Having a buddy system can also help. Given the fact that disabled people are likely to be the only disabled person in their families (Olkin, 2007), they may lack the support that some other minorities, like racial minorities, have within their families. Thus, having a friend to share and get validation of your experiences would prevent rumination and thus the internalization of the negative messages communicated by the ableist microaggressions (Sue et al., 2020). Likewise, establishing or joining a support group would provide encouragement, ideas, and sustenance (Sue et al., 2020).

CONCLUSION

In the microaggression research and literature, less attention is paid to disability-related microaggressions. This chapter provides definitions and examples of common microaggressions experienced by disabled people, including those personally experienced. Counselors and other disability professionals have a responsibility to understand their own disability biases and examine their own behavior to identify when they might commit microaggressions themselves. As most microaggressions are unintentional, it takes conscious work and effort to recognize these behaviors in ourselves. Finally, strategies were presented to respond to and interrupt microaggressions, for those experiencing them as well as allies or bystanders.

DISCUSSION QUESTIONS

1. Consider how a disabled person might experience microaggressions due to their disability, or their race, gender identity, religion, nationality, or other minoritized identity. How might different experiences and interactions result in psychological dilemmas and exacerbated stress?

2. How might a counselor address a situation where they have committed a microaggression targeting a client? What steps could they take to recognize the impact of their behavior and try to mend their relationship?

3. What approaches presented do you feel most comfortable integrating into your daily life if you were to experience or witness a microaggression?

CLASS ACTIVITIES

1. Take the Implicit Association Test (IAT; Project Implicit, 2011) for disability and the Contact with Disabled Persons Scale (Yuker & Hurley, 1987). The IAT is a computerized assessment where the reaction time of test takers is measured, the test taker is presented with positive and negative words primed by disability or not, and is asked to choose if the meaning of the word is positive or negative. Having more implicit bias is indicated by having a longer reaction time for positive words and a shorter reaction time for negative words to be identified correctly when primed with disability. And the Contact with Disabled Persons Scale assesses how often the test taker has been interacting with a disabled person.

   Reflect on your results:

   a. What are your results from both tests?

   b. How do you think your scores are related or not?

   c. Where is this attitude coming from, what are the messages that you were exposed to about disabled people in your family, your social networks like church, neighbors, the school, and in the media? Do you have any disabled family members? If so, how is that person treated in the family? Do you have a disabled friend? If so, how is your relationship with that friend compared to your friends with no disabilities? If it is different, what is different and why? How might all of those experiences be impacting your implicit or explicit attitude toward disabled people?

   d. Do you need to work on your attitudes toward people with disabilities? What steps you can take to identify and address your implicit biases?

   Take both tests and see how you are doing and think about your results. What was your first reaction to your results from those two assessments—any surprises? Please do this exercise even if you have a disability and reflect on your results. The IAP is not accessible for blind people, but in that case, you can still reflect on the third question.

2. A counseling center at a large university decided to run group counseling sessions with freshman students where the main focus is on college transition. Group members

were composed of students having intersectional identities. Mary, the group leader, is a Black, cisgender, lesbian with no disabilities.

Alana, a wheelchair user, shared her struggle with other people on the way to the group meeting. She shared her difficult morning, it was raining and she took the bus to campus. A stranger at the bus stop started to talk to her, "You are so inspirational. I see you every day. What is wrong with your legs? Did you have an accident?" Alana described how the stranger went on and on, making Alana more and more uncomfortable and upset.

Jon, a cisgender White man with no disability, responds: "Hey, what is wrong with that? I mean, I did not get why you are so upset with that lady." Seeing Alana's facial expression, Mary recognized that Jon just committed a microaggression.

Reflect on your results:

a. Identify the microaggressions mentioned in this case.

b. What were the underlying messages received by Alana in this interaction?

c. What kind of message or statement to Alana could have been made that would have validated the microaggressions that she shared?

d. If you were Mary, how might you respond in this moment? After the group?

KEY REFERENCES

Only key references appear in the print edition. The full references appear in the digital product on Springer Publishing Connect™: https://connect.springerpub.com/content/book/978-0-8261-5111-7/part/partII/chapter/ch11

Aydemir-Döke, D., & Herbert, J. T. (2021). Development and validation of the Ableist Microaggression Impact Questionnaire. *Rehabilitation Counseling Bulletin*, 66(1), 36–45. https://doi.org/10.1177/00343552211014259

Conover, K. J., Acosta, V. M., & Bokoch, R. (2021). Perceptions of ableist microaggressions among target and nontarget groups. *Rehabilitation Psychology*, 66(4), 565–575. https://doi.org/10.1037/rep0000404

Davis, D. E., DeBlaere, C., Brubaker, K., Owen, J., Jordan, T. A., Hook, J. N., & Van Tongeren, D. R. (2016). Microaggressions and perceptions of cultural humility in counseling. *Journal of Counseling & Development*, 94(4), 483–493. https://doi.org/10.1002/jcad.12107

Kattari, S. K. (2020). Ableist microaggressions and the mental health of disabled adults. *Community Mental Health Journal*, 56(6), 1170–1179. https://doi.org/10.1007/s10597-020-00615-6

Lee, E. J., Ditchman, N., Thomas, J., & Tsen, J. (2019). Microaggressions experienced by people with multiple sclerosis in the workplace: An exploratory study using Sue's taxonomy. *Rehabilitation Psychology*, 64(2), 179–193. https://doi.org/10.1037/rep0000269

Lett, K., Tamaian, A., & Klest, B. (2020). Impact of ableist microaggressions on university students with self-identified disabilities. *Disability & Society*, 35(9), 1441–1456. https://doi.org/10.1080/09687599.2019.1680344

Mosher, D. K., Hook, J. N., Captari, L. E., Davis, D. E., DeBlaere, C., & Owen, J. (2017). Cultural humility: A therapeutic framework for engaging diverse clients. *Practice Innovations*, 2(4), 221–233. https://doi.org/10.1037/pri0000055

Olkin, R. (2007). Disability-affirmative therapy and case formulation: A template for understanding disability in a clinical context. *Counseling and Human Development*, 39(8), 1–20.

Sue, D. W. (2010b). *Microaggressions in everyday life: Race, gender, and sexual orientation*. Wiley.

Sue, D. W., Alsaidi, S., Awad, M. N., Glaeser, E., Calle, C. Z., & Mendez, N. (2019). Disarming racial microaggressions: Microintervention strategies for targets, White allies, and bystanders. *American Psychologist*, 74(1), 128–142. https://doi.org/10.1037/amp0000296

CHAPTER 12

QUALITY OF LIFE AND PSYCHOSOCIAL ADAPTATION TO CHRONIC ILLNESS AND DISABILITY

MALACHY BISHOP, YUNZHEN (JUDY) HUANG, KAIQI ZHOU, AND MEGAN BAUMUNK

LEARNING OBJECTIVES

After reading this chapter, you will be able to:

- Describe the history and development of quality of life (QOL) as a health and rehabilitation concept
- Explain how QOL has been incorporated into models of psychosocial adaptation to chronic illness and disability
- Define QOL and related constructs, including subjective and psychological well-being and life satisfaction
- Describe and contrast three QOL-based models of psychosocial adaptation to chronic illness and disabililty (CID)

PRE-READING QUESTIONS:

1. How has the meaning and measurement of QOL changed since it was first introduced in modern U.S. history?
2. Can QOL be both an outcome and a framework for psychosocial adaptation to CID in rehabilitation counseling?
3. What constructs are commonly assessed as outcomes in the psychosocial adaptation to CID research?
4. How have models of psychosocial adaptation to CID changed over time?

The purpose of this chapter is to explore the application of quality of life (QOL) and related constructs in the context of rehabilitation counseling and, more specifically, in the psychosocial adaptation to disability and chronic illness research. Psychosocial adaptation to chronic illness or disability (CID) incorporates the wide variety of processes by which people maintain an adaptive balance in the experience of the onset of and living with a CID. This area of research involves the pursuit of understanding of these processes and, ideally, the extension of this understanding to counseling techniques and systemic interventions in practice (Bishop, 2012). Research and theory development in psychosocial adaptation to CID has been characterized as a defining focus of rehabilitation counseling and rehabilitation psychology research and one of the most widely researched areas in rehabilitation and disability studies (Bishop, 2012; Livneh & Thomas, 1997).

For several decades, QOL has been described as an important rehabilitation counseling outcome, an underlying goal of rehabilitation interventions, and the generally accepted philosophical goal of rehabilitation counseling (Crewe, 1980; Fabian, 1991; Fleming et al., 2013; Livneh, 1988; Wright, 1980). The now-ubiquitous sentiment that QOL is an important rehabilitation outcome is examined in this chapter, several decades after it was first suggested in the rehabilitation counseling and rehabilitation psychology literature. This is achieved through a review of the history of the construct and its application. The ways in which QOL has been defined and utilized has developed considerably in this period, and the intersection of QOL with psychosocial adaptation to CID research has provided important new insights and directions.

QOL is a fluid personal, social, political, economic, health, and psychological construct. The modern history of the QOL construct describes a transition from what was primarily a group-based (population or society) perspective to one increasingly focused on the individual's perspective; from a measure used by politicians and government and public health officials to evaluate and guide decisions about public policy to a measure used by clinicians, healthcare consumers, and the general population to consider, describe, and evaluate individual experience. Each step in the ongoing transition of the QOL construct has led to new perspectives, meanings, and approaches to measurement. Frequently, with new stages in this development, earlier definitions were retained and maintained while new offshoots and branches developed within the growing QOL framework. As a result, the construct has become increasingly complex. Conceptual differences between the many QOL-related constructs (e.g., well-being, life satisfaction, health-related QOL, happiness) have been debated and delineated, and research associated with each of these related but distinct constructs has expanded.

In rehabilitation, QOL has been applied (a) clinically, in evaluation and case planning, to inform interventions, and to evaluate outcomes; (b) in rehabilitation research and program evaluation, to assess the impacts of disability at the population and individual levels and to evaluate the effectiveness of rehabilitation programs, services, and interventions; and (c) as we explore in this chapter, in the context of psychosocial adaptation to CID. In this latter context, QOL and related constructs (e.g., subjective well-being, life satisfaction) have been applied as a framework for describing adaptive processes, evaluating outcomes, and understanding the relationships between factors that influence the adaptation process and outcomes (Bishop, 2005a, 2005b; Devins, 1994; Livneh et al., 2014; Livneh, 2001, 2022). To provide context for the discussion of these latter applications, we begin with a discussion of the history and development of QOL in healthcare and rehabilitation. We then review definitions of QOL, explore its application in rehabilitation counseling generally, and conclude with a description of its specific application in three current models of psychosocial adaptation to CID.

HISTORY AND DEVELOPMENT OF QUALITY OF LIFE IN HEALTHCARE AND REHABILITATION

The modern use of the term *quality of life* emerged in the post–World War II era, prompted by efforts by government officials and public health professionals to explore broad questions of public health and policy. These efforts occurred in the context of the postwar recognition that individual health extends beyond the individual's body and is influenced by social and environmental factors (Prutkin & Feinstein, 2002). This perspective is reflected in the 1948 World Health Organization definition of health as "not only the absence of infirmity and disease but also a state of complete physical, mental, and social well being" (World Health Organization [WHO], 1948, p. 69).

In the decades following World War II, large-scale appraisals of the social and environmental factors that influence public health were conducted through large public surveys (e.g., Flanagan, 1978) designed to inform government and health policies. National surveys were designed to examine such aspects of public life as education, health, employment, and population growth (Prutkin & Feinstein, 2002). These objectively measurable, group-based population statistics, characteristics, or variables, also including such indicators as gross national product, wages, cost of housing, and rate of unemployment, were referred to as *social indicators* (Cummins, 1997; Prutkin & Feinstein, 2002; Sirgy, 2021).

The term *quality of life* entered the medical and rehabilitation lexicon in the 1960s and represented a shift from the previous focus on objective population-level indicators to more subjective and personal indicators of well-being. The term's entry coincided with changes in health professionals' perspectives about illness, disability, medicine, and rehabilitation. Specifically, as advances in medicine resulted in increased survival among those with conditions and illnesses that had previously been associated with mortality, there was a change in focus in public health, medicine, and rehabilitation from the "quantity of life" to the quality of life (Pennacchini et al., 2011). This shifting perspective is directly observable in the early uses of the term (QOL) in the rehabilitation counseling and rehabilitation psychology literature in the 1960s and 1970s (see e.g., Lorenze et al., 1974; McAleer, 1975; Vash, 1975). This transition was likely also influenced by the changing priorities and expectations of people with disabilities and their families in the 1960s and 1970s, decades marked by increasing advocacy for equity in access to employment, independent living, education, community participation, and healthcare (Albrecht, 1973; Rubin et al., 2016).

In the 1970s, several highly influential studies spurred the rapid growth of QOL research in medicine, rehabilitation, and the social sciences. These large-scale survey projects (e.g., Andrews & Withey, 1976; Campbell et al., 1976; Flanagan, 1978) dealt with broad conceptual questions and explored the nature, dynamics, and components of QOL, as well as the related constructs life satisfaction and well-being. These questions concerned the relationship between objective and subjective indicators, the valid and reliable measurement of the latter, and the identification of domains important to QOL and life satisfaction (Kerce, 1992; Pennacchini et al., 2011; Prutkin & Feinstein, 2002).

During the 1980s, in mental health, medicine, and the social sciences broadly, there was growing recognition of the potential for the application of QOL concepts in health policy development, program evaluation, and outcome assessment. At the clinical level, however, measures of functional status were still more likely to be employed than measures of QOL. As noted by Prutkin and Feinstein (2002, p. 4) attempts to assess "non-biologic aspects of a patient's daily behavior" continued to be, as they had for decades, based on measurements of functional health status developed for the purpose of classifying functional and other capacities (e.g., occupational skill, mental and emotional status, independence in activities of daily living, rehabilitation potential). Assessment of the impact of CID at the individual level prior to the 1990s, therefore, failed to capture the patient's personal, subjective, or broader psychosocial experience (Fischer et al., 1999). With the desire to obtain a more comprehensive and ecological assessment of the QOL impact of CID and associated treatments came the development of generic health-related QOL (HRQOL) instruments and, subsequently, in the mid-to-late 1990s, condition-specific HRQOL instruments. In the intervening years, the number of general and condition-specific HRQOL measures has grown exponentially.

Patient-reported outcome measures (PROMs) are the most recent iteration of the trend from population-based to person-centered health and QOL assessment and are based on the growing awareness that the validity and relevance of QOL assessment improve when they reflect and incorporate the perspectives and priorities of those being assessed. As a result, QOL instruments are increasingly derived based on patient-reported outcomes (PROs). According to Nowinski et al. (2017), PROs derive directly from patients' reports of their experience with a disease and its treatment. "By their very nature, PROs are patient-centered and their addition to traditionally collected anatomical, biological, and clinical data has resulted in a fundamental shift in how research and clinical practice are conducted" (Nowinski et al., 2017, p. 934).

Many current PRO QOL measures have been developed in the frameworks of the National Institutes of Health (NIH) Toolbox, PROMIS (Patient-Reported Outcomes Measurement Information System) and the Neuro-QoL (Quality of Life in Neurological Disorders) measurement systems. PROMIS has been described as representing "a state-of-the-science model for standardized PRO assessment of health-related quality of life" (Cella et al., 2019, p. 537). The NIH-funded PROMIS initiative is an NIH Roadmap initiative to assess PROs in respondents with a wide range of chronic diseases and demographic characteristics (Hays et al., 2009). Since its development, PROMIS has developed PROMs in physical, mental, and social health for adults and infants, children, and adolescents with chronic conditions (Cella et al., 2015). PROMIS measures can be used with the general population and with individuals with chronic conditions. The PROMIS measures were developed and validated to be psychometrically sound and to be relevant across all conditions for the assessment of symptoms and functions (HealthMeasures, 2022a).

According to Cella et al. (2012) traditional outcome measures of disease status in clinical research have often failed to capture the full impact of disease and treatment, in that the patient's experience of disease symptoms, treatment side effects, functioning, and well-being were excluded. To address these limitations, the National Institute of Neurologic Disorders and Stroke (NINDS) sponsored a multisite project to develop a QOL assessment system for adults and children with neurologic disorders (Neuro-QoL; Cella et al., 2012). The Neuro-QoL system was designed to evaluate and monitor the physical, mental, and social effects experienced by adults and children living with neurological conditions (e.g., stroke, multiple sclerosis, Parkinson disease, epilepsy, amyotrophic lateral sclerosis; HealthMeasures, 2022b). The development of the Neuro-QoL measurement system involved a series of steps designed to ensure both clinical and psychometric validity, involving input from members of the research community, clinical and measurement experts, patients, and caregivers, through a comprehensive process of focus groups, literature review, and large-scale testing to calibrate item response theory (IRT)–based item banks across physical, mental, and social domains of QOL (Cella et al, 2012).

The WHO International Classification of Functioning, Disability and Health (ICF; WHO, 2001) is a classification system of health and health-related domains. Although not designed as an assessment instrument, the ICF is a globally utilized and comprehensive health and functioning framework, and thus is also an important current framework for understanding the relationships between health conditions, the environment, participation, activity, and QOL (Chan et al., 2009; Kennedy et al., 2006; Reed et al., 2005). In an effort to construct a measure capable of validly and reliably measuring QOL, the WHO's QOL Group (WHOQOL, 1994) initiated the development of a multidimensional QOL instrument that would be broadly applicable. The resulting WHOQOL-100 consists of six domains: (a) physical, (b) psychological, (c) level of independence, (d) social relationships, (e) environment, and (f) spirituality (Harper & Power, 1998). Following the development of the WHOQOL-100, the WHOQOL Group (1998) initiated the development of a more widely useful and efficient brief version (WHOQOL-BREF). A disability-specific QOL instrument was also developed (WHOQOL-Dis; Power et al., 2010), which captures additional dimensions relevant to individuals with disabilities.

DEFINING QUALITY OF LIFE

QOL is consistently recognized as ambiguous and difficult to define (e.g., Bishop, Chapin et al., 2008; Haraldstad et al., 2019). It has been defined in a wide variety of ways, by many disciplines, for different reasons, and with different purposes (Bishop, Chapin et al., 2008; Costa et al., 2021). The definitional ambiguity associated with this "umbrella term" (Feinstein, 1987, p. 635) is increased when related constructs, such as HRQOL, well-being, and life satisfaction, are considered, each of which is associated with distinct but overlapping definitions. For the purpose of the focus of this chapter, we will restrict the potentially extensive discussion of definitions of QOL and related constructs to those most frequently employed in the specific context of theories and models of psychosocial adaptation to CID, including subjective well-being (SWB), psychological well-being, and life satisfaction. More extensive discussions may be found in Fleming (this text), Bishop, Chapin et al. (2008, 2009), and Sirgy (2021).

Some researchers have distinguished QOL from SWB and life satisfaction by contrasting the emphasis of the former on external and objectively measurable components, such as environmental conditions and social indicators, with the internal and subjective focus of the latter constructs. Generally, however, there is consensus that QOL incorporates both subjective and objective components (Cummins, 2005) and includes "not only the quality of life circumstances, but also the person's perceptions, thoughts, feelings, and reactions to those circumstances" (Kim-Prieto & Diener, 2005, p. 402). Professional consensus has also been suggested on the following definitional elements: QOL (a) is multidimensional; (b) is influenced by personal and environmental factors and their interactions; and (c) is experienced in terms of commonly shared, universal components, though cultural and individual variables affect the salience of these components at the individual and national level (Cummins, 2005; Haas, 1999; WHO, 1996). These elements are reflected in one of the more widely cited QOL definitions proffered by the WHO (WHOQOL, 1994): QOL is "the individual's perception of his/her position in life in the context of the culture and value systems in which he/she lives and in relation to his/her goals, expectations, standards and concerns" and a "broad ranging concept consisting of a person's physical health, psychological state, level of independence, social relationships, and their relationship to important features of their environment" (p. 153).

Subjective and Psychological Well-Being (Hedonia and Eudaimonia) and Life Satisfaction

HEDONIA AND EUDAIMONIA

Within the well-being literature, a distinction is made between hedonic and eudaimonic definitions. *Hedonia* is often conceptualized as happiness; the pursuit of pleasure, enjoyment, and fun; and the avoidance of pain, and is operationalized as SWB (Diener et al., 1999; Disabato et al., 2016; Giuntoli et al., 2021; Ryan et al., 2008). *Eudaimonia* refers to a way of living, rather than a feeling, and has been conceptualized in terms of the pursuit of meaning, authenticity, excellence, virtue, and being motivated autonomously, and is operationalized as psychological well-being (Disabato et al., 2016; Huta & Waterman, 2014; Ryan et al., 2008).

SUBJECTIVE WELL-BEING

Subjective well-being was described by Diener et al. as a "broad category of phenomena that includes people's emotional responses, domain satisfactions, and global judgments of life satisfaction" (Diener et al., 1999, p. 277). Sirgy (2021, p. 43) summarized SWB as an enduring affective state comprising three components: "(a) actual experience of happiness or cumulative positive affect (joy, affection, pride, etc.) in salient life domains, (b) actual experience of depression or cumulative negative affect (sadness, anger, guilt, shame, anxiety, etc.) in salient life domains, and (c) evaluations of one's overall life or evaluations of salient life domains." High levels of SWB are associated with the frequent experience of pleasant emotions (positive affect), low levels of negative moods (negative affect), and a high level of life satisfaction. Interestingly, researchers have found that the factors that promote negative affect are different from those that promote positive affect, and thus the two are somewhat independent from each other (Diener et al., 2002). As a result, the decreasing of negative mental states does not necessarily increase positive states, or put another way, "the elimination of pain may not result in a corresponding increase in pleasure" (Diener et al., 2002, p. 64). The third component of SWB, life satisfaction, is distinguished from the affective experiences and reflects the cognitive evaluation of life, overall and/or in different areas of life, or life domains. It is one's evaluation of one's own life "determined by an aggregation of evaluations of positive and negative events of important life domains" (Sirgy, 2021, p. 43).

PSYCHOLOGICAL WELL-BEING

Psychological well-being is a broad concept associated with many theoretical underpinnings and is often conceptualized in terms of eudaimonia. Huppert (2009) asserts that psychological well-being is about lives going well and combines subjective well-being with effective functioning. For many years, credible assessment tools evaluating flourishing and psychological well-being were limited, leading to Ryff's (1989) work to identify and use common themes in developmental, clinical, existential, and humanistic psychologies to develop quantitative measurement scales (Ryff, 2017). There are six key components to Ryff's (1989) model of psychological well-being: (a) autonomy, (b) environmental mastery, (c) positive relationships, (d) personal growth, (e) self-acceptance, and (f) purpose in life. The theoretical underpinnings were founded in Aristotle's eudaimonia, as well as Allport's maturity (1961), Jung's individuation (1933), Jahoda's mental health (1958), Frankl's will to meaning (1959), Maslow's self-actualization (1968), Neugarten's executive processes of personality (1973), Bühler's basic life tendencies (1935), Erikson's personal development (1959), and Rogers's fully functioning person (1961; Ryff, 1989; 2017). As we discuss later in this chapter, each of these approaches to understanding QOL have been applied in the context of psychosocial adaptation to CID research.

QUALITY OF LIFE IN REHABILITATION COUNSELING

QOL has been recognized as a philosophically consistent rehabilitation counseling outcome (e.g., Crewe, 1980; Fabian, 1991; Livneh, 1988; Wright, 1980) and underlying goal of rehabilitation interventions (Fleming et al., 2013) since the 1980s. Seminal articles by Crewe (1980), Livneh (1988), Fabian (1989; 1991; 1992), and Roessler (1990) identified QOL as a superordinate rehabilitation counseling outcome and a construct with significant potential for guiding the delivery and evaluation of rehabilitation counseling services (Bishop, Chapin et al., 2008, p. 47). References to QOL as a philosophical and practical construct for application in rehabilitation counseling were evident but sporadic during the 1980s (e.g., Crewe, 1980; Livneh, 1988; Wright, 1980), increased during the 1990s, and by 2001 Bishop and Feist-Price described QOL as the generally accepted philosophical goal of rehabilitation counseling. In the 21st century, rehabilitation researchers have continued to actively explore the application of QOL in rehabilitation services, including in vocational evaluation, rehabilitation planning, counseling, and program evaluation (e.g., Fleming et al., 2013, 2014; Fleming et al., this text; Livneh, 2001, 2022; Rubin et al., 2003, 2016).

It is instructive to consider the reasons these early proponents espoused QOL. Fabian (1991) suggested that the increased use of QOL measures in rehabilitation program evaluation was the result of an increased emphasis on consumer evaluation of rehabilitation programs and a growing recognition that unidimensional program evaluations and interventions were insufficient. Roessler (1990) also noted the benefits of QOL from a program evaluation perspective, suggesting that a QOL perspective on rehabilitation counseling allowed the integration of competing program goals (e.g., client independence and employment) into a higher-order, multidimensional rehabilitation outcome. From the clinical perspective, Roessler also observed the alignment of QOL with established rehabilitation counseling philosophies, including the focus on wellness, a holistic view of the person, and the necessity of considering both the individual and the environment in which the individual lives.

Given the promise of these proposed applications, the extent to which QOL has been applied in vocational rehabilitation outcomes, career counseling, and program evaluation in rehabilitation counseling has, unfortunately, been relatively limited (see Fleming et al., this text; Fleming et al., 2013, 2014). For example, in their comprehensive review, Phillips et al. (2021) found that less than 10% of rehabilitation counseling interventions were aimed at addressing QOL. The full potential of the integration of QOL in client assessment, rehabilitation planning, outcomes measurement, and program evaluation has not yet been achieved. In order for QOL to be effectively and practically applied in rehabilitation counseling, it must be defined, operationalized, and measured in ways consistent with the proposed purpose. Meaningful use of QOL as a clinical tool, or as a measure of clinical outcome, requires awareness of the range of conceptualizations and definitions of QOL for any particular use and consistency between the way the term is operationalized and measured (Costa et al., 2021). Practitioners who would be responsible for the selection, administration, and evaluation of such assessments must have sufficient exposure and practice with the range of options to make informed decisions and use of the construct. Such exposure has not yet reached the requisite level in the educational curriculum, professional settings, or broader systems of rehabilitation counseling.

An exception to the limited integration of QOL in rehabilitation counseling is found in the psychosocial adaptation research, where, beginning with Livneh (1988) and extending to the present, the integration of QOL has proved productive, and, as we review later, has led to a meaningful expansion in the understanding of the processes of psychosocial adaptation. Unfortunately, both the development and application of practical clinical interventions based on these models and the integration of QOL-based outcomes in rehabilitation counseling research have been less robust to date.

To date, researchers have not reached consensus on the choice of outcome indicators to measure psychosocial adaptation/adjustment (Livneh, 2022). In general, two measurement approaches have been used in extant studies: employing an individual measure of adjustment, acceptance, or QOL (e.g., Bishop et al., 2007; Zhang et al., 2019) or employing a combination of measures as indicators of adaptation/adjustment (e.g., Araten-Bergman et al., 2015; Weinert et al., 2011). For the purpose of this chapter, we were curious as to the extent to which QOL has been used as an outcome measure in recent psychosocial adaptation/adjustment to chronic illness and disability. To address this question we conducted a noncomprehensive review of the literature. In this section and in Table 12.1, we summarize and describe the commonly used measures of psychosocial adaptation/adjustment to CID and explore the extent to which measures of QOL are represented.

The measures were summarized from previous reviews (Smedema & Ebener, 2010; Smedema et al., 2009; Smedema et al., 2022). To supplement the previous literature and identify additional psychosocial adaptation/adjustment measures used in research over the past 15 years, the authors also conducted a rapid review of empirical studies on psychosocial adaptation to CID across four databases: CINAHL, APA PsycArticles, APA PsycInfo, and MEDLINE. The search terms were "psychosocial adapt* or psychosocial adjust*" AND "chronic illness or chronic disease or chronic condition or disability," and the search was limited to article titles. The inclusion criteria were as follows: (a) article was published between 2007 and August 2022, (b) study participants were adults with CID, (c) measure(s) of psychosocial adaptation/adjustment to general CID was used, and (d) article was published in English.

The initial literature search resulted in 43 articles. After screening based on the inclusion criteria, seven articles were included for review. A summary of the measures identified from the reviewed articles are provided in Table 12.1. The commonly used measures identified in the previous reviews and the current rapid review are described later.

TABLE 12.1 Psychosocial Adaptation/Adjustment Measures Used in the Reviewed Studies

STUDY	STUDY SAMPLE	PSYCHOSOCIAL ADAPTATION/ADJUSTMENT MEASURES
Araten-Bergman et al. (2015)	Veterans with disability	1. **Acceptance of disability:** Acceptance of Disability Scale (ADS; Linkowski, 1971) 2. **Hope:** The Hope Scale (HS; Snyder et al., 1991) 3. **Social network size:** Social Network Scale (LSNS; Lubben et al., 1988) 4. **Social participation patterns:** Activity Pattern Indicators (Diller et al., 1981)
Bishop et al. (2007)	People with multiple sclerosis	1. **Adaptation to disability:** Ladder of Adjustment Scale (Crewe & Krause, 1990) 2. **QOL:** Delighted-Terrible Scale (Andrews & Withey, 1976) 3. **QOL:** Disability Centrality Scale, domain satisfaction ratings (Bishop & Allen, 2003)
Davison & Jhangri (2013)	Patients with advanced chronic kidney disease	1. **Adjustment to disability:** Psychological Adjustment to Illness Scale-Self Report (PAIS-SR; Derogatis, 1986) 2. **Health-related QOL:** Kidney Dialysis Quality of Life Short Form, Version 1.3 (Hays et al., 1997), includes 43 kidney-disease specific items and the RAND 36-Item Health Survey 1.0 as the generic score
Malcarne et al. (2007)	People with systemic sclerosis	1. **Functioning:** Health Assessment Questionnaire-Disability Index (HAQ-DI; Fries et al., 1982) 2. **Adjustment to disability:** Psychological Adjustment to Illness Scale-Self Report (PAIS-SR; Derogatis, 1986)
Togluk & Çuhadar (2021)	People with chronic obstructive pulmonary disease	**Adjustment to disability:** Psychological Adjustment to Illness Scale-Self Report (PAIS-SR; Derogatis, 1986)
Weinert et al. (2011)	Rural women with chronic conditions	1. **Social support:** Personal Resource Questionnaire 2000 (PRQ2000; Weinert, 2003) 2. **Self-esteem:** Rosenberg Self-esteem Scale (Rosenberg, 1965) 3. **Acceptance of illness:** Acceptance of Illness Scale (Stuifbergen et al., 2000) 4. **Depression:** Center for Epidemiologic Studies-Depression Scale (Devine & Orme, 1985) 5. **Stress:** Perceived Stress Scale (Cohen et al., 1983)
Zhang et al. (2019)	Patients with breast cancer	**Acceptance of disability:** Acceptance of Disability Scale-Revised (ADS-R; Groomes & Linkowski, 2007)

Acceptance of Disability Scale and Its Revision

In the rapid review, the Acceptance of Disability Scale (ADS) and its revision (ADS-R) were used in two of the seven studies (28.6%; Araten-Bergman et al., 2015; Zhang et al., 2019). The ADS (Linkowski, 1971) measures an individual's level of disability acceptance. It was developed based on Wright's (1983) disability acceptance model. The ADS has 50 items rated on a 6-point Likert scale. The ADS generates one summative score, limiting its use in practice (Smedema et al., 2009). In 2007, Groomes and Linkowski (2007) revised the ADS (ADS-R) to improve its utility. The ADS-R contains 32 items rated on a 4-point Likert scale and includes four subscales that, like the ADS, parallel the four value changes proposed by Dembo et al. (1956; Wright, 1983): enlarging the scope of values, containing the effect of disability, subordinating physique to other values, and transforming comparative-status values into asset values. Cronbach's alpha coefficient of the ADS-R was .93 (Groomes & Linkowski, 2007), indicating excellent internal consistency.

Multidimensional Acceptance of Loss Scale

The Multidimensional Acceptance of Loss Scale (MALS; Ferrin et al., 2011) also measures disability acceptance in the context of the Dembo et al. (1956; Wright, 1983) value change model. It has 42 items rated on a 4-point Likert-type scale and has four subscales that parallel the earlier four value changes. Cronbach's alpha coefficients were .80 to .88 for the subscales (Ferrin et al., 2011), indicating good internal consistency.

Reaction to Impairment and Disability Inventory

The Reaction to Impairment and Disability Inventory (RIDI; Livneh & Antonak, 1990) measures an individual's responses or reactions in the adaptation process based on extensive reviews of the rehabilitation literature (Livneh, 1986a, 1986b). The RIDI has 60 items rated on a 4-point Likert scale and contains eight subscales: shock, anxiety, denial, depression, internalized anger, externalized hostility, acknowledgement, and adjustment. Cronbach's alpha coefficients were .69 to .85 for the subscales (Livneh & Antonak, 1997), indicating acceptable internal reliability.

Psychological Adjustment to Illness Scale-Self Report

In the rapid review, the Psychological Adjustment to Illness Scale-Self Report (PAIS-SR) was used in three of the seven studies (42.9%; Davison & Jhangri, 2013; Malcarne et al., 2007; Togluk & Çuhadar, 2021). The PAIS (Derogatis, 1986) measures an individual's psychological adjustment to disease. It has 46 items rated on a 4-point Likert scale and yields seven subscales: healthcare orientation, vocational environment, domestic environment, sexual relationships, extended family relationships, social environment, and psychological distress. Cronbach's alpha coefficients were .63 to .87 for the subscales (Derogatis, 1986), indicating acceptable internal reliability.

Quality of Life Measures

In the rapid review, two of the seven studies (28.6%) used QOL measures as indicators for psychosocial adaptation/adjustment (Bishop et al., 2007; Davison & Jhangri, 2013). The domain satisfaction subscale of the Disability Centrality Scale (DCS; Bishop, 2005a) assesses QOL among individuals with CID. The DCS covers 10 life domains: physical health, mental health, work/studies, leisure activities, financial situation, spousal relationship, family relationships, social relations, autonomy/independence, and religious/spiritual. Cronbach's alpha coefficient was .88 for the domain satisfaction subscale (Bishop et al., 2007), indicating excellent internal consistency.

The RAND 36-Item Health Survey 1.0 (RAND-36; Hays et al., 1993) assesses an individual's health-related QOL. It has 36 items and consists of eight scales: physical functioning, role limitations due to physical health, role limitations due to emotional problems, energy/fatigue, emotional well-being, social functioning, pain, and general health. Depending on the scales, items are rated dichotomously or on a 3-point, 5-point, or 6-point Likert-type scale. Cronbach's alpha coefficients were .78 to .93 for the subscales (Hays et al., 1993), indicating acceptable to excellent internal consistency.

The results of this brief (and limited) review suggest that in the context of psychosocial adaptation research, though not specific to rehabilitation counseling, QOL and related constructs were represented as outcome measures in almost 30% of the studies. In the rapid review, two of the seven studies (28.6%) measured multiple indicators of psychosocial adaptation/adjustment (Araten-Bergman et al., 2015; Weinert et al., 2011), including psychological variables (disability acceptance, hope, self-esteem, depression, stress) and social variables (social network size, social participation, social support). Additionally, functioning has been used as an indicator of psychosocial adaptation/adjustment (Malcarne et al., 2007).

QUALITY OF LIFE IN PSYCHOSOCIAL ADAPTATION RESEARCH

Among the early proponents of greater integration of the QOL construct in rehabilitation counseling, Livneh (1988, 2001; Livneh & Antonak, 1997) introduced, and subsequently expanded, the most comprehensive exploration of the application of QOL in the context of psychosocial adaptation to CID. This integration proved an important impetus in terms of theory development and clinical understanding. Livneh proposed (1988; Livneh & Antonak, 1997), and has since further developed (Livneh, 2001, 2022), a comprehensive framework for understanding the factors that influence "the nature, structure, and outcomes of the adaptation process" and framed these outcomes in the context of QOL (Livneh, 2022, p. 151). Others, either subsequently in the rehabilitation counseling research (Bishop, 2005, Bishop et al., 2007) or in other fields (e.g., Devins, 1983, 1994), have also developed models based on or incorporating a QOL perspective. In this section we review Livneh's framework and two additional models, associated with the work of Devins (1994; 2018) and Bishop (2005a and 2005b).

Livneh's Adaptation to the Chronic Illness and Disability Framework

Livneh's conceptual framework (Livneh, 2001; 2022) describes the components, or the "building blocks that constitute the dynamics of psychosocial adaptation," to CID in terms of a tripart model of sets of variables, including antecedents, processes, and outcomes of adaptation (Livneh, 2022, p. 171). The antecedents include the conditions that existed and events that prevailed prior to and surrounding the time of the onset of CID. Antecedents provide the context to CID onset and include both (a) the medical and environmental causes that trigger CID onset or diagnosis and (b) the contextual and status variables (biological, psychological, sociocultural, and environmental) within which the causally linked events are situated (Livneh, 2022).

These two sets of variables influence the second set of interacting factors, the process component, which includes three overarching elements: (a) specific characteristics of the CID (e.g., medical and functional characteristics, such as severity, course, and duration); (b) the associated psychological experiences and reactions (e.g., anxiety, depression); and (c) the psychological strategies and mechanisms that serve to mitigate, mediate, and filter the psychological impact (e.g., appraisal and initial coping responses; Livneh, 2022). These interacting process sets, in addition to the antecedent sets, to a large extent affect the third and final set, the outcomes.

Livneh (2022) noted that two schools of thought exist about outcome conceptualization: the dichotomous and the continuous. The dichotomous view holds that psychosocial outcome indicators can be classified into either positive or negative, adaptive or nonadaptive outcomes. The continuous approach views outcomes in terms of a continuum, ranging from nonadaptive to adaptive, with numerous states of adaptative levels along this continuum. The latter is the approach adopted in Livneh's model (2022) and is consistent with the view that most human psychological and physical attributes exist in a continuous rather than a dichotomous distribution (Bishop et al., 2023). Livneh identifies QOL as the overarching outcome criterion in psychosocial adaptation to CID and defines QOL for this purpose as consisting of three broad domains: (a) intrapersonal functioning (subjective well-being, life satisfaction, perceived health); (b) interpersonal functioning (e.g., satisfaction with family life, peer relations, and social activities); and (c) extrapersonal functioning (e.g., performance of work activities and/or recreational pursuits, living arrangements, financial status).

Consideration of Livneh's Framework

There are a number of unique elements to Livneh's conceptual framework of psychosocial adaptation. First, among the ecological models of adaptation to CID, it is the among the most thorough and inclusive of the many aspects of both the individual and the environment that may be involved in the psychosocial adaptation process. The understanding of adjustment and adaptation to CID are relatively recent research pursuits. As with QOL, models of adaptation emerged in the post–World War II era as developments in medicine and healthcare prolonged survival and social advocacy movements began to abrogate the medical model in favor of the social model of disability. Early models can be seen as reflecting the views about disability prevalent in the period in which they were conceived. Stage models, models focused on disability as loss, and functional models, while still conceptually relevant today, may be seen as reflecting an outsiders' perspective, and these early models often focused solely on the individual, neglecting consideration of the interaction of the individual with social and built environmental contexts and the impact of these on psychosocial adaptation (Livneh et al., 2014). The introduction of ecological models of adaptation to CID (see Livneh & Bishop, 2012; Livneh & Martz, 2012; Smedema et al., 2009 for reviews) represented a recognition of the inherent importance of person–environment interaction. Livneh's conceptual framework (2001, 2022; Livneh & Antonak, 1997) clearly recognized and more explicitly clarified the role of the environment as a determining factor in adaptation to CID than prior models. Livneh's framework incorporates both past environments (e.g., highlighting the individual's preexisting personality and sociodemographic characteristics, coping strategies, behavioral attributes, and perspectives) and current environmental characteristics "that constantly and dynamically interact with unfolding psychosocial events" (Livneh et al., 2014, p. 133). Thus, like other ecological models, the model clearly integrates both individual and environment, but Livneh's thorough and comprehensive consideration of the relevant elements of each enables a more complete and detailed assessment and understanding of the potential interactions.

Second, in addition to being among the earliest models of psychosocial adaptation to propose QOL as the outcome toward which psychosocial adaptation processes are directed, Livneh's framework delineates and specifies this proposition in terms of specific QOL outcomes across intrapersonal, interpersonal, and extrapersonal functioning. This approach realistically portrays the breadth of psychosocial outcomes while incorporating these under the QOL umbrella in a manner that is consistent with established QOL theories and models. The approach enables one to appreciate the complexity of psychosocial adaptation yet understand this process within an organized and meaningful framework. Finally, framing adaptation in terms of QOL, and then delineating the elements of QOL across the intrapersonal (subjective well-being, life satisfaction), interpersonal, and extrapersonal spheres, gives Livneh's model practical utility in clinical settings. It enables clinicians to evaluate and discuss the client's unique goals, directions, and aspirations and apply the model on an individual basis in clinical practice, based on the unique goals and experiences of each person. In short, the model reflects the complexity of the adaptation process, includes the breadth of factors necessary to understand the influence of person and environmental factors and their interaction, and enables defining and prioritizing outcomes in terms of the hopes and goals and realities of each individual by framing outcomes in terms of the "dynamic nature of the multifaceted and evolving concept of QOL" (Livneh et al., 2014, p. 135).

Devins's Illness Intrusiveness Model

Devins's Illness Intrusiveness Model (Devins, 1994) is a QOL (subjective well-being)-based model describing the nature, determinants, and psychosocial consequences of chronic illness (Devins, 1994). The model has been extensively researched and has been consistently validated among people with a wide range of chronic illnesses (Devins et al., 1983, 1993; Deckert & Devins, 2017; Lebel et al., 2013; Mah et al., 2011).

The term *illness intrusiveness* (II) describes the impact of living with chronic conditions that introduce significant adaptive challenges and coping demands. Specifically, Devins has described II as resulting from "illness-induced interference with valued activities and interests . . . such as disease-related anatomical changes, functional losses, treatment side effects, and disease- and/or treatment-related lifestyle disruptions" (2010, p. 592). II is proposed to compromise well-being indirectly via two pathways: by reducing (a) positively reinforcing outcomes derived from valued activities and (b) personal control by limiting the ability to obtain positive outcomes and/or to avoid negative outcomes (Devins et al., 1983; Devins & Shnek, 2000). These impacts can be assessed in terms of QOL domains. To assess this dynamic, Devins developed the Illness Intrusiveness Ratings Scale (IIRS; Devins et al., 1983), a self-report instrument asking respondents to rate the degree to which an illness or its treatment interfere with each of 13 life domains that were identified by Flanagan (1978) as being important to QOL (Devins, 2018).

The model's components and direction can be conceptualized, based on Devins's published frameworks, as follows: (a) disease and treatment factors to which the person with CID is exposed; (b) II, or the impact of CID on reducing the individual's participation in valued life activities; (c) personal control, or the direct and indirect influence of II on one's perceptions that one is capable of controlling positive life outcomes; and (d) SWB, viewed by Devins et al. as an outcome indicator. The model also recognizes the influence of external factors that could potentially interact with (moderate) the relationships between each of the previously mentioned components, including demographic, psychological, social (e.g., stigma, culture), and contextual (e.g., environmental stressors and facilitators) factors (Livneh et al., 2014). For example, psychological, social, and contextual factors modify both (a) the impact of chronic illness or disease and treatment on II and (b) the effects of II on SWB (Devins, 2018). Similar to Livneh's model, Devins suggests that antecedent factors, such as gender, education, and age, may moderate the effects of illness, conditions, and their treatment on II (Devins, 2010). Additionally, psychological, social, and contextual factors that occur as a consequence of disease and/or its treatment, such as stigma, have been found to moderate the effects of II on SWB (Devins, 2018. 2020).

In his 2018 discussion of II in the context of self-management, Devins describes self-management strategies and interventions that may reduce II. This practical perspective suggests an approach by which rehabilitation counselors may assess and help clients respond to the impact of CID in practice (Devins, 2018).

Consideration of the Illness Intrusiveness Model

The II model is one of the most empirically researched models of psychosocial adaptation to CID and has been extensively validated among an impressive range of populations. The model is based in established theoretical frameworks and models of psychology, behavior, and SWB. It is parsimonious, based on clear, compelling, and well-supported premises, and through three decades of research has been refined and clarified. Devins's framework integrates SWB in a meaningful, clinically useful, and logical framework.

The model is also practical in terms of the ease of translation from the brief assessment to clinical planning. The incorporation of self-management concepts, as described in depth in Devins's 2018 chapter on the topic and elsewhere (e.g., Devins & Shnek, 2000) provides rehabilitation professionals with practical approaches to working to empower clients to increase control and management of their illness. The model emerged within, and to some extent reflects, Devins's professional background in clinical psychology in health and medicine but has direct application in rehabilitation counseling and psychology.

Disability Centrality Model

Bishop's Disability Centrality Model (DCM; Bishop, 2005a, 2005b; Bishop et al., 2007) represents an integration of established theories and concepts from rehabilitation in a QOL-based framework of adaptation. It is designed to provide theoretical understanding and practical implications of the psychosocial adaptation process (Bishop, 2005a). Bishop (2005a, 2005b; Bishop et al., 2007) described the model in terms of the following components.

First, because the impact of CID is usually experienced across multiple domains of life, Bishop suggested that the appropriate framework for assessing and understanding the individual's response is multidimensional and subjective, able to capture the range of experience across life domains, and able to portray the individual's subjective experience across and within those domains. In addition, because individuals are often found to experience positive changes and psychologically beneficial aspects of living with a disability (Livneh, 2021; Livneh & Antonak, 1997; Meuller et al., this text; Smart, 2020; Wright, 1983), negatively valenced measures of psychosocial adaptation to CID that only assess the presence and degree of negative affect are unable to register this aspect of the experience and thus can only provide a limited perspective.

For the purpose of the DCM, QOL is defined as the subjective sense of overall well-being that results from an individual's evaluation of satisfaction with an aggregate of personally or clinically important domains. This specific definition has been alternately referred to in terms of subjective QOL (Cummins et al., 1994; Frisch, 1999; Michalos, 1991), subjective well-being (Ormel et al., 1999), and life satisfaction (Sirgy, 2021).

Second, consistent with Devins's II framework, Bishop posited that the onset and experience of CID frequently, though not universally, compromise psychosocial well-being. This occurs through (a) reduction in opportunities to experience satisfaction in centrally important areas of life, (b) reduction in feelings of personal control, (c) reduction in experiences of positive emotion, and (d) increase in experiences of negative emotions (Bishop, 2005a; Bishop et al., 2007).

An important extension of the II approach in the DCM is based on the recognition, established in the QOL research, that people differ in the importance they place on the different domains of their life (i.e., the extent to which different domains of life are central to their QOL and identity; Cummins, 1997; Jovanović et al., 2019; Sirgy, 2021). The term *centrality* in the DCM represents this concept. The term *psychological centrality* (Rosenberg, 1979) suggests that self-concept, or identity, consists of a set of hierarchically organized components and that for any given individual, some components may be more central to the self-concept than others. Sirgy (2021) described this dynamic as domain salience and, from an energy investment perspective, suggested that domains in which a person has invested effort to attain positive affect or reduce negative affect are likely to be hierarchically elevated compared to those in which there has been less emotional investment. "People have value-laden beliefs directly related to particular life domains . . . some life domains may be more important than others" (p. 696).

A corollary of this dynamic, as identified by Frisch (1999), is that satisfaction in more central areas of life will "have a greater influence on evaluations of overall [QOL] than areas of equal satisfaction but lesser importance" (p. 56). Similarly, an individual whose illness or disability negatively and consistently affects (through the mechanisms identified earlier) domains that are more central or important to his or her QOL would be expected to experience a greater negative impact in terms of overall QOL than one for whom the effects of disability are experienced in more peripheral domains.

For example, an individual with multiple sclerosis whose fatigue, pain, and cognitive and physical limitations make it impossible to continue working would be expected to report a more significant negative impact on their overall QOL if career and work were central to the individual's identity and QOL. These symptoms, and the loss of employment, while still impactful, would be expected to be less significant in terms of overall QOL impact for an individual for whom work was less central to the individual's identity and QOL and who found satisfaction through alternate identities or domains of life.

From a measurement perspective, as described earlier, the DCS (Bishop, 2005b) was developed for the purpose of research and clinical assessment with this model. The scale is a self-report instrument that has been used to assess the model's components. Respondents indicate the degree of CID interference, but also the importance, satisfaction within, and perceived control within each of 10 life domains (physical health, mental health, work/studies, leisure activities, financial situation, spousal relationship, family relationships, social relations, autonomy/independence, and religion/spirituality) derived from the QOL research (Andrews & Withey, 1976; Bishop & Allen, 2003; Frish, 1999; George & Bearon, 1980; Jalowiec, 1990; Padilla et al., 1992).

The additive nature of measuring domain importance has frequently been proposed and incorporated in QOL models and assessments (e.g., Cummins, 1997; Frisch, 1999; Pavot & Diener, 1993) and has been found in research with the Disability Centrality and II models to moderate the relationship between CID impact (or II, respectively) and SWB (e.g., Bishop, 2005b; Bishop et al. 2007; Bishop, Frain et al. 2008; Devins, 2018). It is important to note, however, that the amount of additional information provided through domain importance weighting in QOL measures may be limited, and the value of this approach continues to be debated (Cummins et al., 1994; Hsieh, 2012, 2016; Sirgy, 2021).

The third component of the DCM describes the mechanisms by which people respond or adapt to changes in QOL resulting from the impact of CID. Based on QOL research, Bishop proposed that people seek (and actively strive) to achieve and maintain SWB around an internal set point, which appears to develop through genetic, learned, and socioenvironmental factors (Lykken, 1999; Sirgy, 2021; Stones & Kozma, 1991). This set point is maintained by constantly working to close perceived gaps between one's perceived present and desired level of satisfaction. When QOL is experienced to deviate negatively from the set point, this variance, or disequilibrium, generates motivational feelings of displeasure, prompting the individual to close the gap and restore equilibrium (Sirgy, 2021; Vittersø, 2013).

Interestingly, research suggests that most people (across cultural groups and regardless of objective circumstances; Cummins, 1998, 2000; Diener et al., 1999) rate their QOL as being relatively high (i.e., above average or above the midpoint of measurement scales; Cummins, 1998, 2000). This dynamic has been proposed to be adaptive from evolutionary, health, and social perspectives (Diener & Diener, 1995; Sirgy, 2021) in that it allows for greater opportunities for social and personal advancement, exploratory behavior, and reliable coping resources. Thus, when faced with life changes that reduce SWB, people respond with adaptive changes that allow them to maintain their (relatively high) set point level.

Generally, in response to minor, time-limited variations in SWB, previously learned and previously successful responses (e.g., adopted coping strategies; adjustments in effort, attention, and time commitment) are sufficient to maintain QOL around the set point. The more significant and lasting or permanent changes that may accrue in the context of the onset of CID and other significant life events require more significant and ongoing responses. Such responses are less likely to have been learned or previously developed. Previously adequate resources may be taxed, and the psychosocial impact may be significant. The final component of the DCM proposes the mechanisms by which people adapt to this change in QOL. Three general classes of potential responses are proposed.

The first involves the person making changes in affected domains that allow the person to maintain satisfaction in important domains. Through processes that increase personal control (e.g., self-management; Bishop et al., 2009), the impact in important domains is reduced and the individual can maintain the existing domain structure by maintaining satisfaction in valued areas of life.

Second, in the case of lasting or permanent change, people (either actively and consciously or nonconsciously) alter or shift the relative importance of domains so that previously central but highly affected domains become less central and formerly peripheral but less affected domains become more central (referred to as value change). Conceptually similar approaches have been suggested in the rehabilitation literature by Livneh (1980, 2001) and others (Dembo et al., 1956; Keany & Glueckauf, 1999; Wright, 1960, 1983) and in other health and psychology contexts (Groot & Van Den Brink, 2000; Misajon, 2002; Schwartz & Sprangers, 1999, 2000; Wilensky, 1960; Wu, 2009). In the acceptance of loss theory described by Dembo et al. (1956), adaptation, or acceptance, is described as centering on "changes within the value system" in response to perceived losses associated with the onset of CID (Wright, 1983, p. 163). Value change refers to the idea that individuals respond to perceived losses in one area of life by discovering value in others, representing "an awakening interest in satisfactions that are accessible, and facilitates coming to terms with what has been lost" (Wright, 1983, p. 163).

Third, in what is considered a temporary, interim, or transitional period, neither of these responses occur, and the person continues to experience decreased overall QOL. Further research and development on this proposed transitional phase are underway and exploring the role of acceptance and identity change processes.

A number of testable hypotheses emerge from the DCM. The following hypotheses, based on the model's tenets, have been evaluated and supported in several studies (e.g., Bishop et al., 2008, 2009; Grist, 2010; Mackenzie et al., 2015):

1. QOL and adaptation to CID are significantly and positively correlated.

2. Domain importance moderates the relationship between domain satisfaction and overall QOL.

3. Domain satisfaction and domain control mediate the relationship between impact and QOL.

4. Overall QOL, domain satisfaction, control, and importance are all negatively correlated with the level of perceived impact of the CID.

Consideration of the Disability Centrality Model

The DCM is closely related to Devins's II model, and many of the considerations discussed in the context of that model apply. The model's theoretical underpinnings represent a synthesis of several existing frameworks derived from rehabilitation psychology, social psychology, and the QOL research. The tenets of the DC model have been evaluated empirically to a far more limited extent than those of the II model but have been supported in research among different populations (e.g., Bishop et al., 2008, 2009; Grist, 2010; Mackenzie et al., 2015). Further and expanded research on the tenets of the model is needed. The model is seen as having potential in terms of the development of clinical interventions, but outside the realm of self-management and career counseling (Bishop et al., 2009; Livneh et al., 2014), these have not yet been well developed. The model suggests the importance of multidimensional (multidomain) assessment of satisfaction, perceived control, importance, and the specific impacts of CID in the different domains. The information from this assessment may be informative in rehabilitation planning and in identifying approaches to helping the individuals identify means by which impacts may be reduced, accommodated, or ameliorated.

CONCLUSION

Psychosocial adaptation research reflects the changing paradigms and philosophies of the profession itself, reflecting contemporaneous perspectives on disability and responses to disability. In the relatively brief history of psychosocial adaptation research in rehabilitation, the development of new and diverse models and theories has been rapid. The frequently identified limitations of some historical models (e.g., stage models) is that they were too stringent, too limited in terms of the perspectives of the framers on both process and outcome, reflecting expectations that were inconsistent with the complexity of reality, and too focused on the individual in isolation. They did not reflect the unique and evolving perspectives of the individuals in the experience.

The introduction of the QOL construct has expanded and evolved current understanding of psychosocial adaptation to CID. QOL-based ecological models have developed to incorporate more flexibility and a more realistic recognition of the fundamental role of, and complexity of, environmental interactions. They have also made inherent the perspective of the individual living with CID. The II and DCM models reflect flexibility and a movement somewhat akin to the PCO models of QOL, in that the outcomes are essentially defined by the individual within a multidimensional, subjective framework.

Describing the processes of psychosocial adaptation in an effective manner (i.e., in a way that is valid and consistent with the broad experiences of people living with CID, able to reflect the varying goals of those living through the experiences, and clinically useful) is a particularly challenging endeavor because the range of contexts and variables that must be considered are innumerable. The only consistent and persisting reality is that adjustment to disability "is ever evolving and dynamic (Bentley et al., 2019, p. 81). So, there must be professional understanding of the process. Disability and psychosocial adaptation are evolving because both the individual and the environment (social, cultural, societal, economic, physical, media, demographic, etc.) in which disability is created and experienced are dynamic and ever evolving. Our role, as rehabilitation professionals working with people engaged in the processes of psychosocial adaptation to CID, in various capacities, must be flexible and responsive. The application of QOL to models of psychosocial adaptation has provided a more flexible and positive framework for evaluating and understanding this evolving dynamic. In this chapter we focused on three models, which are themselves continually evolving. We look forward to the further development of new models, and new understanding, increasingly guided by the personal experiences of people living with CID.

CLASS ACTIVITIES

1. As described in this chapter, there are three primary components to psychosocial adaptation to chronic illness and disability (CID) according to Livneh's tripartite model: triggering events, moderating processes, and quality of life (QOL) outcomes. Triggering events include medical condition factors, including psychological reactions, and contextual factors, such as sociocultural, environmental, and personal factors. The moderating processes include coping informed by personal dispositions and experiences. Finally, QOL consists of intrapersonal, interpersonal, and community domains.

   a. Most psychosocial adaptation to CID research focuses on the onset of acquired chronic illness and disability (CID). From this perspective identify and list at least five elements of (1) triggering events, (2) moderating processes, and (3) QOL outcomes of psychosocial adaptation to acquired CID.

   b. How might the elements of the three components change in the following situations?

      • An individual with an acquired disability experiences a secondary health condition.

      • An individual with a congenital disability experiences the onset of a completely new CID.

2. Write a list of five questions you would ask to begin to understand an individual's perception of their subjective and psychological well-being.

3. Consider: What domains of your life are most central for you (as defined by the Disability Centrality Model)? How do you think you would respond (or how have you responded in the past) when satisfaction in important areas of your life was no longer available?

4. In small groups, discuss: How has the meaning of QOL changed since it was first introduced in modern U.S. history? How has the meaning of QOL changed for you personally across your life?

5. Discuss: Think of some other constructs identified as outcomes in the psychosocial adaptation to CID process. Is QOL a more useful and appropriate outcome? Why or why not?

KEY REFERENCES

Only key references appear in the print edition. The full references appear in the digital product on Springer Publishing Connect™: https://connect.springerpub.com/content/book/978-0-8261-5111-7/part/partII/chapter/ch12

Bishop, M. (2005b). Quality of life and psychosocial adaptation to chronic illness and disability: Preliminary *Analysis of a Conceptual and Theoretical Synthes*is. *Rehabilitation Counseling Bulletin, 48*(4), 219–231. http://dx.doi.org/10.1177/00343552050480040301

Bishop, M., Rumrill, P.D., Livneh, H., & Martz, E. (2023). Psychosocial adaptation to chronic illness and disability: Theoretical perspectives, empirical findings, and current issues. In M. Meade, K. Bechtold, & S. Wegener (Eds.), *The Oxford Handbook of rehabilitation psychology* (2nd ed.). Oxford University Press.

Crewe, N. M. (1980). Quality of life: The ultimate goal in rehabilitation. *Minnesota Medicine, 63*, 586–589.

Dembo, T., Leviton, G. L., & Wright, B. A. (1956). Adjustment to misfortune—a problem of social-psychological rehabilitation. *Artificial Limbs, 3,* 4–62.

Devins, G. M., & Deckert, A. (2018). Illness intrusiveness and self-management of medical conditions. In E. Martz (Ed.), *Promoting self-management of chronic health conditions: Theories and practice* (pp. 80–125). Oxford University Press.

Diener, E., Suh, E. M., Lucas, R. E., & Smith, H. L. (1999). Subjective well-being: Three decades of progress. *Psychological Bulletin, 125*(2), 276–302. https://psycnet.apa.org/doi/10.1037/0033-2909.125.2.276

Fleming, A. R., Fairweather, J. S., & Leahy, M. J. (2013). Quality of life as a potential rehabilitation service outcome: The relationship between employment, quality of life, and other life areas. *Rehabilitation Counseling Bulletin, 57*(1), 9–22. https://doi.org/10.1177/0034355213485992

Livneh, H. (2001). Psychosocial adaptation to chronic illness and disability: A conceptual framework. *Rehabilitation Counseling Bulletin, 44*(3), 151–160. http://dx.doi.org/10.1177/003435520104400305

Livneh, H. (2022). Psychosocial adaptation to chronic illness and disability: An updated and expanded conceptual framework. *Rehabilitation Counseling Bulletin, 65*(3), 171–184. http://dx.doi.org/10.1177/00343552211034819

Livneh, H., Bishop, M., & Anctil, T. M. (2014). Modern models of psychosocial adaptation to chronic illness and disability as viewed through the prism of Lewin's field theory: A comparative review. *Rehabilitation Research, Policy, and Education, 28*(3), 126–142. http://dx.doi.org/10.1891/2168-6653.28.3.126

Ryff, C. D. (2017). Eudaimonic well-being, inequality, and health: Recent findings and future directions. *International Review of Economics, 64,* 159–178. https://doi.org/10.1007/s12232-017-0277-4

III

FAMILY ISSUES IN ILLNESS AND DISABILITY

In this section, the authors draw on the most current research related to people with disabilities and their families. Issues, such as involvement, support, and coping of family members (parents, children, spouses, and partners), must be addressed to promote optimal medical, physical, mental, emotional, and psychological functioning of the loved one with a disability. Coping, resiliency, and psychosocial adjustment draw from the individual's support system. Hence, the attributes of family members cannot be separated from those of the loved member with a disability. Indeed, as families heal, so do their loved ones with disabilities. The authors in this section look deep into relationships within the family, such as the attachment of children and adolescents with disabilities and their parents. The literature examining relationships between parents with disabilities and their children, including those of adult age, is sparse, and cultural differences are seldom discussed. Among the strengths of this section are chapters discussing the unique aspects and personal experiences of parenting children with disabilities, being an adult caregiver for a partner or child with a specific disability, and the related adjustment, stresses, and rewards of caregiving as well as best practices for teaching coping skills and resilience. The authors give voice to parents who describe their experiences caring for a loved one with a disability and coping in a family system thrown into crisis mode by the introduction of disability—an event that may threaten family members' health if not dealt with appropriately. In addition, family member's concerns surrounding support systems, health care and services, insurance, education, and having a voice in policy making legislation. This section also explores grief, death, and dying of terminal or elderly family members with a disability and the emotional decision in having to place a loved one into a nursing home.

MAJOR HIGHLIGHTS IN PART III

- Chapter 13 offers qualitative research that demonstrates unique cultural differences, demands, and responsibilities of families parenting children with disabilities. There is no doubt that parenting with a disability or being a parent of a child with a disability can be stressful. It is interesting to note that many authors view the overall impact as not necessarily negative. Family reactions are discussed in relation to family adjustment models and effective coping strategies. Different variations are explored such as when a parent has a disability, when a sibling has a disability, and parenting a child with a disability. Cultural differences are also explored regarding how various racial and ethnic groups view and treat disability, and the impact of those cultural beliefs when a disability is introduced to a family.

■ Chapter 14 presents an empowered and empowering perspective on the experience of parenting a child with a disability. Throughout the chapter are woven the experiences and perspectives of a mother of an adult son with Down syndrome. The authors review the historical context and current research on families' experiences related to disability, explore the important role of families in the disability advocacy movement, discuss the variability in parents' experiences, and provide examples of parental leadership in health care, education, and policy.

■ Chapter 15 delineates concepts, models, and practical applications for counselors dealing with issues of grief, loss, death, and dying. This section provides empirical support for addressing issues early on in various stages of grief. The new *Diagnostic and Statistical Manual of Mental Disorders* (DSM-5; American Psychiatric Association, 2013) category of Persistent Complex Bereavement Disorder is discussed, laying the foundation for clinical interviews, standardized assessments, and treatment strategies for families dealing with this form of complicated and complex grief. In addition, the author discusses the range of mental, emotional, and physical exhaustion experienced by some caregivers. Newer research is offered suggesting that the caregiver role can be quite satisfying despite the sometimes-devastating effects on family members. The reader is directed to studies that have advanced the understanding of families in relation to grief, death, and dying. This newer research highlights elements of the caregiving role that can increase spiritual growth, meaning, and purpose, which ultimately assists in the grieving process. Finally, the emotional decisions of making end-of-life decisions and the need to place a loved one into a nursing home are explored.

■ Approximately 53 million Americans provide care to a family member with a disability or chronic illness, this translates to about 1 in 5 adults. The authors of Chapter 16 explore the pros and cons of caregiving, noting the mental and physical stress associated with having few resources or perceiving that one is alone, and conversely the rewards of having a purpose, doing something meaningful, and providing unconditional love through caring. The authors explore special issues for caregivers of children with disabilities, those in mid-life, and older adults, as well as the concepts of resilience and post-traumatic growth as buffers against caregiving strain. The authors also present best practices for supporting family caregivers, through family psychoeducation, respite, and other services. The chapter finishes with perspectives on future research to better address the needs of family caregivers leading to improved family support for people with disabilities and chronic illness.

REFERENCES

American Psychiatric Association. (2013). *Diagnostic and statistical manual of mental disorders* (5th ed.). American Psychiatric Publishing.

CHAPTER 13

FAMILY ADAPTATION ACROSS CULTURES TOWARD LOVED ONES WITH DISABILITY

NOREEN M. GRAF AND JACQUELINE MERCADO LOPEZ

LEARNING OBJECTIVES

After reading this chapter, you will be able to:

- Define family and recognize the characteristics of a healthy family
- Identify and recognize common reactions to disability in the family, including coping mechanisms
- Analyze reactions to disability based on the specific family member with the disability
- Analyze reactions to disability based on the familial relationship to the family member with the disability
- Sifferentiate between reactions to disability in the family based on cultural influences

PRE-READING QUESTIONS

1. What are the characteristics of a healthy family? How do healthy families deal with crisis?

2. How do we differentiate reactions to disability based on cultural influences? How do culturally assigned roles and expectations impact family reaction to disability?

3. Describe your experience (or projected experience) with disability in your own family. How has your culture impacted how your family functions in relation to the family member with a disability? How has your role in the family been impacted by disability in the family?

The first experiences of supportive and social units come, most often, from the family: "a group of two people or more (one of whom is the householder) related by birth, marriage, or adoption and residing together; all such people (including related subfamily members) are considered as members of one family" (U.S. Census Bureau, 2021, para. 28). Here, parents are obligated to provide adequate basic care for their children by supplying food, shelter, medical care, and schooling. The onset of disability in the family creates challenges for them, sometimes even to basic care obligations, depending on the resources available to, and the unique characteristics of, the members. Today, more than 65 million Americans care for a family member with a disability or illness; two-thirds of them are women (American Psychological Association, 2017). This chapter discusses the impact of disability on family by examining the reactions of family members to disability, factors that influence adjustment to disability in the family, adjustment models, parenting reaction perspectives, effective family coping, the impact of disability based on the family role of the person with a disability, and cultural influence on family adaptation to disability.

DEFINING *FAMILY*

Much of the literature related to families and disability is written from the framework of the traditional family model: married parents living with children. But only about 18% of American households are made up of a married man and woman and their children, and another 15% are persons living alone, many of them elderly and young unmarried persons. The remaining households are single-parent households, mixed families, same-sex-parent households, extended family households, cohabiting unmarried partners, and numerous other combinations of persons living together. In the United States, an average of 2.6 persons lives in a household; the average income for the household is about $67,500. The percentage of persons below the poverty level in 2020 was 11.4%, approximately 37 million people. Compared with families without members with disabilities, families with members with disabilities are more likely to live in poverty and have a lower median income (U.S. Census Bureau, 2022). They are also more likely to have increased medical expenses in addition to childcare expenses, further taxing the financial resources of these families.

Because families are the primary support systems of persons with disabilities, it is important to understand the characteristics of healthy and well-functioning units. A healthy family depends less on the structure of the family and more on characteristics of its members. With this in mind, families of any makeup—traditional, single-parent, extended family households, or otherwise—can be healthy families; however, a lack of financial, social, and personal resources will certainly make it more difficult to remain so. Six characteristics of healthy families dealing with a disability among its members are described next (DeFrain & Asay, 2007; Lin, 1994):

1. Commitment that involves the prioritization of family over self, coordination of family roles and responsibilities, working together toward mutual goals, and supporting one another.

2. Togetherness, which refers to the family planning for family time as in eating, playing, and celebrating together; it is less important what activities are shared as long as they are performed together.

3. Appreciation and admiration of an individual's strengths, talents, and interests as well as encouragement of individual pursuits.

4. Good communication that establishes a sense of belonging, diminishes frustrations, and improves marital relations; this involves listening and conflict resolution rather than avoiding a problem situation.

5. Spiritual well-being that involves the family sharing a common faith or spiritual belief that increases family cohesion.

6. Coping with crisis and stress that involves the family's willingness to face the reality of difficult situations and cope effectively, systematically, and rationally.

REACTIONS OF FAMILY TO DISABILITY

Emotional Reactions

In 1962, Olshansky described *chronic sorrow* as the regret and sorrow experienced by parents at the birth of a child with a disability caused by the loss of the expected child. It was seen as an understandable sorrow that could last indefinitely, as parents would reexperience sorrow at each of their child's developmental milestones. Twenty years later, Wolfensberger (1983) alternatively described *novelty shock crisis*, a state of confusion resulting from lack of information and societal reaction. This term illustrated the shift in thinking from disability as the problem in the family to understanding that a lack of social supports was also a hindrance to caregivers. Today, the term *caregiver burden* is frequently used to assist in the understanding of the amount of responsibility placed on caregivers that can result in extraordinary stress (Zarit et al., 1980). Caregivers may need to provide assistance with daily activities even to the extent that they feel they are missing out on life, which can lead to feelings of anger, resentment, and depression. They may become emotionally drained and physically exhausted due to increased financial responsibilities and may need to take over all or part of the disabled member's family responsibilities while maintaining their own.

Stress Reactions

Stress occurs when any demand placed on an individual or system exceeds the coping capacity. Initially, stress is inevitable at the onset of significant changes of any type. The stress created by disability in the family can cause it to collapse and struggle, or it may lead the family to become stronger, closer, and a better functioning system. Stress is more evident in families with disability than those without it (Hodapp & Krasner, 1995; Taanila et al., 2002; Wallander & Noojin, 1995) and in parents of children with disabilities, no matter the category of disability (Hsiao, 2018). A number of difficult family challenges may contribute to stress, including repeated medical and emotional crises, financial hardships, difficult schedules, modification of activities and goals, societal isolation, difficulty in educational placements, and marital discord (Lavin, 2001; McCubbin & Patterson, 1983). Other factors that increase stress for parents include having a greater number of children, behavior problems of the child, ineffective coping strategies, and having difficulty accessing reliable childcare (Hsiao, 2018; Warfield, 2005). In a study to look at the everyday lives of families with children who have chronic illnesses, families reported daily stresses as including chronic preoccupation with making health decisions, restricted social lives, and overall low vitality (Martin et al., 1992).

As a result of the medical costs of chronic illness and disability and the need for caretaking that can cause one family member to decrease or give up work, there can be considerable stress caused by the financial impact of disability to families. According to the 2019 U.S. Census Bureau, American Community Survey, children living in poverty are considerably more likely to have disabilities as those living above the poverty level (6.55 versus 3.85%). Park et al. (2003) determined that among children with disabilities who are 3 to 21 years old, 28% are living below the poverty level, affecting their health, living environment, family interactions, productivity, and emotional well-being. In addition, mothers of children with disabilities tend to have lower incomes and work fewer hours than mothers of children without disabilities (Neely-Barnes & Dia, 2008). Higher family income has been found to allow for increases in parents' coping options and adaptability, satisfaction, and ability to spend time supporting and nurturing their children, as well as to better afford costs associated with care (Mcleod & Shanahan, 1996; U.S Census Bureau, 2019; Wang et al., 2004; Yau & LiTsang, 1999).

Although stress has been noted as high in families, there is generally a decline in stress over time as the family adapts to their circumstances. In a longitudinal study that examined stress among parents of children with intellectual disabilities over a 7-year period, stress declined significantly over time in the areas of worry about speech deficits, intelligence deficits, behavior at home, behavior in public, and obtaining help. Parents in this study also had additional children without disabilities and rated the amount of stress due to the child with a disability as twice that of the amount of stress caused by a child in the home without a disability (Baxter et al., 2000).

Marital Discord

Marital difficulties are frequently discussed in the literature as problematic when families experience disability. In a meta-analysis of studies related to parents of children with disabilities, these parents had a higher rate of divorce than parents without children with disabilities (Risdal & Singer, 2004). Taanila et al. (1996) investigated the long-term effects of chronic illness, severe intellectual impairment, and physical disability on parents' marital relationships and found that 25% of the parents reported that their child's disability was a contributing factor to their marital impairment. Specifically, the intense demands of daily caretaking, unequal division of daily task labor, and insufficient available time for leisure activities were identified as contributing to marital discord.

Although preexisting marital discord can serve to increase family stress, severe childhood disability may also contribute to the onset of marital difficulties and be responsible for the higher rates of divorce among couples. Divorce is more likely to occur in families where one of the parents acquires a disability or a child is born with or acquires a disability. In families with children with developmental disorders, this increase is generally small, with only a 5.35% greater chance of divorce (Hodapp & Krasner, 1995). In a study of children with a chronic illness and variety of disabilities, the percentage of increase in divorce was even lower at 2.9% (Witt et al., 2003). Contrarily, Singer and Farkas (1989) found that families with infants with disabilities reported greater closeness.

FACTORS THAT INFLUENCE ADJUSTMENT TO DISABILITY IN THE FAMILY

Families have a great impact on the recovery/adjustment, well-being, and success of an individual with a disability (Degeneffe & Lynch, 2006; Kosciulek, 1994), and family competence is considered by many to be a key factor in adjustment to disability (Alston & McCowan, 1995). Parents who believe they are competent in their role as parents feel they are more in control of their behaviors, are more efficient, and are more satisfied with their parenting (Rybski & Israel, 2017; Sevigny & Loutzenhiser, 2010). Power and Dell Orto (2004) noted seven family characteristics that will influence how a family reacts to disability:

1. *Risk factors* will contribute to poor functioning in a family; these include a lack of support systems, family compositions that may add to stress such as single-parent households, stressed families, or families in conflict.

2. *Protective factors*, identified as strong family connections, effective communication, and problem-solving, will increase the likelihood that families will successfully adapt.

3. *Belief systems* that are moderated by religious and cultural values impact how the family manages the demands of disability, makes sense of the disability, and communicates with health professionals.

4. *Access to coping resources* includes personality strengths, previous life experiences, positive attitudes, values and religious beliefs, extended family support, and community and financial resources.

5. *Family history* involves the previous experiences in dealing with illness and disability and managing losses.

6. *Family relationships and communication styles* involve the members' ability to be open and honest with one another, to nurture each other, and to function in a well-structured manner versus members acting in isolation.

7. *Who in the family is disabled* plays a role in that dreams and expectations are affected differently based on if the member is a caretaker or dependent. Caretaker impairment will have a more detrimental impact on the family.

ADJUSTMENT MODELS

A number of models have been used to describe the process of family adaptation to disability. The family stress theory was propounded by Reuben Hill in 1949 after his work with families of soldiers. His ABCX model explained how a stressor event, the family's perception of that event, and the available resources interacted to avoid or create a crisis reaction. McCubbin and Patterson (1983) expanded this model in the double ABCX model by incorporating the use of family coping mechanisms to deal with a crisis event, recognizing an accumulation of stress on families over time and a need to use existing and new resources and coping skills to reach positive adaptation, termed *bonadaptation*.

The family resilience model has also been utilized to examine family adjustment. *Resiliency* is the ability to adapt, adjust, and thrive in difficult times. In rehabilitation, resiliency refers to the ability to adapt and adjust to disability and then to achieve a successful outcome (Kosciulek, 1994; Lustig, 1997). *Family resiliency* refers to the family's ability to make successful adaptations. The resiliency model of family stress, adjustment, and adaptation (McCubbin & McCubbin, 1993; McCubbin et al., 1996) focuses on how families can positively adjust and cope to maintain their quality of life. The model places emphasis on the functional capacity and strengths of the family rather than on deficits. It builds on the positive assets of the family, specifically what the family is good at, and then works toward increasing problem-solving, coping, and adjustment. Thus, instead of assessing only the deficits and needs of the family, the counselor would assess family strengths in terms of existing resources to deal with the family crisis, views, and attitudes toward the crisis, and the family's coping and problem-solving skills

Following this assessment, the counselor assists the family in building and utilizing resources and prepares the family to the extent possible for what to expect from the rehabilitation process and assists in developing realistic expectations for recovery. Counselors will also make efforts to help the family review and reframe the occurrence of disability in the family. Families are assisted in coming to understand that their reactions to disability and feelings of stress, being overwhelmed, or being angry are all normal reactions to a crisis. By reframing the event as an opportunity to work as a family to overcome obstacles, the family can become stronger, more efficient, and closer. Finally, counselors build on existing coping skills, including communication skills and work history, moving toward open family communication so that fears, misconceptions, and apprehensions about family roles can be resolved and long-term goals can be established. With open communication, family members can make decisions about who will be a caretaker and what role changes will occur. If these issues are not dealt with openly, anger and resentment may result (Frain et al., 2007).

Stage models have been used to describe the adjustment of persons to disability (Livneh & Antonak, 1990) over time. Blacher (1984) described three stages of adjustment of parents: First, an initial emotional crisis in which parents experience feelings of denial and shock; a second stage of fluctuating emotions that include anger, depression, guilt, shame, rejection of the child, and overprotection of the child; and a final stage of acceptance. A revision of this model by Anderegg et al. (1992) that emphasizes the grieving process consists of three stages: confronting, adjusting, and adapting.

A number of researchers have moved beyond the notion of adjustment and adaptation phases as being the final stages or end goal and have come to incorporate an additional growth phase, recognizing that families may grow closer as a unit due to the challenges and rewards brought on by disability (Bradley et al., 1993; Laufer & Isman, 2021; Naseef, 2001). In a sample of 257 parents of children with various disabilities, growth was indicated in life appreciation, personal strength, and spiritual change (Laufer & Isman, 2021).

Although stage theories have the benefit of attempting to explain how people proceed toward adjustment, they have been criticized for insufficient attention to the unpredictable or recurrent and complex aspects of adjustment to disability (Kendall & Buys, 1998). Likewise, Snow (2001) and Esdaile (2009) found that mothers of children with disabilities find these theories condescending and meaningless because they do not take into account the variety of positive experiences, insights, and understandings gained from caring for a child with a disability.

PARENTING REACTION PERSPECTIVES

In reviewing the literature related to reactions of parents of children with disabilities, Ferguson (2002) described five approaches to conceptualizing parental reactions: *psychodynamic, functionalist, psychosocial, interactionist,* or *adaptational.* For a number of decades, a *psychodynamic approach* was the only lens used to describe parental reactions to disability. This led to viewing parental reactions from a pathological standpoint, viewed as either apathetic or involved and either angry or accepting. From this standpoint, parents' reactions were framed as unhealthy and neurotic. Even involvement with the child could be interpreted as resulting from underlying guilt. Justifiable anger at a lack of appropriate care could be seen as displaced anger and a lack of adjustment.

With a shift to behavioral treatment approaches in the 1960s, a *functionalist* approach frequently labeled parents' reactions as dysfunctional, and children's parents were often seen as additionally disabling to the child. With the advent of the 1970s, the *psychosocial* approach to viewing disability focused on the interplay of the environment and the emotions of the parents. The emotions of shock, loneliness, stress, and grief became the focus. The work of Olshansky (1962) in the area of chronic sorrow and Wolfensberger (1983) in the area of shock and grief are examples of using the psychosocial approach to conceptualize parental reactions. From this standpoint, parents are viewed as suffering from loss. The *interactionist* standpoint, which is an infrequent approach, views parental reactions as a function of societal stigma, fatigue, disempowerment, and poverty, leading parents to feel powerless. Finally, a more recent approach to viewing parental reaction is the *adaptational* approach that emphasizes supportive social policy and cultural values as essential components of parental reaction to disability. It emphasizes the continued process of adaptability and resiliency of families and recognizes coping skills and positive aspects of raising a child with a disability, including the potential of marital and spiritual growth and family harmony. From this standpoint, families can be viewed as empowered, cohesive, and adapted.

EFFECTIVE FAMILY COPING WITH DISABILITY

The emotional, financial, and social impact of disability on the family will be determined largely by how the family responds to crisis and how effectively the members manage and resolve conflict, make decisions, and meet role expectations. Families that avoid or seek to escape dealing with disability will likely experience greater disorganization and stress, whereas families that demonstrate competence in reorganizing and actively addressing issues by changing their behaviors and attitudes to meet new demands will likely have greater positive adjustment (Alston & McCowan, 1995; Sevigny & Loutzenhiser, 2010).

In order to determine what family qualities are most helpful toward the effective adjustment of disability, McCubbin and McCubbin (1988) identified three family types: balanced, midrange, and extreme. The balanced family possesses two characteristics that render it most resilient and functional: rhythm and regenerativity. Rhythm in a family refers to established rituals, rules, and routines that allow children to have a clear understanding of what is expected of them and allows for increased closeness and bonding among family members. These families also report greater flexibility and satisfaction. Regenerativity in families refers to family coherence and hardiness. Coherence involves the emphasis placed on caring for one another, respect, loyalty, trust, pride, and common values. Hardiness involves internal control of events, activity involvement, and willingness to explore and challenge themselves (McCubbin & McCubbin, 1988).

Similarly, Walsh (2003) reflected this description of resilient families, listing three factors that assist them to succeed. First, families need to be able to make sense and meaning of the difficulties they face. Second, they need to affirm their strength and maintain a positive perspective. Finally, they need a shared spiritual belief system. In addition to these characteristics, families must also be flexible, connected, and resourceful to persevere.

Expanding further on resilient families, the National Child Traumatic Stress Network website (NCTSN, n.d.) identifies four characteristics of resilient families, including (a) they have beliefs and attitudes that facilitate coping; (b) they do their best to maintain routines and rituals but with flexibility; (c) they use effective communication about both information and feelings; and (d) they show adaptive problem-solving. Families are more resilient when they view a traumatic event as a family crisis that will be faced together, when they take care of each other's needs, accept distress as a normal reaction, and maintain reasonable hope.

While many studies look at the variables that make up resilient families as being present or absent, Stuntzner and Hartley (2014) view resilience as "an evolving process in which a person's ability to feel and demonstrate resilience continually or sporadically improves with conscious and mindful awareness and practice" (p. 5). This outlook allows for improvement through practice and awareness. In a study, Knestrict and Kuchey (2009) investigated resiliency among families who had children with severe disabilities and found a strong connection between socioeconomic status (SES) and family resiliency. Of the families they determined to be resilient, all were in the upper family income categories. Likewise, the lowest-functioning families were in the low-income category. The effect of higher SES was that families were more likely to have health insurance benefits, additional income provided for a better level of care, and the ability to access information and services. They found that more money was available to provide for respite care, home remodeling, and additional activities, such as aquatic and equine therapy, and more leisure time. The authors acknowledge the potential for state and federal programs to equalize disability services across SES levels, but point to continued funding cutbacks that limit available services.

Families have expressed a number of other needs that, if provided, could assist in family functioning, including family and social support, medical information, financial information and assistance, help explaining the disability to others, childcare, and professional support and services (Sloper & Turner, 1992; Walker et al., 1989). In a study of needs for families with a child with cerebral palsy (CP), parents desired information on services, help planning for the future, help finding community activities, and more respite time. Parents whose children used wheeled mobility expressed needing help paying for home equipment and home modifications and finding childcare workers, respite care providers, and community recreational activities (Palisano et al., 2010).

DISABILITY IMPACT AND THE FAMILY MEMBER WITH A DISABILITY

When a Child Has a Disability

The extent of the physical impairment, the predictability of the course of the illness, and whether or not it is life threatening affect the reactions of families and children to disability. The more severe and difficult the management of the disability is, the greater the family's susceptibility to stress reactions, frustration, and feelings of being overwhelmed (Lyons et al., 2010). In examining the influence of predictability of symptoms in young children with chronic illnesses on parents' stress levels, Dogson et al. (2000) found that childhood illness with unpredictable symptoms caused significantly higher levels of distress.

In addition to the disability's severity and predictability, the child's age will have an impact on emotional adjustment. Children who are very dependent on their parents, who do not have an opportunity to socialize with friends, or who are frequently absent from school due to medical conditions may be delayed in emotional and social development. If children are less socially mature or if they have experienced rejection from peers, they may have difficulty making friends, feel rejected, and become isolated. Adolescents who are unable to achieve sufficient independence or explore friendships and intimate relationships or whose body image is negative may become frustrated and depressed (Falvo & Holland, 2018).

Other emotions that children and adolescents with disabilities may have are fear, grief, anger, and denial. Anger can be experienced as loud outbursts as well as moodiness, pouting, and silence. Grief may be experienced as sadness but can also be masked behind hostility and resentment toward others. Uncertainty related to medical procedures or returning to school or other social environments may trigger lingering fear and apprehension. Denial and unreasonable expectations may initially serve to protect the child from emotionally dealing with difficulties related to the disability, but they can also serve to keep the child from making efforts to adjust to the condition (Power & Dell Orto, 2004).

As with other crises, parents' initial reactions to disability onset may present as shock and denial, a time of numbness, and disbelief. These reactions are productive in that they provide psychological protection until the family members work up to psychological coping but may also interfere with rational decision-making if the parents refuse to accept the diagnosis or the permanency of a condition. Parents may then experience a number of emotions as a result of having a child with a disability, including being overwhelmed, confused, and profoundly sad (Power & Dell Orto, 2004). They may experience guilt, believing that something they did or failed to do may have caused the disability or may become depressed (Norton & Drew, 1994). Parental depression and feelings of helplessness and stress may then contribute to additional restrictions or limitations on the child with a disability (Tomasello et al., 2010).

A number of studies have compared the impact of a birth of a child with a disability to a death in terms of adjustment because families have been noted to progress through the grief stages of shock, realization, defensive retreat, and acknowledgment (Norton & Drew, 1994; Wolfensberger, 1983). These studies suggest that parents grieve the death of the child that they anticipated, and they grieve the loss of dreams they had for their child. Depending on the disability, parents may need to alter their physical, emotional, or cognitive expectations of their child. For example, for children with significant mobility impairments, parents who wished to play sports with their children may initially grieve that perception of a future loss. In addition, parents may experience anger or look to place blame on hereditary causes in themselves or their partners. If poor nutrition, drug use, or other controllable factors are suspected to have contributed to the child's disability, such as in fetal alcohol syndrome, intense guilt and societal scorn may also result (Vash & Crewe, 2004).

In a study of parents of children with intellectual disabilities, Gallagher et al. (2008) found parents to have high levels of anxiety and depression that were most influenced by the amount of caregiver burden and their feelings of guilt. Another study by Norton and Drew (1994) identified the family hardships associated with raising a child with autism as difficulty with communication and bonding, sleep disruption, behavior problems, a need for consistent routine, respite care and problems, and future financial planning needs. The inability to effectively communicate and the child's rejection of physical contact and a seemingly noncaring attitude toward the family create difficulty in parental bonding. The child's behavior and need for consistency make traveling outside the home difficult. Children may sleep for only a few hours at night, causing sleep deprivation for parents. In addition, any disruption in routine may lead to screaming outbursts and prolonged crying. Because of the constant caregiving demands, respite is important, particularly for the primary caregiver, and siblings may be called on to provide care that can either be seen as positive role modeling or, if used to excess, may have a negative impact.

In examining caregiving burdens of families with a member with intellectual and behavioral/psychiatric problems, Maes et al. (2003) concluded:

> *Psychiatric and behavioral problems are often incomprehensible and unpredictable, which causes the parents to feel dissatisfied, inadequate to cope, insecure and reticent to act. But feelings and motivations of parents on the other hand may also have profound effects on the behavioral difficulties of their child. Parents consider the psychiatric or behavioral problems of their child to be an extra burden and feel it more difficult to raise and manage such a child in the family situation. This forces them to change the situation and to call on the help of external services.* (Maes et al., 2003, p. 454)

These authors conclude that families need more resources for respite, extended social support groups for emotional support, specialized training, and recognition of negative feelings.

Not all parents react in the same way to having a child with a disability; whereas some report continued discomfort with their child, others find the child has strengthened their marriage and family life (Scorgie & Sobsey, 2000). In comparing differences in the mother's and father's reactions to a child with a disability, some studies have found that mothers react with greater depression, express greater caregiver burden, and feel higher levels of stress than fathers do. They spend more hours caring for the child with a disability than fathers do. However, Hastings (2003) found that stress and depression levels were similar in mothers and fathers of children with autism, but mothers exhibited higher levels of anxiety. In an additional study, Hastings et al. (2005) reported that despite race or ethnicity, mothers report experiencing both greater depression and greater positive effects from parenting a child with a disability than fathers do.

In addition to parents, grandparents are increasingly being called on to care for their grandchildren with disabilities. This is especially true for African American and Latino families. Grandparents may have unique problems associated with caregiving because, unless they are the legal guardians, they have more difficulty accessing services and information (such as medical and school records) necessary for caretaking. In addition, they may have financial concerns; they may have difficulties due to aging and a need for respite; they may have problems associated with the child's parents, particularly if they have exited their child's life due to addictions or legal problems; and they may have problems navigating social service, judicial, and educational systems (McCallion et al., 2000). It is not surprising that grandparents have also been found to be susceptible to depression in some studies, but results vary and this remains unclear. What may be the most important to determining the amount of stress and caregiver burden experienced by grandparents may be strongly impacted by their beliefs and attitudes related to disability (Neely-Barnes & Dia, 2008). Positive effects of caretaking for a grandchild with a disability have been noted as creating better relationships and a greater sense of connectedness, meaning, and personal growth (Gardner et al., 2004).

The Decision to Place a Child Outside of the Home

The decision to place a child with a disability outside of the home is difficult for many parents. Several studies have demonstrated that increased stress is related to the extent of behavior problems (Maes et al., 2003) that may in turn affect the family's decision to place the child in residential care. This decision generally occurs at birth and in the transition out of high school. In a study to examine outside placement decisions of parents of young adults with severe intellectual disability, McIntyre et al. (2002) found that outside home placement could be predicted by the extent of behavior problems and mental health problems of the young adult.

When a Partner Has a Disability

Because most of the caregiving falls on the spouse, the impact of disability can be overwhelming for couples. Researchers have found that among couples in which one of the partners had a spinal cord injury (SCI), the caregiving partner had equal or higher levels of stress, fatigue, resentment, and anger when compared with the partner with the disability (Chan et al., 2000; Weitzenkamp et al., 1997). Parker (1989) reviewed the impact of disability on the partner's caregiver and concluded that they have higher levels of stress than any other caregiver due to the psychological and social effects of caring for their partner.

When a partner acquires a cognitive disability, such as traumatic brain injury (TBI), stroke, or Parkinson disease, the caregiver loses the equitable relationship and assumes a parenting role for their spouse, and they often feel as if they have gained a child and lost a spouse. The spouse caregiver must take on many of the duties of the afflicted spouse and may need to assume all of the financial burden as well and is frequently forced to make difficult financial cuts that may involve liquidating assets. In order to provide sufficient care, the caregiver may need to reduce social time with friends and family, creating social isolation. Even if the caregiver finds time to socialize, socializing may be difficult because he or she will not fit well into either the couple's socializing world or the single world. Ultimately, the strain of caretaking, financial struggles, and social isolation may lead to a marital relationship that is void of sexual relations. For some, this overwhelming change in living conditions and relations leads to separation or divorce (Parker, 1989).

Multiple sclerosis (MS) is a progressive disorder that will involve increasing reliance on others for activities of daily living (ADLs) and social interactions. Hakim et al. (2000) identified a number of issues related to living with MS that could affect partner relationships, including the reduction of social interactions and a shrinking number of friends, particularly as the disease progresses. In addition, the partner with MS frequently retired early, and many partners believed that their own careers were inhibited due to the spouse's illness. Partners also experienced higher levels of anxiety and depression associated with greater severity of MS. Even so, the authors did not find a greater incidence of divorce among couples with MS when compared with the general population.

For persons with SCI, the divorce rates are higher than the general population whether they marry before or after they are injured, and the likelihood of marriage after injury is decreased (Brain and Spinal Cord.org, 2010). Aside from the individual's adjustment to physical changes and pain, those in partner relationships will encounter a number of lifestyle changes that affect their relationships, such as changes to sexual intimacy, independence, raising children, job security, financial security, and recreational activity involvement. The emotional responses to these changes will also affect the relationship and may include depression and anxiety, suicide ideation (an initial suicide rate of four to five times that of the general population), and alcohol and drug abuse (Craig & Hancock, 1998). In a review of the literature on partner relationships and SCI, Kreuter (2000) found that divorce rates from 8% to 48% have been reported in the literature, depending on the time since injury for participants. In general, it appears that divorce rates are higher in the first 3 years and then decline to a normal rate. DeVivo and Richards (1992) noted a number of factors that put persons with SCI at greater risk for divorce, including being nonambulatory, being female, not having any children, being young, having a previous divorce, and having an injury less than 3 years old. In a study that interviewed 55 couples with preinjury or postinjury marriages, Crewe et al. (1979) and DeVivo et al. (1995) found more stability and life satisfaction in postinjury marriages. Kreuter et al. (1994) studied marriage stability following SCI and found differences based on the age of the couple; older couples had greater emotional attachment or relationship satisfaction than younger couples.

Despite the negative public perception that persons who date people with disabilities are deviant or desperate (Olkin, 1999), in a qualitative study to examine females who were dating men with SCI, Milligan and Neufeldt (1998) found that maladaptive motivations were not present. They identified a number of factors related to the disability that influenced the development of the relationships. Nondisabled participants described their partners as well adjusted to their SCI and exhibiting autonomous attitudes. These elements in combination with individual personality traits were described as important features of their attraction. Attributes of the nondisabled female partners included open-mindedness about a relationship with a person with SCI, previous experiences with disability, role flexibility, acceptance of the partner's need for assistance, commitment to foster independence, and resiliency against social disapproval.

In relation to cognitive and mental health disabilities, studies have also shown high rates of divorce. Lefley (1989) identified problem behaviors in families of persons with severe mental illness, including persons with disabilities abusing family members, conflicts with neighbors, noncompliance with medications and other interventions, unpredictable reactions, and mood swings. Butterworth and Rodgers (2008) reported that a number of studies have demonstrated that divorce frequently follows the acquisition of mental illness in couples where one partner has a mental illness. Causes of marital termination have been attributed to relationship dissatisfaction, marital conflict, and social causes. In couples where both partners have a mental illness, divorce rates have been shown to be eight times that of the general population.

Studies related to couples in which one partner acquires a TBI have reported varying rates of divorce ranging from 15% to 54% and dependent on factors such as the length of the relationship preinjury and how much time has elapsed since the injury. In a study that examined 120 persons with TBI, people who were more likely to stay married had been in longer-term preinjury marital relationships, were older, had less severe TBI, and their injuries were not due to violent crimes (Kreutzer et al., 2007).

When a Parent Has a Disability

Early speculation related to children being raised by persons with disabilities suggested that children were in danger of negative emotions and behaviors, such as anxiety and depression, and developmental issues, such as dependency, helplessness, overcompliance, social alienation, and isolation. However, the empirical literature presents no definitive evidence of these negative parenting effects. Buck and Hohmann (1983) reported that children raised by a father with SCI showed no difference from other children in terms of physical health measures, personality disturbance, body image or sexual orientation, or interpersonal relationships. The differences noted in male children were that they were more conventional, practical, and tough-minded but less secure than other males. Female children were found to be more self-assured, imaginative, and unconventional, but were less tough-minded and realistic than other females. Coles et al. (2007) studied children of parents with MS and noted that often these children assume caregiving roles by cleaning, cooking, shopping, budgeting, and giving emotional support. Children with a parent who has MS have also been shown to have higher levels of anxiety dysphoria, somatization, interpersonal difficulties, and hostility and less satisfaction with life (Pakenham & Bursnall, 2006). The fact that positive and negative effects are present is to be expected because children who have parents with disabilities have different growing-up experiences and challenges. However, negative differences may be directly related to a lack of financial and social supports to alleviate overburdening children.

Parents with mental retardation (MR) face problems such as poverty, lack of parenting models, isolation from families, lack of public resources, and limited experiences. For these parents, providing adequate parenting depends on long-term support (Whitman & Accardo, 1993). Incidences of neglect and abuse are due to a lack of support and resources more than cognitive deficit (Tymchuk & Andron, 1990). In a study of children whose parent(s) had MR, two-thirds were diagnosed with MR or developmental delays. Most of the delays were corrected with intervention, pointing to the need for additional resources and supports. In addition, a number of studies have demonstrated the need for and efficacy of parenting skills training for parents with MR (Feldman et al., 1992; Whitman & Accardo, 1993).

Parents with sensory impairments reported difficulty in assisting children with school work and a need to rely on children as interpreters (Strom et al., 1988), and hearing children of deaf adults (CODA) often grow up in the Deaf culture, learning sign language and acting as interpreters for parents. These children grow up with distinct advantages but can also feel caught between two worlds; they sometimes describe being raised as a deaf child (Malik & Jabeen, 2016).

When a Sibling Has a Disability

Depending on the age of the child, siblings may have a number of reactions to a sister or brother with a disability. Young children may experience some fear that they may catch the disability, or they may believe they are responsible in some way for the disability due to wishful or magical thinking (Batshaw, 1991), or they may feel jealous or embarrassed of their sibling, causing abusive behaviors (Havens, 2005; Pearson & Sternberg, 1986). Poor adjustment of siblings has been attributed to high levels of family conflict, poor parent functioning, low family adaptability and cohesion, and deficit problem-solving skills and communication.

In a study of 49 siblings, Giallo and Gavidia-Payne (2006) found that they had significantly higher overall adjustment difficulties, more emotional and peer problems, and lower levels of socialization compared with the normative sample. In order to investigate how family characteristics, family routines, and problem-solving influence sibling adjustment, these authors determined that (a) sibling adjustment to disability was not significantly impacted by sibling level of daily stress and coping skills, (b) level of parent stress was a predictor of sibling adjustment, (c) siblings in households with regular and consistent family routines exhibited fewer adjustment problems, and (d) siblings had better adjustment in households that demonstrated great problem-solving strategies and more effective communication.

Research involving siblings has also described some positive benefits (Hannah & Midlarsky, 1985), but siblings are often expected to assume additional responsibilities, such as providing for the inclusion, socialization, and physical care of their sibling with a disability (Skrtic et al., 1984; Swenson-Pierce et al., 1987). Parents of nondisabled siblings who can provide care and socialization may benefit from the additional assistance, but some studies have determined that nondisabled siblings may be given too much responsibility for their maturity level. Charles et al. (2009) discussed the negative impact for young caregivers as including the loss of their childhood and increased stress. However, siblings report both positive and negative effects related to caregiving. In a study of school-aged siblings' stressors, siblings identified being the most stressed when they felt embarrassed in the presence of their friends, they felt the happiest when they played with their sibling, and they felt the most uplifted when their sibling expressed affection through hugs and kisses (Orfus & Howe, 2008).

Most of the literature related to siblings of persons with disabilities focuses on the childhood relationships between the disabled and nondisabled siblings. However, as the person with a disability ages and parents become too old to care for their children, the sibling may be called on to provide extensive care. Although some persons with disabilities may move into group homes, the demand for residential care far exceeds availability, and waiting lists for group homes may be prohibitively long.

Perspective on Family Impact From the Person With the Disability

Previously scantly addressed in the literature on family impact has been the perspective of the person with the disability. In a study of over 400 persons with disabilities (PWD), Jenkins and Graf (2020) found that PWD disagreed with much of the family impact literature. They disagreed that disability frequently affect the family in terms of guilt, loneliness, or jealousy. Their study concluded that while most PWD felt family was happy to help, about a third of participants believed their families were never to rarely happy to help. Overall, the participants disagreed that their families experienced a social impact due to the disability. Participants did agree that maintaining intimate relationships and finding partners was made difficult due to their disability. In terms of spiritual impact, half the participants reported their families believed God could make their disabilities better. The authors conclude that disability is not a consistent familial experience, but impacted by gender, marital, living, and parental status.

CULTURAL IMPACT ON FAMILY ADAPTATION

For the purposes of this section, I briefly address culture in relation to family dynamics and responses. Although it is difficult to imagine how odd U.S. culture might seem to others, examination of documents intended to explain our culture to migrating persons highlights cultural differences in family behavior and practices:

- Americans will invite strangers (people they have never met) into their homes.
- Visitors to an American home might be allowed or even encouraged to see any room of the house. It is not unusual for people who visit a home in the winter to use the bed in the master bedroom as a place to deposit their coats.
- Some entertaining might take place in the kitchen. The kitchen is not the exclusive territory of the female of the house. Men might be seen helping in the kitchen, cooking and/or cleaning up. Men might even be seen wearing aprons.
- Children may get more attention than they would in some other countries. The children might be included in a social activity, particularly if the activity entails dinner. Children may take a fairly active role in the conversation and may even get more attention than some of the adults.
- The host might have pets, usually dogs or cats, who live in the house along with the human inhabitants and who may be permitted to enter any part of the house and use any item of furniture as a resting place.
- The social interaction might entail much mixing of the sexes. Although it sometimes happens that women will form their own conversation groups and men theirs, there is no rigid sexual segregation at American social gatherings.

■ Although they will make certain accommodations for guests, particularly for guests at a formal gathering, Americans do not have the idea that their normal lives should be entirely devoted to guests during the time the guests are visiting them. Thus, if they have other obligations that conflict with hosting, they may turn their attentions to other commitments, such as providing transportation for young children who have obligations or answering a telephone call and engaging in an extended conversation. (University of Missouri–St. Louis, 2013)

Disability is defined differently across cultures in terms of the meaning of experience, family values, and interaction with social systems. Understanding cultural differences in family function is essential to understanding the adjustment process, as well as understanding the strengths of family systems. Living as a minority family in the United States differs from living in the majority culture in a number of ways identified by Sue and Sue (1999). Families must frequently deal with racism, and there is a greater likelihood of living in poverty. Family values, although not in conflict with the majority values, place greater emphasis on family and less emphasis on the individual. Values and dreams related to wealth, occupation, and status may differ in their meaning to minorities. They are also likely to be transitioning into assimilation and juggling two cultures. They may have come from histories that include slavery, immigration, and refugee status, and may have been forced from their countries or made difficult decisions to leave. They may also be in the process of learning or using English, which may not be a good substitute for expression.

African American Families

The African American family differs in that it uses extended family members as primary caretakers, has great flexibility in family roles, is intensely religious, and has developed coping skills to stressors brought on by racism, poverty, and unemployment (Hines & Boyd-Franklin, 1982). In addition, African American families may face healthcare provider diagnostic bias in terms of delayed diagnoses and experience substantial differences in healthcare sought and received (Burkett et al., 2015). In a study of disparities among African American and Caucasian children with autism spectrum disorder, Mandell et al. (2007) found African American children were more likely to be misdiagnosed than Caucasian children. They were five times more likely to be improperly diagnosed with adjustment disorder and two and a half times more likely to be misdiagnosed with conduct disorder. This suggests healthcare providers may have race-based preconceived notions when approaching assessment, which may result in critical delays of child development and treatment.

Alston and Turner (1994) examined African American family strengths, noting strong kinship bonds that include immediate, extended, and even fictive kin. They suggest that one reason African American families do not access rehabilitation services may be that they have the capacity to support a family member with a disability through the process of adjustment to the disability. Greater role flexibility is present in African American families for a number of reasons, including the fact that Black women frequently are in a head-of-household position by choice or because a disproportionate number of men in the Black community are incarcerated, unemployed, or living out of the home. When the mother is employed, extended family members or older children are enlisted to provide for childcare and household duties. Unlike families that adhere to rigid roles, the African American family has adapted to avoid overload through role flexibility. In the case of disability in the family, members may be accustomed to assuming a variety of family roles and duties.

In addition to role flexibility, studies have found that African American family caregivers find greater satisfaction and feel less anxious and less burdened than Caucasian caregivers. In a qualitative study of 22 Black family caregivers who were caring for relatives with dementia, Lindauer et al. (2016) identified the two themes of *Hanging On* and *Changed but Still Here*. These themes illustrated the high value of caring for the family member as long as possible. One participant stated, "Way back when . . . even in the struggles, and slavery, all we had is each other. So that's why we hang on to each other" (p. 5). In the second theme, participants focused on what remained of their loved one's personality as opposed to dementia-related losses. Ancestral values were seen to influence the belief that no matter how changed a person, what remained was worthy of both compassion and respect.

Religious orientation has also been noted as a strength for African Americans because it offers spiritual inspiration, social support, and an opportunity for ventilation of distress and other emotions. The church is viewed as a further extension of the family that emphasizes positive outlook and increases self-esteem. It also assists in providing for basic needs, such as shelter, food, clothing, childcare, and assistance in locating work (Alston & Turner, 1994). In a study, Chatters et al. (2015) examined the influence of attendance at religious services on depression and stress among Black participants. They found social support offered through church networks acted as a protective factor against psychological distress and depressive symptoms. Thus, religion appears to serve as both emotionally and physically assistive and as a protection against psychological impairment.

Other family strengths noted by Alston and Turner (1994) are education and work ethics. African Americans value education and encourage children to succeed academically because this is considered one of the pathways to social and economic upward mobility. Unfortunately, this is all too often an uphill battle. In their examination of special education placement in elementary and middle schools, Morgan et al. (2015) found:

> Minority children were consistently less likely than otherwise similar White, English-speaking children to be identified as disabled and so to receive special education services. From kindergarten entry to the end of middle school, racial- and ethnic-minority children were less likely to be identified as having (a) learning disabilities, (b) speech or language impairments, (c) intellectual disabilities, (d) health impairments, or (e) emotional disturbances. (p. 278)

Thus, similar to the healthcare system, disparities are evident early on in educational institutions, which result in a lack of appropriate educational accommodation. If behavioral disturbances are misdiagnosed, focus may be misdirected to behavioral modification and discipline.

Alston and McCowan (1995) determined that African Americans who adjust well to disability have families that are close and supportive, have strong emotional support, and have members willing to assist with ADLs. These authors suggested that Black families are not easily disrupted by disability and can accommodate disability while maintaining stability, humor, and generosity. They also suggest that African American families benefit from a lack of traditionally defined roles and are able to redefine and reassign family roles as needed to meet the needs of the family. Interestingly, perhaps one of the obvious cultural differences is that conflict was not predictive of poor adjustment. Black families did not view the expression of family conflict as an obstacle to adjustment. Rather, the expression of disagreement and emotions was seen as natural and acceptable.

Asian American Families

Asian Americans are a homogeneous population whose relatives have descended from a number of geographic locations, including Cambodia, China, India, Japan, Korea, Malaysia, Pakistan, the Philippine Islands, Thailand, Vietnam, and the Asian/Pacific Islander population.

According to Miles (2000), U.S disability culture and traditional Asian beliefs and traditions do not align well. The core values of Asian families are duty to family, family welfare, family reputation and avoidance of shame, respect, harmony, education, wisdom, knowledge, humility, work, obedience, and self-sacrifice. Their parenting style is generally more patriarchal and controlling (Kim et al., 2017; Lynch & Hanson, 2004). The Chinese are highly interdependent and very willing to sacrifice for family members. They seek assistance within the family context first and find seeking government assistance is intimidating, as it is frequently difficult to find translators when needed or desired (Liu, 2001).

Canfei is the traditional Chinese word for disability. Its interpretation is handicap and useless. Another common word used is *canji*, which translates to handicap and illness (Liu, 2001). In traditional Chinese culture, two main philosophical principles govern Taoism which are following natural laws and being humanistic (i.e., considerate, kind). Taoism stresses duality, or the yin and yang, and the importance of responsibility, balance, and harmony. Disabilities may be viewed as disharmony and therefore subject to discrimination and marginalization. Significant differences exist in the Asian American outlook related to disability. Depending on the level of acculturation, Asian parents may view children with disabilities as shameful or humiliating and may believe that they are to blame for the disability. They may also shelter their children from societal integration in order to protect them from discrimination (Yan et al., 2014).

In a study of Chinese families in New York, Ryan and Smith (1989) determined that language barriers caused almost half the parents not to understand their child's diagnosis. Parents were also inclined to view disability as a temporary condition, and many exhibited reactions of denial, guilt, and only partial acceptance. Parents attributed disability to either natural, supernatural, or metaphysical causes. Supernatural causes resulted from a belief there had been a religious or ethical violation that caused a deity to become angry. One-third of the parents surveyed believed in a metaphysical cause for their child's disability and attributed disability to a lack of balance between the yin and yang, considered essential for health. Imbalances were felt to produce fever and chills in children, which were seen as having the potential to lead to disability. These parents used alternative medicine that included incense to remove evil spirits, acupuncture, and wearing silver bracelets.

As the family becomes more acculturated, negative attitudes are replaced with attitudes of hope and acceptance (Cho et al., 2003). In a study of first-generation Chinese families with a child with a disability, Parette et al. (2004) noted that parents were involved, valued education, were concerned about social stigma, and did not express shame about their child's disability.

Latinx Families

The Latinx population of the United States has increased by 50% since 1990. Because of poor healthcare, exposure to violence, and work in settings that expose them to greater physical risks, disability is prevalent in Latinx communities (World Institute on Disability, 2004). Although every culture and every family is different and they come to the United States from a number of Central American and South American countries, some common themes are present in Latinx families, including religion, family, and gender roles. Religion is important to community and family life, and most Latinxs practice Catholicism, but many also have additional beliefs that are related to their countries of origin. Many Latinxs believe that things that happen in their lives are beyond their control and are meant to be; they also may engage in magical thinking and have a strong belief in miracles and the power of prayer. They may believe in positive or negative spirits that can cause difficulties or bad luck in their families and marriages (de Rios, 2001; Falicov, 1998).

For Latinxs, the purpose of marriage is to have children, and there is little separation between the two. Family is frequently the top priority, and couples tend to include children in nearly all activities and outings. Extensive interaction with large and extended families is common, and extended family is frequently relied on for social, emotional, and financial support. Perhaps due to the high value placed on family interaction, Skinner et al. (1999) found that many of the 150 Latinx mothers in their study believed that having a child with disabilities made them better mothers. Latinx families with disabilities have long been credited with viewing disability as a punishment from God (Falicov, 1998; Vega, 1990), but in a study of Mexican and Mexican American beliefs about God in relation to disability, Graf and Blankenship (2007) found that only a small minority of Mexicans and Mexican Americans believed disability to be a punishment from God. This study, and others, point to the importance of reexamining cultural values over time.

In a study of Latinx elders, Ruiz and Ransford (2012) cautioned that there has been a decline in the ability of Hispanic families to measure up to the traditional obligations, known as *familismo*. Hispanic families have previously relied on large extended family networks to dutifully provide care for their own. Ruiz and Ransford's study revealed family self-reliance "may no longer be attainable" (p. 56). Elders in this study reported infrequent family contact and experiencing hardships that went unnoticed by younger family members. It is essential that health professionals examine family circumstances without making cultural assumptions. "By perpetuating an over-romanticized notion [of familismo], communities may inadvertently be contributing to a shortage of formal support services for older Latinos" (p. 56; Carrillo et al., 2001).

Disability that affects gender roles may be particularly difficult for Latinxs because gender roles tend to be traditional, with the male expected to be the financial provider, to be physically and emotionally strong, and to be a protective authority figure. Women are expected to provide for the children and elderly family members and to be self-sacrificing; they are in charge of the home and children but are expected to defer to their husbands. Although these traditional roles have begun to change for many Latinxs, these traditional beliefs and roles are the foundation for current practices and beliefs (Vega, 1990). In a study to examine the influence of gender on Spanish family caregiving, Casado-Mejía and Ruiz-Arias (2016) noted that males became caregivers if there was not an available female to meet this role. Women caregivers experienced greater strain than males, especially if they tried to maintain employment. Women were also less likely to receive outside help than males who became caregivers.

Arab Families

An estimated 3.7 million Arab Americans have migrated from 22 countries and are one of the fastest-growing ethnic minorities in the United States. Despite differences in religion, professions, and education, they share a common language: Arabic (Zidan & Chan, 2019). As one of the oldest cultures on Earth, the Arab culture is associated with the Islam religion and centers around the Quran, the central religious text. Muslims believe in one God (Allah) and revere Muhammad as his prophet. They also believe in other prophets associated with the Jewish and Christian faiths such as Abraham, Moses, and Jesus. Tenets of Islam include prayer, almsgiving, fasting, and a pilgrimage to Mecca (Al Khateeb et al., 2014).

Arab culture is collectivist, patriarchal, and interdependent. In Muslim communities, family is frequently the most important social unit. Even into adulthood, Muslims may turn to family members to provide food, clothing, and housing assistance. Maintaining family harmony is especially important, and family interests outweigh individual interests. Family hierarchies are observed, and the elderly are held in the highest regard. Within traditional family structures, mothers are the primary caregivers and fathers participate less in parenting but hold higher status. (Hasnain et al., 2008). Genders are segregated to varying degrees in Arab societies, and women are expected to dress modestly and wear a veil (jihab). As parents age, children are obligated to care for them (Al Khateeb et al., 2014).

Influenced by Greek philosophers such as Plato (who considered disability harmful) and Aristotle (who advised against raising a child with a disability), some Arab countries imposed oppressive conditions for PWD, who were excluded from society and mistreated. Even today, PWD may experience discrimination and intolerance, which are extended to the family. In the past, and to some extent today, mothers are sometimes blamed for the child's disability, which is seen as imposed due to her sins. While attitudes are slow to change, with the establishment of the Arab Labor Organization in 1965, changes in attitudes led to persons with disabilities being cared for; however, stigmatization remains prevalent, and parents often experience feelings of guilt. (Saad & Borowska-Beszta, 2019).

A number of distinctions are apparent in Arab cultures which impact the prevalence of disability, such as the presence of consanguineous marriage, which is marriage between blood relatives (i.e., cousins), which may increase the presence of congenital anomalies. Early marriage is also prevalent in some Arab countries, with between one-seventh and one-third of girls marrying before the age of 18, depending on the country. Other non-Arab countries such as South Sudan have a rate of over 50% child marriages. This phenomenon is tied to values, traditions, and social and economic conditions. However, when youth give birth, they are not biologically or psychologically mature, which increases the likelihood of giving birth to children with special needs. This is compounded by a high infant mortality rate and compensated for by increasing the number of pregnancies (Saad & Borowska-Beszta, 2019).

As in other faiths, Islam emphasizes protection and care for those who need assistance and encourages inclusion of all members of the community. Despite this, disabilities are sometimes seen as punishment from God (Armstrong & Ager, 2005). Many Muslims view disability as preordained or qadar/kismat, a belief in fate. However, Muslims also acknowledge a balancing of fate with free will, where one must do what is responsible and necessary (Hasnain et al., 2008). Despite attribution of disability to God or evil spirits, Arab American families express typical reactions to a diagnosis of disability, including shock, anger, guilt, and so on. However, due to the stigma associated with disability, they may experience greater stress reactions than some other cultures (Al Khateeb et al., 2014).

In one qualitative study (Endrawes et al., 2007), the researchers found most of the seven Arab families interviewed believed that the social stigma prevented their loved ones from seeking treatment for mental illness. The author concluded that families hide mental illness because of the damage to family reputation. Shame and embarrassment may accompany mental illness in the family along with a belief that bad blood was passed to them by previous generations or that an evil spirit possession has taken place, known as *Zar*.

For many Arab families, concern over caring for family members and reliance on family, coupled with distrust of institutions aimed at social services and support, may lead families to refuse external services. This can lead to delays in services and delayed early interventions for children with disabilities. Typically, Arab families rely on extended family to determine the most appropriate plan and provide emotional and material resources, but for immigrants, this may not be possible. When service providers are in contact with a person with a disability, they should include extended family, when possible, in treatment planning (Al Khateeb et al., 2014; Hasnain et.al., 2008). It is also important to be aware of communication styles of Arabs, which include repetition of themes, elaboration, and exaggeration to emphasize importance of a topic and close proximity and frequent touching among, but not between, genders. Also noteworthy are patterns of speaking fast and loud and patterns of intonation and silence (Al Khateeb et al., 2014).

Acculturation is an important issue to consider, as Arab Americans have an extensive history of unique cultural practices and immigration. Level of acculturation is frequently associated with length of time in a new place, and thus values and attitudes prevalent in the United States may become more acceptable as time goes on (Zidan & Chan, 2019). However, "Arab Americans with a strong sense of ethnic identity will likely struggle with adopting Western culture and U.S. views regarding people with disabilities" (Zidan & Chan, p. 3). Specific recommendations for working with Arab Americans include understanding language and communication differences, level of acculturation, consideration of religious affiliation, appreciation of family response to disability as potentially stigmatizing and shameful, and placing great emphasis on confidentiality (Al Khateeb et al., 2014).

Indigenous American Families

The term *Native American* has recently fallen out of favor with some indigenous groups who would ideally like to be called by their tribal names. The National Conference of State Legislatures (2020) reports there are 574 federally recognized tribes. Other preferred terms are *Indigenous Americans* or *American Indians* (National Museum of the American Indian, n.d.). In the United States, Indigenous Americans and Alaska Natives have grown from 2.9 million (0.9% of the population) in 2010 to 3.7 million, accounting for 1.1% of the population (U.S. Census Bureau, 2020). Indigenous Americans may be citizens of their tribes and the states in which they live (National Museum of the American Indian, n.d.). As sovereign nations, tribes uphold the right to self-govern and the mandate to protect the safety and well-being of the individuals in their communities (Lucero & Leake, 2016). More than half of Indigenous Americanslive in rural or small-town communities, and 68% live directly on or close to their tribal lands (Dewees & Marks, 2017).

Understanding the health disparities within the Indigenous Americanpopulation has been historically limited due to the difficulties in sampling this isolated, diverse, and culturally distinct population (Sarche & Spicer, 2008). Martin and Yurkovich (2014) explored American Indians' perceptions of a healthy family and stated that the most significant health disparities occurred among this population. Indigenous Americans have considerably worse health outcomes, including higher infant mortality rates, more disease and disability, and shorter life expectancies (Westmoreland & Watson, 2006). Currently, the life expectancy of Indigenous Americans is 5.5 years less than all other U.S racial and ethnic groups (Indian Health Services, 2019). Other prevalent health issues among this population include chronic liver disease and cirrhosis, diabetes mellitus, unintentional injuries, assault/homicide, intentional self-harm/suicide, and chronic lower respiratory diseases (Indian Health Service, 2019).

Cultural trauma is an issue that has long been present in this group as a consequence of generations of violent colonization, assimilation policies, and general loss. Under the circumstances, the effects of generational trauma among Indigenous Americans have resulted in changes to traditional ways of child-rearing, family structure, and relationships. Poor emotional health, low self-esteem, depression, substance abuse, and high suicide rates have been observed in the population (U.S. Department of Health and Human Services, 2014) and may result, in part, from cultural trauma.

Indigenous Americans have the highest poverty rate compared to other minority groups and account for the highest rate of disability rates compared to the general population (Martin & Yurkovich, 2014). Many of the issues faced by Indigenous American communities are misunderstood or unknown because they are often left out of significant data-collection efforts (Dewees & Marks, 2017). Due to these inequities, Native reservations, especially rural ones, struggle to provide adequate housing, safe communities, and quality healthcare (Pathak, 2021).

Indigenous Americans' unique perspectives and worldviews differ from mainstream America (Peweardy & Fitzpatrick, 2009). In the same way, Indigenous Americans have disparate views regarding disability. The disability constructs that influence Indigenous American culture are said to vary on factors such as:

> *The social construct of disability (within and outside native cultures); 2) the stigma associated with certain disabilities within the majority society and how this stigma influences public policies and practices that affect native communities; and 3) the apparent priority given to disability within Indian [sic] communities.* (Joe, 1997, p. 251)

The social construct of disability provides a framework for society's understanding and interactions with individuals who are different (Dray, 2009). To further emphasize the impact of culture and disability, Joe (1997) denotes that acculturation in Indigenous American communities living within a bicultural world has greater effects on the family's perceptions and responses to disability. One barrier associated with seeking necessary services within IA culture is stigma; a social phenomenon that often stems from a lack of understanding or fear associated with negative attitudes and internalized shame (Borenstein, 2020). In efforts to increase culturally responsive care and mental health equity within indigenous mental health professionals, O'Keefe et al. (2021) found that stigma emerged as a consistent barrier across several Native studies. Therefore, Indigenous Americansmay neglect to seek services for fear of being labeled as weak or hesitant about how others may view them due to the negative perceptions attached to seeking services (Duran et al., 2005; Freitas-Murrell & Swift, 2015; Johnson et al., 2010; Venner et al., 2012). Instead, it is customary for Indigenous American families to prioritize seeking help within their own culture rather than seeking modern remedies (Joe, 1997).

LaFromboise et al. (1990) describe the Indigenous American tribes' extended family as the central organizing unit, emphasizing interdependence, reciprocity, and obligation to care for one another. Indigenous American tribes' value systems are primarily influenced by culture and language (Allison & Christine, 1999). Specific health beliefs and cultural practices are learned within the family system (Martin & Yurkovich, 2013). Given their unique cultures and languages among tribes, they may have significantly different perspectives on child-rearing, intervention, medicine, and healing. "Language, kin structure, religion, land, and health behavior impact family culture and affect their perceptions, beliefs, and practices about prevention, and cause and treatment of illness and disability" (Allison & Christine, 1999, p. 197). Indigenous American rituals and ceremonies, such as death ceremonies, healing rituals, Native American medicine, peyote worship, and dances, played a crucial role in traditional culture (Alexander, 2021). The use of humor and laughter is also customary and preserved among Indigenous American culture. For some, humor is unique and is considered the heart of their resilience and survivability, as laughter is believed to heal and help with the recovery of many ailments (Lindquist, 2016).

Indigenous American values are deeply rooted in family ties. There is a deep respect for people and strong respect for elders (Weaver & White, 1997). The extended family system is of core value in tribal communities. The extended family includes mothers, fathers, grandparents, aunts who are often referred to as the child's mother, uncles who may be referred to as the child's father, and cousins who are often referred to as brothers and sisters (Allison & Christine, 1999). Indigenous American families are often intergenerational households as they extend to family and nonfamily members who are incorporated into the family by formal or informal means (Horse, 1980). Grandparents typically fill leadership positions and hold vital decision-making roles regarding health and family crises (Weaver & White, 1997). Traditional parenting roles hold value in child-rearing practices. The custom of storytelling is a traditional parenting role used to teach and help uncover a sense of identity, purpose, and guidance in their children (Ramirez, 2004; Wark et al., 2019). Interactions between parents often involve nonverbal communication known as "silent language," which involves gestures, body language, touch, and facial expressions, to communicate with their children (Taylor et al., 2006). At large, parents serve as the first and primary guide to shaping their child's morals and values (Killsback, 2019).

Across the Indigenous American culture, children are considered gifts to be honored and cherished. In the family unit, children are celebrated for their developmental milestones by providing them with a sense of belonging through the practice of naming ceremonies in which the child is given a meaningful Indian name (LaFromboise & Low, 1989). However, Indigenous American children face high systemic disadvantages and health inequities. The disproportionate health disparities among Indigenous American children are injury (Wong et al., 2014), preterm birth (MacDorman, 2011), and other risk factors (Cappiello & Gahagan, 2009). Indigenous American children also experience higher special education rates than other racial groups (Murry & Wiley, 2017). Indigenous American families encounter unique barriers to education. For example, tribes upholding a sovereign status may "impede the delivery of disability services since they are not obligated to comply with disabilities-related legislation in the same way as private and public entities" (Murry & Wiley, 2017, p. 8). Additional barriers Indigenous Americanstudents with disabilities encountered, as seen in a 2021 study, were teacher shortages in the rural communities; unmet needs for basic food, water, and shelter; and access to high-speed internet (Running Bear et al., 2021). Therefore, Indigenous Americanstudents' learning is hampered by educational gaps resulting in poor health literacy and health behaviors (Sarche & Spicer, 2008).

In a qualitative study defining healthy Indigenous American families, the authors found that having a cultural link or identity is integral to maintaining a healthy family (Martin & Yurkovich, 2014). The perceptions and reactions to disability vary within the family context. Some families may identify with a "traditional" way of life and may interpret the cause of the illness and disability from this perspective, which influences the decisions related to the course of treatment. Other families may reject traditional tribal beliefs and practices. Nontraditional forms of practice may be accepted by families as well as spiritual and personal support and attending their place of worship (Allison & Christine, 1999).

Generations of atrocities, mistreatment, inequalities, and health disparities may explain Indigenous Americans' mistrust of outsiders and government providers (U.S. Department of Health and Human Services, 2014). However, as this population grows, so will the demand for services. It is important to note that rehabilitation counselors view Indigenous Americans from their unique and cultural context; without consideration of Indigenous Americans' culture and beliefs, they may be reluctant to accept interventions (Sarche & Spicer, 2008). Counselors must develop trust and respect the sovereign status of Native American nations and their clients' individual and tribal identities (Running Bear et al., 2021).

CONCLUSION

Understanding the role of the family and how it functions to enhance or to detract from the lives of people with disability is imperative because this basic social unit can provide a lifetime of love, support, encouragement, and care. It is important to assess family needs and support services so that the family does not become overwhelmed or feel isolated in their endeavors to assist their loved one and to integrate into the larger community. This involves understanding numerous differences in family reactions and functioning based on the resilience of the family, who in the family has the disability, the extent of the disability, the resources available, and cultural beliefs and practices.

CLASS ACTIVITIES

1. Ask students if any of them have experienced disability or chronic illness in their family and if they are willing to share how culture plays a role in family functioning in relation to the disability.

2. Compare and contrast how different cultures or ethnic groups may deal with disability within the family.

3. Considering the family characteristics identified by Power and Dell Orto (2004), which family characteristics do you believe have the greatest impacts on family adjustment to disability, and why?

KEY REFERENCES

Only key references appear in the print edition. The full references appear in the digital product on Springer Publishing Connect™: https://connect.springerpub.com/content/book/978-0-8261-5111-7/part/partIII/chapter/ch13

Al Khateeb, J. M., Al Hadidi, M. S., & Al Khatib, A. J. (2014). Arab Americans with disabilities and their families: a culturally appropriate approach for counselors. *Journal of Multicultural Counseling & Development, 42*(4), 232–247. https://doi.org/10.1002/j.2161-1912.2014.00057.x

Alston, R. J., & Turner, W. L. (1994). A family strengths model of adjustment to disability for African American clients. *Journal of Counseling and Development, 72,* 378–383.

Blacher, J. (1984). Sequential stages of parental adjustment to the birth of a child with handicaps: Fact or artifact? *Mental Retardation, 22*(2), 55–68.

Campbell, E. M., & Smalling, S. E. (2013). American Indians and bullying in schools. *Journal of Indigenous Social Development, 2*(1), 1–15

Coles, A. R., Pakenham, K. I., & Leech, C. (2007). Evaluation of an intensive psychosocial intervention for children of parents with multiple sclerosis. *Rehabilitation Psychology, 52,* 133–142.

DeFrain, J., & Asay, S. M. (2007). Strong families around the world: An introduction to the family strengths perspective. *Marriage & Family Review, 41*(1/2), 1–10. https://doi.org/10.1300/J002v41n01_01

Dogson, J. E., Garwick, A., Blozis, S. A., Patterson, J. M., Bennett, F. C., & Blum, R. W. (2000). Uncertainty in childhood chronic conditions and family distress in families of young children. *Journal of Family Nursing, 6,* 252–266.

Frain, M. P., Lee, G. K., Berven, N. L., Tansey, T., Tschopp, M., & Chronister, J. (2007). Effective use of the resiliency model of family adjustment for rehabilitation counselors. *Journal of Rehabilitation, 73*(3), 18–25.

Hasnain, R., Shaikh, L. C., Shanawani, H. (2008). *Disability and the Muslim perspective: An introduction for rehabilitation and health care providers.* Center for International Rehabilitation Research and Exchange. http://cirrie-sphhp.webapps.buffalo.edu/culture/monographs/muslim.php#copyright

Liu, G. Z. (2001). *Chinese culture and disability: Information for U.S. service providers.* http://cirrie.buffalo.edu/culture/monographs/china.php

MacDorman M. F. (2011). Race and ethnic disparities in fetal mortality, preterm birth, and infant mortality in the United States: an overview. *Seminars in Perinatology, 35*(4), 200–208. https://doi.org/10.1053/j.semperi.2011.02.017

McCubbin, H. I., & Patterson, J. M. (1983). Family transitions: Adaptation to stress. In H. I. McCubbin & C. R. Figley (Eds.), *Stress and the family: Coping with normative transitions* (Vol. 2, pp. 5–25). Brunner/Mazel.

Ryan, A. S., & Smith, M. J. (1989). Parental reactions to developmental disabilities in Chinese American families. *Child and Adolescent Social Work, 6,* 283–299.

CHAPTER 14

GIVING PARENTS A VOICE: CHALLENGES EXPERIENCED BY PARENTS OF CHILDREN WITH DISABILITIES

KATHY SHEPPARD-JONES, STEPHANIE MEREDITH, AND CONSTANCE RICHARD

LEARNING OBJECTIVES

Throughout the chapter, perspectives of one family will be provided through the voice of Stephanie, a mother of an adult son with Down syndrome. After reading this chapter, you will be able to:

- Understand the historical context of family experiences related to disability
- Give examples of family advocacy organizations
- Understand the variability of family experience
- Give examples of how families can have positive and negative experiences in health-care, education, and policy

PRE-READING QUESTIONS

1. How many children in the United States have a disability?
2. How does culture influence the experience of parenting a child with a disability?
3. What is family engagement, and what is an example of how families can be engaged?

THE EXPERIENCE OF PARENTING A CHILD WITH A DISABILITY

Families have long played a critical role in the history of disability rights. Parent movements have influenced policy and legislation for children with disabilities, demanding that their children not be hidden from their communities in institutions, but rather remain in the family home. Parental influence is found in changes in healthcare, education, community living, and employment. Parents recognized the inaccuracies of systems indicating that their children with disabilities were uneducable, unfixable, and "less than" with no prospects of contributing to society. Families have spurred education legislation that gave children the right to a free and appropriate public education through the Individuals with Disabilities Education Act and its amendments. Disabilities can be experienced at any point across the life span. For the purpose of this chapter, we will focus on the experience of families where a child is born with or acquires a disability before adulthood. Disabilities can occur prenatally, or before birth. Disabilities may also happen during or around the time of birth. These are considered congenital disabilities. Disabilities can also take place at any point during childhood. In terms of emerging disabilities that are increasingly found in U.S. families, the prevalence rate of autism has increased markedly over the last two decades. Nationally, the most recent estimate for the prevalence in American children is 1 in 44 (Centers for Disease Control and Prevention [CDC], 2022). It is further estimated that one in six children has been diagnosed with developmental disability, including:

- Autism
- Intellectual disability (ID)
- Learning disability
- Hearing impairment
- Cerebral palsy
- Attention deficit hyperactivity disorder
- Blindness (Zablotsky et. al., 2019)

In the United States, approximately 14.1 million children have, or are at risk of, a chronic physical, developmental, behavioral, or emotional condition (U.S. Census Bureau, 2021). The range of disabilities and adaptations to them varies widely. What is clear is that families where at least one family member has a disability are extremely common.

The way in which a disability occurs can also influence adaptation to the disability. This is true for the individual and for the family. Disability stigma can have a significant impact on families, especially when considering the myriad social and political placements within which families exist. The role of culture is also extremely powerful and is embedded within development for all children. A child with a disability can be seen as bringing shame upon a family. Children may be hidden or avoided. Various religions also see disability as a result of some sin perpetrated by the parents. The response of families to the presence of disability can have long-lasting implications for a child.

Regardless of culture, socioeconomic status, and the multitude of factors that influence child development, a thread of hope and optimism of all that is possible often accompanies the expected birth of a baby. The reality of a baby being born with a disability can change some of the emotions and expectations for everyone involved. When a baby is born with a disability, parents must decide how to share the news with family and friends, how to prepare other children in the family, learn about medical issues, find services, and plan for the future (Iannone & Meredith, 2020).

The conclusion of this chapter includes an update that answers the four questions that Stephanie and Justin wrote down when Andy was born.

Misconceptions of parent experiences are pervasive, and the approach taken by professionals in interacting with families can play a role in parent experiences. A family-centered approach puts the well-being of families and children first. It is a partnership between families and the professionals who serve them. Because parent expectations are also influenced by access to accurate and timely resources and supports, a family-centered approach includes positive communication and information sharing. Disability and family organizations can advocate on behalf of individuals and families and provide meaningful connections that can help build a network of support around a family. Supports and services that are family-centered can also foster family engagement. Family engagement happens when families are active collaborators. It is a continuous process across settings, where families and

CASE STUDY 14.1. STEPHANIE'S FAMILY STORY

When my son was born on January 30, 2000, I was 23 years old. My husband, Justin, was 24. We were fresh out of college, and Andy was our first baby. After Andy was born, we learned that he had some complications, so the doctors and nurses whisked him off to the neonatal intensive care unit (NICU) for treatment. He looked so vulnerable lying in an isolette with IV and oxygen tubes and his hands raised above his head in the position of field goal posts. About 4 hours later, our pediatrician pulled us into a room off the side of the NICU and listed the characteristics that made him think Andy had Down syndrome: low muscle tone, almond-shaped eyes with an extra inner fold, Brushfield spots in his eyes that make them sparkle, a "sandal-gap" between his big toe and the second toe, and a broad, flat nose. Our doctor was fairly matter-of-fact and then left us to process the information together.

After the doctor walked out of the room, Justin and I cried and took the time to write down everything that made us feel worried:

1. How could we possibly afford the resources he might need as young parents?
2. Would other kids make fun of him?
3. Would he live with us forever?
4. Would our identity always be tied to being the parents of a child with Down syndrome?

The hospital where Andy was born was also fairly progressive in 2000 and actually had three parent support specialists on staff in the NICU. The day after Andy was born, one of those parent support specialists met with us and shared the book *Babies With Down Syndrome* and showed us a photo of her own son with Down syndrome on a bike. She spoke with such pride about her outgoing and energetic son. That was such a transformational moment for us when we realized that life with a disability could still be fun. Receiving accurate and up-to-date information right away was also crucial to helping us understand the medical and social issues and being empowered with information and the available supports and services at the first point on the life course.

Our bishop from church also gave us the best advice as we sat in the NICU and asked him about what the Down syndrome diagnosis would mean from a spiritual perspective. He said, "Well, you will be responsible for teaching him as much as he can learn, and he will be responsible for what he knows." Looking back on it, I love this response because many in our religion just say all people with intellectual disabilities go to heaven. Our bishop's response meant that Andy was capable of learning and making decisions but that God would also be merciful where Andy's understanding might be limited. That was a really empowering expectation to be told in those early days.

professionals work together to actively support children's development and growth. When families are effectively engaged, children with disabilities and their families can thrive.

The State of the Research on Parents' Experiences and Perspectives

The presence of disability has long been associated with inequities in key areas that are generally associated with quality of life. Children with disabilities in the United States are also more likely to live in poverty (Fujiura & Yamaki, 2000), and families are less likely to have healthcare access and stable housing and more likely to be food insecure (Parish et al., 2008). In recent years, research on parental experiences has shifted toward resiliency-based models and away from the "tragedy metaphor" in which there was a foregone conclusion that families existed within a constant state of crisis (Maul & Singer, 2009). A resiliency approach takes stressors into account and reconciles them through ongoing adaptations. While early research emphasized chaos and catastrophe for all involved family members, a strong base of emerging literature paints a more balanced picture of family experiences.

In a national study of families in the United States that included a child with Down syndrome (DS), most respondents reported positive emotions toward that child, including love (87%) and pride (83%). While complex challenges were described among siblings without DS (Skotko et al., 2016), Skotko earlier found that 96% of brothers and sisters who responded to the survey expressed affection toward their sibling with DS, and 88% felt that they were better people because of their siblings with DS (Skotko et al., 2011).

Similar to the majority of behavioral science research, parental adaptation research has been centered in developed countries. As such, parental adaptation and caregiving research is an emerging area in less developed countries and their corresponding cultures (Bizzego et al., 2020; Grove et al., 2022; Henrich et al., 2010; Maulik et al., 2011). What is known is that culture influences parental involvement and adaptation and thus outcomes for parents and children with disabilities (Acar et al., 2021). Interventions are currently being conceived and culturally adapted to address and include parents of children with disabilities.

Grove et al. (2022) reviewed parental participation in intellectual and developmental disability (IDD) research in seven of the most prominent IDD journals between 2010 and 2019, focusing on the diversity of location and research methods. They found that close to 20% of the studies had at least one parent measure. Close to a quarter of the studies focused on parents only, 42% of the studies focused on both children and parents, and roughly one-third concentrated solely on children. The social roles of parents and the parent–child relationship tended to be the center of the research. The top five countries that produced the highest numbers of parental articles were the United States, followed by the United Kingdom, Australia, Canada, and China. The top five countries accounted for 68% of all the articles found, and no other country accounted for more than 2.3%.

A 2017 study of Taiwanese mothers of children with autism provided an example of how the influence of extended family, disability stigma, ignorance, and/or practitioners/educators' lack of disability knowledge have affected outcomes for children with disability and the well-being of the parents/caregiver (Hsu et al., 2017). The themes they found were (a) taking the blame, (b) my world was turned upside down, (c) to live a child-centered life, and (d) two lives as one. Stigma was also prevalent, and the researchers found that contrary to typical Taiwanese cultural family systems where the husband's family is the primary support, mothers found their own birth families more supportive. Parents-in-law would blame their daughter-in-law's "bad genes" or caregiving as the cause of autism. This finding may stem from the cultural and familial stigma reflected in the themes of taking the blame and my world was turned upside down. Hsu et al. concluded their study by stressing the need for interventions that strengthen familial bonds when working with parents of children with autism in Taiwan.

High-quality, culturally responsive interventions are crucial when working with culturally diverse parents. Bernal's framework (Bernal & Sáez-Santiago, 2006) asks interventionists to consider ecological validity when adapting, creating, and implementing interventions. The framework mandates researchers to (a) culturally match the client and therapist; (b) use the preferred language of the client; (c) use examples, narratives, symbols, and figurative language that are culturally relevant; (d) use culturally specific content and knowledge; (e) use specific social roles or norms and problems; (f) consider cultural values and norms when creating intervention norms; (g) culturally address how the intervention is given and presented; and (h) consider the contextual aspect of the intervention (e.g., the social and economic environment and its impact on the acceptability, accessibility, and thus feasibility of the intervention).

In a systematic review of the cultural adaptation of psychosocial interventions for parents and their children with intellectual disabilities in low- and middle-income countries, Susanty et al. (2019) found 13 studies between 1981 and 2020 that met their eligibility criteria of focusing on cultural adaptation of psychosocial interventions that were targeted at parents of children with IDD. Four of the studies focused on the connection between parental psychological well-being and improved parenting skills. The other nine explored parental training and its effect on the development of children with disabilities. All the studies pointed to positive outcomes from the cultural adaptations. However, the reviewers concluded that none of the studies carefully integrated Bernal's framework (Bernal & Sáez-Santiago, 2006).

Ultimately, Susanty et al.'s review showed that cultural adaptation of psychosocial interventions centered around parents is a promising avenue of research, but more rigorous methodological studies are needed. In recent years, the Patient-Centered Outcomes Research Institute has devoted attention and funding to address strategies for adapting research and providing research to families of children with disabilities from different racial and cultural backgrounds.

Religion and spirituality play an integral role in shaping society, and thus the individual's and family's response to a child's disability. In order to create and provide culturally competent support and services, knowledge and understanding are critical to understanding the family's beliefs, values, and community connections (Boehm & Carter, 2019; Gaventa, 2018; The Joint Commission, 2010). However, there is a shortage of literature in the United States and elsewhere that examines the influence of religion and spirituality on parental adaptation. Numerous scholars and researchers have called for a focus on the impact of faith on family adaptation (Carter, 2013; Reynolds et al., 2016).

Boehm and Carter (2019) examined four dimensions of faith that they posited are fundamental to understanding the impact of religion and spirituality on parent adaptation. The four dimensions were (a) religious community involvement, (b) social support, (c) level of religiosity, and (d) spiritual practices and beliefs. They found that faith is notable in the lives of parents and caregivers. In their study of 530 participants, the strength of religion was found to be moderately strong, 92% believed in God or a higher power, and most meditated or prayed daily. Over three-quarters believed that their faith influenced their decisions and that they found emotional or social support in their faith practices or community. Yet the study also underscored the diversity of caregivers' active engagement with their faith communities. The frequency of attending services, activities, belief traditions, denominations, and use of social supports varied widely in the study population. Boehm and Carter also pointed out that a modest proportion of caregivers did not find religion or spirituality important.

Furthermore, Boehm and Carter (2019) inferred from their data that spirituality or religious engagement may positively influence the well-being of parents and caregivers. Yet social support via religious engagement was found to be lacking. Close to two-thirds, 64%, of their participants, said they would not be able to name an individual from their faith community that they'd seek out for help, and only 35% of the participants reported that they sought help from their community. The study did not assess the reasons for the lack, but posited that it could be because it was unavailable, seen as unhelpful, or not sought after by the participants. Since less than half the participants reported engaging in religious or spiritual activities (classes, groups, or service opportunities) other than attending services, the researchers also theorized that perhaps greater engagement with religious and spiritual activities would strengthen the support the participants received due to establishing new supportive relationships, access to supports, and enhancing their own beliefs. Since the researchers did not ask about the caregivers' desired engagement, they could not define whether or not participation in the faith community was "encouraging or concerning." Previous studies have shown that a lack of accessibility and hospitality were barriers for parents (Jacober, 2010; O'Hanlon, 2013). The research underscored the need for future studies to understand desired engagement, spouses' alignment on religion and faith (since the study only looked at one parent and most participants were mothers), and how parents' and caregivers' religious faith practices and beliefs impacted their children with disability.

Looking at the research on how religion and spirituality influenced coping and adaptation to having a child with a disability (Bennett et al., 1995; Pearce, 2005; Poston & Turnbull, 2004; Selway & Ashman, 1998), Kamei (2014) posited that to understand the influence of religion and spirituality on caregivers and family coping and adaptation, one could understand religion and spirituality as a family resource and/or family perception components in the double ABC X model of family stress (McCubbin et al., 1982), which has often been used as a framework to understand caregivers' adaptation processes. The model theorizes that the amalgamation of the pre- and post-family stressors, resources, and perceptions will create the family's experience of the "stress" or the response to their child's disability when applied to parental and family adaptation or whether or not it turns into a crisis. With enough resources and positive perception, stress may never turn into a crisis. Conversely, low resources and negative perceptions can fuel the fire of crisis. Kamei, citing Turnball et al. (2010), pointed to how religion can provide explanations and definitions surrounding a child's disability, the treatment of the child, and the function of each family member; in addition, faith communities can be seen as resources due to the social support caregivers receive from them. By comparing Christianity and Buddhism, Kamei underscored how different faith practices may function in the model by either accelerating or alleviating the stress. Kamei concluded that it was vital that service providers, educators, and other professionals understand the role of religion within the family, for it could be a positive or negative factor in parental and family adaptation.

While families are the major conduit to connecting children with disabilities to needed services, their involvement as valued members of the service delivery team is often overlooked (Smart, 2021). King et al. (2017) pointed out that parent and family-centered practices and interventions are not as common as one may assume. Their scoping review detailed services and supports provided to parents by professionals and created a framework for parent/family wellness in a family-centered continuum of services. Parent/family wellness springs from a need to ameliorate parent-specific needs, assist parents with managing and delivering therapy, and provide disability-specific education. Service coordination and psychosocial interventions support addressing parent-specific needs; training and instruction on services and therapy are the services and support for managing care and treatment delivery; and providing information, resources, and educational services is the outcome of education. The researchers posited that this framework could be used to address existing gaps in providing interventions. Furthermore, King et al. concluded that there was a need for more longitudinal research on family adjustment and well-being focused on family-centered practices because there's little existing data on long-term outcomes.

Directions in Parental Leadership

History has not been kind to people with disabilities. Aristotle wrote, "As to the exposure and rearing of children, let there be a law that no deformed child shall live" (Minnesota Governor's Council on Developmental Disabilities, 2022, para. 2). This thinking was largely perpetuated over many centuries. The rise of Christianity did lead to better treatment of people with disabilities, but families were the primary determinants of survival. Institutions (or asylums) began in 787 CE. Survival here was not likely. While the idea that people with disabilities were "children of God" in Western culture, there was a strong economic divide, with children and adults with disabilities generally living impoverished lives. The popularity of institutions grew significantly between 1800 and the 1950s, when parents began mobilizing in response to serious concerns about lack of appropriate care of professionals for their children. A national movement led by parents declared, "The Retarded Can Be Helped."

Parent groups began forming in the 1930s; the first was the Cuyahoga County Council for the Retarded Child. In the 1950s, parents of children with IDs formed The Arc (initially known as the National Association of Parents and Friends of Retarded Children). Families wanted their children to be raised at home instead of in institutions. Families wanted their children to go to school, just like any other child without IDD. With over 600 local chapters and over 1,000 programs, the Arc is a long-time advocate for the rights of individuals with IDD and their families (https://thearc.org). The Arc and other advocacy organizations advocated for research and funding that led to Medicaid and Medicare legislation. National condition-specific organizations started forming between the 1970s and 1980s to further unify families in advocating for research, funding, and policy support.

The work of Dr. Wolf Wolfensberger (1934–2011) helped to further set the stage for higher expectations for individuals with disabilities and their families. Wolfensberger promoted the idea of "normalization" in the 1960s for individuals with ID. This was central to the deinstitutionalization movement, where congregate and segregated facilities were largely replaced by community-based residences. The notion of normalization became more broadly used in terms of cross-disability service provision.

CASE STUDY 14.2. STEPHANIE'S FAMILY STORY

Just a few days after Andy was born, we were connected with our local Down syndrome organization and the early intervention parent support group. I was so grateful—and also nervous—to connect with other families. The idea of family advocacy felt very intimidating at first, but when I started to learn about some of the injustices that people with disabilities face, I dove into the world of advocacy. Before Andy was born, I was somewhat of a doormat and didn't stick up for myself much, but I soon realized that I developed a spine when advocating for my son and people that I care about.

A story that motivated me early on was a trip made by our local Down syndrome organization leaders to Russia, where the institutionalization rate of people with Down syndrome was very high at the time. These leaders worked alongside a nonprofit disability organization in Russia to share their stories of raising their children at home in order to inspire the parents in Moscow to also give their children the opportunity to grow up in their communities. When I learned about the 95% institutionalization rate at the time in Russia and the tragically outdated information received by the parents, my first instinct was to try and adopt a child. However, I realized we could help many more children if we focused instead on disseminating accurate and up-to-date information about Down syndrome to those parents, and my husband and I were in an ideal position to help, between my background as a technical writer and his work at a translation company.

So, we set out to connect with the nonprofit organization in Moscow in 2001 and asked what books would be most helpful to parents in Russia at the moment of diagnosis. Over the next several years, we negotiated the rights to translate and distribute the book, *Babies with Down Syndrome* in Russia and raised the funds to translate the book. Meanwhile, the organization in Moscow raised funds to print the book locally and distribute it to local birth hospitals.

By the time I was able to visit Russia in person in 2011, the institutionalization rate for children with Down syndrome had dropped to less than 50% in Moscow (according to the local charity, Downside Up), thanks to the work of the local parents, local nonprofit organizations, and the dissemination of resources that we worked on. By working together, we were able to empower parents to raise their children at home and advocate for their place in the community.

Giving Parents a Voice in Healthcare and Health Services

Accessible, affordable healthcare is a crucial ingredient for the healthy growth of children. However, families are less likely to receive appropriate medical care for their children who experience a special healthcare need (Health Resources & Services Administration [HRSA], 2022). For most parents, healthcare providers are the first line of defense for a medical issue involving their child. Physicians are seen as the experts and the healers. But for a parent of a child with a disability, medical providers can convey vital first impressions about disabilities and the potential of their child. In the best circumstances, physicians can promote hope and optimism. Yet it was not that long ago that physicians would advise parents of a newborn with IDD to institutionalize the child immediately, and some families continue to experience trauma today when the diagnosis is presented in ways that further stigmatize disabilities. As one parent shared:

> In 1967, when I was born, had I been born with Down syndrome, doctors would have told my parents to institutionalize me, tell family and friends that I had died, and to live their lives as if I had never been born. Parents were told that their baby with Down syndrome would ruin their marriage, cause siblings to be neglected, and would ruin them financially. I am so very thankful for the parents who didn't listen. Those who brought their babies home, defied the odds, and listened to their hearts. Imagine the courage that took, considering there was no public education access, medical care was not always given, and therapies such as occupational therapy, physical therapy and speech language therapy were not provided. Because of these brave parents, organizations such as Down Syndrome Association of Central Kentucky (DSACK) were founded. Now I see our DSACK community surrounding families who are struggling, celebrating every milestone with one another, and forming lifelong friendships. DSACK walks beside families by offering support, social opportunities, lifelong learning programs, and more free to all families who have a child born with Down syndrome.

An example of an institution as described earlier was the Willowbrook State School, which opened in 1947 in New York City. Residents lived in deplorable conditions: neglected, dehumanized and forgotten. As public outrage over the abuse, underfunding, and warehousing of those living at Willowbrook grew, more parents began rejecting institutionalization en masse. In many ways the parent advocacy movement was the outgrowth of a rejection of the medical and institutionalization models and is sometimes reflected in continued tensions between the medical and disability advocacy communities. For example, research shows that many parents have experienced trauma that can last decades when receiving a diagnosis of Down syndrome, particularly when parents feel like clinicians demonstrate a lack of compassion, pressure them to terminate their pregnancy, convey pessimistic expectations about outcomes for their child and family, or provide limited or no additional resources or support systems (May et al., 2020).

Moreover, parents often relay that clinicians convey ableism when discussing a diagnosis at the first point on the life course or diagnostic journey (Carroll et al., 2018). One mother of a child with cerebral palsy recounts,

> I was just listening to all these so-called experts. And so my way of thinking was, "Oh, my gosh, now he's a child with cerebral palsy." But really he was the same kid. He had cerebral palsy the day before and he had it the day after. We just didn't know what to call it. And all of a sudden we started treating him differently. (Snow, 2013)

Research about parent preferences has led to a better understanding of how clinicians can best support families on their diagnostic journey when they discuss the medical issues, the life outcomes, psychosocial supports, and other supports and services (Sanborn & Patterson, 2014; Sheets, Best et al., 2011). Clinicians can empower the trajectory of the family when they show compassion as the family processes information while also giving up-to-date information and a progressive vision of life with disability, such as the resources found at the National Center for Prenatal and Postnatal Resources at lettercase.org (Levis et al., 2012; May et al.).

The important role of parents cannot be underestimated in the ongoing health of children with special healthcare needs and developmental disabilities. When exploring health and wellness outcomes for children with a disability, family influence is considered more important than that of any provider of healthcare (Elliott & Mullins, 2004). Family-centered healthcare is an approach to healthcare services that can improve health outcomes and interactions between families and healthcare providers (Goldfarb et al., 2019). Indeed, beyond making a difference at the individual level, parents have mobilized in ways that influence systems and amplify critical knowledge for other families and expectant parents.

CASE STUDY 14.3. STEPHANIE'S FAMILY STORY

When Andy was born, my husband was just starting a new business, and we learned very quickly that we could not purchase a private health insurance policy for Andy because Down syndrome was considered a preexisting condition. Ultimately, we ended up spending one-third of our income on healthcare expenses in 2002—even without a major incident—and were forced to move to another state where we were able to access Medicaid for children with disabilities. We shared our story with any legislator who was willing to listen—as did many other families. It was through this family advocacy in healthcare systems that the law fundamentally changed with the passage of the Affordable Healthcare Act so that individuals with preexisting health conditions could purchase private policies.

CASE STUDY 14.4. STEPHANIE'S FAMILY STORY

When Andy was about 16 years old, he sat on a pencil one day, and we feared that some of the lead had broken off into his backside. We rushed down to our local urgent care where we waited for care in triage. Andy was calm and polite but definitely uncomfortable after sitting on a sharpened pencil. Eventually, the urgent care doctor walked into the waiting room and told us that he did not treat patients like Andy and that we should drive another half an hour to the children's hospital. At first, I thought he meant that the urgent care didn't treat puncture wounds, but when I later checked with other friends in the field, they said puncture wounds are often treated at urgent care. It was then that I realized that Andy had been turned away—not because of the type of injury he had—but because of his disability diagnosis. Unfortunately, these types of experiences are not uncommon among people with disabilities.

THE LEADERSHIP EDUCATION IN NEURODEVELOPMENTAL AND OTHER RELATED DISABILITIES TRAINING PROGRAM

Parents can be important allies in advocating for better training among medical providers. Fundamentally, when parents, providers, and self-advocates work together to shape policy, train clinicians, and inform best practices, the outcomes for the entire team improve as clinicians are better able to meet the needs of their patients. Successful models of this are found in the national Leadership Education in Neurodevelopmental and Other Related Disabilities (LEND) training program, funded by the HRSA Maternal and Child Health Bureau (https://mchb.hrsa.gov/training/projects.asp?program=9). LEND programs train graduate- and advanced-level student trainees across disciplines. Trainees receive concentrated courses and rotations in an effort to improve health outcomes for children with disabilities and their families. Each LEND training program includes multiple professional disciplines, including a family faculty member to ensure that future professionals recognize, seek out, and learn from the perspectives that parents and family bring to healthcare settings.

Giving Parents a Voice in Education

When both parents and educators work as a team in educational decisions, outcomes are better. An array of professionals can be involved, including general and special educators, therapists, counselors, and a variety of interventionists. Each brings expertise, but no one knows a child better than the family. Ultimately, parents need educators to listen to their vision of the future for their child and help them achieve their goals. Of course, those goals may need to be customized based on the observed needs of the child, but parents and their children with disabilities need to be provided support and encouragement to pursue their dreams. Moreover, parents and teachers who are empowered can be important allies in providing strategies for teachers to help students be successful in the classroom.

The Partnership Capacity Matrix (Pleet-Odle, 2017) introduced the concept of four quadrants in which family and professional interactions may occur. The quadrants fall along a continuum of knowledge, skills, and resources held by professionals and families. When both family and professional capacities are low, one finds "distrustful isolates," where there is little ability to accomplish much or communicate well. Both sides do not trust the other, and each side feels overwhelmed and isolated. When family capacity is high and professional capacity is low, families are perceived by professionals as difficult or "demanding customers." However, when professional capacity is high but family capacity remains low, professionals believe they, as professionals, have the tools to manage the situation best. This leaves out families as an important part of the decision-making process. In the fourth quadrant, both professionals and families have high capacity and create an empowered alliance. In this ideal situation, both personal relationships and the ability to problem-solve together are highly valued, and the parents and educators share decision-making and power to work toward a set of common goals.

CASE STUDY 14.5. STEPHANIE'S FAMILY STORY

When Andy was little, I anticipated that he would be included all day, every day when he started school. I had gone to conferences to learn that inclusion was the best model, and everyone loved him, so that was my expectation. When we moved from New York to Georgia, we were unable to find an inclusive preschool setting through the school district, so we compromised and sent him to a typical preschool in the morning and the special education preschool in the afternoon. I had occasionally gotten the vibe that his special education preschool teacher didn't adore him like his other teachers did, but I never expected what came next when I experienced the crushing reality of our kindergarten Individualized Education Plan (IEP) meeting.

I was overwhelmed when I walked in the room, and there were about 15 people seated around the table at our IEP meeting. The reason the room was so full was because his preschool special education teacher had invited the principal and teacher from another school with a self-contained room. Fortunately, I had my husband and another parent friend who came along with me, so we were only outnumbered five to one.

This preschool teacher started the meeting by listing all of Andy's challenges. She said he couldn't respond to his own name, follow directions, or draw a circle—things I knew he had been able to do for years—and she recommended that he be placed in the self-contained room at the other school. I'm sure she followed up with his strengths, but I was so gutted that I couldn't hear anything else. Our neighborhood school principal and teacher, who had seemed enthusiastic about Andy when we first introduced ourselves, began to retreat, fearing they wouldn't have the resources to serve our son.

I was crushed. They didn't believe in my boy. They weren't even going to give him a chance to go to school with his neighborhood friends and learn from them. Fortunately, my other mom friend caught my eye and slightly shook her head to let me know I shouldn't agree. So I told them that before we agreed to anything, we would need to observe him in all the proposed and current learning environments.

What ended up happening is that I videotaped him in his current settings—at therapy, the special education preschool, and the typical preschool. When he was at the typical preschool, I took video of him responding to his name when called for singing time, coloring a picture among other children, and engaging with the class to find Easter eggs. I took video of him drawing circles with his occupational therapist at private therapy. And then I took video of him at the special education preschool where the teacher was reading a book to the small group. She asked Andy, "What's this?" when pointing to a dog and he patted his leg to answer her in sign language. She didn't recognize it and looked up to shake her head at me as if to say, "He can't even recognize a dog."

In our follow-up meeting, I showed this video footage, and the teacher from the typical preschool (who was a certified teacher) shared that Andy was engaged and happy in her class. And with that combination, we won our first advocacy battle for Andy to attend our neighborhood school and be included in the regular classroom at least 50% or more of the time with some pull-out for resource services.

It was a rough start, and I don't think we would have prevailed without the video and teacher from his typical preschool class, but that first battle paved the way for a more inclusive education. While there were still bumps in the road along the way, our school was tremendously supportive in hosting disability awareness campaigns, giving Andy opportunities to shine in extracurricular activities, modifying assignments in the regular education classrooms, and treating him just like any other kid. In response, he blossomed and made friends who have invited him to dances, participated in sports with him, and even showed him how to get a job in high school at the local grocery store.

Those friends Andy has made over the years have taught him the most important lessons: to be social and independent—critical soft skills for employment. Since that first IEP meeting, we've started every other IEP meeting with the same mantra: Our goals for Andy are for him to be able to navigate the world independently; read, write, and do math to the best of his ability; and get a job. Therefore, inclusion is critical because he needs to be able to get along with everyone, and those kids who are his friends today will be his employers and coworkers of the future.

When parents and individuals with disabilities are empowered to shape their own vision of the future in education, they can carry through on that motivation as the child grows to pursue job and career goals. When families have high expectations for success, their child with a disability is also more likely to have positive postschool outcomes, including employment and higher education (Carter et al., 2012). Family engagement can also result in:

- More opportunity to develop self-determination skills
- More employment experiences while in high school

EXHIBIT 14.1. Vision Statement Template and Example

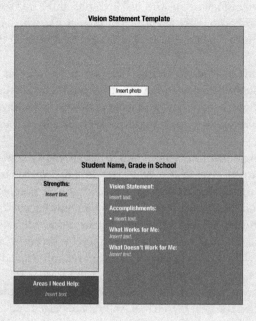

Families and children can develop a vision statement that indicates what the child wants for their future. Professionals can work with families to support the development and updates to the vision statement over time. This strengths-based process is a way that families can plan for the future for a child from a young age.

Vision Statement Example

John, 11th grade

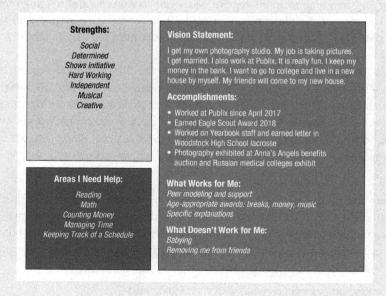

- Increased understanding of how benefits and employment are related
- Greater access to higher education
- Improved collaboration with educators and other professionals
- Increased participation and engagement
- Decreased use of inappropriate guardianship

A vision statement is a powerful tool that identifies strengths, accomplishments, and what does and does not "work" for a child with a disability. A vision statement is a map of the future. The act of creating a vision statement can help families plan for the future and determine what is needed to support that future. Vision statements can be updated over time and can help parents learn how to share their voice and the voice of their child with others.

CASE STUDY 14.6. STEPHANIE'S FAMILY STORY

One day when Andy and I were driving home from school, he told me he wanted to get a job at our local grocery store because many of his other friends at school were working there. I told him I'd look into it, thinking I'd need to set up a job coach, talk to vocational rehabilitation, and set up a meeting with his IEP team. In Andy's mind, he was telling me what he was planning to do that day.

After I finished cooking dinner that night, I sent my daughter upstairs to tell Andy that dinner was ready, but he was nowhere to be found. When we checked outside, we noticed his bike was missing, and I had a message on my phone from Andy saying, "Mom, I go to Publix. I go get a job. You come help me."

Sure enough, he had ridden his bike to the grocery store, found a friend who worked there to show him where to apply for a job, and he called me for help when he ran into a roadblock when entering his information on the computer application. The store was so impressed with his initiative that they said they'd be happy to hire a young person with that level of initiative, and he's now worked there for over 5 years.

This level of motivation is gathered from social incentives, an investment of talents and skills, self-empowerment, and a vision of the future shaped by individuals with a disability and their families. To discover these talents, skills, and incentives, educators and professionals must work together as a team to empower the individual with a disability to shape their own destiny.

Family engagement and leadership can drive positive change, not only for an individual student but also at a systems level. One example is found in a Partnerships in Employment state systems change grant for youth with significant disabilities. These 5-year projects are intended to improve employment and higher education outcomes for youth with disabilities. One state project assembled a statewide leadership team including a family member and family advocacy organizations. It also hosted an active family advocacy work team that developed both a family engagement curriculum (available at https://hdilearning.org) and other resources targeting families and professionals. Because family expectations have been shown to be malleable over time (Doren et al., 2012), the family advocacy work team also developed a set of "Top Ten Lists" to identify those most salient pieces of information needed for families at certain ages in their children's lives. This mechanism highlighted the power of families' lived experience and resulted in resources for parents and caregivers with children age 3 and up. The complete list of Employment Checklists are available at https://hdi.uky.edu/employment-checklists.

Giving Parents a Voice in Policy

The Kennedys are perhaps the family that has most shaped U.S. federal policy and awareness. The Kennedys had nine children: including Rosemary, who had an ID. A *Saturday Evening Post* article written by Eunice Kennedy about her sister Rosemary and their family provided a positive portrayal that helped combat the stigma associated with having a family member with ID.

During his presidency, John F. Kennedy moved forward an agenda that funded research and services for people with developmental disabilities and their families. He convened a President's Panel on Mental Retardation in 1961. The final report of the panel led to federal legislation in the form of Public Law 88-164 that created university-affiliated programs and Community Mental Health Centers. Public Law 88-156 brought an increase in services for maternal and child health and began funding IDD research at the state level. Leadership of and by families continued to grow, with gains in education and employment in the 1970s and 1980s. The emergence of Partners in Policymaking in the 1990s created a replicable model that has helped provide a foundation of knowledge and mentoring that continues to build leaders today (Schuh & Dixon, 2000).

PARTNERS IN POLICYMAKING

Parent voices are found in national, state, and local advocacy groups. A model program, Partners in Policymaking, launched in Minnesota in 1987 (https://mn.gov/mnddc/pipm), provides leadership and advocacy training for adults with disabilities and parents of children with disabilities. The program's focus is on building capacity for system change. The core curriculum topics include content that provides a historical perspective, foundational knowledge around services and supports in education, employment and independent living, policy and advocacy. This approach is intended to drive positive change at the individual and systems level. Partners in Policymaking recognizes participants' life stories are testimonies that can influence policy makers. Participants gain knowledge and leadership skills to successfully partner with local, state, and federal policy makers to effect change.

Over 27,000 advocates nationwide have gone through this training, which meets one weekend a month for 8 months. Advocacy efforts of Partners in Policymaking alumni have reached every level of government. From school boards to the White House, alumni of Partners in Policymaking have been empowered to advocate and tell their stories. There are innumerable examples of alumni making a difference. Washington, DC, Partner in Policymaking alumni Teriana Cox was on the dais when President Obama signed the Workforce Innovation and Opportunity Act of 2014 (WIOA). U.S. Senator Maggie Hassan, an alumnus of the New Hampshire Partners in Policymaking, credits the program as the first step in her career.

RECOGNIZING THE GAPS IN OUR UNDERSTANDING

In a 2017 systematic review of disability and family research, Shurr and Hollingshead found that an overwhelming majority of research emphasized mothers as the primary reporters. Additionally, the diversity categories around gender identity and sexual orientation were largely absent. Further research is needed that is reflective of multiple identities. At the same time, we must continue to recognize that, just as the experience of disability is individualized, so too is the experience for families. There are family-specific needs that go along with having children who have disabilities. The social model of disability views disability as a result of society's inaccessibility and lack of usability. This "mismatch" can also exist for families related to a lack of needed environmental supports (Resch et al., 2018). This could be considered one way to recognize and address the needs of families that are not being

CASE STUDY 14.7. STEPHANIE'S FAMILY STORY

Federal Policy. When Congress proposed to cut Medicaid in 2017, advocates where I live in Georgia mobilized to share our stories with legislators to let them know how much Medicaid means to parents in the disability community.

We sent emails to parents of children with disabilities throughout the state inviting them to share a photo of their family and one paragraph about the difference Medicaid had made for their child and family. We ended up collecting over 40 stories that we printed and shared with federal legislators. Our strategy was very low tech, and the low production quality actually emphasized even more that our effort was led by families and not a professional entity. The compilation of these stories was powerful in sharing a unique lens that some legislators had not considered when they proposed cutting Medicaid and shined a light on our financial challenges that needed to be addressed through federal policy. While we appreciated that legislators were responsive to our concerns, the situation could have been avoided if parents and individuals with disabilities were included as stakeholders in conversations when policy changes are in the developmental stage.

State Policy. Later in 2021, we again enlisted our social media groups and mailing list of parents of children with disabilities to advocate for Georgia to increase the vaccine prioritization of people with disabilities. When the vaccine prioritization plan was announced in late 2020, people with disabilities and significant comorbidities were placed in the last phase of rollout behind essential workers like grocery store employees. We again reached out to our network of parents to share their stories about the impact of COVID-19 on their families with their legislators via email and their communities via social media. We also contacted the local press about our concerns because Andy had to significantly limit his available work hours to stay safe as a high-risk person, and Heidi's son faced potentially dire medical consequences as a person with Down syndrome, autism, and cancer survivor. Fortunately, after two rounds of public pressure in January and February, the state did respond and raise the vaccine prioritization of people with disabilities. However, these types of efforts require a significant amount of time, energy, and worry from an already stressed population, so inviting people with disabilities and their families to provide input as valued stakeholders when developing policies through entities like the Governor's Developmental Disabilities Council could significantly alleviate the advocacy stress faced by families.

Local Policy. When my son was in third grade, our local school district proposed cutting one-third of the paraprofessionals serving students with disabilities in our school district to balance the budget. Upon hearing this news in the local newspaper, I sent an email to the parents I knew who had children with disabilities and posted a message on Facebook. We created an email template and advised our network of parents to send this email to the superintendent and school board to inform them of our concerns about the proposed staff cuts. The number of paraprofessionals serving students with disabilities should be determined by IEPs, and over 80 parents sent the district leadership emails about our concerns. We subsequently organized a small team of parents to speak during the public comment section of the local school board meeting. At the time, the district wasn't responsive to our needs, so we had to individually address the impact of these staff cuts at stressful IEP meetings. Therefore, the lack of attention to parent voices in setting policy caused significant stress multiplied exponentially times each IEP meeting for both parents and education professionals in the district.

met by the myriad of formal and informal systems. Research that assesses the impact of supports and services, community inclusion, family coping mechanisms, and interventions that provide the most promising outcomes for families continue to be needed. This will enable families to seek the most effective supports and settings and also to have data to support their advocacy efforts.

It is also virtually impossible to disentangle the impact of individual systems on the voices of parents and families, as there is interplay across healthcare, education, and other social service systems with which families may interact. It is the combination of these experiences, both positive and negative, that can shape the voices of families.

CASE STUDY 14.8. STEPHANIE'S FAMILY STORY

Where we have genuinely struggled has been getting access to healthcare and therapies that Andy needed to meet his developmental milestones and stay healthy. In addition, we spent hours formulating arguments and engaging in conversations to convince educators to include Andy in school, and I have awakened in a panic in the middle of the night, writing legislators and policy leaders about services Andy and his friends needed to achieve their potential and get the support they deserve. The disability diagnosis has not been at the core of our challenges as a family—the core challenges have centered around discriminatory attitudes about people with disabilities, assumptions about where Andy belongs, and a lack of commitment to providing the supports and services for our son to thrive in the most inclusive settings.

CONCLUSION

A family that includes a child with a disability is, first and foremost, a family. Each family's journey is different. Parents can be powerful voices in all areas that impact their family, including healthcare, education, and policy. Access to practical research findings, resources, mentors, and advocates can build a community of well-informed parents of children with disabilities. This, in turn, can ensure that voices of families are included in decision-making at an individual and systems level and thus improve transition and quality-of-life outcomes for people with disabilities. While parents have made many strides forward, there is much work to be done. As history shows us, the voices of parents are valuable and necessary to continuing and accelerating this progress.

CASE STUDY 14.9. ANSWERS TO STEPHANIE AND JUSTIN'S QUESTIONS

What we ultimately learned is that Andy's disability has not been the biggest challenge. While he certainly has experienced some frustration related to his disability, especially when trying to learn in school and some early bouts with respiratory infections, Andy is a joy to be around and lives a fulfilling life. He's sarcastic, thoughtful, loyal, loving, witty, and determined. Down syndrome is part of his unique identity as an individual. The biggest challenges for us, in fact, have been access to supports and services and discrimination based on his diagnosis.

The questions that Stephanie and her husband, Justin, posed when Andy was born are answered for readers here:

1. How could we possibly afford the resources he might need as young parents?

    Update: Andy was able to receive early intervention services like speech therapy and physical therapy right away free of charge. The therapists taught me how to feed him, how to build up his strength to sit up and walk, and how to sign his first words before he was able to speak. I soon wondered how any parent raised a kid without these wonderful specialists by their side.

2. Would other kids make fun of him?

Update: Andy was much cooler in school than my husband or myself ever were. To be fair, that's not a high bar, but he was genuinely cool. He went to every school and church dance with a date, he played lacrosse, and he earned his Eagle Scout award. Usually, any kids who were unkind to him were unkind to everyone.

3. Would he live with us forever?

Update: Andy has had his bags packed to move out since he was 13 years old. He has every intention of moving out, and I'm working hard on building the scaffolding to make that possible for him in a few years as he starts college this fall. My husband, meanwhile, is trying to bribe him with a large-screen TV to stay with us longer so that he doesn't lose his best friend.

4. Would our identity always be tied to being the parents of a child with Down syndrome?

Update: It's strange that this was a concern, but it was. I imagine it's similar to feeling that you don't want to be defined entirely by a disability. However, the community and work that I've been introduced to because of Andy's diagnosis has been one of the greatest gifts in my life. I've been able to travel around the country and to Japan and Russia to teach about Down syndrome advocacy, and I couldn't be prouder than to be recognized as Andy's mom.

DISCUSSION QUESTIONS

1. Describe some concerns families might have upon learning that their child has a disability.

2. Why is it important that more parental adaptation research is conducted in both Western and non-Western countries?

3. If you were asked to design a research study on families and disability, what would you focus on and why?

4. What does the research say about the role of religion in parental adaptation? Why is it important that service providers, educators, and other professionals understand how religion influences parental and family adaptation?

5. Why is ecological validity important to adapting and creating parental adaptation interventions? Use Bernal's framework to support your answer.

6. Resiliency is now being used to understand parental adaptation. What examples of resiliency can you find in Stephanie, Justin, and Andy's story?

7. Summarize approaches professionals can use to build partnerships with families.

8. Compare areas where research initiatives have progressed for families of children with disabilities and where research still needs to improve.

9. How might life be different today for people with disabilities without parental advocacy in the 20th century?

10. Describe measures educators can take to create an empowered alliance, according to the Family Partnership Matrix, to develop educational priorities and practices for students with disabilities.

CLASS ACTIVITIES

1. Conduct a search to find the family advocacy organizations in your state. Are there local chapters near you? Learn about the mission and activities of each.

2. Create a list of 10 questions that you would like to ask a parent or family member about their experience having a family member with a disability. Reach out to a family advocacy organization to ask if you can interview one of the members.

3. Find the Parent Training and Information Center (PTI) in your state. The list of PTIs is available at www.parentcenterhub.org/find-your-center/

4. List five things that professionals can do to promote family engagement and five things that can keep families from being engaged.

5. Review disability legislation prompted by parent advocacy in the 20th century through today.

6. Watch *Including Samuel*, a documentary by Dan Habib. This film provides a glimpse into the lives of five families who have a child with a disability.

KEY REFERENCES

Only key references appear in the print edition. The full references appear in the digital product on Springer Publishing Connect™: https://connect.springerpub.com/content/book/978-0-8261-5111-7/part/partIII/chapter/ch14

American Association on Intellectual and Developmental Disabilities. (2015). *Self-determination and self-advocacy by people with IDD*. https://www.aaidd.org/docs/default-source/National-Goals/self-determination-and-self-advocacy-by-people-with-idd.pdf?sfvrsn=9d3a7f21_0

Carter, E. W. (2013). Supporting inclusion and flourishing in the religious and spiritual lives of people with intellectual and developmental disabilities. *Inclusion*, 1, 64–75. https://doi.org/10.1352/ 2326-6988-1.1.064

Iannone, N. M., & Meredith, S. H. (2020). *Diagnosis to delivery: A pregnant mother's guide to Down syndrome*. (10th anniversary ed.). https://downsyndromepregnancy.org/book/diagnosis-to-delivery/

Maul, C. A., & Singer, G. H. (2009). "Just good different things": Specific accommodations families make to positively adapt to their children with developmental disabilities. *Topics in Early Childhood Special Education 29*(3), 155–170. https://doi.org/10.1177/0271121408328516

Minnesota Governor's Council on Developmental Disabilities. (2022). *Parallels in time*. https://mn.gov/mnddc/parallels/

Snow, K. (2013) *Diagnosis does not define a person* [Video]. Minnesota Governor's Council on Developmental Disabilities. https://mn.gov/mnddc/kathie-snow/kathie-snow-01.html

CHAPTER 15

PSYCHOSOCIAL COUNSELING ASPECTS OF GRIEF, DYING, AND DEATH

MARK A. STEBNICKI

LEARNING OBJECTIVES

After reading this chapter, you will be able to:

- Identify and recognize the unique aspects of psychosocial counseling issues related to persons with life-threatening illnesses and disabilities
- Analyze specific family member and caregiver stress associated with the dying and death of their loved one with a life-threatening disability
- Differentiate the clinically significant symptoms related to the *Diagnostic and Statistical Manual of Mental Disorders, Fifth Edition,* and *Diagnostic and Statistical Manual of Mental Disorders (text revision)* description of Persistent and Complex Bereavement Disorder as well as the newer category of Prolonged Grief Disorder.
- Recognize the unique cultural attributes of grief, dying, and death that will assist in facilitating culturally focused psychosocial counseling approaches

PRE-READING QUESTIONS:

1. What are the unique psychological and emotional impacts on family members and caregivers who must deal with issues related to grief, dying, and death of a loved one?

2. How do we differentiate psychosocial counseling issues related to dealing with persons who have chronic illnesses and disabilities versus those with life-threatening illnesses?

3. Describe your experience with grief, dying, and death of a family member and how this has impacted your life. What unique losses have you experienced versus other losses you have experienced throughout your life?

George Engel's (1961) classic work on grief has challenged researchers and practitioners alike in the medical and psychological community with the perplexing question of "Is grief a disease?" The idea that grief should even be considered within the classification of a medical condition helped launch the foundational work in the fields of psychosomatic medicine and the development of biopsychosocial models of significance by Engel and others that followed this research agenda (Stroebe, 2015).

Despite newer models of grief and the associated symptomatology as described by the diagnosis of Persistent Complex Bereavement Disorder (PCBD) in the *Diagnostic and Statistical Manual of Mental Disorders, Fifth Edition* (*DSM-5*; American Psychiatric Association [APA], 2013) and the 2022 *DSM-5* text revision (*DSM-5-TR*) inclusion of the diagnostic category of Prolonged Grief Disorder (PGD), the nature, experience, and expression of grief may not be expressed and experienced universally. Indeed, there is a cultural significance by which grief is both experienced and expressed. Accordingly, the cultural expression of grief itself complicates the psychosocial assessment, mental health diagnosis, and treatment interventions of grief. Thus, there are many challenges for counselors as they attempt to understand the meaning of their clients' multiple losses amid the constructs, definitions, and theories that surround psychosocial adjustment to the nature of grief.

Worden (2009) reminds practitioners that grief itself is a multidimensional or a multidetermined phenomenon. Some grievers express very little emotion after critical events of death, dying, or loss, while others are overwhelmed to the point of total mental and physical incapacity. Grief is basically what the person says it is, how the person describes it, expresses it (verbally and nonverbally), and experiences it. Despite that, some authors define grief as the psychological and emotional reaction that is experienced after a person dies (Brinkmann & Kofod, 2018); others describe a unique anticipatory grieving process that occurs before an individual's death that is culturally experienced and expressed (Jones-Eversley & Rice, 2018; Rando et al., 2012; Stebnicki, 2018, 2021a, 2021b). For example, African Americans are disproportionately impacted by grief, dying, and death because of higher morbidity and mortality rates than other racial-ethnic groups (Jones-Eversley & Rice, 2022). The epidemiological concerns and public health impact of African Americans are well documented in studies of health disparities, particularly during phases of the COVID-19 pandemic (Stebnicki, 2021b).

The grief experienced by the military culture also has some unique psychosocial characteristics not experienced by civilians due to severe wounds and mortality sustained during combat operations and training exercises (Stebnicki, 2021a). Active-duty service members, veterans, veterans with disabilities, and military families experience loss, grief, and bereavement at higher rates than civilians. This is due to the nature of the occupational risk involved in combat deployments and humanitarian missions. Many times, major depressive disorder, posttraumatic stress symptoms, and psychosocial issues pose clinical concerns for military service personnel due to the chronic and persistent nature of repeated exposure to extraordinarily stressful and traumatic events experienced during military and veteran life.

As many seasoned grief counselors share, establishing a person-centered and culturally focused rapport is essential in developing an optimal working alliance with a diverse range of individuals and groups. First and foremost, earning the circle of trust is essential in dealing with the psychosocial aspects of grief counseling during therapeutic interactions. Thus, it is essential that counselors facilitate a high level of compassion and empathy. Therapeutic approaches facilitated by professionals must extend beyond treating the purported mental and physical health effects that accompany grief by looking at the underlying complex factors.

Overall, the skills of working with the psychosocial aspects of grief, dying, death, and loss are essential, particularly in working with persons who have acquired chronic illness and disability. It is beyond the scope of this chapter to provide a comprehensive discussion of grief theories, models, and interventions. However, this chapter helps elucidate important psychosocial issues in death and dying as they relate to how individuals experience and express grief within the context of the person's physical, psychological, cognitive, emotional, social, cultural, and spiritual well-being.

Grief is defined most parsimoniously as the emotional response to loss (Stebnicki, 2018; Stroebe et al., 2008). However, many languages and cultures have no word for the term and constructs related to grief (Klass, 2014). The word *grief* is from the Anglo-French *gref,* which is derived from the Latin word *gravis,* which means heavy, painful, important, and the carrying of burdens. Overall, the definition itself appears to be grounded in cultural meaning (Rosenblatt, 2012).

The idea that grief should be considered within the context of a specific mental health condition has spurred debate among the disciplines of medicine, psychology, mental health, and thanatology over the last 25 years. Grief may occur in non–death-related events that involve extraordinarily stressful and traumatic events, which typically include multiples losses (e.g., medical-physical-mental health, divorce, job loss). Critical incidents, such as person-made (e.g., warfighting, terrorism, school shootings) and natural disasters (e.g., hurricanes, floods, wildfires) all have an accumulation of losses and should be considered within the grieving process. The psychological, emotional, physical, and spiritual costs to such critical incidents complicate the healing process but also help clarify the definition of grief (Stebnicki, 2017). Cultural and spiritual sensitivity are also critical aspects in understanding how grief is defined, expressed, and experienced during therapeutic relationships with persons grieving (Klass, 2014; Murstori & Haynes, 2020; Rando et al., 2012; Stebnicki, 2018, 2021a; Strupp et al., 2021).

In search for a definition of grief, it may be helpful to understand how grief is measured. To assist in the constructs of measuring grief, Prigerson et al. (1995) developed a comprehensive research questionnaire, the Inventory of Complicated Grief (ICG), that measures the individual's experience of persistent grief that goes beyond the normal healing period. The ICG and its accompanying research may assist counselors in understanding the characteristics and symptomatology of *complicated grief* (Igarashi et al., 2021). Subsequent revisions of the ICG include the ICG-R (Prigerson & Jacobs, 2001) and the current PG-13 (Prigerson et al., 2009), which is now commonly used to measure complicated grief.

Indeed, grief and loss are mutually shared across all cultures and experienced by nearly all individuals over one's lifetime (Murastori & Haynes, 2020; Stebnicki, 2016c, 2018). Despite the healing aspects of grief, it is of paramount importance to note that prolonged pathological grief can become dysfunctional in one's life (Craig, 2010; Rando et al., 2012; Stroebe, 2015). The early work related to grief, dying, and death by Kübler-Ross (1975) appeared to lay some of the critical underpinnings that gave legitimacy to the experience of grieving. Kübler-Ross defined the experience of grief in terms of a model of linear progression that occurred in five stages: denial, anger, bargaining, depression, and acceptance. The underlying assumption is that grieving is a natural event, and as one progresses through this process, it should result in personal and psychological growth, as well as emotional healing. Although there may be shortcomings with stage models because they represent an artificial linear progression of the grieving and mourning process, the benefits of early work in this area prepared the groundwork for the modern hospice movement (Balk, 2014; Hospice Foundation of America, 2022).

Bereaved individuals going through the grieving process, regardless of stage model, have many serious expressed and nonexpressed thoughts and questions that confront them physically, emotionally, psychologically, and spiritually. Questions such as "What will my life look like now?" "What did the deceased's life mean to me?" "How can I possibly feel safe and secure in a world such as this?" "Who am I now that this death has occurred?" "Why do bad things happen to good people?" and/or "Why do good things happen to bad people" (Kushner, 1980; Neimeyer et al., 2002; Worden, 2009) suggest such existential and spiritual questions challenge the personal meaning in death and dying in fundamental ways.

PERSISTENT COMPLEX BEREAVEMENT DISORDER AND PROLONGED GRIEF DISORDER: CRITERIA IN THE *DSM-5* AND *DSM-5*-TR

Historically, the APA's *DSM* has not cited grief as a specific psychiatric disorder. Rather, grief has been clinically defined as a condition that can be triggered by loss and bereavement, which primarily manifests as major depressive disorder or adjustment disorder, which does not adequately cover the psychological condition itself (Murray Parkes, 2005). With the inclusion of PCBD in the *DSM-5* in 2013, complicated grief and its co-occurring syndromes related to grief have helped lay the foundation for structured interviews, standardized assessments, and a path for the diagnosis and treatment of grief. After years of debate concerning the individual's experience of grief in mental health and related fields, the 2022 text revision of the *DSM-5* (*DSM-5-TR*), PGD has become an official diagnosis and has replaced the earlier diagnostic category of PCBD. This change allows clinicians to bill insurance for treating this condition (APA, 2022a; Advisory Board, 2022). This diagnostic category also has accumulated research on measuring the associated clinical mental health symptoms that hinder one's healing in the grieving process.

For many years, there has been a call for a diagnostic category in the *DSM* that reflects the symptomatology related to the grieving process (Rando et al., 2012). Accordingly, there have been systematic attempts in the research to identify, delineate, and assess grief and its co-occurring mental health conditions. Generally, the literature commonly describes other grief syndromes using the terms *absent, abnormal, complicated, distorted, morbid, maladaptive, atypical, intensified and prolonged, unresolved, neurotic, dysfunctional, chronic, delayed,* and *inhibited grief*. It is beyond the scope and intention of this chapter to comprehensively discuss each of the syndrome's clinical features. However, there appears to be an emphasis for the counseling profession to understand that syndromes related to *complicated and prolonged grief* cannot be confined to one syndrome or disorder, but rather includes multiple phenomena for consideration when measuring one's experience and expression of grief (Nielsen et al., 2017).

The earlier work of Prigerson et al. (2008; as cited by Rando et al., 2012) provides some of the foundational work underlying the category of PCBD (APA, 2013) and the current PGD (APA, 2022a). More recently, Lenferink et al. (2022) have studied the psychometric properties of instruments that measure PCBD with the intention to accurately diagnose and treat this unique condition. For instance, associations between grief symptoms, posttraumatic stress disorder, and depression have been elucidated and speak to issues related to the challenges confronting clinicians providing the most accurate and complete diagnostic category before implementing therapeutic grief-related treatment modalities.

The *DSM-5* has five criteria that consider the individual's reactive distress associated with the loss and grief in close relationships. The abbreviated criterion are (a) the individual's experience of the death; (b) the clinically significant symptoms that persist for at least 12 months after the death of an adult and 6 months for children in which there is persistent yearning, sorrow, emotional pain, and preoccupation with the deceased; (c) the presentation of at least six clinically distressing symptoms on more days than not; (d) the bereaved individual's clinically significant distress is exhibited by disturbance in social, occupational, or other important psychosocial areas; and (e) the bereaved individual's reaction is out of proportion to or inconsistent with the cultural, religious, or age-appropriate norms.

In addition to criterion a to e, the *DSM-5* measures the significance of symptoms as they relate to disruption in one's social and interpersonal life. There is also the inclusion of one specifier, *traumatic bereavement*, and four differential diagnoses (i.e., normal grief, depressive disorders, posttraumatic stress disorder, and separation anxiety disorder), that assist professional counselors in comprehensively identifying the underlying cause or etiology of the *persistent and complex bereavement* such as bereavement because of homicide, suicide, degree of suffering, mutilation, injury, and the overall nature of the death as experienced by the bereaved. Given the seriousness of these clinically significant symptoms, as well as the high risk for suicide ideation, attempts, and completions, it is understandable that more therapeutic attention is required than dealing with the primary emotion of grief itself.

In the newer text revision of the *DSM-5-TR*, PCBD is replaced by the category of PGD. Boelen et al. (2020) point to two separate distress criteria ("Intense yearning/longing for the deceased person" and "Preoccupation with thoughts or memories of the deceased person") and eight co-occurring clinically significant psychological symptoms (e.g., intense loneliness) that are identified. A closer examination of the *DSM-5-TR* is required by licensed clinicians to diagnose and treat the complex array of clinically significant symptoms relating to treating PGD and co-occurring disorders more accurately. The counseling professional already has a natural means for professional and personal growth opportunities acquired through continuing educational training as it relates to one's area of specialty. Besides graduate training, there are postgraduate workshops and seminars for licensed professionals that relate to the newer *DSM-5-TR* diagnostic category of PGD. The APA (2022b) offers multiple resources for counselors to better understand how to diagnose and treat this and other co-occurring conditions.

PSYCHOSOCIAL COUNSELING ASPECTS OF COMPLEX GRIEF

The literature related to grief, dying, and death is clear that most forms of grief syndromes are complex in nature (Murray Parkes, 2005; Prigerson et al., 2008; Rando et al., 2012; Stebnicki, 2018; Stroebe, 2015). Counselors must reach beyond the person's primary emotion of grief in therapy to achieve optimal psychosocial therapeutic benefits with their clients. Indeed, complicated grief itself can be debilitating because complex co-occurring clinical conditions tend to develop as the result of death and loss (Prigerson & Jacobs, 2001). In fact, the *DSM-5* and *DSM-5-TR* delineate how the functional psychological consequence of complex and prolonged grief presents with co-occurring conditions such as major depressive disorder, posttraumatic stress disorder, substance use disorders, and separation anxiety disorders (Nielsen et al., 2017; Stebnicki, 2021a; Valentine et al., 2016). The complexity of the grieving and mourning process itself lies in many other factors such as one's past experience of grieving, culturally specific issues related to the expression of grief, pre- and co-occurring mental health conditions related to the grief scenario or critical incident, and other clinical symptoms that present during therapeutic interactions (e.g., suicide ideation, persistent thoughts and preoccupation with the deceased, excessive use of substances, feelings of hopelessness, detachment, and social isolation). Accordingly, many authors recognize the complex variation within the mourning and grieving process in therapy (Nielsen, 2017; Rocco & Shuck, 2019; Stroebe et al., 2017).

Worden (2009) suggests that the goal of grief therapy is to resolve conflicts of separation to the deceased and for the therapist to assist the bereaved in adjusting and adapting to life without their loved one. Developing a therapeutic relationship with the bereaved is the key to achieving a strong working alliance. Skilled and competent counselors understand that acknowledging the person's loss, normalizing the experience of loss and grief, dealing with other issues of complex grief at the appropriate time, and approaching clients with a compassionate and empathetic energy assist in gaining optimal therapeutic and trusting relationships.

In cases of chronic and persistent grief reactions as seen in the PGD diagnostic criteria, counselors want to identify risk factors that are related to their client's (a) medical/physical functioning (e.g., life-threatening illness, newly acquired catastrophic disability); (b) psychiatric/mental health functioning (e.g., presence of depression, anxiety, substance use, or other co-occurring conditions); and (c) level of psychosocial adjustment, support, and resources. Symptoms of clinical significance include flashbacks of the death experience; emotional and social detachment; isolation; avoidance of intrusive thoughts related to the death experience; cognitive and emotional feelings of numbness, detachment, and confusion; intense levels of bitterness, anger, and hostility; and feelings related to severe hopelessness, helplessness, and suicidal ideation.

In many models of grief and bereavement therapy there is a growing acceptance that attachment, remembering, and continuing bonds with the deceased are both natural and healthy (Koblenz, 2016; Worden, 2009). The manner in which "continuing bonds" therapy is facilitated varies. However, many proponents suggest it is important to have clients (a) connect with the deceased by making efforts to locate the deceased (e.g., heaven), (b) experiencing the deceased in dreams, (c) communicating with the deceased (e.g., speaking with them in silence, visiting the cemetery), (d) remembering the deceased often (thinking about them), and (e) attaching through a variety of objects (e.g., clothing, jewelry, home videos; Normand et al., 1996; Rando, 1984; Worden, 2009). The absence of such approaches can lead to a lack of information about the deceased, unresolved feelings, frustration, and chronic and persistent feelings of sadness. Overall, continuing this bond with the deceased is instrumental in the mourning process and helps in assisting with increased coping and resiliency after the loss (Neimeyer, 2001).

TRAUMA AND GRIEF

The human spirit and soul are at stake for professionals at the therapeutic epicenter of mental health disaster relief and dealing with the loss and grief associated with person-made and natural disasters. The stench of death in hospitals and tent cities lies motionless on the battlefield of a coronavirus pandemic. Gun violence that erupts in our communities reminds us of how fragile and vulnerable human life can be as we are assaulted by both known and unknown assailants. Providing therapeutic services to individuals, groups, and communities that have sustained significant losses requires that psychosocial grief counselors learn how to mend the fragmented self as we place the "do not disturb" or "in session" sign on our metaphoric exterior door while recognizing that we may need to heal our own empathy fatigue before we can competently serve others who have experienced trauma and grief.

The horrific terrorist attacks of September 11, 2001; the attack on the U.S. Capitol by pro-Trump supporters and insurrectionists on January 6, 2021; and the COVID-19 pandemic are examples of extraordinarily stressful and traumatic events that left emotional, physical, spiritual, and environmental scars on the minds, bodies, and spirits of many in the United States. The medical, physical, psychological, social, and emotional devastation left in the aftermath of these and other critical events have created a type of historical trauma among Westerners that has prompted a consciousness shift within the counseling profession (Stebnicki, 2016a, 2021b). It is of particular interest how we can apply models of loss, grief, dying, and death to inimitable cultural events that occur on large-scale disasters such as virial pandemics, forest fires, catastrophic floods, school shootings, gun violence in our communities, earthquakes, and other critical incidents that spark the primary emotion of loss and grief (Stebnicki, 2017, 2021b).

There are multiple opportunities for professional counselors to prepare for, plan, and intervene in a variety of critical incidents that result in catastrophic loss of life. It is beyond the scope of this chapter to compare and contrast theories, models, and interventions in grief counseling; critical incident stress debriefing; or disaster mental health response. This would certainly be a fruitful area for researchers to explore in a meta-analysis as well as other research designs. The results, discussion, and conclusion of such purported studies on catastrophic loss of life have common factors that relate to the symptomatology, clinical features, standardized and functional assessments, and therapeutic interventions to facilitate with individuals grieving multiple losses. Presently, the literature appears to mix concepts, theories, and interventions as they relate to grief counseling and trauma response.

The *DSM-5* and *DSM-5-TR* may be a bridge for practitioners and researchers alike dealing with issues of grief, loss, dying, and death given the new diagnostic category of PGD. Given that trauma creates a chronic, persistent, and sometimes delayed grief reaction, the diagnostic and associated clinical features may help support a diagnosis of such a mental health condition. Indeed, there are various definitions and models of disaster mental health response out of which some appear the same as, similar to, and different from models of grief counseling and interventions. However, competent and ethical counselors are aware of the appropriate application for diagnosing, triaging, and intervening across different settings, cultures, and types of traumatic experiences. In other words, competent mental health professionals understand the cultural and clinical differences between intervening in a rural Arkansas tornado, a California wildfire, or a Chicago neighborhood exploding in gun violence. Likewise, the seasoned grief counselor knows how to facilitate grief therapy with children, adolescents, and adults across a variety of losses that spark persistent and complex feelings of bereavement (e.g., sudden death of a child, dying of AIDS, or death by suicide).

CHRONIC ILLNESS AND DISABILITY: A COMPLEX GRIEF RESPONSE

One particular area that has been studied a great deal is the grief and loss reaction associated with chronic illnesses and disabilities (CIDs). Persons with CID are served at a much greater frequency than ever before. This is particularly relevant for military veterans with CID (Stebnicki, 2021a). Indeed, there are medical advances extending the life expectancy of person-made (e.g., terrorism, community-based gun violence) and natural disasters (e.g., hurricanes, floods, earthquakes) and injuries sustained by the recent wars in Iraq, Afghanistan, and multiple other geographic hotspots outside the United States (Stebnicki, 2017, 2021a). Overall, persons with physical, cognitive, emotional, and psychiatric disabilities seek counseling services in much greater numbers than previously reported (Smart, 2016).

The Centers for Disease Control and Prevention (CDC, 2022) estimates that 6 in 10 adults in the United States have a chronic disease such as heart disease, cancer, chronic lung disease, stroke, Alzheimer disease, diabetes, and/or chronic kidney disease. The World Health Organization (WHO, 2020) reports about 1 billion persons, or one in three adults worldwide, live with one or more disabilities. Besides chronic diseases, many disabilities are caused by motor vehicle accidents; falls causing catastrophic injury; acts of physical, sexual, and intimate partner violence; and war. Other commonly occurring medical-physical conditions include traumatic brain injury, traumatic amputation, spinal cord injury, musculoskeletal injuries, and chronic pain conditions. Counselors could benefit greatly from having the awareness, knowledge, and skills in working with the unique psychosocial aspects of loss, mourning, and grief as they relate to persons with CID.

Many individuals who experience permanent medical-physical disabilities experience a complex level of psychosocial adjustment because of the loss of their residual functional capacity. In essence, there is a grieving and mourning process that individuals and family members go through as individuals with CID progress through the physical rehabilitation process (Marini, 2016; Smart, 2016; Stebnicki, 2017). Skilled and competent counselors understand that persons with CID experience losses in many different ways such as:

- Loss over the control of one's life and overall independence
- Loss in a sense of fairness and justice
- Loss of emotional and mental security
- Loss of mental capacity to make decisions independently
- Loss of physical capacity, body image, and ability for sexual or intimate relationships
- Loss of career identity, vocational opportunities, or ability to progress academically

Processing the multiple losses with clients can bring meaning and purpose to clients living with CID. Many individuals are empowered by understanding that they are people first and that their *dis*-ability does not define the boundaries of their mental and physical capacities.

The literature related to how persons with CID cope with loss is quite immense. Coping has been viewed as a psychological strategy to decrease, modify, or diffuse the impact of stress-related life events (Livneh & Antonak, 2012). The defining characteristics of coping with a CID include how the person

(a) exhibits and experiences coping as a state or trait; (b) controls or manipulates his or her coping strategies; (c) organizes his or her coping style on a range of internal-external characteristics; and (d) responds from an affective, cognitive, and/or behavioral style of coping. Falvo and Holland (2018) describes *coping strategies* in relation to CID as a subconscious mechanism to deal and cope with stress. The intent is for the person to reduce his or her level of stress and anxiety. Coping styles (e.g., denial, compensation, rationalization) are particularly relevant for persons coping with CIDs. This is because in psychosocial adjustment to disability, there is a strong need for the person to bring balance, normalcy, productivity, and a certain quality of life back to optimal functioning.

From a counseling perspective, it is important to choose goals with clients and family members that relate to the person's (a) stability, (b) progressive nature, (c) episodic nature, (d) degenerative nature, and (e) periods of exacerbation and remission of the individual's CID. Counselors who bring meaning to the loss of mental and physical capacity have opportunities to gain therapeutic leverage with their clients. Cultivating coping and resiliency skills while allowing the person to grieve and mourn the loss of his or her medical/physical and mental health can assist in empowering persons with CIDs for optimal wellness across multiple life areas.

OLDER ADULTS AND GRIEF

The "baby boomer" generation, born between 1946 and 1964, is clearly in a unique developmental life space than other generations as they journey through the 21st century and attempt to retire from their primary occupation. (Bruyere et al., 2017). There are multiple financial, social, emotional, mental, and physical health concerns among this generation. Due to cost of living, reduced retirement benefits from their primary occupation, and other financial burdens, there are more persons 65 years of age and older who continue to work at least part-time. In fact, one in every five American workers is more than 65 years old, and by 2024, persons aged 55 years and older will comprise approximately 20% of the workforce. Thus, as the number of individuals surviving into older adulthood increases, the number of medical, physical, and mental health stressors have a potential to lead to diminished independence and functional capacity (Falvo & Holland, 2018).

The Pew Research Center social and demographic trends show that baby boomers report an over-all quality of life rating lower than other generations (Pew Research Center, 2008). As a natural part of the aging process, older individuals experience multiple losses because of mood dysregulation, neurocognitive decline, loss of sensory capabilities, medical and physical conditions, and loss of independence (Eisenberg et al., 1999; Falvo & Holland, 2018; Garfield, 1979). Veterans with chronic illnesses and disabilities are at a much greater disadvantage than those who have not served due to the complex and co-occurring medical, physical, and mental health conditions sustained during their military service (Stebnicki, 2021a). Prime examples can be seen in veteran homelessness, where well over 37,000 veterans remained homeless in 2019 (Hayden, 2018). Additionally, there are over 700,000 veterans who fought in the Gulf War (1991–1292) and other Southwest Asia theaters of operation who have been diagnosed with Gulf War illness, a newer category of service-connected disability instituted by the Veterans Administration in 2020 (U.S. Department of Veterans Affairs, 2022). As a result of the aging process, acquired chronic illness and disability, stress and trauma, and overall decline in mental and physical health, grief itself becomes a complicated process and is difficult to define (Parks, 2007; Prigerson et al., 2008; Rando et al., 2012) and diagnose, such as in clients who present with clinically significant symptoms of PGD. Consequently, grief as a psychosocial and psychiatric condition is complicated when older individuals experience the full range of medical, physical, psychological, cognitive, social, and emotional health issues. Thus, grief places older persons at risk for any number of losses in daily functioning and independence.

Indeed, preexisting mental and physical health conditions before CID contribute much to one's wellness and resiliency (Shannonhouse et al., 2016), especially in the case of older individuals. It may become an asset or protective factor in dealing with issues of loss and grief during older adulthood. Persons who age successfully have a better acceptance of past losses, griefs, conflicts, and a good mastery of some level of independence and control over their environment (Falvo & Holland, 2018; Kampfe, 2015; Weil, 2005). Counselors who have had training related to negative stereotypes about persons with disabilities, aging (ageism), prejudice, and attitudinal barriers against older persons (gerontophobia) can reduce the stigma, misconceptions, and fear of addressing psychosocial issues with older persons and issues related to the aging process. Thus, infusion of content related to counseling older persons within the counselor education curriculum can increase the knowledge, awareness, and skills of professional counselors to build rapport and facilitate an optimal therapeutic relationship with older individuals (Bruyere et al., 2017; Kampfe et al., 2005).

CAREGIVER STRESS IN THE GRIEVING PROCESS

Based on the record numbers of aging baby boomers, one of the fastest-growing occupations in the United States is that of home health care aide. Family members are oftentimes caregivers for persons with CID; despite that, nearly 70% to 80% of all Americans are transferred to and die in an institution such as a hospital or a nursing home (CDC, 2005; Stanford School of Medicine, 2022). Statistically the number of deaths increased significantly during the COVID-19 pandemic, where many cases were undetected or underreported (Shen et al., 2021). Family member and caregiver stress can be deeply wounding and complex, as a roller coaster of emotions are experienced. Some family members and caregivers bring meaning to the anticipatory grieving and bereavement process, which has therapeutic benefits through one's self-guided or professionally facilitated journey (Wagner, 2020). Additionally, there are cultural implications that require certain rituals, core values, and other bereavement issues that benefit both the family member and caregiver as well as the dying person (Chen et al., 2021).

For the first time in more than half a century more Americans are dying at home rather than in hospitals or nursing homes. Cross and Warriach (2019) report that the number of deaths due to chronic illness and disease at home has increased from 24% in 2003 to approximately 31% in 2017. However, there is limited data that require further research to address issues related to the patient's quality of life experienced at home as they are living with a CID. Despite the fact that institutions are designed to meet the acute primary medical needs of persons with CID, most institutions cannot offer what a concerned family member can in terms of emotional and psychosocial support. In some hospitals and nursing homes, family members are viewed as a nuisance, getting in the way, rather than allies in caring for the patient (Jones, 1979). In addition, some institutional environments restrict visitation by children or the patient's friends and extended family. This can add to a source of family and caregiver stress because of the inability to provide essential emotional and psychosocial support. The American hospice movement has advocated for and increased the quality of life for both patients, family members, and caregivers providing palliative care for those with serious illnesses with a focus on practical, emotional, and spiritual support.

The stress on family members and caregivers is immense. The average nonprofessional unpaid caregiver in the United States is 45 to 64 years of age and is typically caring for a spouse or family member who is aged more than 65 years (Bureau of Labor Statistics, [BLS] 2019; Lee & Carr, 2011). Many caregivers have families of their own and try and maintain educational and career endeavors while providing frequent caregiving activities to their family member with a CID. The Pew Research Center reports that 6 in 10 adults report having a parent over 65 years of age where they provide assistance with errands, housework, and home repairs (Pew Research Center, 2015). The intense person-centered nature of caregiving itself creates an emotional, physical, and spiritual exhaustion that can result in empathy fatigue (Stebnicki, 2008, 2016b). The research under certain circumstances supports the notion that family caregivers can endure a significant amount of stress (Marini, 2016). In Marini's (2012) meta-analysis of research related to caregiver stress, he found a significant number of studies that report poor health and psychosomatic conditions associated with being a caregiver. The primary factors linked to caregiver stress occur when (a) there is little or no respite or backup assistance to perform the essential tasks and functions in the caregiver role, (b) persons with CID are verbally or physically abusive toward the caregiver, and (c) a greater number of hands-on direct care hours are spent caring for the disabled loved one. These factors increase the risk for poor health among caregivers themselves.

In Marini's (2016) review of the literature on the psychosocial impact of caregiving on caregivers, he notes the significant number of empirical and anecdotal studies in which the act of caregiving can provide meaning and purpose in one's life. Despite the impact of this demanding work, lengthy hours, and the stress associated with caregiving, it has been reported by some to be rewarding. In other words, there appears to be a life lesson learned in the mental-emotional process of both family and professional caregiving. There are positive experiences of caregivers, particularly when the loved one with a disability reciprocates in appreciation and gratitude. This appears to minimize the caregiver stress and burden.

When the stress of caregiving itself becomes mentally, physically, and emotionally exhausting, some caregivers may require the support of a professional counselor. Counselors working with caregiver stress can assist by offering services that are focused on (a) respite care services; (b) processing caregiver emotions that are associated with negative feelings toward their loved one; and (c) advocacy related to fragmented medical and mental health services, support groups, financial support, and managing end-of-life services and resources (Lee & Carr, 2011; Marini, 2016; Worden, 2009). Overall, minimal attention has been given to sources of caregiver stress in terms of the caregiver's reaction and experience of this highly stressful job that many times cannot be fulfilled by any other person or institution. The lack of resources for emotional, physical, and financial respite provides multiple opportunities for counselors who work with issues of death and dying to integrate family members as a natural part of psychosocial counseling.

TRANSITION TO DIFFERENT LEVELS OF CARE

The transition from home to a different level of care (e.g., assistive living, acute/long-term rehabilitation facilities, intermediate/skilled nursing home, state-operated institutions) is a difficult choice for individual(s) and family members. They leave the comforts and safety of their home, many times letting go of memories, familiar environments, friends, and neighbors, and sometimes leaving behind their adult children whom perhaps they have lived with, as well as a spouse, partner, and/or pets. Establishing new living arrangements and routines in a more restrictive environment translates into less independence for the person and in some cases an overwhelming amount of debt for families in terms of healthcare costs not covered by federal, state, and/or private insurance programs. With the significant growth in populations such as older Americans, veterans, and persons with CIDs, counseling professionals who assist caregivers and family members are presented with a formidable challenge. Professionals working with individuals can begin the helping process by exploring the rationale and justification that initially prompted the transition to a different level of care. Consequently, the decline in the individual's medical, physical, and mental health conditions must be weighed alongside issues such as quality of life, healthcare benefits, ongoing treatment for chronic health conditions, affordable medical care, caregiver support systems, and many other factors.

Besides skyrocketing financial costs in healthcare, transition to a different level of care brings a cascade of psychosocial stressors and traumas for many. Older individuals and persons with CIDs are identified in the literature as one of the most vulnerable and at-risk populations for mistreatment by a caregiver, spouse, and/or partner (Lachs & Pillemar, 1995; Lee & Carr, 2011). These critical incidents are characterized as physical, emotional, psychological, sexual abuse and neglect, abandonment, and financial exploitation. Despite the fact that these psychosocial stressors and traumas may occur outside one's home setting such as a long-term care setting, the transition to a different level of care may bring about family crisis. Consequently, it is of paramount importance that helping professionals plan, organize, and involve family members, healthcare professionals, and peer support systems that can assist the individual(s) during this transition so that goals related to optimal wellness can be met.

As noted in the psychosocial literature, one of the prominent psychological and emotional features associated with placing a loved one into another level of care outside of their home are the feelings of guilt (Roach et al., 2021). Fundamentally, guilt is triggered by a variety of sources, including the caregiver's or family member's relationship with the person impacted by a chronic illness and/or disability, the level of perceived care required to maintain health and wellness, the rationale and circumstance which prompted the transition to another level of care, and the perceived stress of the caregiver or family member. The experience of guilt is most closely related to the clinically significant conditions of major depressive and prolonged grief disorders. If these become chronic and persistent conditions, family members and caregivers could benefit from the therapeutic assistance of a qualified counselor. Indeed, family members take on the roles as surrogate decision-maker, healthcare power of attorney, and advocate, which can create high levels of stress and anxiety. Thus, normalizing these experiences without pathologizing the psychological and emotional stressors is a good place to begin healing caregiver stress and patterns of burnout.

One of the most critical aspects of caregiver stress and burnout is the experience of guilt that can create negative emotions toward a family member's loved one. If guilt becomes a chronic and persistent pattern as it relates to the loved one's transition to a different level of care outside their home, it can create a pattern of unhealthy communication and relationships among family members (Prunty & Foli, 2019). There are other issues that complicate transition to a different level of care such as the family member's negative attitudes and perceptions about how to substantially improve their loved one's quality of life, addressing therapeutic decisions related to end of life, dying and death issues, and overall having to place the loved one into a hospice or palliative care setting (Chen et al., 2021; Krigger et al., 1997; Strupp et al., 2021). Ultimately, these issues complicate the psychosocial aspects of issues related to grief, dying, and death of a loved one who may be in transition to a different level of care. Caregivers who include their loved ones in the decision-making process throughout this transition can enhance optimal family communication and therapeutic partnerships. Additionally, caregivers and family members who reach out for professional assistance from medical, physical, psychosocial, and mental health care providers can enhance and optimize quality of life and end-of-life decisions and outcomes.

Not all caregivers and family members' experience guilt with regard to making critical healthcare decisions during transitions to another level of care outside the home (Lopez, 2009). Most of what is known in the literature relates directly to end-of-life decision-making tasks by family members as caregivers. Consequently, doing what is in the best interest of a loved one should not translate into caregiver abandonment or a family member's lack of feelings. Rather, the psychosocial issues that arise during caregiving decision-making responsibilities relate to protecting the quality of life, creating comfort, relying on religious/spiritual beliefs for guidance, honoring wishes, and seeking professional guidance on behalf of their loved one. When acute or chronic illness and disability arises within the family, major decisions must be made with regard to medical placement, healthcare treatment options, and all other medical, physical, and mental health resources that could potentially benefit their loved one. Worden (2009) suggests that the death of a family member has long-term psychological effects on the surviving spouse, partner, or adult children. This is particularly relevant when feelings of guilt arise among family members as surrogate decision-makers regarding healthcare and residential placement issues. The long-term psychological impact experienced by family members are complicated issues for professional counselors to deal with because transition to different levels of care and the death event are multidimensional in nature. No two persons grieve alike. For instance, there are multiple issues to consider in the death of an infant, child, adolescent, younger person, or an older adult. The nature and events surrounding the death (e.g., stillbirth, motor vehicle accident, disease, suicide, battlefield mortality) create a plethora of psychological, emotional, cognitive, and behavioral responses of the surviving family members. The emotional integration of the family, how they come together to support each other, and their level of coping and resiliency all determine how grieve is expressed and communicated during the healing process.

For some family members, the transition to a more restrictive or institutional environment itself signals an anticipatory grief response. If healthy grieving begins early on, whereby the family member anticipates the death event, there is potential for the healing process to begin (Stebnicki, 2018). In other words, family members who begin the healthy grieving process prior to the death of their loved one typically begin developing coping resources and resiliency skills that will eventually assist them at the time of death with a loved one. However, the death and dying event can create both a healthy and unhealthy psychological, emotional, cognitive, and behavioral response. For instance, an unhealthy response in the anticipatory grieving process may be seen as a family member who withdraws, isolates, and detaches from their dying loved one. This unhealthy response pauses healthy grieving because of the overwhelming psychological response where the family member suppresses or represses their grief experience. In effect, being in the presence of the dying family member, particularly if it is outside their loved one's home environment, can create a range of emotions such as denial of the illness, anger related to perhaps past relational conflicts and/or traumas, feelings of abandonment, and guilt for not developing greater communication and intimacy throughout the dying family member's life.

Conversely, in the healthy anticipatory grieving process, the family member, spouse, or partner exhibits strong verbal and nonverbal communication with the dying family member. There is unconditional love, compassion, and open communication characterized by memorializing both negative and positive past events that is essential for bringing meaning, closure, and healing. There is an understanding and reality of what the next few days, weeks, or months may bring for the dying family member. The emotional integration of these thoughts, feelings, and experiences brings about a coping and resiliency response that deals primarily with issues in the here-and-now. Overall, the recognition and acknowledgement of the impending loss bring about a healthy resolution with a unique healing that brings comfort to the surviving family member.

In a systematic review of the literature on interventions to prevent or delay placement of adults into long-term care facilities, Duan-Porter et al. (2020) found that successful case management interventions (e.g., high-frequency contacts, early intervention) may offer the greatest benefits to individuals with CIDs. Successful case managers who deal with persons with CIDs first and foremost intervene early on prior to the individual's medical, physical, or mental health crisis. Other interventions besides case management that have shown mixed and inconsistent results (Duan-Porter et al., 2020) in terms of success with preventing or delaying placement into a long-term care facility include caregiver support, respite care and adult day-care programs, and preventative home visits.

Overall, successful case managers can assess, screen, evaluate, and triage individuals with the most critical needs. They have access to multiple community and healthcare resources to provide optimal benefits to individuals inside or outside of their home. Successful case mangers work competently with persons transitioning to multiple levels of care outside their home. Competent counseling professionals who address persons with CIDs working therapeutically in the here-and-now, involving the person themselves in the decision-making process, and inviting family participation can assist during this transition period to different levels of care outside the individual's home environment.

END-OF-LIFE DECISIONS

Perhaps one of the most overlooked areas in the grief, dying, and death literature is bereavement and anticipatory grief as they related to assisted suicide and end-of-life decisions that challenge family members. Researchers have demonstrated the significant clinical features (e.g., clinical depression, panic and anxiety, financial stress) of family members struggling with their loved one's suffering mentally, physically, and spiritually as a result of a life-threatening disability and/or anticipated death (Kevorkian, 2016; Koblenz, 2016; Lee & Carr, 2011; Michler Detmer & Lamberti, 1991; Valentine et al., 2016; Werth, 2002). Chronic and persistent mental health conditions that continue without psychosocial support and treatment place the dying individual at risk for suicide attempts or completion. Thus, these psychosocial issues should be of paramount concern for counseling professionals. Some research supports the notion that counseling clients in decisions of assisted suicide may lead to positive outcomes for the survivor (Worden, 2009). If the person's family is not involved in issues of assisted death, then they may have grief reactions more similar to a family survivor of someone who died alone by self-inflicted suicide (Werth, 1999).

Several issues deserve attention before counselors move forward with discussing end-of-life decisions with clients. This is because (a) oftentimes, issues related to suicide ideation and assisted suicide arise naturally within a therapeutic context; (b) counselors may have strongly held religious/spiritual beliefs and values related to end-of-life decision-making issues that may manifest as countertransference, which ultimately may harm the therapeutic relationship; and (c) there are well-defined state laws, counseling ethics, and healthcare policies that dictate and guide one's decision-making to discontinue life or prolong treatment decisions, which can become overwhelming for clients, counselors, and family members (Kevorkian, 2016; Lee & Carr, 2011; Werth, 2002).

Counselors who provide services to the terminally ill have an ethical obligation to understand the applicable laws and healthcare policies that govern the termination of treatment and end-of-life decisions. First and foremost, the American Counseling Association's (ACA) *2014 Code of Ethics*, Section B.2.b.-Confidentiality of End-of-Life Decisions states that counselors must maintain client confidentiality of any discussion related to termination of treatment, physician-assisted suicide, and issues related to end-of-life care (ACA, 2016). The 2014 ACA *Code of Ethics* and the newer proposed guidelines indicate that, depending on the circumstance, counselors must consult with supervisors, colleagues, and/or others regarding the client's disclosure of end-of-life decisions and termination of medical treatment issues. Additional ethical considerations apply to end-of-life decisions and discontinuation of medical treatment because these issues do not constitute a direct threat or act of suicide. At the time of this writing, "physician-assisted suicide," now more commonly referred to as "physician-assisted death," is recognized by law and court ruling in 10 states (California, Colorado, Hawaii, Maine, Montana, New Jersey, New Mexico, Oregon, Vermont, and Washington) and the District of Columbia. The case law and ethical concerns related to these issues are quite extensive and go beyond the scope of this chapter related to psychosocial concerns of grief, dying, and death.

Overall, counselors can be of value to clients and family members when discussing issues related to end-of-life decision-making. They can assist clients in exploring the risks and benefits of medical treatments, make future plans regarding their family's emotional and financial well-being, and assist clients in getting emotional and psychological closure to other critical end-of-life decisions (Corey et al., 2019). Foundational counseling skills, such as the facilitation of compassion, empathy, and family support, honor the person's decision to discontinue medical treatment or prolong life. Indeed, clients with life-threatening disabilities experience a roller coaster of emotions in dealing with the multiple losses associated with the debilitating conditions of chronic and persistent medical, physical, emotional, and spiritual pain. Some of the anticipated emotions that clients may experience related to end-of-life decisions are guilt, anger, confusion, anxiety, fear, panic, isolation, detachment, and the search for meaning (Kevorkian, 2016; Rando, 1984; Worden, 2009). Resources that are commonly used in end-stage diseases and terminal illness include but are not limited to caregiver support, palliative care and hospice services, mindfulness meditation, financial counseling, one-on-one religious/spiritual services, and many types of complementary and alternative therapies (Lee & Carr, 2011; Murastori & Haynes, 2020).

CONCLUSION

The psychosocial aspects of grief, dying, and death are overlooked in the fields of counseling and psychology. These issues are multidimensional by nature and require therapeutic attention so that the process of grieving and dying can be humanizing for the client and his or her family members. More recently, it has been recognized that the grief and loss experienced by extraordinarily stressful and traumatic nondeath events such as person-made and natural disasters have similar clinical characteristics and patterns of mourning losses. Recognition of the new *DSM-5-TR* diagnostic category of PGD provides legitimacy for the individual's sense of loss and mourning based on multiple events related to death and dying. It is essential that counselors address such psychosocial concerns with clients because of the added therapeutic value and ethical obligation to guide the individual and his or her family in important decisions regarding death and dying.

CLASS ACTIVITIES

1. Ask students if any of them have experienced loss such as that described in this chapter and if they would be willing to share some of their own and their families' experience. Have them identify what were the strengths that the family used to pull them through this very difficult time in their lives.

2. Discuss how different cultures or ethnic groups may deal with the impending death of a family member.

3. In contemplating the impending death of a loved one, discuss the financial and legal issues that behoove surviving family members to consider, including their loved one's will, power of attorney, executor, type of burial and funeral arrangements desired by the dying loved one, and the financial costs to be prepared for.

KEY REFERENCES

Only key references appear in the print edition. The full references appear in the digital product on Springer Publishing Connect™: https://connect.springerpub.com/content/book/978-0-8261-5111-7/part/partIII/chapter/ch15

Boelen, P. A., Eisma, M. C., Smid, G. E., & Lenferink, L. I. M. (2020). Prolonged grief disorder in section II of the DSM-5: A commentary. *European Journal of Psychotraumatology, 11*(1), 1–4. https://doi.org/10.1080/20008198.2020.1771008

Duan-Porter, W., Ullman, K., Rosebush, C., McKenzie, L., Ensrud, K. E., Ratner, E., Greer, N., Shippee, T., Gaugler, J. E., & Witt, T. J. (2020). Interventions to prevent or delay long-term nursing home placement for adults with impairments: A systematic review of reviews. *Journal of General Internal Medicine, 35*(7), 2118–2129. https://doi.org/10.1007/s11606-019-05568-5

Igarashi, N., Aoyama, M., Ito, M., Nakajima, S., Sakaguchi, Y., Morita, T., Shima, Y., & Miyashita, M. (2021). Comparison of two measures for complicated grief: Brief Grief Questionnaire (BG) and Inventory of Complicated Grief (ICG). *Japanese Journal of Clinical Oncology 51*(2), 252–257. https://doi.org/10.1093/jjco/hyaa185

Kevorkian, K. A. (2016). Counseling the terminally ill and their families. In I. Marini & M. A. Stebnicki (Eds.), *The professional counselor's desk reference* (2nd ed., pp. 469–473). Springer Publishing Company.

Lopez, R. P. (2009). Doing what's best: Decisions by families of acutely ill nursing home residents. *Western Journal of Nursing Research, 31*(5), 613–626. https://doi.org/10.1177/0193945909332911 PMID:19321882

Marini, I. (2012). Implications of social support and caregiver for loved ones with the disability. In I. Marini, N. M. Glover-Graf, & M. J. Millington (Eds.), *Psychosocial aspects of disability: Insider perspectives and strategies for counselors* (pp. 287–310). Springer Publishing Company.

Nielsen, M. K., Neergaard, M. A., Jensen, A. B., Vedsted, P., Bro, F., & Guldin, M-B. (2017). Predictors of complicated grief and depression in bereaved caregivers: A national prospect of cohort study. *Journal of Pain and Symptom Management, 53*(3), 540–550. http://dx.doi.org/10.1016/j.jpainsymman.2016.09.013

Normand, C. L., Silverman, P. R., & Nickman, S. L. (1996). Bereaved children's changing relationships with the deceased. In P. R. Silverman & S. L. Nickman (Eds.), *Continuing bonds: New understandings of grief* (pp. 87–111). Taylor & Francis.

Stebnicki, M. A. (2021b). *Counseling practice during phases of a pandemic virus.* American Counseling Association.

Wagner, K. (2020). Storying grief: A familial performance of death and dying. *Liminalities: A Journal of Performance Studies, 16*(3), 1–14. http://liminalities.net/16-3/grief.pdf

Worden, J. W. (2009). *Grief counseling and grief therapy: A handbook for the mental health practitioner* (4th ed.). Springer Publishing Company.

CHAPTER 16

PSYCHOSOCIAL ISSUES FOR FAMILY CAREGIVERS

GLORIA K. LEE, EUN-JEONG LEE, KRISTIN M. RISPOLI, AND TRISHA L. EASLEY

LEARNING OBJECTIVES

After reading this chapter, you will be able to:

- Understand the impact on caregivers when family provides care for their loved ones with a chronic illness and disability
- Recognize the role of resilience when a family takes care of a family member with a chronic illness and disability
- Identify different types of strategies and services available for family caregivers of individuals with a chronic illness and disability across the life span
- Understand the role of caregivers as collaborators with providers in the service of caregiving

PRE-READING QUESTIONS

1. How do family members care for each other when someone needs assistance?
2. How might approaches to care differ based on cultural values?
3. What are the differences between short-term care and longer-term care needs?
4. How might the situation be different for an adult caring for a parent versus a partner?

WHO ARE CAREGIVERS?

The Family Caregiver Alliance defines a *family caregiver* or *informal caregiver* as an unpaid individual (e.g., spouse, partner, family member, friend, or neighbor) involved in assisting individuals with a chronic illness and disability (CID). The National Alliance for Caregiving (NAC) and the American Association of Retired Persons (AARP) conduct research roughly every 5 years on caregiving in the United States. The most recent report, *2020 Caregiving in the U.S.*, surveyed 1,392 caregivers ages 18 and older and found that the number of people in the United States providing unpaid care to a family member or friend 18 years or older has increased by over 8 million—an increase from 39.8 million in 2015 to 47.9 million in 2020. Today approximately 53 million Americans (i.e., one in five adults) are caregivers, having provided care to an adult or child with a CID at some time in the past 12 months (NAC & AARP, 2020). The demographic characteristics of caregivers represent all generations, racial/ethnic groups, income and educational levels, family types, gender identities and sexual orientations. The *Caregiving in the U.S.* report (2020) indicated the demographic distributions are as follows: 61% are women, 61% are non-Hispanic White, 17% are Latinx, 14% non-Hispanic African American or Black, 5% Asian American and Pacific Islander, and 3% other race/ethnicity. Eleven percent are students enrolled in college or other classes, 9% have served active duty in the U.S. Armed Forces, and 8% self-identity as lesbian, gay, bisexual, and/or transgender (LGBTQ; NAC & AARP, 2020). Caregiving spans all generations. On average, caregivers of adults are 49.4 years old; however, male caregivers are more often younger (42% are of 19 to 49 years of age). Older caregivers tend to take care of someone of similar age, while younger caregivers often provide care to someone older. Compared to the 2015 survey, there is an increase in young people providing care, including 6% are Gen Z and 23% are Millennials. As much as one-quarter of caregivers were considered "sandwich" caregivers, defined as persons who care for a parent and have a child under 18 years of age (Alzheimer's Association, 2016). Adult siblings who assume a caregiving role when aging parents no longer are able to take care of an adult child with a disability become a "compound caregiver" (Smith et al., 2007).

The average duration of caregiving is 4.5 years, although 29% of caregivers provided care for 5 years or longer. The three most common problems or illnesses reported by caregivers as reasons for care were old age (16%), mobility issues (12%), and Alzheimer disease or dementia (11%; NAC & AARP, 2020). Caregivers provide an average of 24 hours of care per week. Typical caregiving tasks include the following breakdown: transportation (80%), grocery or other shopping (78%), housework (76%), preparing meals (64%), managing finances (58%), medication management (50%), and arranging outside services (35%). Six in ten caregivers help with daily living activities such as getting in and out of bed and chairs, dressing, toilet assistance, bathing, feeding, and incontinence. Caregivers' responsibilities often extend beyond the traditional direct care of these daily living activities and instrumental activities to communicating and interacting with various healthcare professionals on their behalf, monitoring the severity of their condition so that care can be adjusted accordingly, and advocating for them with healthcare providers, community services, and government agencies (NAC & AARP, 2020)

Diversity of Caregiving Across the Life Span

The International Alliance of Carer Organizations (IACO, 2021) acknowledged and valued the fundamental role of the caregiver. Though caring responsibilities are in the fabric of existing family roles, caregivers are often unpaid family members or friends who assume caregiving responsibilities following a diagnosis or long-term illness or are thrust into the caregiver role immediately following a traumatic event such as a catastrophic illness.

Conceptualizing the impact of disability and the role of caregiver within the family dynamic necessitates an understanding of the diversity of family caregivers and their unique needs. Family members who may be called to carry out care tasks can include a diverse group, including but not limited to diverse roles in the family, age, socioeconomic status, gender, sexuality, race/ethnicity, religions, and other cultures.

The predominant providers of informal care are women, and in most cases, spouses or adult daughters (NAC & AARP, 2020), with spouses acting as the primary caregiver and daughters entering the role when the spouse is deceased or unable to function as caregiver (Dwyer, 1992). Spouses often are with their family members throughout a CID trajectory. They act as important sources of emotional support, while providing the necessary caregiving tasks needed to assist the family member in need. A spouse may unexpectedly become a caregiver after an intensive care unit discharge (Agard et al.,

2015), through a progressive dementing illness (Alzheimer's Association, 2016), and during the last years of life (Ornstein et al., 2019). A spouse's transition into caregiving and the effects of multiple years in a caregiving role can have individual, couple, and family effects. Maintaining relationship quality (e.g., intimacy, role changes), family functioning (e.g., childcare, finances, career), and psychological and physical health while navigating disability (Capistrant et al., 2014; Gordon & Perrone, 2004; Perrone et al., 2006; Seltzer & Li, 2000) underscores the multiplicity of challenges to be considered with spousal caregiving.

Gender differences show to be a predictor of caregiver strain in spousal caregivers (Lee et al., 2015; Lee et al., 2021). A meta-analysis showed that women reported having higher levels of burden and depression and lower levels of subjective well-being and physical health (Pinquart & Sorensen, 2006). Lee et al. (2013) assessed the gender difference of spousal caregivers of individuals with multiple sclerosis and reported that female caregivers were more likely to use criticism and coercion (i.e., controlling pattern) as a way of coping, highlighting the importance of noting gender differences when developing coping strategies to reduce caregiver strain.

As aging individuals with a CID outlive their parents, siblings are often handed the baton to assume caregiving responsibilities for their brothers and sisters (Bittles et al., 2002; Hodapp et al., 2017). Most families expect that adult siblings will become future primary caregivers for their family member with a disability (Smith et al., 2007). There is also the potential for caring for multiple family members, a situation referred to as being a "compound caregiver." Compound caregivers simultaneously care for a sibling, parent(s), and/or biological children—a responsibility that requires time, energy, resources, and support that can be difficult and overwhelming, cause family conflicts, and impact family relationships (Lee et al., 2021; Lee et al., 2022; Perkins & Haley 2010). This relational dynamic necessitates an understanding of the unique needs of family caregivers, including navigating service systems, identifying economic resources, and conceptualizing the impact of disability within the family dynamic (Timmons et al., 2004).

The caregiving role naturally evolves across the developmental life span, which can require a shift or adaptation of caregiving responsibilities. As the life span of individuals with CID increases (Thomas & Barnes, 2010), caregivers typically attempt to meet higher caregiving needs and to provide longer hours of caregiving (Williamson & Perkins, 2014). Caregivers who fall into providing intensive caregiving needs and duration are more vulnerable to experiencing emotional stress, physical strain, financial strain, and negative health impact. Furthermore, they have the greatest needs to reach out to professionals for their own self-care, resources for stress management, and information to provide care to their loved one and respite service (NAC, 2015).

Counselors and other related professionals should pay attention to family support practices that not only work on establishing a therapeutic alliance in the family community but also attends to each family member's individual role, needs, and desired outcomes. There is a mutually beneficial relationship between family-focused services and positive outcomes at both the family and individual level (e.g., Gore et al., 2019; Marshall & Ferris, 2012). Unique circumstances translate to unique needs of the caregivers and the family members with a CID. The collaborative process of building the family into the rehabilitation process requires a strong working alliance with the family community and each individual family member (Millington & Marini, 2015).

UNIQUE CHALLENGES OF CAREGIVERS

Caring for a family member with a CID frequently brings a range of challenges that impact psychosocial adjustment and may lead to negative outcomes among caregivers. Multiple risk factors for poor family adjustment to CID have been identified, including specific demographic characteristics, disease-related factors, psychosocial factors, and environmental factors. Because family caregivers can take many forms of relationship, such as parents, spouses, siblings, and/or other relatives, the adjustment process may present differently with unique challenges depending on the relationship the individual has to the person with CID. The following is a description of unique challenges according to caregiving responsibilities for people in different developmental stages.

Caregiving of Young Children With a CID

For young children with CID and their families, disability status is likely to be an integral part of life for the child and/or the family. However, there may be a period of uncertainty regarding the diagnosis or prognosis. Take autism spectrum disorder (ASD) as an example. The diagnosis may be a lengthy process with the need to rule out other conditions due to the wide spectrum of symptoms, complexity and overlapping with other diagnoses, and the ever-changing conceptualization of the condition (Rutter, 2011). The diagnosis itself may cause relief for some parents as the potential course of treatment may become clear. However, other parents may also be dissatisfied, particularly if they felt dismissed by professionals and discouraged from involvement in the diagnostic process (Lee et al., 2021; Shyu et al., 2010). Caregivers need to learn about the new diagnosis and the management of the CID on top of the disruptions of school, daily, and family lives. Furthermore, many factors associated with the child's symptoms contribute to parenting stress, such as a child's functional levels (Brown et al., 2011; Hall & Graff, 2011; Ingersoll & Hambrick, 2011) and severity of their behaviors (Lecavalier et al., 2006). At an early stage of CID, parents may question their parenting ability because of the steep learning curve and adjustment of family life. This adds to parenting stress, leading to subsequent negative outcomes for the family (Karst & Van Hecke, 2012). In addition, it is not uncommon to have a primary caregiver often take the main responsibilities in providing care for the child with a CID. As a result of this demand, it is more difficult to meet the needs of other family members such as spouse and siblings, thus affecting the family functioning and dynamics as a system (Gordon & Perrone, 2004; Jellett et al., 2015; Karst & Van Hecke, 2012).

Caregiving of Emerging Young Adults and Adults With a CID

As school-age students transition to adulthood, the fragmented services, lack of support in the community related to work, independent living, community integration, romantic relationships, and future caregiving causes youth and their families to experience the "falling off the services cliff" phenomenon (Roux et al., 2015). There is often a disconnect between the service needs of young adults and the services provided by adult agencies. For the services that do exist, families struggle to understand the diverse eligibility requirements in the adult service system—a process that can be quite problematic for autistic youth compared to other disability groups, for example, given the heterogeneity of their support needs (Havlicek et al., 2015). When a family member with a CID becomes an adult, caregiving responsibilities often shift from parents to other family members, often siblings, as parents become older and may not be in the capacity to provide care (Smith et al., 2007). It is during this transition that guardianship issues and how taking on caregiving responsibilities may affect siblings' life can be a challenge, particularly in the context of the siblings' other responsibilities or desires for their own adult life. During this stage, it is also common that spouses take on the role of a caregiver of adult-onset CID such as in cases where a person experiences unexpected injury or onset of a chronic condition such as multiple sclerosis. Unique challenges faced by this type of caregiving situation include role ambiguity. Role ambiguity happens when expected roles are not incomplete and the existing role responsibilities become even more demanding because an individual with CID no longer keeps up with tasks (Usita et al., 2004).

Caregiving of Aging Adults With a CID

On the other spectrum of the life span, caregivers of individuals with CID such as dementia are often called the "unexpected carer of caregiver" because they often face multifaceted, complex caregiving demands. Spousal caregivers of patients with terminal or palliative cancer or dementia, due to the nature of CID, face the progression of the illness that is associated with a sense of grief and loss (Treml et al., 2021). When seeing a loved one at advanced stages of dementia, caregivers are also experiencing the loss of their loved one the way they have known them (Abby et al., 2005). For young caregivers, negative consequences occur as they must balance their caregiving role with child rearing, their own careers, and relationships (Connidis, 2010). The term *sandwich caregivers* describes the responsibilities of people who are caring for an older relative as well as raising their own children because they have responsibilities to both.

CAREGIVING CHALLENGES AND ITS NEGATIVE IMPACTS ON CAREGIVERS

Despite the growing understanding and appreciation of the impact of a CID on family members, the needs of family caregivers continue to be underrecognized. Research on how cultural factors interplay with family adjustment to CID is particularly necessary, in addition to more feasible and comprehensive assessment methods for assessing family adaptation in clinical rehabilitation settings. While family adjustment has been shown to impact individuals with CID, caregivers continue to be "hidden patients" as the person with a CID continues to be the focus of most interventions (Palmer, 2017). Given the complexity of caregiving and the family system, family caregivers continue to undergo tremendous stress. The barriers that these family caregivers experience are further compounded by limited access to resources and systemic societal issues (e.g., marginalization, systemic racism). These barriers include poverty, unemployment/underemployment, lack of education, limited access to healthcare services, health insurance, and public stigma. These not only affect family caregivers' physical and mental health but also have significant impact on individuals with CID and their intervention outcomes (Buchanan et al., 2010; Finlayson & Cho, 2008). The following sections will address specifically the negative outcomes associated with caregiving. In the *Strategies and Best Practices* section, intervention outcomes will be addressed.

Health and Psychological Impact

Caregiving comes with health risks. An early meta-analysis on caregivers of a family member with dementia identified 23 studies comparing the physical health among caregivers with non-caregivers across 11 health categories and showed that caregivers showed a slightly greater risk for health problems than did non-caregivers (Vitaliano et al., 2003). Caregivers showed higher stress hormones, antibodies, and global reported health as indicators of poor health. In addition to chronic stress induced stress hormonal changes through primarily cortisol (Steptoe et al., 2000), caregivers also are likely to be engaging in risky behaviors such as diet change, substance use, smoking, sedentary lifestyle, and general poor self-care, which then leads to a decreased immune system and increased cardiovascular and metabolic dysregulation (Family Caregiver Alliance, 2006; Kannel & Vokonas, 1986). A meta-analysis showed that mothers of young children with developmental disabilities experienced poorer health than mothers of typically developing children (Masefield et al., 2020). Another meta-analysis also showed that older caregivers tend to have more negative effects on their physical health when they are faced with dementia-related stressors (Pinquart & Sorensen, 2007). In a population-based study, non-White caregivers often provide more care services than their White counterparts and show worse problems in physical health (McCann et al., 2000).

With respect to mental health and wellness, depression and other distressed emotional responses are commonly reported among caregivers. For example, elevated levels of depressive symptoms have been identified in samples of mothers of children with developmental disabilities and caregivers of people with neurological disorders, traumatic brain injuries, and cancer (Ikiugu et al., 2021; Miyashita et al., 2008; Pan & Lin, 2022; Treml et al., 2021). Specific to those caring for people with cancer, Pan and Lin (2022) reported in their meta-analytic study of over 25 countries that the prevalence rate of depression was 25% among caregivers, with prevalence being higher in those in the eastern countries than in the western countries, possibly due to the filial piety and obligatory care that is influenced by the Eastern culture (Lim et al., 2014). Further, a higher prevalence rate of depression was found in caregivers who provided care for patients with terminal or palliative cancer due to the sense of grief and loss (Treml et al., 2021).

More alarming, mental health problems among family caregivers are associated with an elevated risk for suicidal thoughts (as high as 55%) due to the many overwhelming psychological strains and negative changes in interpersonal relationships associated with caregiving (Piscopo et al., 2016; Vasileou et al., 2017). Several studies on caregivers of emerging young adults with neurodevelopmental disabilities show they tend to exhibit poor adjustment outcomes, including anxiety, depression, marital adjustment, quality of life, life satisfaction, mental health, and family dynamics (DaWalt et al., 2018; Jellette et al., 2015; Khanna et al., 2011; Lee et al., 2019; Lee & Shivers, 2019). Ikiugu et al. (2021) conducted a meta-analysis study on the mental health and well-being of caregivers of individuals with traumatic brain injuries and reported general negative outcomes in depression, anxiety, satisfaction, burden, self-esteem, disruption of daily schedule, social isolation and bodily pain resulting from psychosocial strain, and care recipient activities of daily living.

Psychosocial Impacts of Caregiving

Caregivers often face issues with family dynamics and isolation from other family supports (Roberts & Struckmeyer, 2018). A systematic review of the impact of dementia on informal caregivers (Lindeza et al., 2020) concluded that caregivers experienced social and emotional consequences mainly due to inappropriate medical/formal care support, cost of the illness, and the natural progress of dementia that contributed to the negative appraisal of the caregivers. Younger caregivers may experience disruptions to their personal life, including putting on hold or changing course entirely on their careers and education, marriage, saving for their own family, and caregiving for their own family (Hughes et al., 2017; NAC, 2009; National Academies of Sciences, Engineering, Medicines, 2016; National Opinion Research Center, 2014; Roberts & Struckmeyer, 2018). Caregiving can also result in considerable financial strain (Capistrant, 2016).

While there are many associated challenges and negative impacts on caregiving, many family members still report positive experiences associated with caring for a family member with CID despite encountering challenges. Certain personality traits, personal characteristics, psychological factors, and social factors can buffer adversities, thus propelling caregivers into healthy outcomes. Though this chapter does not cover theories of adjustment, readers can refer to other literature for an overview of family adaptation models (Lee et al., in press; Rosenthal et al., 2009).

BENEFITS OF CAREGIVING

Researchers have been interested in exploring positive outcomes of caregiving (e.g., Li & Loke, 2013). Positive factors identified include greater insights into illness/hardship, personal growth, strengthened relationships, increased appreciation of life, health gains, and changes in priorities/personal goals (Pakenham, 2005). In addition, perceiving rewards to family caregiving, such as feeling useful, needed, and important due to taking on the caregiving role, has been related to decreased feelings of burden among caregivers of individuals with spinal cord injury (SCI; Rodakowski et al., 2012). Though this is a relatively newer area of research, initial findings suggest there may be positive benefits to caregiving which may be leveraged to promote positive adjustment to CID and may help to develop the caregiver interventions. For instance, Lindeza et al. (2020) concluded that positive aspects of caregiving include personal accomplishment and stronger relationships, often connected with good medical counseling and formal care support, as well as support from family and friends. Other specific protective factors that may support caregiver adjustment to CID have also been identified. Social support may play a protective role in not only supporting caregivers' emotional needs and addressing risk for increased isolation related to taking on the caregiving role but also through providing instrumental, tangible support to assist with caregiving (Hawken et al., 2018). This is one example of how culture may be viewed as playing a protective role, as some cultures may place a higher value on social support and interconnectedness, and therefore these resources may be more readily available. Other aspects of culture, such as how health and disability are viewed, perspectives on death and dying, and spirituality, can also play protective roles, though more investigation is needed to fully understand these factors. Use of problem-solving strategies and problem-focused coping to address challenges associated with caring for a family member with CID has also consistently been related to positive family outcomes, such as improved general caregiver health and quality of life (Grant et al., 2006; Lynch & Cahalan, 2017). Use of these types of strategies has been associated with decreased psychological distress and increased positive outcomes across caregiver groups, particularly when compared to use of emotion-focused coping strategies (Hawken et al., 2018). Caregiver personal characteristics, such as resilience, self-compassion, and posttraumatic growth, have also been found to play a protective role against caregiving stress. Finally, the concept of acceptance, as well as benefits-finding or sense-making, has also been documented as a way to adjust to adversities and is considered a resilient trait (Pakenham, 2005; Roberts & Struckmeyer, 2018).

Resilience

Resilience is defined as a construct that includes individuals' ability to adapt in the face of hardship and life stress (Connor & Davidson, 2003). Resilience is defined as the ability to effectively deal with stressful events and rebound from crisis (Luthar et al., 2000), and it is an important personality trait for promoting positive adaptation. In addition to strong relationships between resilience and positive outcomes such as quality of life and positive affect, resilience has also been shown to play a protective role against stress, anxiety, and depression among caregiver populations (Anderson et al., 2020; Hawken et al., 2018). Park et al. (2018) found that caregivers who are more resilient may be better able to overcome the emotional and physical challenges associated with parenting a child with a CID and thus are more adept at managing stress.

Self-Compassion

Self-compassion represents a form of emotion-based coping, one that specifically involves how an individual relates to himself or herself when facing difficult experiences (Neff, 2003). Self-compassion has previously been shown to predict psychosocial outcomes for parents of children with ASD over and above predictions based on children's symptom severity alone (Neff & Faso, 2014). Furthermore, self-compassion has been associated with caregiver well-being (Bazzano et al., 2013). Self-compassion may also serve as a buffer against other challenges caregivers face, such as courtesy stigma in autism (Liao et al., 2019)—a concept by Goffman (1963), or stigma by association. Self-compassion is associated with greater well-being and lower distress among parents of young children with ASD even after accounting for stigma, social support, and a child's symptom severity (Neff & Faso, 2014). Another study found out that self-compassion mediated the relationship between stigma and depressive symptoms among parental caregivers of transition- age youth with intellectual and developmental disabilities (Ivins-Lukse & Lee, 2021). As self-compassion is accessible to anyone and also amenable to change, it is worth developing interventions to improve self-compassion for caregivers to reduce the mental health consequences associated with caregiving.

Posttraumatic Growth

Posttraumatic growth (PTG) is defined as positive psychological changes experienced after successfully dealing with the consequences of trauma (Tedeschi & Calhoun, 2004). In addition, PTG posits that following a traumatic event or personal crisis individuals may not only return to their baseline but also grow personally in new positive ways due to finding new meaning in their experience. Tedeschi and Calhoun (2004) also identified five domains related to PTG, including (a) new possibilities, (b) appreciation of life, (c) personal strength, (d) relating to others, and (e) spiritual/religious change. Previous studies have shown that PTG has been related to other protective factors such as social support and hope among family caregivers (Nouzari et al., 2019). In addition, Bayat (2007) found that spiritual and personal growth was found because of caring among caregivers of children with ASD.

STRATEGIES AND BEST PRACTICES IN SUPPORTING CAREGIVING FAMILIES

Interventions for families who provide care and support for a family member with CID is unique because services and support must equip the caregivers to provide the necessary care for the family member with a CID. However, equally important are the support for the caregiving families themselves due to the caregiving tasks and the impact associated with it. The literature has supported the transactional aspects of caregiving in different disability groups such as ASD (e.g., Karst & Van Hecke, 2012) and dementia (e.g., Hughes et al., 2017). Thus, when a family provides care and support for a family member with a CID, caregivers must be provided with the knowledge, skills, and resources so that they have the know-how and resources to do the job of caretaking. In addition, the caregiving role and process itself may contribute to unexpected consequences to the caregivers in terms of disruption, delay, or opportunity of their life course, which affects their overall adjustment. Therefore, services and support that address the needs for both the person with a CID and the caregiver must be tailored and attended.

Different types of intervention strategies serve different purposes. In this section, we will provide information about common strategies and interventions that support caregivers with a family member with a CID, as well as trends and effectiveness. These include (a) parent management training or any kind of training that involves the caregiver actively learning and/or delivering the skills, (b) family psychoeducation, (c) family school partnership, (d) respite support, and (e) peer support. While the first three types of caregiver services have established some merits of evidence-based support, respite support and peer support remain an emerging trend of caregiving services. The last section consists of a section on meta-analytic studies in synthesizing studies on interventions that may not have identified a content theme of strategic approach, but these studies are noteworthy to mention.

Parent Management Training

Parent management training (PMT) is more traditionally available for young children and adolescents because of the direct and relatively intensive parent teaching skills to the children. PMT is a family of treatment programs that aims at changing parenting behaviors and teaching parents positive reinforcement methods for improving behavior problems in children. Ample research supports its efficacy for young children and adolescents with and without disabilities, including those with attention deficit hyperactive disorder (e.g., Fabiano et al., 2012; P. Lee et al., 2012) and developmental disabilities (Tellegen & Sanders, 2013). A meta-analysis (Skotaczak & Lee, 2015) showed that PMT demonstrates a large effect size on positive parenting practices and parenting style and a medium effect size on maladaptive behaviors, ability to work as a team, and ability to manage children's behavioral issues. However, no effect was demonstrated on parenting stress, satisfaction, and efficacy. Examples of PMT programs that have strong empirical support include *the Triple P Positive Parenting Program* (Whittingham et al., 2009), *the Incredible Years* (McIntyre, 2008), *the Autism Spectrum Conditions-Enhancing Nurture and Development* (ASCEND; Pillay et al., 2011), *the Parent-Child Interaction Therapy* (http://www.pcit.org/what-is-pcit.html), and the Research Units in Behavioral Intervention (RUBI) Autism Network (https://www.rubinetwork.org/).

The concept of parent-directed intervention is often less common when working with individuals of older age. However, certain programs are highlighted here such as the Program for the Education and Enrichment of Relationship Skills (PEERS; Laugeson et al. 2009), a parent-delivered cognitive behavioral social skills program. Though more comprehensive in scope than most interventions, the Treatment and Education of Autistic and related Communications handicapped Children) program (TEACHH; Schopler & Reichler, 1981) is notable for its systemic approach and inclusion of parents in the treatment of children with ASD. TEACCH emphasizes individual differences and strengths, structure and visual learning, a focus on psychoeducation across systems, and a high level of collaboration with parents and families in that parents should be involved in both the assessment and implementation of a teaching program for children with ASD, with parents often included as co-therapists as part of the TEACCH curriculum. The TEACCH program had been shown to significantly improve mothers' teaching skills and the management of the children's problematic behaviors. In a systematic review, Yasmeen et al. (2020) identified the effect of caregiver-facilitated pain management intervention and concluded that caregiver outcomes such as pain knowledge were improved by inform–activate engagement strategies, that is, strategies that encompass the provision of education and the prompt of playing an active role in patient care. However, interventions did not improve provider (e.g., satisfaction) or health system (e.g., hospital length of stay) outcomes.

Family Psychoeducation

Family psychoeducation (FPE) is an intervention approach that involves individuals and families to support recovery. FPE has a long-standing evidence that stemmed from psychiatric rehabilitation (McFarlane et al., 2003). Evidence showed that FPE demonstrated positive client outcomes as well as caregiver outcomes, which include better caregivers' health, emotional well-being, family interaction, knowledge of mental illnesses, and service utilization, and can reduce their perceived stress and isolation (Fristad et al., 2003; Sanford et al., 2006). FPE educates families for resource building, skills training, and problem-solving and gives social and emotional support. The Schizophrenia Patient Outcomes Research (Kreyenbuhl et al., 2010) reports on best practices for individuals with schizophrenia. Among the 16 psychopharmacological and psychosocial interventions, FPE is recommended as one of the best practices, thus attesting to the importance of psychoeducation for families as an evidence-based intervention.

FPE has also been applied to family intervention for adolescents and transition-age youth with ASD. Examples include *Transitioning Together* (DaWalt et al., 2018), *the Volunteer Advocacy Program* (Taylor et al., 2017), and *the Specific Planning Encourages Creative Solutions* (Hagner et al., 2012). These interventions have undergone randomized controlled trial studies showing effective outcomes not only on parental variables, including parental depressive symptoms, caregiving burden, improved problem-solving, empowerment and advocacy skills, improved parent–child relationships, and transition knowledge, (DaWalt et al., 2018; Hagner et al., 2012; Taylor et al., 2017) but results also showed improvement in youth and family expectations, as well as student self-determination and career decision-making ability.

Family–School Partnerships

There is a wealth of research supporting active engagement of families in the process of designing and implementing supports for children and adolescents with disabilities. For instance, improved postschool outcomes are observed for youth with ASD when families are more engaged with the school during the transition process (Lee & Carter, 2012). A longitudinal study by Van Ingen and Moore (2010) showed that parents who maintained active involvement with the comprehensive services of their adult children tended to trust and work openly with professionals, accepted the reality of needing help, engaged in advocacy efforts, lived a balanced life, maintained supportive contact, and gave and received support from other parents. Results from this study highlighted the importance of collaborative efforts between families and service providers to better the lives of caregivers and their adult children with intellectual and developmental disabilities (IDDs). Alternatively, professionally driven planning and processes distance students and their families from active participation (Thoma et al., 2001).

Family–school partnership (FSP) models are defined as person-centered approaches through which families and schools engage in a cooperative, coordinated, and collaborative process to support positive outcomes in social, emotional, behavioral, and academic functioning of students in general (Christenson & Sheridan, 2001; Moorman Kim & Sheridan, 2015). Specific components that characterize FSP models are shared roles and responsibilities, active collaboration between families and school professionals, targeting both home and school settings through intervention strategies, and multidirectional communication between all parties (Garbacz et al., 2015). Largely studied in the child and school literature, concepts employed in FSP models are also useful for understanding possible avenues for similar partnerships between caregivers and the organizations serving individuals with disabilities across the life span.

Positive effects are evident for children/youth and their families following participation in FSP and similar models. Recent meta-analyses examining FSP programs for children with social and behavioral concerns found positive effects on social-behavioral competence, mental health, and academic achievement, particularly when strategies were also implemented in the home setting (Smith et al., 2020). Family engagement in education and FSP are crucial for autistic students to have positive work and education outcomes (Moorman Kim & Sheridan, 2015; Rispoli et al., 2019) and improved outcomes for children with disruptive disorders (Garbacz et al., 2015). Positive family support is associated with a greater likelihood of students participating in their own Individual Education Program (IEP) transition meetings (Roux et al., 2015), employment (Carter et al., 2012), and postsecondary education attainment (Chiang et al., 2012).

The emphasis on the transactional aspects of intervention, that is, these positive effects on family caregivers will also lead to improvement on the child or student with disabilities, cannot be underscored. Thus, although student outcomes pertaining to the FSP model will not be discussed at length here, we would like to briefly highlight some positive outcomes. Family engagement facilitates setting reasonable goals and expectations that foster autonomy for youth with disabilities (Simonsen & Neubert, 2013), youth active participation in their transition planning meeting (Griffin et al., 2014), and better outcomes in employment, residential independence, social participation (Kirby, 2016) and well-being, and overall transition to adulthood outcomes (e.g., Dieleman et al., 2018; Lee & Carter, 2012) for autistic youth and other types of disabilities (Smith & Anderson, 2014).

Respite Support

Although not unique to aging, *respite care* often can be associated with caring for aging individuals. The National Academies of Sciences, Engineering, and Medicine (2016) define respite interventions as the type of therapeutic services that encompass any care delivery models or programs that support family caregivers of older adults, which can include but are not limited to adult day center–based programs, group counseling, individual counseling, voucher programs for household chores, and short-term and long-term care.

According to the Alzheimer's Association (2016), about 5.4 million Americans have aging-related disabilities such as Alzheimer disease or dementia, and as much as 96% of them are cared for by a family member. Respite care can be provided by professionals, volunteers, businesses, and organizations and can be in-home care nonmedical services for the patients or for transportation or preparing meals. Respite care can also be center-based services where patients with a CID attend a secure and social environment or for specific support (e.g., medication administration, social or recreational activities). Caregiving that involves more complex decisions can be supported by a life care professional with specialty training in geriatrics and/or disability or by hospice service and advocates. All these resources are imperative in providing the necessary knowledge, support, and relief for caregivers and care recipients.

A recent meta-analysis investigating the effectiveness of the different types of services for caregivers of patients with dementia (Cheng & Zhang, 2020) showed that evidence existed supporting the use of psychoeducation for quality of life. Furthermore, psychoeducation, occupational therapy, and multicomponent interventions also increased the mastery of caregiving, and communication training was shown to be effective in improving communication skills. However, support groups and respite were shown to not be effective, and treatment in general showed weak results in terms of anxiety, burden, and social support. This study also showed that there were no differences in terms of delivery, that is, whether intervention was provided to both the patient and the caregiver or the caregiver only, whether service is delivered individually or in groups, or whether intervention was multicomponent or single component (Cheng & Zhang, 2020).

There is a wealth of literature supporting that home-based services that address disability education, problem-solving strategies, and skills training in managing behavioral symptoms, as well as communication, environmental modifications, respite care, and community resources, are effective in improving the quality of life of caregiving families of individuals with dementia. See the work of Gitlin and researchers (e.g., Gitlin & Hodgson, 2015; Gitlin et al., 2016; Zarit et al., 2017). However, researchers criticized that a lot of the programs may not have been evaluated at the level of scientific rigor to show its effectiveness, that is, the application of the service that is external to or outside the service contexts (Gitlin et al., 2017, Glasgow et al., 2012; Nichols et al., 2016). There is a movement from the National Alzheimer's Plan (U.S. Department of Health and Human Services, 2016) and the National Academy of Medicine's Families Caring for an Aging Society (Schulz & Eden, 2016) to call for the need to integrate and evaluate services and programs when delivered in the community settings and to understand the impact on families of diverse backgrounds. Such examples include the Memory Care Home Solutions (MCHS) program, a community-based dementia care program for caregivers that incorporates both a basic (dementia education, care strategies, and social support) and an enhanced option (additional hands-on practice on the care strategies; Gitlin et al., 2017). Results showed that caregivers in the enhanced program were performing better than those in the basic program in terms of age and being a spouse, reported greater perceived distress with behavioral symptoms of the patient with dementia, and reported the need to manage a higher number of activities of daily living tasks. At the 3-month follow-up, a reduction from 53.4% to 27.2% of caregivers reporting having more than one adverse health-related event of persons with dementia was reported. Families managing high functional dependence opted for more assistance.

Another example of an evidence-based practice of respite- care psychosocial intervention that has proven support for caregivers of aging individuals with dementia and Alzheimer disease is the Community Resources for Enhancing Alzheimer's Caregiver Health (REACH) II program (Czaja et al., 2018). This program is a collaboration with the United Home Care Services (UHCS) that provides support for caregivers with personal care, home health, companion, and respite services. It consists of six individual face-to-face and six individual phone sessions and phone supports. Czaja et al. studied the program's effectiveness among 146 Latinx caregivers in terms of perceived social support, burden, depression, and caregiving self-efficacy. Results showed a decrease in depression and burden at both the 6-month and 12-month follow-up, and there was an increase in perceived social support at the 12-month follow-up.

Peer Support

Peer support has not been perceived as formal care. However, emerging literature has brought attention to the value of its utilization (Carter et al., 2020; Greenwood et al., 2013; Jones et al., 2021). For instance, Carter et al.'s scoping review (2020) on peer support interventions on caregivers of individuals with dementia offers a general understanding of the unique contribution of how information sharing, non-healthcare provider support, skill development, personal coping skills, healthcare provider support, and self-management can contribute to improve the burden, anxiety, depression, health, and well-being for caregivers of people with dementia. Greenwood et al. (2013) conducted a qualitative study to summarize the essence of the benefits of having peer support from the perspectives of caregivers. Themes emerged, revealing benefits described as understanding that they were "not alone" in their experiences and emotions, opportunities to talk freely about difficult experiences, and learning how others cope. A preliminary study of a peer mentoring program was evaluated for caregivers of individuals with traumatic brain injuries. Participants in the peer mentor intervention group reported significantly greater improvement in caregiver stress at discharge and 30 days postdischarge than participants in the usual care group. Reported depressive symptoms were also lower for the intervention group, but change scores did not achieve statistical significance at discharge or 30-day follow-up (Jones et al., 2021).

In a large-scale study the effectiveness of the National Alliance of Mental Illness (NAMI) Basics (2022), a peer-led family support program for caregivers of children with mental health illness, was evaluated in a sample of caregivers of five NAMI affiliates with over 100 caregivers randomly assigned to the Basics and waitlist control groups. Compared with caregivers in the waitlist condition, NAMI Basics participants reported significant increase in parent engagement or intention to engage with mental health services and decrease in their child's intrapersonal and interpersonal distress, although no significant differences were found in parenting stress, attitudes toward mental health services, or stigma.

When a parent focuses on providing care for another child with disability, other family members' needs may not be attended to, or they may not understand the changes due to the added demands of caregiving. This is particularly true for other children in the family, and if not given the support, they are likely to be at risk of having poor development and functioning (e.g., Wolff et al., 2022). Support thus has begun to focus on this group. In a systematic review of 16 interventions aimed at siblings of youth with IDDs, Tudor and Lerner (2015) supported some benefit to sibling outcomes, including a sense of support and knowledge and other outcomes such as sibling relationships, self-esteem, behaviors, and mood symptoms, though substantial variability in the methodology and outcomes may contribute to the undocumented or mixed findings. A more recent mixed-methods systematic review evaluated quantitative and qualitative evidence on the mental health and well-being outcomes on 24 psychosocial interventions among siblings of individuals with neurodevelopmental disabilities. The largest immediate improvements include self-esteem, social well-being, and disability knowledge, while the most sustainable outcomes were emotional and behavioral adjustment, as well as disability knowledge. The authors concluded that though small, the effect was positive for siblings in the intervention groups as compared to waitlist control groups.

CULTURE AND FAMILY

Family is considered a small cultural unit because the family develops its own rules and norms and shares values over many years. Contemporary composition of the concept of family certainly has extended beyond a traditional father and mother role, such that other types of family compositions must be considered, such as adoption, same-sex couples, or blended families. Adding disability into the context adds another layer of "culture" and can be defined and perceived differently across the values shared within the family and the cultural norms in the community where the family lives and the sanctions of the cultural society (Glover-Graf, 2018). This chapter does not address culture and its combination with disability and/or family but would encourage readers to other resources for information (e.g., Glover-Graf, 2018; Millington & Marini, 2015). However, we would like to highlight a few examples of the complexity of this multiple intersectionality and provide selected examples of services that are available for different cultural caregivers of individuals with a CID. For example, if the community strongly believes psychiatric disabilities are a punishment from God, individuals with psychiatric disabilities and their families are more likely to face public stigma, and in turn, the family may decide to hide psychiatric disability, which will impact the acceptance for individuals with psychiatric disabilities. In addition, the rigidness of role changes in the family can be different based on cultural orientation. For example, Latinx cultures typically hold less rigid family roles (Sue & Sue, 2015). Therefore, if a father who used to be a main income source for the family is no longer employed due to a new disability, it is more culturally acceptable for the mother to step into the father's role and become a decision-maker for the family. Although these examples are limited within racial and ethnic groups, these illustrate cultural differences in family function, and it is important to note that there are more differences depending on the cultural/social contexts to understanding the adjustment process in rehabilitation.

Living as a minority family can bring many stressors such as discrimination, immigration/refugee status, economic situation, cultural identity/acculturation, and language proficiency (Gee et al., 2020; Thomson et al., 2015). These factors may create new challenges and needs for support for family caregivers in the rehabilitation process. For example, African American families often report mistrust toward service providers due to the issues related to misdiagnosis and overdiagnosis (Mandell et al., 2007). In addition, family involvement is less valued in the United States, while many Asian patients living in America may wish to involve their family members in treatment decision-making efforts (Corrigan & Lee, 2021). Research shows, for example, that filial piety impacts self-care concerns among Chinese people with aging issues (Dong et al., 2014). Research has shown that African American, Hispanic American, and Native American parents are active in the transition process as much as, or more than, European American parents (Geenen et al., 2001). Yet, educators continue to hold common misconceptions that culturally and linguistically diverse (CLD) parents do not want to be involved in the transition process. Kim et al. (2007) found Korean American parents of youth with disabilities used their social networks and religion-affiliated ethnic organizations to obtain information about services, including emotional and financial support, for their children.

Shared decision-making (SDM) is a highly valued concept that is encouraged for service providers to communicate with patients in the United States. Yet, this patient autonomy approach may not necessarily be as valued in Eastern or collectivist societies (Markus et al., 1996; Oishi & Diener, 2016). Cultural values for autonomy in other ethnic groups may be contrary to relatedness and group cohesion (Iyengar & Lepper, 1999).

Family-centered decision-making (FCDM) has been posed as an alternative to SDM among ethnic minority families. Many cultures and subgroups tend to practice stronger family values. For example, in traditional Asian American culture, one's identity is defined within the family constellation (Sue & Sue, 2015). One study showed a group of Korean American patients with cancer significantly preferred active family involvement in care-seeking compared to European Americans (Blackhall et al., 1995). In addition, a more recent study examined preferences of SDM versus FCDM when comparing services for people with psychiatric disabilities using the vignette study design (Gao et al., 2019). The study found Chinese participants preferred FCDM significantly more than European American participants (Gao et al., 2019).

These examples in the United States are a snapshot of the diverse experiences people may have based on racial/ethnic minority status. Considering these factors may increase awareness and generate discussion regarding how culture impacts families in rehabilitation, the challenging part for rehabilitation professionals is that culturally adaptive family-based interventions are extremely limited. Lack of multicultural training for rehabilitation professionals is another issue, and cultural competence may be associated with rehabilitation outcomes.

CLINICAL IMPLICATIONS

Given the prominent issues faced by caregivers, practitioners must play an important role in bringing attention to caregivers' needs in order to facilitate healthy outcomes.

In addition, to understand the complex challenges that caregivers face, whether the challenges are for the care recipient or for themselves, caregiver needs assessment must be at the forefront of another clinical implication. The Recognize, Assist, Include, Support and Engage (RAISE) Family Caregiver Act (2018) created an advisory council to develop the country's first Family Strategy. The council provided five goals with 26 recommendation strategies to help caregivers do better outreach and support family caregivers in engaging in evidence-based healthcare services. Furthermore, the Family Caregiver Alliance (2006) suggested that a comprehensive needs assessment is imperative in order to determine the appropriate kind of intervention or resources to be provided and should be standard practice and family-centered and culturally competent, resulting in a care plan with clear outcomes that must be reassessed on a regular basis. They provided guidelines that a comprehensive assessment should include information about employment status, family relationships, home environment, health of the care recipient, caregiver values, caregiver physical and mental health and quality of life, knowledge and skills related to caregiving, finances, and available social support and resources. Understanding unmet needs can then lead to a caregiving plan with appropriate resources and support, provision of caregiver education and support programs, respite care to reduce caregiver burden, financial support to alleviate economic stress, and primary care interventions that address directly the caregiver needs. Thus, the comprehensive treatment of physical and psychosocial intervention should be a public health priority in order to maintain the long-term healthcare system, and importantly so, given the rapidly growing aging population, but this practice, unfortunately, is not as common as it should be (Hughes et al., 2017).

Organizations serving individuals with disabilities across the life span (e.g., schools, community mental health centers, hospitals, primary and specialty care facilities) need to recognize the unique and complex needs of caregivers. Support in the form of resources, psychoeducation, training, and peer support groups should be made available across the diverse contexts through which individuals with disabilities receive care. Often, these kinds of interagency or intersystemic collaborations are imperative, especially when patient care transitions from one stage to another (e.g., medical stage) or when a student transitions from one life stage to another (e.g., grade schools, postsecondary; Lee & Carter, 2012).

RESEARCH IMPLICATIONS

Even though research in caregiving needs, supports, and services have improved, much effort still needs to be made to advance in this area to improve the knowledge, services, and outcomes. A better understanding of direct resources and caregiver programs in tandem with caregiver needs continues to be understudied. The heterogeneity of caregiver demographics has remained a major challenge. The benefits of different programs can vary depending on different demographics (e.g., gender, race/ethnicity, cultural differences, relationship to the care recipient, living situation, urban versus rural locale), but more research is needed to confirm findings and determine how to best use this information. There are also gaps in knowledge related to specific demographic groups of dementia caregivers, including men, minorities, rural, and long-distance caregivers (Gitlin & Hodgson, 2015). Another concern is that many studies have relied on convenience samples that have skewed to spousal caregivers being White, with a higher income and more education; these results may not be generalizable to other caregivers (Pruchno et al., 2008), especially those who are underserved and marginalized.

Research also points to the fact that improvements are needed in the reporting of intervention studies and in making the classification of interventions more transparent and consistent. We further recommend fewer and larger-scale reviews and more attention to positive outcomes in order to better inform the field. Developing interventions with broader impacts and packaging them to meet caregivers' changing needs in the course of CID and the family cycle should be a priority for researchers and practitioners.

Another important question is whether results from randomized controlled trials translate to success in "real-world" community settings. The Administration on Aging/Administration on Community Living has funded translation studies in recent years, but additional research is needed to test other interventions and strengthen conclusions (Gitlin & Hodgson, 2015; Hughes et al., 2017). Enrollment and attrition continue to be an issue even when effective programs are introduced to the community for no cost (e.g., Mavandadi et al., 2017). Thus, understanding reasons for low engagement and strategies to improve buy-ins would enhance the utilization of effective services to benefit families.

Implementation science calls for the needs to involve stakeholders and the incorporation of contextual factors when implementing services and programs for caregivers. Furthermore, innovative methods of evaluating program effectiveness must be considered and used. Zarit et al. (2017) identified that although randomized controlled trials are considered the gold standard in evaluating program efficacy, such efforts often lead to reduction of use or ineffective outcomes when applied to community settings, as shown in the autism literature (Boyd et al., 2021; Dingfelder & Mandell, 2011). This research–practice gap occurs in part because efficacy trials often do not consider the social contexts, perceived needs, values, and beliefs of key stakeholders. Thus, researchers need to involve stakeholders' values and understand the local context when conducting adaptation research (Aarons et al., 2011; Fixsen et al., 2005) and to use other designs in evaluating programming, such as quasi-experimental design, reserved quasi-experimental design, within-person design (Zarit et al., 2017).

One solution to increasing the likelihood of success when interventions are brought to scale and reducing attrition is to have caregiver involvement in research from the beginning. One common approach that facilitates systematic end-user involvement is participatory action research, which seeks to build collaboration between researchers and those who will use the research in all aspects of the research project (International Collaboration for Participatory Health Research, 2013). Innovative approaches using a participatory action research (PAR) paradigm are emerging in the literature, such as developing app-based technology to encourage participation in physical activities among children with disabilities (Shikako et al., 2019), developing stress reduction practices for caregivers of individuals with developmental disabilities (Bazzano et al., 2015), and welcoming parents as part of the grassroot effort in building a web-based resource for parents of young children who are newly diagnosed (Rabba et al., 2020) for future parents to use.

CONCLUSION

Professionals tasked with managing care and providing direct care to individuals with CID must have training in recognizing and responding to the needs of caregivers. For instance, preservice special education teachers should complete coursework addressing caregiving needs and methods for facilitating collaborative relationships with parents/caregivers of the students with whom they work. Likewise, counseling and mental health professionals should receive similar training prior to being licensed for independent practice and continuing education throughout their careers. The topic of caregiving is often overlooked in curricular standards, such as those set forth by large accreditation bodies including the American Psychological Association and the Council for Accreditation of Counseling and Related Educational Programs.

Professionals who are working with caregivers should recognize and validate the diversity in experience—both the positive and the negative—that is often central to the caregiving experience. They should seek to validate the feelings experienced by caregivers and support caregiver attainment/maintenance of physical and mental wellness. Key phenomena to be considered include resilience, self-compassion, and posttraumatic growth. There should be opportunities for caregivers to build their social support system, such as offering caregiver support groups at a long-term care facility specializing in the treatment of patients with dementia and similar cognitive challenges.

CLASS ACTIVITIES

Activity 1

Identify two caregivers who provide care for two individuals representing very different profiles of disabilities (e.g, young versus aging person with disability; adult-onset versus developmental disability). Interview them and find out about their experiences in terms of:

  a. Challenges their family member with a disability faces

  b. Challenging aspects of caregiving

  c. Positive caregiving experiences

Activity 2

Identify a setting (e.g., school, vocational rehabilitation facility, psychiatric center, Veterans Affairs) in your area and gather information by researching through the website or by interviewing a clinician working in the agency. Find out about the types of services and supports that are available for the family caregivers. Discuss among your group whether you think the service is adequate to address the needs of the caregivers.

Activity 3

Pick two types of intervention strategies that are discussed in the chapter. List the pros and cons of each strategy. Provide your rationale for the pros and cons as you have conceptualized them.

KEY REFERENCES

Only key references appear in the print edition. The full references appear in the digital product on Springer Publishing Connect™: https://connect.springerpub.com/content/book/978-0-8261-5111-7/part/partIII/chapter/ch16

Cheng, S.-T, & Zhang, F. (2020). A comprehensive meta-review of systemic review and meta-analyses on nonpharmacological interventions for informal dementia caregivers. *BMC Geriatrics, 20*, 137. https://doi.org/10.1186/s12877-020-01547-2.

Fixsen, D. L., Naoom, S. F., Blase, K. A., Friedman, R. M., & Wallace, F. (2005). *Implementation research: A synthesis of the literature.* University of South Florida, Louis de la Parte Florida Mental Health Institute, The National Implementation Research Network (FMHI Publication #231).

International Collaboration for Participatory Health Research. (2013). *Position paper 1: What Is participatory health research? Version: Mai 2013.* International Collaboration for Participatory Health Research. http://www.icphr.org/position-papers/position-paper-no-1

Karst, J. S., & Van Hecke, A. V. (2012). Parent and family impact of autism spectrum disorders: A review and proposed model for intervention evaluation. *Clinical Child and Family Psychology Review, 15*(3), 247–277. https://doi.org/10.1007/s10567-012-0119-6

Lee, E.-J., DeDios-Stern, S., Lee, G. K., & Wilson, C. (in press). Families in rehabilitation psychology. In M. Meade & S. Wagener (Eds.), *Oxford university handbook of rehabilitation psychology* (2nd ed.), Oxford University Press.

Li, Q., & Loke, A. Y. (2013). The positive aspects of caregiving for cancer patients: A critical review of the literature and directions for future research. *Psycho-Oncology, 22*, 2399–2407. https://doi.org/10.1002/pon.3311

Millington, M. J., & Marini, I. (2015). Family care and support. In M. J. Millington & I. Marini (Eds.), *Families in rehabilitation counseling: A community-based rehabilitation approach* (pp. 87–107). Springer Publishing Company.

Moorman Kim, E., & Sheridan, S. M. (2015). Foundational aspects of family–school connections: Definitions, conceptual frameworks, and research needs. In S. M. Sheridan & K. M. Kim (Eds.), *Foundational aspects of family-school partnership research* (pp. 1–14). Springer International.

Treml, J., Schmidt, V., Nagl, M., & Kersting, A. (2021). Pre–loss grief and preparedness for death among caregivers of terminally ill cancer patients: A systematic review. *Social Science & Medicine, 284*, 114240. https://doi.org/10.1016/j.socscimed.2021.114240. https://doi.org/10.1016/j.socscimed.2021.114240 https://doi.org/10.1016/j.socscimed.2021.114240

Wolff, B., Magiati, I., Roberts, R., Skoss, R., & Glasson, E. (2022). Psychosocial interventions and support groups for siblings of individuals with neurodevelopmental conditions: A mixed methods systematic review of sibling self-reported mental health and wellbeing outcomes. *Clinical, Child and Family Psychology Review*, online first. https://doi.org/10.1007/s10567-022-00413-4.

Sidebars on Selected Websites or Resources on Evidence-Based Practice

The National Alliance for Caregiving (NAC; https://www.caregiving.org/). The NAC is a nonprofit coalition of national organizations. The website provides a wealth of information on building health, wealth, and equity for family caregivers through research, innovation, and advocacy.

Family Caregiver Alliance (FCA; https://www.caregiver.org/). The FCA provides a broad range of information about caregiving, including the identification of resources in the Bay Area, caregiving resources for family caregivers of adults with physical and cognitive impairments, such as Parkinson disease, stroke, Alzheimer disease, and other types of dementia. The FCA also provides information about best practices and research reports.

The ARCH National Respite Network and Resource Center (https://archrespite.org/).

The NRC website provides resources for caregivers by providing locators to identify respite services in their communities, services to advocate for promoting policy and programs, and research and training centers.

National Clearinghouse on Autism Evidence and Practice (NCAEP; https://ncaep.fpg.unc.edu/). The NCAEP is a clearinghouse website that provides evidence-based behavioral, educational, clinical, and developmental practices and service models used with individuals on the autism spectrum from birth through age 22. Information is for families, practitioners, and researchers.

Karst and Van Vancke's article (2012) describes comprehensive information on assessment and evidence-based interventions for family caregivers of individuals with autism spectrum disorder across the life span.

The Family Caregiving Advisory Council's recommendation serves as the foundation for the National Family Caregiving Strategy for the Congress in 2021 for the planning of services and support at federal, state, and local communities: https://acl.gov/sites/default/files/RAISE_SGRG/RAISE%20RECOMMENDATIONS%20FINAL%20WEB.pdf

IV

SPECIFIC TRAUMA AND STIGMATIZED POPULATIONS

Since the first edition of this book was published in 1977, the literature related to topics in this section has grown significantly. Chapters included for this edition reflect the growing need in counseling, psychology, rehabilitation, and other social sciences to prepare professionals for diagnostic, treatment, and preventive interventions, and the coordination of important resources to help persons with chronic illnesses and disabilities achieve optimal levels of independent functioning. In this section, we focus on specific traumatized as well as stigmatized groups.

Authors in Part IV reflect on the all-important topic of substance use disorders, for which treatment has continued to evolve since the implementation of the *Diagnostic and Statistical Manual of Mental Disorders* (DSM-5; American Psychiatric Association, 2013) as the number of opioid overdose deaths continue to rise. In addition, an ongoing contemporary counseling need relates to the veterans from Afghanistan and Iraq who continue to face physical and mental health issues since returning. It is also important to realize that we must not only work with returning veterans, but their families as well during and after the adjustment process as they attempt to return to civilian life. People with disabilities who are abused comprise another traumatized population, and abuse is particularly prevalent among those with developmental disabilities. Counseling strategies are provided to assist those who are abused; and community and social supports for these survivors are explored. There has also been a growing increase in immigrants, refugees and asylum seekers, either from violence, war, or climate change and other natural disasters. Guidelines for mental health screening and best practices counseling with these vulnerable groups are discussed. Finally, another growing trend is the increase in older workers either needing to continue working out of financial necessity or because they wish to stay engaged because they find it pleasurable and rewarding. The authors explore various models of aging, employer discrimination issues, and provide counselors with strategies on how to best work with this population.

MAJOR HIGHLIGHTS IN PART IV

■ Substance use disorder (SUD) is a complex, uniquely stigmatizing chronic condition associated with significant negative consequences for individuals living with SUD, their friends and family, and their communities. Chapter 17 offers current information on the health and psychosocial impacts of SUD at the individual and the broader social level, examining the systemic impact on families, the social determinants of health and SUDs, and the causes and consequences of the current overdose and opioid epidemics. The authors describe the high rate of co-occurrence of SUD with other chronic conditions and disabilities, and the intersectionality of SUD and other marginalized identities. Evidence-based treatment practices, effective vocational rehabilitation strategies, and relevant community resources are presented along with the barriers to accessing healthcare/treatment, employment, housing, and civil rights.

- The military population, including those currently serving and Veterans, have disproportionate rates of disability and can experience a variety of mental health and wellness challenges related to their service. Counseling services may be needed by Service Members, Veterans, and military-connected families and significant others at any stage of military service- for example, during basic training, deployment, or after leaving military service. In chapter 18, the authors discuss the cultural context of relationships, issues, and trends in relation to Veteran and family reintegration; present current literature on effective theories, techniques, and interventions that can be utilized when working with Veterans and their families; and highlight community resources that are available to support military Veterans and their families as they assimilate into the civilian community and workforce.

- Individuals with disabilities experience abuse and intimate partner violence at higher rates than non-disabled people. Parents, caregivers, partners, and other relatives are the most common perpetrators of abuse. Abuse includes physical, emotional, financial, sexual, and neglect, and much goes unreported. In chapter 19, the author presents an intersectional discussion of abuse and neglect among individuals with disabilities, raising specific issues for women, men, and those in the LGBTQIA+ community. She uses Bronfenbrenner's bioecological model to illustrate how a variety of factors can influence one's ability to leave abusive relationships and situations. The author concludes the chapter with a discussion on how counselors and related professionals can respond well, beginning with learning deeply about subcultures, listening carefully, and providing culturally sensitive, client-centered and disability-related accommodations in safety planning.

- In Chapter 20, the author discusses the growing global humanitarian efforts to work with immigrants, refugees, and asylum seekers due to climate change, war, violence, and other natural disasters. This vulnerable population comes to the US typically under dire circumstances, where many have fled their country in order to survive, with the hopes of having their basic needs met such as safety, warmth, food, and the chance for a better life. The author discusses who these populations are, the sociocultural and familial impact of war and climate refugees, and counselor guidelines on how best to provide mental health screenings and counsel this vulnerable population.

- The authors of Chapter 21 also discuss the growing trend in America; the increase of aging and once retired workforce who will have either continued to work past the retirement age due to the rewards of remaining active or have returned to the workforce out of financial necessity. Various developmental models of aging are discussed as well as the need for effective functional assessments of aging workers with or without a disability. The authors discuss the practical implications of clinicians and counselors in providing guidance to this population, and provide areas for future research.

REFERENCE

American Psychiatric Association. (2013). *Diagnostic and statistical manual of mental disorders* (5th ed.). American Psychiatric Publishing.

CHAPTER 17

LIVING WITH SUBSTANCE USE DISORDER: FROM STIGMA TO RECOVERY

MYKAL LESLIE AND STUART RUMRILL

LEARNING OBJECTIVES

After reading this chapter, you will be able to:

- Define substance use disorder (SUD) and differentiate SUD from other similar terms and ideas
- Understand the wide-ranging individual, familial, and societal impacts of SUD in the United States
- Identify some of the unique characteristics of SUD-related stigma and the systemic negative impact of SUD-related stigma to a person's recovery
- Understand the various components of the recovery process, including the barriers to and impacts of employment and housing for individuals living with SUD

PRE-READING QUESTIONS

1. What is a substance?
2. What is the difference between addiction and a substance use disorder?
3. When does substance use become a substance use disorder?
4. What are the symptoms and consequences of SUD?
5. What are some legal protections for people with SUD?
6. What are some treatment options for people with SUD?

INDIVIDUAL, FAMILIAL, AND SOCIETAL IMPACT OF SUBSTANCE USE DISORDERS

What Are Substance Use Disorders?

Many people are familiar with the term *substance use disorder* (SUD), but it can be difficult to understand how SUD is similar to, or different from, other terms such as *alcoholism*, *drug addiction*, *substance abuse*, and *substance misuse*. In this section, we will define both the term *substance* (or *drug*) and *SUD*. We will discuss ideas about what an SUD is, what causes SUD, and how someone is diagnosed with an SUD.

What Is a Substance?

Much like the term *drug*, *substance* refers to any psychoactive compound with the potential to cause health and social problems, including SUD. Substance does not only refer to illegal drugs such as heroin or cocaine but also to legal substances (e.g., alcohol and tobacco) and drugs that are controlled for use by licensed prescribers for medical purposes (e.g., Ritalin and Vicodin; McLellan, 2017). There are many categories of substances that are commonly used to differentiate various substances based on the effects they have on the brain and body, along with the behavioral changes they can cause in a person. We will briefly define each of the seven main categories of substances.

- Depressants
  - □ Effects: slow down, "downers," relaxation, tiredness, euphoria
  - □ Examples: alcohol, benzodiazepines (e.g., Valium and Xanax), and barbiturates
- Stimulants
  - □ Effects: "uppers," increase energy, concentration, wakefulness, "rush"
  - □ Examples: nicotine (from tobacco products), caffeine, cocaine (including "crack" cocaine), amphetamines (e.g., Ritalin and Adderall), and methamphetamine (also known as "meth")
- Opioids
  - □ Effects: pain killers, intense pleasure, euphoria
  - □ Examples: heroin, morphine, fentanyl, codeine, Vicodin, and oxycontin
- Cannabinoids
  - □ Effects: feelings of elation (a "high"), can negatively affect mental and physical functioning
  - □ Examples: marijuana, hashish, Dronabinol, and other forms of THC (e.g., edibles or "dabs")
- Hallucinogenics
  - □ Effects: alter the user's perception of reality, auditory and visual hallucinations, "tripping"
  - □ Examples: LSD, psilocybin ("shrooms"), mescaline, peyote, and DMT
- Dissociatives
  - □ Effects: inhibit pain, "out of body," "floaty," disconnected, relaxed mental state
  - □ Examples: phencyclidine (PCP), ketamine, dextromethorphan (DXM), and *Salvia*

- Empathogens
  - Effects: emotional communion, oneness, relatedness, emotional openness, warmth, belonging
  - Examples: MDMA (known as "ecstasy" or "molly"), ethylone, and PMA/PMMA (Hart & Ksir, 2017; McLellan, 2017).

The Blurry Line Between Substance Use and Addiction

Throughout human history, substances have been integrated into society to help people relax, stay awake or alert, cope with pain, and aid in religious rituals to experience the supernatural. Throughout the course of a typical day, you might observe others going to a café in the morning and having a cup of coffee to wake up (caffeine), taking a cigarette break to relax during the work day (nicotine), or going out to a bar after work to have a few drinks and "unwind" with friends (alcohol). Even substances that have become infamous in our culture are used or have previously been used for helpful medicinal purposes (e.g., opioids as painkillers, cocaine as a local anesthetic, amphetamines to treat attention deficit hyperactivity disorder [ADHD]; Hart & Ksir, 2017).

The point at which the use of a substance becomes an "addiction" or a "substance use disorder" has long been a widely debated topic in the medical and psychological fields. The use of substances escalates into "substance misuse" or "substance abuse" when someone (a) uses an illicit or nonprescribed substance or (b) uses any substance in relatively high doses or in situations that can cause health or social problems, either immediately or over time (McLellan, 2017). A common example of substance abuse/misuse is binge drinking, wherein a person has four (five for males) or more standard alcoholic drinks in one sitting (within a few hours). The consequences of substance abuse/misuse can be direct, such as immediate health consequences or even death (overdose), or can be indirect, such as an automobile crash from impaired driving, intimate partner violence, or suicide attempts (McLellan, 2017).

A small proportion of individuals (estimated to be around 10%–15% depending on the substance; Sussman et al., 2011) who abuse/misuse substances repeatedly and over prolonged periods may develop an SUD or a substance addiction. In addition to the consequences of substance use/abuse mentioned previously, SUD involves the development of a psychological dependence on the substance, sometimes called an *addiction* (McLellan, 2017). In this process, the individual abusing the substance experiences cravings for it and has significant difficulty reducing or stopping use of the substance despite significant health, social, or psychological consequences (Rubin et al., 2016).

Some substances are believed to be more addictive, or more likely to result in a person developing an SUD as a result of prolonged use. Though we still do not fully understand the complexity of what causes someone to develop an SUD, scientists have pinpointed one specific area of the brain that likely plays a significant role in this process. The area, sometimes referred to as the *reward center* of the brain, releases chemicals, called *neurotransmitters*, that reinforce certain behaviors in people by producing a feeling of pleasure. Many of the substances believed to be "highly addictive" have a strong direct or indirect impact on this area of the brain, which may result in the cravings for the substance as well as the extreme "highs" or the euphoria associated with the use of the substance. As a result of prolonged use, this area of the brain adapts and stops producing the reward feeling for everyday tasks and behaviors, leaving the person more dependent on substances to feel any type of pleasure (Hart & Ksir, 2017; Rubin et al., 2016; Sellman, 2010). In addition, SUD is known to impact an individual's learning and memory, motivation, and decision-making ability, making it a truly complicated biopsychosocial phenomenon (Bettinardi-Angres & Angres, 2011).

Is Substance Use Disorder a Disease?

Whether SUD is a disease, a disorder, or a behavioral choice has long been a topic of debate. With mounting evidence of the complex genetic, biological, and social factors that contribute to SUD, the American Medical Association (AMA) officially identified SUD as a disease in 1987 (Bettinardi-Angres & Angres, 2011). Heshka and Allison (2001) proposed a four-point definition of "disease" to consolidate various definitions from medical literature.

1. Disease is a condition of the body, its parts, organs, or systems or an alteration thereof.

2. It results from infection, parasites, nutritional, dietary, environmental, genetic, or other causes.

3. It has a characteristic, identifiable, marked group of signs or symptoms.

4. It deviates from normal structure or function (variously described as abnormal structure or function; incorrect function; impairment of normal state; interruption, disturbance, cessation, disorder, derangement of bodily or organ functions; Heshka & Allison, 2001).

Based on this definition, SUD appears to meet all criteria to be considered a "disease." Research using brain imaging has demonstrated various alterations in brain structure and chemistry as a result of prolonged substance use, which addresses the initial prong of the definition (Sellman, 2010; Sussman et al., 2011). In terms of the second prong, resulting from "environmental, genetic, and other causes," SUD has been shown to have both environmental and genetic components (Sellman, 2010; Thombs & Osborn, 2013). As to the third prong, SUD has long been diagnosed based on a group of similar signs and symptoms (such as cravings, loss of control, tolerance, withdrawal, continued use despite significant negative consequences, etc.; American Psychiatric Association [APA], 2013). Lastly, SUD is perhaps most commonly defined by disruption of "normal functioning," as stark changes in behavior and personality are often seen in individuals who have been diagnosed. Although there is no one widely accepted definition of the term *disease*, SUD appears to qualify even using the more stringent definitions.

Regardless of its disease classification, SUD is perhaps best described as a chronic-relapsing condition that can be managed or controlled through treatment but not necessarily "cured." After treatment, less than 10% of people with SUD will achieve continuous abstinence, but many will experience significant periods of functional stability and improvement over time (Sellman, 2010). Within the literature, SUD has been compared to other chronic medical illnesses with substantial behavioral components such as type 2 diabetes, hypertension, and asthma. All four of these conditions/diseases have similar rates of symptom recurrence and relapse and are largely dependent on lifestyle changes such as diet and behavioral modifications to improve the individual's health condition (Sellman, 2010).

Individual Response to Substance Use Disorder Diagnosis

The definition of how SUD is diagnosed has varied over time, but the most recent accepted definition of SUD was released by the APA in the latest (fifth) version of the *Diagnostic and Statistical Manual of Mental Disorders* (*DSM-5*). According to the *DSM-5*, a person can be diagnosed with an SUD if they demonstrate a significant level of distress or impairment over the previous year, as evidenced by at least two of the following symptoms:

- Taking the substance in larger amounts or over a longer period than was intended
- Inability to control or cut down on substance use
- Spending a great deal of time trying to get, use, or recover from using a substance

- Having a craving or strong desire to use a substance
- Failing to fulfill responsibilities/duties at work, school, or home due to substance use
- Continuing to use a substance despite significant social or interpersonal problems
- Giving up or reducing social, work, or recreational activities due to substance use
- Continued use of substances in physically hazardous situations
- Continued use of substance despite known physical or psychological consequences
- Experiencing tolerance effects (i.e., needing more and more of a substance to achieve desired effects)
- Experiencing withdrawal (i.e., physical symptoms that vary depending on the substance as a result of reducing or stopping use of the substance; APA, 2013)

The higher number of symptoms experienced by the individual, the more severe the SUD is considered to be.

In the disability literature, we often discuss the idea of "onset of disability/condition" as well as the individual's corresponding "response" to the diagnosis/condition/impairment. As we conceptualize SUD within this disability framework of diagnosis and response, several aspects of the experience of SUD differentiate it from other conditions. First, there is rarely a clear-cut onset of symptoms. Onset is generally insidious (meaning that the symptoms develop over time and with prolonged use and may not be apparent for some time), although there have been cases where individuals develop addictive symptoms immediately or shortly after using a substance for the first time (Sellman, 2010; Thombs & Osborn, 2013). Another separating feature of SUD is observed in how the diagnosis process occurs. In a typical disease process, it may be expected that a person experiences signs and symptoms or has some sort of emergency issue that results in them seeing a physician and being diagnosed. Although these processes can certainly occur in SUD (e.g., a person is concerned about their well-being and seeks assistance or is evaluated due to a medical emergency caused by substance usage), there are several other "routes" by which an SUD may be diagnosed. Due to the legal implications of substance use, a person may be legally mandated to be evaluated for an SUD based on a driving under the influence (DUI) arrest or on an illicit substance possession charge. Another example would be an individual referred to SUD treatment/evaluation as a result of having a positive drug screen at work. Regardless of the scenario, it is common for an individual to be evaluated or diagnosed with an SUD involuntarily and, similarly, it is common for individuals with SUD signs/symptoms not to seek treatment of their own volition and for SUD- related issues to go undiagnosed.

In fact, data from the National Survey on Drug Use and Health (NSDUH; SAMHSA, 2021) indicated that only 6.5% (or 2.6 million people) of those with SUDs (41.1 million people) received any SUD-related treatment in 2020. Stated another way, throughout the year 2020 93.5% (38.4 million people) of those who met criteria for SUD did not receive any type of SUD treatment. "Any SUD treatment" includes attending self-help groups such as Alcoholics Anonymous (AA) or Narcotics Anonymous (NA). Almost all (97.5%) of those who did not receive any treatment, despite meeting the criteria for SUD, reported they did not feel they needed it. For the other 2.5% who felt they needed treatment but did not receive it, the most common reasons given were cost/no healthcare (19.1%), not finding the type of treatment they wanted (14.4%), and being concerned about stigma from neighbors and the community (11.9%; SAMHSA, 2021).

The staggering statistic regarding the 37.5 million Americans who had SUD issues but indicated they did not need treatment beckons a discussion of one of the commonly cited psychosocial responses to SUD issues, namely, "denial." Addiction researchers have estimated that denial in those with SUD is present in between 30% and 55% of cases (Schuckit et al., 2020). Denial includes falsely reporting nonuse as well as downplaying or ignoring use-related issues.

Research into the underlying causes of denial has generally concluded that a combination of factors leads individuals to demonstrate some of these hallmark features of denial. These include a desire to avoid negative consequences and attitude from others, not appropriately appraising the risks of substance use, and the expression of subconscious defense mechanisms (Schuckit et al., 2020). Tied into our later discussion regarding the stigma of SUD, many individuals have beliefs about what "substance abusers" or "addicts" look and act like that are heavily stigmatized and often not in line with how these individuals view themselves, whether intentionally or adaptively as a means of preserving self-image (Akdağ et al., 2018; Forchuk, 1984).

Once a person is confronted with SUD issues or an SUD diagnosis, the path of least resistance from a cognitive appraisal standpoint may be to disregard or diminish the severity of the issues or the diagnosis, rather than having to either view oneself as a stigmatized "addict" or challenge long-held stigmatized beliefs about people with SUD. In essence, the stigma and life-threatening nature of substance use lend themselves to individuals experiencing cognitive dissonance between how they view themselves and the reality and consequences of some of their behaviors (Forchuk, 1984). It is no coincidence, therefore, that admission of problems and being "powerless" to the substance of choice are central tenets of the 12-step program that is utilized in many popular self-help groups for SUD (AA, 2022).

Health Impact

The negative impact of substance use on a national level has led the U.S. Department of Health and Human Services (HHS) to label this situation a public health emergency (HHS, 2022) and the Centers for Disease Control and Prevention (CDC) to identify the current opioid problem as an "epidemic" (CDC, 2022). The NSDUH from 2020 revealed that prevalence of SUD in the United States is 14.5%, or 40.3 million people (SAMHSA, 2021). This data was surprising given the previous year (2019), which indicated that 20.4 million Americans met criteria for SUD, suggesting a nearly 100% increase in prevalence. It is important to note that 2020 was the first year that the NSDUH utilized the updated *DSM-5* criteria for SUD, designed to diagnose the condition more accurately than the *DSM-IV TR* criteria relied on in the 2019 data. It is also likely that a real surge was consistent with the general increase in mental health and substance use issues seen as a result of the COVID-19 pandemic. Of the 40.3 million people who met criteria for SUD, 28.3 million reported an alcohol use disorder (AUD), 18.4 million had a drug use disorder (DUD), and 6.5 million experienced both AUD and DUD comorbidly. Among illicitly used substances, cannabis, opioids, and stimulants were the most frequently abused drugs (SAMHSA, 2021).

In terms of the national health impact of SUD, 95,000 Americans die of alcohol use each year, making it the third leading cause of preventable death. Alcohol contributes to about 18.5% of emergency room visits and 22.1% of overdose deaths related to prescription opioids. Over 91,000 American lives were lost due to drug overdose in 2020, the leading cause of unintentional injury death in the United States (CDC, 2022; Lockwood, 2018). In addition to the intangible human cost of substance use, the economic impact of substance use is estimated to cost over $440 billion annually, including healthcare costs, lost productivity, and criminal justice costs.

The Overdose Epidemic

Nearly 1 million Americans have died from drug overdoses since 1999, constituting a massive public health concern. It also remains an intruging psychosocial phenomenon tied to SUD, as statistics demonstrate that the states with the highest substance usage rates are not necessarily the ones with the highest overdose rates. Drug overdoses appear to be a complex public health issue that is impacted by a variety of factors, including but not limited to joblessness, poverty, lack of housing, social support, mental health comorbidities, and access to treatment (CDC, 2022). Over 91,000 drug overdose deaths were reported in 2020, a 31% increase from 2019 data (CDC, 2022). Most recently, for the first time in recorded history, 2021 saw over 100,000 deaths from drug overdose in one calendar year (April 2020 to April 2021; CDC, 2022). Opioids are the most dangerous illicit substance, involved in three-quarters of all overdoses in the United States, but deaths due to stimulants (methamphetamine and cocaine) are also on the rise. Drug overdoses have surpassed motor vehicle accidents as the leading cause of unintentional injury deaths (Lockwood, 2018). Drug overdose rates are up across all genders, races/ethnicities, and ages for adults, and an average of 252 Americans die every day from overdoses (CDC, 2022).

THE OPIOID CRISIS

The origins of the current opioid epidemic are complex, but they can be traced, in part, to pain management treatment and prescription patterns in the 1980s and 1990s (CDC, 2022; Dasgupta et al., 2018; HHS, 2022; Lockwood, 2018). As the number of opioid prescriptions increased throughout the 1990s, marketing efforts reassured the medical community and patients alike of the low-risk benefits of drugs such as OxyContin, resulting in a growth in prescription rates from 670,000 in 1997 to 6.2 million in 2002 (CDC, 2022). The combination of mass marketing and lenient prescribing practices was further complicated by the rise of "pill mills" in areas hit the hardest by poverty and unemployment in the collapses of the manufacturing and coal industries in areas such as the Ohio Valley, Appalachia, Maine, and Alabama, where rates of OxyContin abuse were five to six times the national average (Lockwood, 2018). This is often referred to as the first "wave" of overdose deaths in the current opioid crisis.

The second distinct wave of overdose deaths began in 2010 and was marked by a rapid increase in heroin overdose deaths, which tripled between 2010 and 2015 (CDC, 2022; Dasgupta et al., 2018; Lockwood, 2018). This wave coincided with the peak of opioid prescriptions in 2011 at 206 million and the subsequent national crackdown on lenient prescription practices and pill mills, greatly reducing access to prescription opioids (Dasgupta et al., 2018; Lockwood, 2018). The unfortunate consequence of the reduced access to prescription opioids in concordance with an increased illegal supply of heroin was that heroin became a much more potent and affordable alternative for those who had developed a dependency and tolerance for opioids but had no legal means of accessing the drugs (Dasgupta et al., 2018).

The third and most recent wave began in 2013 and is tied to significant increases in overdose deaths involving synthetic opioids, specifically illicitly manufactured fentanyl (IMF) and its analogs (CDC, 2022; Dasgupta et al., 2018). Overdose deaths attributed to IMF increased nationally by a staggering 540% from 2013 to 2016 (Dasgupta et al., 2018). In 2016, synthetic opioids were the leading cause of opioid overdose deaths (19,413), followed by death attributed to prescription opioids (17,087) and overdose deaths attributed to heroin (15,469; HHS, 2022). Another notable shift in the third wave is that individuals presenting for treatment are now more likely to report beginning opioid use with heroin (Dasgupta et al., 2018).

Currently, 2.7 million Americans have an opiod use disorder (OUD). An estimated 9.3 million people misused opioids in 2020, and just over 900,000 reported using heroin in that same year (SAMHSA, 2021). Roughly a quarter of individuals who are prescribed opioids for chronic pain end up misusing them, and between 8% and 12% of those who use any type of opioid develop an OUD (NIDA, 2022).

THE "SILENT" STIMULANT EPIDEMIC

Although opioid overdoses have been at the center of the conversations about this national crisis over the past two decades, deaths involving stimulants such as methamphetamine and cocaine are becoming an increasing problem (Volkow, 2020). Overdoses involving methamphetamine and cocaine have steadily risen over the previous decade, with overdose deaths involving methamphetamine increasing more than 10-fold since 2009 and overdoses involving cocaine showing a similar pattern. Cocaine-involved overdoses now account for nearly one in five overdose deaths in the United States. Meanwhile, psychostimulant-involved overdoses (including methamphetamine) account for around 23% of total overdose deaths (CDC, 2022).

Several explanations for the increases in stimulant use and corresponding overdose deaths have been proposed. It is important to note that the increase in stimulant-involved overdoses has not necessarily corresponded to increases in the sheer use of these substances. In fact, it is likely that more individuals are either intentionally using stimulants in combination with other dangerous substances, such as opioids, or that many individuals are using products that have been, knowingly or unknowingly, laced with other potent high-risk substances such as fentanyl (Volkow, 2020). Data shows that more individuals are combining opioid and stimulant use and that individuals with OUD are substituting stimulants such as methamphetamine due to them being perceived as safer, as well as being less costly or easier to obtain (Volkow, 2020). Further, recent studies have indicated that the COVID-19 pandemic coincided with an uptick in stimulant usage, making this a resurgent concern that we can ill-afford to ignore (Volkow, 2020).

Social Determinants of Health and Substance Use Disorders

Social determinants of health are the economic and social conditions that influence individual and group differences in health status (Braveman & Gottlieb, 2014). In the context of SUDs, social determinants encompass economic and social conditions that influence the SUD experience and outlook among individuals and groups; for instance, does birth order affect SUD prevalence in young adults? Do people from a lower socioeconomic status (SES) experience more severe SUDs than those of a higher SES?

When examining social determinants of health, it is important to consider environment in the context of individual, interpersonal, community, and society. At the individual level, there are factors such as gender, race, ethnicity, incarceration, and age; at the interpersonal level, adverse childhood experiences such as abuse, neglect, and parental substance abuse; at the community level, neighborhood violence and social capital; and at the societal level there are the broader and/or overarching policies such as the Americans with Disabilities Act (ADA) of 1990 and its protections of people with disabilities and SUDs (Henry, 2019). Each of these factors across all levels has been studied and/or shown to be relative to SUD and within/between group health differences.

For example, at the individual level, employment status is often shown to be related to SUD. In a 2017 study, Ronka et al. found that those with long- and short-term unemployment status, along with those who were retired, had the highest hazard ratios for total drug- related mortality compared to those who were employed. Some studies have found drug and alcohol use being major barriers to employment (Bakken-Gillen et al., 2015; Miguel et al., 2019; Pete et al., 2015), with unemployment being associated with poor quality of life and SUD outcomes (Lee et al., 2018; Lee et al., 2019; Luhmann et al., 2014; Schauss et al., 2019; Sumner & Gallagher, 2017) and employment being shown to be associated with higher quality of life, lowered rates of SUD (Bakken-Gillen et al., 2015), and more positive treatment/recovery outcomes for those who do have SUDs (Bowden & Goodman, 2015; Harrison et al., 2020; Lusk, 2018; Miguel et al., 2019; O'Connell et al., 2007; Sahker et al., 2019; Walton & Hall, 2016).

At the interpersonal level, there are several social relationship and home status factors shown to be related to SUD, such as being divorced, separated, or widowed; not living in a private household; and living alone. These situations have been shown to be associated with drug-related mortality, drug-induced poisonings, and drug-related illnesses (Ronka et al., 2017). Interpersonal trauma and adverse experiences have also been observed to play a role in poorer mental health, SUDs, and violence (Henry, 2019). Some of these trauma and adverse experiences may include, for instance, adverse childhood experiences (abuse, neglect, parent divorce/separation, domestic violence exposure, parental mental illness, and household member incarceration; Henry, 2019). Finally, victim blaming, which is the tendency to place sole responsibility for one's negative life circumstances on the individual in question due to their attitudes, behaviors, and lifestyle choices, while ignoring the influence and impact of external environmental factors (Otu et al., 2020), is another interpersonal concept that may have a negative impact in terms of SUDs.

There are also many factors at the community level that can impact SUD. In addition to unstable housing, unreliable income sources, immigration status, transportation, poor neighborhoods, and lack of social amenities (Cook et al., 2021; Langlois et al., 2020; Otu et al., 2020; Sugarman et al., 2020), SES and its relation to SUD has been studied extensively. SES is the perceived and/or actual social standing or class of an individual, family, or group that can be measured by a combination of education, income, and occupation (American Psychological Association [APA], 2022). Langlois et al. (2020) and others have examined this variable through the lens of subjective social status (which measures perceptions of relative social standing and addresses perceived inequality through mediums such as economic wealth, racial/ethnic discrimination, and level of occupational power or control) and objective social status (which addresses actual inequality). Examining these two variables and their influence on many SUD outcomes, Langois et al. found that objective social status was only associated with cigarette smoker status or level of nicotine dependence, whereas subjective social status was associated with drug use severity. Social disadvantage or lower SES and objective or subjective social status have been widely found to be associated with poor SUD and drug use outcomes such as (illicit) drug use, drug-related mortality, and drug overdose (Ronka et al., 2017).

Finally, at the broader societal level, there are factors that may influence SUD in individuals. People can modify, flee from, move to, or adapt to an environment and, at the same time, they are influenced by the environment, which may facilitate or inhibit modification, movement, or adaptation. Arguably, the factors that begin at the societal level that then "trickle down" and negatively influence individuals at community, interpersonal, and personal levels may be most influential. Ostensibly, starting from the bottom up (going from personal to societal), responses to problems are more clearly outlined as the problems themselves are more readily apparent. As in the case when addressing "personal" problems, there is only one individual perspective at stake and, for instance, a practitioner could propose an intervention such as recommending that the individual attend a self-help group such as AA or come up with a list of alternative habits to drinking or using drugs that they can rely on in times of cravings. However, when addressing interpersonal factors or problems, at least one other individual is now involved. The nature and solution to the problem are now more complex, and this complexity can exponentially evolve as one climbs to community barriers and then to societal ones. Problems become more pervasive, yet also more difficult to identify and address.

Co-Occurrence With Other Conditions

Compared to the general population, individuals with disabilities are particularly susceptible to experiencing SUDs (Sprong et al., 2014). SUDs occur at rates 200% to 400% higher in people with disabilities than in people without disabilities (Sprong et al., 2014). The rate of SUDs has been found to vary depending on the type of disability. The rates among persons with spinal cord injury, vision impairment, amputation, and traumatic brain injury range from 40% to 50%. Approximately 40% of persons diagnosed with SUDs have been diagnosed with active mental health disorders. In turn, between 20% and 50% of consumers presenting for mental health treatment have experienced an SUD in their lifetime. Over 50% of those with SUDs have, at some point in their lives, been diagnosed with a mental health disorder (Padwa et al., 2013). Sellman (2010) cited multiple studies indicating that the comorbidity of psychiatric disorders for individuals with SUDs ranged from 75% to 90% with the most common diagnosed mental disorders being social phobia, major depression, and posttraumatic stress disorder (PTSD).

Research suggests several reasons why people with disabilities are at an increased risk for SUD. The high prevalence of SUDs in people with disabilities is associated with (a) medication and health problems, (b) societal enabling, (c) lack of identification of problems, and (d) lack of identification of accessible and appropriate prevention and treatment services (Sprong et al., 2014, p. 4). For example, due to higher rates of pain-associated conditions, people with disabilities are more likely than other people to be prescribed opioid pain relievers (NCHS, 2016). In a systematic review and data synthesis, Vowles et al. (2015) found that rates of opioid misuse averaged between 21% and 29% among patients with chronic pain and rates of addiction averaged between 8% and 12%. Similarly, Martell et al. (2007) reported that up to 25% of patients using opioid medications exhibited some signs of medication misuse. In a nationally representative study by Katz et al. (2013), controlling for sociodemographic confounds, the presence of a physical condition, a mental condition, the combination of a physical and mental condition, and an existing SUD all significantly increased the odds of substance abuse/dependence.

Chronic pain conditions, including different musculoskeletal, digestive, and nerve pain conditions, impact over 100 million Americans each year (Bilevicius et al., 2018, Vest et al., 2016). Although pain management was previously believed to be a protective factor for preventing OUD, recent studies have shown that is not necessarily the case, and with the prevalence of opioid use to manage both acute and chronic pain, these disabilities are central to the discussion of disability and SUD (Bilvicius et al., 2018; Katz et al., 2013; Vest et al., 2016).

A growing body of research emphasizes the role of trauma and anxiety-related conditions, such as PTSD, in the comorbid development of SUD (Bilevicius et al., 2018). PTSD also has a crossover presence with chronic pain conditions. PTSD is present in as many as 30% of American adults with chronic pain conditions and in 50% to 80% of the military veteran population (Bilevicius et al., 2018).

Additionally, unintentional death through overdose has repeatedly been found to be more likely among people who have experienced a serious traumatic injury, such as spinal cord injury or traumatic brain injury (TBI; Clark et al., 2017; Hammond et al., 2015; Krause et al., 2017; Krause et al., 2018; O'Neil-Pirozzi et al., 2018). The high rates of narcotics prescribed to this population make these individuals particularly susceptible to SUDs, a risk further increased by comorbid physical, cognitive, and psychosocial factors (Clark et al., 2017; Hammond et al., 2015; O'Neil-Pirozzi et al., 2017). In fact, recent National Institute on Disability, Independent Living, and Rehabilitation Research (NIDIL-RR)–funded project findings indicate that people with TBI are 11 times more likely to die from an overdose than those without TBI (Administration on Community Living, 2019).

Systemic Impact on Families

Any discussion of the psychosocial impact of SUD would be incomplete without a conversation on the systemic impact of substance use on the family unit. The impact of having a family member with an SUD is bidirectional, as the negative impact of the SUD can have devastating consequences for each family member; however, a family unit that is supportive and actively involved in treatment can be a key component in the recovery process for a person with an SUD. Thus, involving the family in the treatment process can be critical for the family members' well-being, as well as for the person with the SUD (Lander et al., 2013).

Being a child of a parent with an SUD can have a lifelong negative developmental impact and can have a multigenerational impact, leading those individuals to struggle with developing meaningful relationships with their children. Over 10% of children live in homes where at least one parent has an SUD (Lander et al., 2013). These children are at high risk for experiencing emotional and behavioral problems and have an increased risk for developing their own SUD-related issues. Children of a parent with an SUD are three times more likely to experience physical or sexual abuse and to experience a severe disruption in attachment, roles, communication, social life, and finances (APA, 2010). These children are more likely to experience issues establishing trusting relationships with others, to deal with issues of fear and anxiety likely as a result of unpredictable parental behaviors, and to experience "role reversal" early on in life, having to "parent" their parent who is experiencing the SUD-related issues (Lander et al., 2013).

Having a parent with an SUD can also lead children to experience severe loss through parental divorce, incarceration, loss of role functioning as parent, and even death, which brings about further emotional and behavioral consequences (Daley et al., 2018). Daley et al. indicated that rates of removal from the home for children of a parent with an SUD were 34.4% in 2015 (an increase of nearly 100% from the 2000 rates) and that around 37% of parents with SUD in a quality improvement study indicated they had relatives or grandparents caring for their children (Daley et al., 2018). Further, maternal substance use while the child is in utero is associated with premature birth, fetal alcohol syndromes, and neonatal abstinence syndromes, leading to higher risk for developmental and psychological issues across the life span (Daley et al., 2018).

In general, family members of individuals with SUD have an increased prevalence of illness and domestic violence, as well as psychological and interpersonal issues, conflict, stress, and financial and legal problems (APA, 2010). Resilient family members who use positive coping mechanisms; have strong social skills; and have positive connections with parents, other relatives, teachers, or other adults tend to be more protected from these negative consequences (Daley et al., 2018). Research has confirmed that, though treatment options for family members are limited, they can benefit from receiving treatment and, by doing so, can positively influence the family member with the SUD (APA, 2010).

Partners and spouses of individuals with SUD-related issues are at risk for intimate partner violence, emotional abuse, financial issues, interpersonal stress, and ultimately divorce or separation (Lander et al., 2013). Emotional difficulties such as anger, frustration, and a general sense of helplessness contribute to conflict and division between partners/spouses. Treatment provided to spouses and partners is effective in helping the partner with the SUD achieve abstinence or reduce relapses. Couples counseling can improve communication and relationship health while also supporting recovery for both members of the couple (APA, 2010; Daley et al., 2018).

UNIQUENESS OF SUBSTANCE USE DISORDER STIGMA

Overall, people with disabilities, whether SUDs or other mental or physical impairments, have experienced more stigma than any other group in human history (Corrigan, 2014; Smart, 2016). SUDs are among the most stigmatizing of chronic conditions (Schomerus, 2014; Smart, 2016). In fact, Smart (2016) identified three different continua of stigmatization of prejudice toward individuals with disabilities, including a continuum for visibility of disability, one for cause of disability, and another for type of disability.

Regarding visibility, Smart (2016) proposed that visible disabilities with stable courses are typically the least stigmatizing, followed by visible disabilities with episodic courses, invisible disabilities with stable courses, and finally, the most stigmatizing, invisible disabilities that are also episodic in nature. In terms of ambiguity and visibility of disability, SUDs, being classified as invisible, episodic, and psychiatric in nature, are highly stigmatizing.

Smart (2016) also described the continuum of prejudice related to the cause of disability. Generally, disabilities that are acquired later in life, as opposed to being present at birth, are perceived to be more preventable, therefore increasing the perception of accountability for the individual with the disability. The exception to this rule is when the acquisition of a disability is perceived to be a result of a "noble endeavor" such as a combat or an industrial injury, making those disabilities less stigmatizing than congenital disabilities, followed by acquired disabilities not of "noble" causes. The most stigmatized in terms of perceived cause are those acquired disabilities in which the person is thought to have contributed to the acquisition process (e.g., HIV/AIDS, obesity, SUDs; Smart, 2016).

Stigma of Substance Use Disorder

Research supports Smart's (2016) continua of stigma in that invisible, episodic, and acquired conditions such as SUD are the most highly stigmatized by the general public (Schomerus, 2014). In a survey of the U.S. population (Link et al., 1999) found that SUDs evoke a higher desire for social distance when compared to other mental health diagnoses. Ninety percent of respondents in the survey were unwilling to have contact with an individual with cocaine dependence, followed by 70% for those with alcohol dependence, 63% for individuals diagnosed with schizophrenia, and 47% for individuals diagnosed with depression (Link et al., 1999). A replication study by Pescosolido et al. (2010) revealed that this pattern of public opinion remained unchanged over the course of a decade. This same social distance effect has been identified in studies examining SUDs relative to medical conditions including cancer, diabetes, and other highly stigmatized conditions such as AIDS (Schomerus et al., 2006).

The perception of the general public that SUD is a behavioral and controllable "choice" contributes to the degree of stigma related to these disorders (Schomerus, 2014). In the Link et al. (1999) survey described earlier 44% and 49% of respondents viewed case vignettes of cocaine dependence and alcohol dependence, respectively, as depicting "mental illness" compared to 88% for schizophrenia and 68% for depression (Link et al., 1999). Almost identical results were obtained by Schomerus et al. (2013), suggesting that this phenomenon has remained relatively durable across time. In fact, a decade-long epidemiological study by Chartier et al. (2016) revealed that substance use stigma has remained stable over time in the United States.

Further evidence for the uniqueness of the stigma attached to SUDs can be found by studying public attitudes regarding the cause of SUDs relative to other mental health conditions and behavior-related medical diseases. Despite research revealing commonalities in behavioral adherence to treatment between SUDs and other chronic medical conditions, the same patterns of causal attribution can be observed when examining attitudes toward substance use in comparison to behavior-related medical diseases (Schomerus, 2014). In a 2006 study, Schomerus et al. found that an overwhelming majority of Americans (85%) believed a person with AUD to be at fault for their condition, even more so than people living with HIV (68%), myocardial infarction (45%), and diabetes (33%). In summarizing decades of relevant public opinion research, Schomerus (2014) noted that the two most impactful stereotypes held toward people living with SUD are that they are "weak-willed" and "unpredictable and dangerous."

In a similar vein, Livingston et al. (2012) proposed three main reasons for the high degree of stigma people living with SUD encounter. First, SUDs are symbolically linked to other stigmatized health conditions such as HIV/AIDS, hepatitis C, other mental health conditions, unsafe behaviors such as impaired driving, and social problems like poverty and criminality. Second, SUDs are treated as a moral and criminal issue, which is particularly the case in the United States, as some substances (e.g., heroin) are more highly criminalized and are treated with more punitive measures. Use of illegal substances increases the degree of stigma experienced as opposed to use of legal substances, such as alcohol, especially in the United States (Schomerus, 2014). Third, people with SUDs are perceived as having control over their condition. Making a causal attribution to the person with an SUD dictates the social response of viewing substance use as a moral deficit in which the person has corrective control (Livingston et al., 2012).

PROCESS OF STIGMATIZATION

An understanding of the process of stigmatization is necessary to examine the effects of public stigma on structural discrimination and self-stigma. Stigmatization starts when a person or group of persons is labeled due to differences. Then, the person or group of persons is linked with undesirable characteristics and consequently experiences loss of status and/or discrimination (van Boekel et al., 2013). Stigmatization can occur on a personal level due to prejudiced beliefs, stereotyping, and discriminatory action, but it also can be embedded into institutional practice and policies, which is known as *structural discrimination* (Jones & Corrigan, 2014). Public stigma has a reciprocal effect on structural discrimination, as both can serve to increase the other (van Boekel et al., 2013). For example, widely held beliefs, such as people with SUDs should be punished rather than helped, can impact structural-level policies, thereby lowering support for public health–oriented drug control policies, including funding for treatment and harm reduction practices (Kulesza et al., 2016). This structural discrimination based on moralistic and punitive attitudes toward individuals with SUDs can be both intentional and unintentional. Even though some policies and practices are grounded in research and not intended to discriminate, they increase stigma and barriers to treatment and recovery for people with SUDs nonetheless (Kulesza et al., 2016; Schomerus, 2014).

One area affected by structural discrimination against people with SUDs is access to healthcare and treatment. For example, many private insurance plans exclude substance use–related conditions, which seemingly is related to health-risk assessment but embodies the underlying moral stance on the degree of self-responsibility and controllability of the SUDs (Schomerus, 2014). Within mental health care, SUDs can be a contraindication of mental health treatment, and many countries choose to separate mental health care and substance use treatment (Rubak et al., 2005). Thus, many people with co-occurring symptoms have substance use issues that are undiagnosed and untreated (Albanese et al., 2006). Another example of seemingly unintentional healthcare structural discrimination is the lack of access to organ transplants and medical treatment for people with hepatitis C, a policy not shown in research to be clinically necessary (Rehm et al., 2003).

Another area of structural discrimination related to substance use is healthcare spending. Lack of available financial resources related to substance use can reduce availability and quality of treatment options and reduce public funding available for harm reduction programs. Examples of these programs include housing assistance, employment assistance, and other harm reduction measures such as overdose prevention and syringe/needle exchange programs (Kulesza et al., 2016; Schomerus, 2014; van Boekel et al., 2013). A survey in Germany revealed that, when asked for which of nine medical conditions funding could best be cut, the highest percentage of participants (78%) selected alcohol use. Similarly, when asked for which conditions should funding on no account be cut, alcohol use was selected least frequently by participants (Beck et al., 2003). A replication study in 2004 supported the presence of these attitudes toward healthcare funding for SUDs (Schomerus et al., 2006).

Some forms of structural discrimination pose a direct threat to the autonomy of individuals with SUDs. Compulsory treatment policies wherein individuals are mandated to treatment are one specific example. A 1996 survey of attitudes toward compulsory treatment in the United States showed that, regarding substance use treatment, 41% of participants supported mandatory hospital treatment, 39%

agreed with mandatory outpatient treatment, and 25% approved of mandated medication (Pescosolido et al., 1999). Follow-up surveys in the United States a decade later showed no significant changes in attitudes toward this legally coerced treatment for individuals with SUDs (Schnittker, 2008; Schomerus, 2014).

Whereas many research studies have examined explicit sources of stigma such as public stigma and structural discrimination, Kulesza et al. (2016) suggested that examining implicit sources of stigma may be a more accurate reflection of actual substance use stigma. The main reason for this recommendation was the impact of social desirability bias inherent to explicit measures of stigma. Implicit stigma, or self-stigma, can be greatly affected by the explicit sources of public stigma and structural discrimination. Self-stigmatization involves both emotional and cognitive components as the person applies negative beliefs about his or her disease or disorder, in this case substance use, to herself or himself (Schomerus, 2014). In fact, as an acquired disability, many individuals who develop substance use issues internalize previously held biases related to substance use in addition to experiencing outside sources of stigma (Smart, 2016). As Corrigan et al. (2006) reported, many individuals are aware of the stereotypes regarding their disability, and most even agree with them.

Self-stigma has an adverse effect on an individual's well-being, treatment efficacy, and willingness to seek treatment, and is thus a major barrier toward recovery (Kulesza et al., 2016; Mak et al., 2015, Schomerus, 2014). As the negative stereotypes about the disorder are integrated into the individual's sense of self, both self-esteem and self-efficacy are decreased, leading to consequences such as depressive symptoms, loss of morale, and an increased need for inpatient treatment (Link et al., 2001; Rusch et al., 2009; Schomerus, 2014). As noted by Mak et al. (2015), self-stigmatization often deters individuals from help seeking, treatment participation, and medication adherence while also increasing the risk for premature service termination.

In terms of wellness and quality of life, those with higher self-stigma demonstrate high levels of depression, emotional discomfort, and more severe psychiatric symptoms and demonstrate lower overall well-being, life satisfaction, attainment of personal goals, and levels of personal life meaning (Mak et al., 2015). High levels of shame, a construct relating closely to level of self-stigma, are positively associated with perceived stigma and sense of rejection and negatively associated with mental well-being and quality of life (Luoma et al., 2007). Further, if a substance is used as a coping strategy for shame, it can negatively affect recovery by increasing substance use, which in turn increases the level of experienced shame (Dearing et al., 2005; Luoma et al., 2012). Interestingly, Schomerus et al. (2011) linked the formation of these negative self-stereotypes with the individual's perceptions of the prevalence of negative stereotypes in the public. This aggregation of evidence suggests that the issue of self-stigma may be less of a dysfunctional cognition as it is typically perceived and more of a product of the societal and institutional stances taken on substance use (Mak et al., 2015; Schomerus, 2014).

Intersectionality of Substance Use Disorder and Other Marginalized Identities

When examining intersectionality and SUD, SUD itself (a type of disability) is one of the identity categories that leads to experiencing oppression, stigma, and discrimination. Further, when coupled with the status of another stigmatized group/minority identity, outcomes can be worse. Disability itself does not discriminate; anyone can acquire a disability at any point in life (regardless of age, race, gender, religious background, etc.) However, now that in the professional realm the currently adopted disability model is of a biopsychosocial nature, we understand that the prevalence or instance of disability for many conditions and categories occurs irrespective of one's (marginalized) identity(ies), but it is the actual lived experiences of a person with a disability that occur within and are informed by society that are sensitive to such identities.

Some intersecting identities that have been researched for people living with SUDs include race/ethnicity, gender, sexual orientation, old age, and socioeconomic position. In a 2016 study of implicit and explicit addiction stigma and how they differed among race/ethnicity and gender groups, Kulesza et al. found that gender was not associated with addiction-specific stigma in explicit or implicit forms. They did find, however, that race/ethnicity was. Specifically, Latinx and White people who injected drugs were more likely to be on the receiving end of implicit stigma (i.e., implicitly judged more often as "deserving punishment" than "deserving help"). This stigma was not evident in explicit measures (i.e., one of the items asked, "Do we punish this person or offer help?"). Meyers et al. (2021) did find evidence of gender being related to greater drug use–related stigma in a systematic review. They reviewed over 75 studies total, with 53% being quantitative by design and 47% qualitative. Interestingly, and perhaps somewhat like Kulesza et al.'s (2016) findings, the quantitative literature was inconsistent regarding associations between gender and drug use–related stigma: 55% of studies found no association between gender and drug use–related stigma, whereas 10% showed that women were more stigmatized and 5% showed it was men who were more stigmatized. The qualitative literature was far more consistent; 97% of the studies demonstrated that women experienced greater stigma.

Those who identify as lesbian, gay, or bisexual (LGB) have been found to experience higher suicidal ideation and SUD diagnoses than their heterosexual counterparts, and these disparities are often found to be greater when LGB individuals are Black or Hispanic. In their 2021 study, Kelly et al. found that White, Black, and Hispanic LGB men and women showed higher odds of suicidal ideation, SUD, and suicidal ideation coupled with SUD (occurring at the same time) than their same-race heterosexual peers—by rates of three times higher. Additionally, they found that Black and Hispanic LGB women had greater odds of SUD than White heterosexual women. These differences were not found among men.

Criminal Justice System Involvement

People with SUDs are much more likely to be involved with the criminal justice system, and many involved in the criminal justice system have drug and/or alcohol abuse histories (Moore et al., 2020). When offenses are drug- or alcohol-related (e.g., driving while intoxicated, selling drugs), offenders have an overwhelmingly higher chance of current or lifetime SUD diagnoses: approximately 22 times and 15 times, respectively (Moore et al., 2020). In a longitudinal study of over 1,200 African Americans, Green et al. (2020) found that long-term drug use (i.e., *duration* rather than *age of onset*) significantly predicted criminal offending over the life course. The individuals with long-term drug use had twice the risk of being arrested for property and violent crimes relative to those who "experimented" with drugs, and the long-term users had 4.5 times greater risk of being arrested for a drug-related offense compared to the experimenters.

People with SUD and women involved in the criminal justice system independently face many community participation and quality-of-life barriers, many of which may be due to stigma. This may certainly also be the case for women involved in the criminal justice system who also have a history of substance abuse. Between 40% and 72% of women involved in the criminal justice system have drug or alcohol abuse histories (Kopak & Smith-Ruiz, 2014). Many of these individuals claim that they were under the influence of some sort of substance when they committed the crimes that led to their imprisonment. Drug use has also been found to be implicated in approximately 25% of property offenses and 32% of drug-related offenses among incarcerated women who were under the influence of substances at the time of their arrest (Kopak & Smith-Ruiz, 2014).

People with SUDs who have a criminal background may be doubly disadvantaged when it comes to stigma, especially regarding seeking employment, where it is routine for employers to ask applicants about criminal history and require that they pass a drug test. Even if one does overcome the initial hurdle of securing a job, there may be stigma and legal barriers involved in maintaining it.

In summary, people with SUDs face many challenges, and stigma may be one of the most significant. Stigma can arise from many sources and manifest itself in many ways and settings. Individuals from certain minoritized and/or underprivileged backgrounds may be disproportionately impacted. Therefore, it is important to combat stigma to the maximum extent possible, and both legal protections and social justice/advocacy-oriented approaches may be useful in this.

CIVIL RIGHTS AND PROTECTIONS FOR AMERICANS WITH SUBSTANCE USE DISORDER

Federal civil rights laws prohibit discrimination against qualified "individuals with disabilities" in many areas of life. Individuals experiencing SUD or who are in recovery are, under specific conditions, considered individuals with a "disability" protected by the ADA (SAMHSA, 2007). In order to be protected under ADA, an individual must demonstrate that her or his SUD substantially limits or has substantially limited major life activities. The ADA also protects those who have been falsely believed to have or have had an SUD (Leslie et al., 2019; SAMHSA, 2007).

Limitations in the Protections for Individuals With Substance Use Disorder

SUD is considered a disability under the ADA, but under specific conditions. Section 104 of the ADA excludes all individuals who are actively using illegal drugs, but the ADA protects those who have gone through, or are currently in rehabilitation, as well as those who have been erroneously identified as substance users (ADA National Network, 2019). Additionally, people whose use of alcohol or drugs poses a direct threat—a significant risk of substantial harm—to the health or safety of others are not protected. People whose SUD does not, or has not in the past, significantly impaired a major life activity are also not covered (SAMHSA, 2007).

Legal and illegal substances are treated differently under the ADA. In the case of alcohol use, a person with an AUD is covered under the ADA and entitled to consideration of accommodation if they are qualified to perform the essential functions of the job but are not protected for any use of alcohol that affects job performance or renders the employee not "qualified" (ADA National Network, 2019; EEOC Technical Assistance Manual, 2002; Leslie et al., 2019). Similarly, someone taking a prescribed medication (such as opioid "painkillers") is protected so long as they are legally using the drug as prescribed for the underlying condition. If the person misuses or abuses the prescription, they may not be covered by the ADA. The ADA also covers those with a legal prescription for medication-assisted treatment, such as Suboxone, methadone, or Vivitrol (ADA National Network, 2019).

Active use of illegal substances is always excluded from ADA coverage; however, those who are "recovering," as defined by those not "currently" using substances and receiving treatment, and those who have successfully completed treatment are protected under ADA on the basis of their past SUD (ADA National Network, 2019; EEOC Technical Assistance Manual, 2002; Leslie et al., 2019). "Current" use has been legally defined as (a) testing positive on a drug test, so long as the test is accurate; (b) illegal use of drugs that has occurred recently enough to justify an employer's reasonable belief that involvement with drugs is an ongoing problem; and notably, (c) "current" is not limited to the day of use, or recent weeks or days, but is determined on a case-by-case basis (ADA National Network, 2019; EEOC Technical Assistance Manual, 2002).

Another group of laws are designed to target workplace substance use, an example of which is the Drug-Free Workplace Act of 1998 (Safety Management Clinic, 2008). This act applies to public entities and any private companies or individuals who are federal contractors and grantees, as well as "safety-sensitive industries." These industries include fields pertaining to public safety and national security, including employees in aviation, trucking, railroads, pipelines, and other transportation industries (Safety Management Clinic, 2008). Under the ADA, employers are legally prohibited from firing, refusing to hire, or promoting someone due to a history of substance use or if she or he is actively enrolled in a drug or alcohol program (Safety Management Clinic, 2008). Employers may not single out employees for drug testing due to an appearance of being under the influence of a substance, and employers may not ask employees about legal prescription drug use as part of a prehiring or prepromotion drug test (EEOC Technical Assistance Manual, 2002; Safety Management Clinic, 2008).

Legal Guidelines for Employment of Persons with Substance Use Disorder

Employers cannot deny a job to or fire a person because she or he is in treatment or in recovery for an SUD, unless the person's disorder would prevent safe and competent job performance (SAMHSA, 2007). An employer must, however, be willing to provide reasonable accommodations to employees with SUD, unless the accommodations would cause an "undue hardship" on the employer. Employers must also remember to maintain and ensure confidentiality with any medical-related information they attain regarding an employee, which includes information about past or present SUD (SAMHSA, 2007).

It is important to note that in the hiring process an employer cannot inquire about whether a person has or has had a disability and about the nature or severity of a disability. An employer is also restricted from asking if a job applicant has ever abused or been addicted to drugs or alcohol, or if an applicant is currently in or has previously been in an SUD treatment program (SAMHSA, 2007).

On the other hand, an employer is entitled to inquire if an applicant is currently using illegal drugs, drinks alcohol, or can perform the duties of the job. An employer is also entitled to make medical inquiries after making a job offer that include examinations that may reveal a past or present SUD, so long as all applicants offered employment are required to undergo the same examinations. Employment can be conditional based on the results of such inquiries and exams (SAMHSA, 2007).

TOWARD A PROGRAM OF RECOVERY

To assist individuals in managing SUD, treatment is critical. In this section, we review some of the available treatment options for SUD and discuss the idea of recovery as a holistic journey toward SUD management and overall wellness. Treatment programs can range from short-term, one-on-one outpatient counseling, to long-term residential treatment programs. The following is a brief explanation of the main types of available drug treatment programs in the United States (NIDA, 2018).

Types of Treatment Programs

A variety of treatment settings and modalities are regularly utilized to address SUD. Inpatient programs provide people living with SUD a temporary respite from their natural environments, which may be contributing factors in their ongoing substance use. Inpatient programs can be divided into long-term and short-term residential programs. Long-term facilities are often nonhospital based and provide 24/7 care, and the planned length of stay is generally between 6 and 12 months. Short-term facilities generally utilize 3- to 6-week treatment programs and are commonly found in hospital-based settings (NIDA, 2018).

Outpatient programs can provide a less costly alternative to residential facilities and can vary in length and intensity. The more intensive programs may last for several hours each day and are often referred to as intensive day treatment or partial hospitalization programs (PHPs). PHPs can be an entry point for individuals who then progress through treatment to frequent/intensive programs. Intensive outpatient programs (IOPs) are often the next "step" down from PHPs and meet for several hours, several times each week. Finally, outpatient treatment programs may offer an aftercare component where treatment is conducted less frequently (e.g., one session a week for 2 hours) to be a final "step down" from more intensive services. Outpatient programs often rely heavily on the use of group counseling, and many encourage or require participants to simultaneously attend peer support groups such as AA, NA, or Self-Management and Recovery Training (SMART) recovery (NIDA, 2018).

Principles of Effective Treatment

The National Institute on Drug Abuse (NIDA) has proposed many "Principles of Effective Treatment" for treating SUD (NIDA, 2018). Many of these principles speak to common misunderstandings or misperceptions about the origin of SUD and what constitutes effective treatment. These principles (available online at https://nida.nih.gov/publications/principles-drug-addiction-treatment-research-based-guide-third-edition) provide a basis for understanding what research has shown works and what does not necessarily work in SUD treatment (NIDA, 2018). There is no "one size fits all" approach to SUD, and even the best individualized treatment programs do not always work the first time around. The good news is people are capable of recovering and, despite occasional setbacks, individuals tend to find strategies for recovery that work for them over time.

What Is Recovery?

The concept of recovery often reflects the spectrum of beliefs about what it means for an individual with an SUD to "manage or control" SUD symptoms through treatment and/or abstinence. For example, SAMHSA's working definition of recovery as it pertains to the "health" domain is as follows:

> *Overcoming or managing one's disease(s) or symptoms—for example, abstaining from use of alcohol, illicit drugs, and non-prescribed medications if one has an addiction problem—and for everyone in recovery, making informed, healthy choices that support physical and emotional wellbeing.* (SAMHSA, 2012, p. 3)

The original definition of recovery, developed by those in recovery within AA, described a program that included abstinence from alcohol and/or the drug of choice and developing a new lifestyle via the 12-step program (Kaskutas et al., 2014). It is common to see abstinence as the ultimate goal of recovery, although recovery almost always also includes a restoration of functioning and a positive movement toward maximizing functioning and reaching one's "potential." Sobriety could be conceptualized as "remission" of SUD symptoms, meanwhile "recovery" should emphasize an individual's path to maximizing wellness and functioning (NIDA, 2022).

Whether an individual with an SUD can fully "recover" or achieve long-term remission continues to be debated. Several brain imaging studies provide support for the utility of abstinence in the recovery process. Studies of the effects of substance use on the brain have indicated that prolonged use can have detrimental consequences in cognitive functioning, neurotransmitter functioning, and general neurophysiological functioning. However, through sustained abstinence, some aspects of cognitive functioning can significantly improve within even the first 14 days, while other deficits tend to be more enduring and irreversible (Mon et al., 2014; Rosenbloom & Pfefferbaum, 2008; van Eijk et al., 2013). Evidence of neurophysiological recovery supports the notion of some form of recovery, whereas the lasting deficits further substantiate the disease model of addiction.

The Affordable Care Act (ACA) of 2010 encourages two major paradigm shifts in SUD treatment, including moving from a symptom/pathology focus to a recovery process that has a wellness orientation, as well as reconceptualizing SUD with chronic care models rather than using acute care measures (Kaskutas et al., 2014). These shifts reflect important movements to make treatment more holistic, destigmatize the recovery process and set much more realistic expectations for individuals in the recovery process (Kaskutas et al., 2014; SAMHSA, 2012).

These modern recovery models not only encourage individuals to manage SUD symptoms over their life span but also emphasize co-occurring condition management and overall physical wellness and nutrition, have a strength-based focus, encourage employment and access to stable housing, and utilize systems approaches that include family members in the treatment process. These models also emphasize multiple pathways to recovery (NIDA, 2022; SAMHSA, 2012), which leaves room for individuals who are engaged with treatment programs outside of the traditional 12-step treatment with AA/NA/CA (Cocaine Anonymous) involvement and leave room for including successful recovery programs that may not be total abstinence based or that emphasize elements of the hard reduction approach. Research on SUD has demonstrated that relapses are, unfortunately, common, and to view recovery from a binary success or failure lens reinforces feelings of guilt, shame, and failure associated with relapses and decreases chances that individuals will reengage with treatment and recovery in a timely manner (Sellman, 2010). Setbacks are part of the process, and having realistic expectations (both the individual with the SUD and their support system) is a critical element to a sustainable recovery program.

Evidence-Based Practices

There have been extensive research efforts to identify SUD treatment practices that are most likely to result in positive recovery outcomes. In the following paragraphs we list and discuss both medication-assisted treatments (MATs) and psychotherapy options that have been strongly supported by research to treat various types of SUD.

MEDICATION-ASSISTED TREATMENT

MAT is an effective strategy for treating individuals diagnosed with OUD. MAT is Food and Drug Administration (FDA) approved to assist individuals dealing with addiction to opioids, helping to normalize brain chemistry, block the euphoric effects of the drug, reduce cravings, and avoid negative withdrawal symptoms. Specific medications used in MAT for opioids include methadone, buprenorphine, and naltrexone. Research has consistently shown that these medications are most effective when administered in combination with counseling and other behavioral interventions. Several medications have also been FDA approved to treat AUD. Medications that have been approved to treat alcohol addiction include naltrexone, acamprosate, disulfiram, and topiramate (SAMHSA, 2022).

PSYCHOTHERAPIES

Several psychotherapeutic treatments have been identified as "evidence-based" either for the general population of those with SUDs or for specific subsets, such as for alcohol or tobacco use. To gain the "evidence-based" designation, these interventions have to show significant benefits to individuals with SUD through large series of randomized clinical trials (RCTs) across a broad base of representative population samples. These interventions include cognitive behavioral therapy (CBT), relapse prevention (RP), community reinforcement approach (CRA), contingency management (CM), motivational enhancement therapy (MET), motivational interviewing (MI), and brief interventions (BIs) for alcohol and tobacco use (Jhanjee, 2014; SAMHSA, 2022). While it is not within the purview of this chapter to go into detail about any of the specific evidence-based practices (EBPs) to treat SUD, the authors encourage professionals planning to work with consumers with SUD to pursue further training in one or more of these valuable modalities.

The Role of Housing in Recovery

Access to stable housing is a critical element of any comprehensive recovery plan. Unfortunately, homelessness continues to be an ongoing social concern in the United States, with over half a million Americans experiencing homelessness at any given time (SAMHSA, 2020b). Among those who are homeless in the United States, one-third are actively experiencing SUD-related issues and around two-thirds have a history of SUD (Dickson-Gomez et al., 2011; Wittman et al., 2017). Those who do not have access to stable housing are at risk for relapse of substance use and mental health concerns, increasing risk of HIV and other health problems, and have an increased mortality rate that is three times higher than individuals who have stable housing (Wittman et al., 2017). From an economic perspective, the U.S. Department of Housing and Urban Development (HUD) estimates that each individual who is homeless costs U.S. taxpayers an estimated $40,000 per year (over $200 billion in total) in costs associated with healthcare, criminal justice, and other expenses (Wittman et al., 2017).

Although there is a notable negative impact of homelessness on recovery, the inverse is also true; that is, access to stable housing is associated with many positive recovery outcomes, including fewer relapses, reduced criminal justice recidivism, better employment outcomes, and overall higher quality of life (Dickson-Gomez et al., 2011; SAMHSA, 2020b; Wittman et al., 2017). As many pathways to recovery exist, there is also no "one size fits all" model of affordable housing. Next, we will review the most widely cited affordable housing models, including Permanent Supportive Housing (PSH), Housing First (HF), and abstinence-based recovery housing, also known as Sober Living Homes (SLHs; SAMHSA, 2020b; Wittman et al., 2017).

PSH is a community-based approach that is specifically designed to assist individuals and families with chronic illnesses, disabilities, mental health issues, and/or SUD who have experienced long-term or repeated homelessness. PSH does this by offering long-term rental assistance and supportive case management services to those in the program (NAEH, 2022). PSH is part of the larger HF movement, which prioritizes finding access to stable housing for individuals regardless of the status of their current behavioral health concerns, including substance use. HF is based on the general idea that people's basic needs, like food and shelter, must be met before other issues can be addressed. As such, HF emphasizes consumer choice and service participation in an effort to increase consumer "buy-in" to services and improve recovery outcomes (NAEH, 2022; SAMHSA, 2020b; Wittman et al., 2017).

HF relies on extensive and individualized case management and supportive wrap-around services to meet each consumer's variety of personal and health-related needs. The HF model has shown promise in being a long-term solution; between 75% and 91% of individuals and families remain housed a year after engaging with the HF program (NAEH, 2022). Importantly, many of the participants in the HF programs engage with available supportive services, which have been shown to increase participation in job training programs, increase school attendance, reduce overall substance use rates, decrease instances of domestic violence, and reduce number of days hospitalized (NAEH, 2022; SAMHSA, 2020b; Wittman et al., 2017).

Recovery housing programs differ from HF approaches in that they are often grounded in the abstinence-based recovery paradigm and they tend to require attendance at self-help groups such as AA or NA. Other requirements may include participation in community and employment services in addition to SUD treatment. The four levels of recovery houses described by the National Association of Recovery Residences (NARR) include Oxford Housing, monitored SLHs, supervised housing, and residential treatment housing (SAMHSA, 2020b). These programs are often used as individuals transition out of residential or inpatient treatment back into the community. They focus on peer support, with many being run by individuals who themselves are in recovery, and they provide a social environment that emphasizes a "recovery lifestyle" and allows residents to "work their program" (Wittman et al., 2017).

Evidence generally supports the effectiveness of recovery housing programs. For example, studies examining the communal housing options, Oxford Houses, have shown that when compared to those who transition directly back into the community, those who lived in Oxford Housing had lower rates of substance use and criminal justice recidivism (SAMHSA, 2020b). Further, those living in SLHs have demonstrated positive rates of employment relative to those not in recovery housing (SAMHSA, 2020b; Wittman et al., 2017).

In 2020, HUD launched the Recovery Housing Program as part of the Support for Patients and Communities (SUPPORT) Act. This program is designed to provide stable, temporary housing for individuals in recovery from SUD. This provides additional federal funding and support to assist in development and continuance of housing programs for up to 2 years until the individual with the SUD is able to secure permanent housing (HUD, 2022). While these programs continue to show promise, there are several barriers and challenges that still need to be addressed. For example, there remains a strong social stigma toward housing supports as evidenced by NIMBY (not in my back yard) groups who seek to prevent local housing programs for individuals with SUD. Further, there remain zoning and transportation issues, particularly for the housing options that do not require sobriety, that place barriers for residents to accessing healthcare, employment opportunities, and other needed services (Wittman et al., 2017).

Harm Reduction Programs

Harm reduction is a term that encompasses programs and interventions whose goals are to minimize the negative consequences of health issues, including SUD. The caveat to harm reduction is that these programs do not require that the "problem behavior," substance use, for example, be ceased completely or permanently (Hawk et al., 2017; Marlatt, 1996). The idea is to meet the individual "where they are at" in order to minimize harmful impacts and restore as much functioning as is feasible as soon as possible. The foundation of modern harm reduction programs lies in responses to the hepatitis B and HIV outbreaks of the 1970s and 1980s (Hawk et al., 2017; Marlatt, 1996). Harm reduction programs for SUD include syringe exchange programs, safe injection facilities, overdose prevention programs and policies (e.g., NARCAN), HF programs, and opioid replacement therapies (Hawk et al., 2017).

Given the traditional abstinence-only approaches of SUD treatment in the United States, the presence of harm reduction programs has often been hotly debated. Those who oppose the programs argue that any programs that do not prioritize full sobriety do more harm than good to the individuals with substance issues and to the greater communities (Hawk et al., 2017). It is important to note that harm reduction programs do not discourage abstinence and also do not "attempt to minimize or ignore the real and tragic harm and danger that can be associated with illicit drug use" (NHRC, 2022, p. 2).

Over the years, studies examining the impact of harm reduction programs have generally affirmed their place within the SUD treatment framework. Harm reduction programs are feasible, effective, and cost-effective (Hawk et al., 2017). These interventions, which vary widely in target populations (e.g., teenagers, intravenous [IV] drug users, those at risk of opioid overdose) and goals (e.g., access to stable housing, reduction in overdose rates, reduction in public tobacco or alcohol use, reduction in transmission of bloodborne pathogens) are useful for reaching broad sections of the population and from an overall public health standpoint, improve public health and well-being and save lives (Huhn & Gipson, 2021).

Employment in the Recovery Framework

Alongside stable housing, employment has been consistently identified as one of the most critical factors in determining an individual's overall well-being and quality of life. Obtaining and retaining employment is especially important to individuals with SUD in the "recovery" process, as it has been shown to have a positive impact on quality of life, life satisfaction, overall health, social well-being, and personal acceptance of disability (Dunigan et al., 2014; Gold, 2004; Kerrigan et al., 2004; Roessler & Rumrill, 1998; Sprong et al., 2014). Maintaining employment decreases the chances of relapse for individuals in recovery and can provide vital supports to the recovery process.

Although structural discrimination, personal factors, and disease factors play a role in the high unemployment rates of individuals with SUD, the assumption that poor employment outcomes are strictly a result of these factors is insufficient (Baldwin et al., 2010). An advanced labor market analysis for individuals with SUDs shows that 20% of the employment gap and 30% of the wage gap relative to those without SUD is not explained by functional limitations and other productivity-related variables (Baldwin et al., 2010). This means that there are still workplace barriers that are preventing this largely underutilized workforce resource, people in recovery, from maximizing their potential. The stress, anxiety, and other affective and psychological consequences of workplace discrimination can also be triggers for relapse, compounding the problem even further (Sigurdsson et al., 2012).

Individuals with SUD may choose to file allegations of workplace discrimination with the Equal Employment Opportunity Commission (EEOC). A review of the workplace discrimination allegations under Title I of the ADA to the EEOC by Leslie et al. (2019) revealed that Americans with SUD report disproportionately higher numbers of allegations in the areas of discharge, hiring, and suspension relative to individuals with other disabling conditions.

STIGMA IN THE WORKPLACE

Individuals with substance use histories, or even those who merely report using alcohol or other drugs sometimes and recreationally, may be perceived as not having the necessary skills and competencies to be good employees. They may be perceived as dangerous and/or criminals who are untrustworthy, self-destructive, and lacking in job potential (Niewegloski et al., 2017; Roche et al., 2019). These concerns and stereotypes typically arise from false understandings and misperceptions about drug and alcohol use/abuse, value judgements about substance use, and potential future consequences for the workplace (Roche et al., 2019). Most of these notions are unfounded assumptions, but others may have some merit and be derived from credible sources. In his now-dated 1986 executive order to create a drug-free workplace, U.S. President Ronald Reagan wrote "federal employees who use illegal drugs, on or off duty, tend to be less productive, less reliable, and prone to greater absenteeism than their fellow employees who do not use illegal drugs" (Roche et al., 2019, p. 180).

SUD-related stigma can affect potential and current employees in several domains such as hiring, promotion, benefits, and everyday social interactions, and they affect more people than one would think. Consistent with overall SUD prevalence rates, Bush and Lipari (2015) reported that nearly 1 in 10 (9.5%) of full-time employees met the criteria for SUD in the previous year, and, among American workers, 15% reported using illicit drugs, 34% reported engaging in recent binge-drinking, and 9% reported heavy alcohol use in the past month (SAMHSA, 2016). McMahon (2012) reported that the "overwhelming" majority of cases of workplace discrimination are not related to job acquisition, but rather job retention or the (perceived) quality of one's work. In other words, people with SUD or those who use and/or abuse (il)licit drugs are more likely to lose their jobs due to stigma rather than be denied the opportunity for a job, even though some may still encounter the barrier of a job interviewer thinking "if they're an addict then they're already disqualified" (Leslie et al., 2019; Leslie et al., 2022; Nieweglowski et al., 2017, p. 5).

SUD-related stigma on the job, when employers and/or coworkers know about one's substance use history, can directly lead to one losing their job—for example, the employer fires them—but also indirectly. For someone with an SUD who is already working, the SUD-related stigma can negatively impact their overall work experiences, performance, mental health, social interactions, promotional opportunities, pay/salary, and broader career trajectories (Roche et al., 2019). Further, there are certain work cultures/environments where substance use/abuse is accepted or encouraged: areas such as food service; arts, entertainment, and recreation; and management have been found to have the most prevalent illicit drug use rates (Leslie et al., 2022), while other workplace conditions may lead to greater use, such as stressful and isolated environments, low levels of supervision and work visibility, high mobility, and low job satisfaction (Roche et al., 2019).

There are many workplace policies that address SUD, and some are fair and just, whereas others focus on punishing users. The latter is likely to lead to higher overall workplace SUD stigmatization, whereas other policies that emphasize and embrace methods for sensitively and appropriately addressing SUD, along with providing information on treatment and resources for users (Roche et al., 2019), are less likely to lead to stigmatization. In addition to these approaches, other ways to combat stigma include educating employers and employees on SUD, being open and willing to explore and provide reasonable accommodations to employees with SUD, and exposure, such as asking employers to provide testimonials on former individuals with SUDs they hired who turned out to be quality employees.

IMPORTANCE OF EFFECTIVE WORKPLACE POLICIES

Having an effective system in place to get employees who need treatment headed in the right direction requires an organized and systematic approach to employing individuals with SUD and training both employees and supervisors to "buy in" to the proactive culture. The Substance Abuse and Mental Health Services Administration (SAMHSA; an agency within the U.S. Department of Health and Human Services) provides free and extensive resources and toolkits to employers on how to build effective drug-free workplace programs.

SAMHSA's (2020a) step-by-step process begins with building a representative drug-free workplace team, holistically assessing workplace needs and culture around substances, developing a detailed workplace policy, implementing the program on multiple organizational levels, continually evaluating the program for effectiveness, making quality improvements, and finally providing support and guidance along the way. It is critical to remember that, based on an organization's specific workplace needs, every drug-free workplace policy and program will need to be customized to specifically fit the needs of all the stakeholders. With that in mind, we want to make some universal recommendations for identifying and addressing substance use in the workplace.

One of the biggest takeaways from research on drug-free workplace programs is that employers who invest in a program (Employee Assistance Program [EAP], mental health programs, etc.) that provides screening and referral services consistently see better results for employees and increased cost savings over time. Ideally, this service provides both confidential screening and brief interventions for SUD. The confidentiality of the screenings should be reinforced. The screenings can be short in nature, such as using the four-item CAGE-AID screener (SAMHSA, 2020a). Based on the screening, brief interventions can be provided or referrals to more intensive, in-network services can be made. Brief interventions have shown high success rates for catching alcohol abuse early on and have shown promising results for preventing drug abuse from progressing into a full-blown disorder (SAMHSA, 2020a). Confidential aftercare follow-ups can be an effective tool for checking in with employees and ensuring that their long-term needs are being met.

Drug testing can also be a critical resource for identifying substance use in the workplace and maintaining a safe work atmosphere. Several studies have shown that drug testing can significantly lower the incidence of workplace injuries (NSC, 2020). If you are required or choose to make drug testing an integral part of your workplace policy, we recommend using a lab that is certified by HHS, consulting with a legal team and staying current with implications of the changing legislative landscape, using testing that respects employee confidentiality and integrity, having an established written policy about substance use in the workplace, ensuring that results are absolutely confidential, and being consistent with response to workers who test positive (NSC, 2020). Given the current impact of prescription opioids, it is recommended that the tests use more than the traditional five-panel tests to ensure prescription drugs, like oxycontin, can also be identified. Finally, it is important to educate employees on the rationale behind drug testing and develop a culture around drug testing being a critical component of maintaining a safe and injury-free workplace that is beneficial to all employees.

Just having a program in place or utilizing an EAP is not enough. Many employers with EAPs struggle to get individuals into treatment, even with services. This is where decreasing stigma and raising awareness in the workplace becomes critical to employees being willing to ask for help and understanding where to go for help. It is worth reiterating that if an employee fears disciplinary action or retaliation for substance-related issues, they are more likely to attempt to conceal any signs. This goes hand in hand with having a confidential process set up for employees to seek help and ensuring that employees and supervisors are educated on appropriate channels to report any potential warning signs they observe.

It is recommended that, as part of this education process, supervisors and employees be trained on the signs or warning indicators that someone may be experiencing SUD-related issues. The best way to create a drug-free workplace is by instituting more preventative measures to catch potential SUD issues before they happen. The Job Accommodation Network (JAN, 2022) has provided a guide to accommodation and compliance for employees with SUD. This includes an extensive list of behaviors that can be considered "warning signs" for potential SUD-related issues (https://askjan.org/disabilities/Drug-Addiction.cfm).

When signs are recognized, broaching the subject of substance abuse with an employee can be a daunting task. The Society for Human Resource Management (SHRM) recommends addressing performance or conduct concerns, perhaps within the context of a performance review if timely, as this can open the door for more candid discussions about substance-related struggles an employee may be having. It also allows the supervisor an opportunity to understand the context of what is being observed. For example, an employee might disclose that she or he has been dealing with the loss of a loved one or stressful family issues at home. At this point the employer or supervisor can have conversations about available options for treatment, accommodations, or even potential leave options. Employers and supervisors should be clear about expectations going forward and potential ramifications of the employee maintaining current behavior patterns (SHRM, 2020).

DISCLOSURE AND WORKPLACE ACCOMMODATIONS

Despite having reassurances of confidentiality and available treatment, employees may still be reluctant to disclose SUD-related issues for fear of punitive measures or retaliation or, in many cases, because they may be in denial of the symptoms they are experiencing. Unfortunately, lack of acceptance or awareness of symptoms is a common barrier to treatment for individuals with SUD. Further, if the individuals are aware of their own symptoms, they may still be sensitive to the stigma of being labeled an addict or an alcoholic.

Employers who create a culture of confidential and fair treatment of employees, as well as an awareness and acceptance of SUD as a disease, rather than a moral failing, are the most likely to have employees who are willing to disclose SUD and utilize treatment options (SAMHSA, 2020a; SHRM, 2020). Once again, when an employee discloses an SUD diagnosis, they should be presented with options for treatment, accommodations, and clear and reasonable expectations for behaviors and consequences for any continued performance issues or substance use.

In terms of accommodations, JAN (2022) provides a list of questions they recommend that employers looking to accommodate employees with SUD consider. Accommodations for employees for SUD may address specific cognitive/neurological limitations, such as inattention, stress intolerance, or other executive functioning deficits. Accommodations for people with SUD commonly include time flexibility that allows attendance to counseling and support meetings, which may include extended lunch breaks or time off. Building in natural supports within the workplace facilitates workplace success, and one idea for doing so is setting up a peer support program for employees who are in recovery.

Part of developing an employee accommodation plan is determining if any transitional work opportunities are available to the employee. This is especially relevant for safety-sensitive work positions where fitness to return to work may be considered a liability and safety concern. If an employee is out of work to complete intensive training, the goal should be to get them back onto the worksite as soon as feasible, even if on a part-time or transitional basis. This information can be outlined in a written return-to-work agreement plan clarifying expectations and any consequences. Spending time off work and off-site is generally not helpful in advancing employee recovery efforts (National Business Group on Health, 2009; SAMHSA, 2020a).

CONCLUSION

In conclusion, SUD is a chronic-relapsing condition that can significantly impact an individual's physical and mental functioning, their relationships with family and friends, and their communities as a whole. A pervasive component of SUD is substance-related stigma. People living with SUD experience high degrees of stigma from themselves, others around them, the general public, and public policy and legislation. This stigma manifests itself in the form of stereotypes and discrimination, and it is these negative attitudes and stereotypes toward those living with SUD that contribute to the multitude of barriers they face in attempting to manage SUD symptoms and enter "recovery." Recovery itself is a complex idea that encapsulates both direct symptom management and other life activities directed at preventing future relapses. Effectively treating SUD and assisting someone in their recovery involves utilizing evidence-based individual and group counseling practices, emphasizing social and peer support, assisting individuals in securing access to stable employment and housing, and removing barriers to recovery through advocacy and psychoeducation.

CLASS ACTIVITIES

1. Explore the interactive web page "Mouse Party" (https://learn.genetics.utah.edu/content/addiction/mouse) to learn about the ways different substances affect the brain.

2. Watch a film that depicts someone with an alcohol or drug problem. If the film includes multiple people who have one, choose one character. Watch their behavior in

the film closely. Review the *DSM-5* diagnostic criteria for SUD provided in this chapter and determine if you would diagnose this person with an SUD. How many of the criteria would you say that they meet? How severe is their SUD? Some film suggestions (instructors may want to review content of film on the Internet Movie Database website [IMDb] before choosing what to show/assign):

a. *28 Days* (2000)

b. *Basketball Diaries* (1995)

c. *Crazy Heart* (2009)

d. *Days of Wine and Roses* (1962)

e. *Everything Must Go* (2010)

f. *Flight* (2012)

g. *Leaving Las Vegas* (1995)

h. *The Lost Weekend* (1945)

i. *Requiem for a Dream* (2000)

j. *Scarface* (1983)

k. *Smashed* (2012)

l. *Trainspotting* (1996)

m. *When a Man Loves a Woman* (1994)

3. Explore SUD stigma. Ask students to write down on a small slip of paper one or more biases they may hold toward people with SUD. Assure them that there is nothing wrong with holding these biases. Ask students to write their comments anonymously and then drop their slips of paper into a hat. Draw papers out of the hat and discuss them with the class as a whole, or you may wish to assign students homework to explore a stereotype or bias further, perhaps even asking them to search for any evidence that refutes a stereotype.

4. Encourage students to attend an Alcoholics Anonymous (AA) or Narcotics Anonymous (NA) meeting. (May be for extra credit, or consider having this be an assignment for the class.) Students may be asked to discuss or write about their perceptions.

KEY REFERENCES

Only key references appear in the print edition. The full references appear in the digital product on Springer Publishing Connect™: https://connect.springerpub.com/content/book/978-0-8261-5111-7/part/partIV/chapter/ch17

ADA National Network. (2019). *The ADA, addiction, and recovery.* ADA National Network: Information, Guidance, and Training on the Americans with Disabilities Act. https://adata.org/factsheet/ada-addiction-and-recovery

Gold, P. B. (2004). Some obstacles to employment for persons with chronic substance use disorders inadequate federal-state vocational rehabilitation (VR) services. *Substance Use & Misuse, 39*(14), 2631–2636. https://doi.org/10.1081/LSUM-200034674

Lusk, S. (2018). Predictors of successful vocational rehabilitation closure among individuals with substance and alcohol use disorder: An analysis of Rehabilitation Services Administration data from 2010-2014. *Alcoholism Treatment Quarterly, 36*(1), 1–14. https://doi.org/10.1080/07347324.2017.1420433.

Sellman, D. (2010). The 10 most important things known about addiction. *Addiction, 105*(1), 6–13. https://doi.org/10.1111/j.1360-0443.2009.02673.x

Sprong, M. E., Melvin, A., Dallas, B., & Koch, D. S. (2014). Substance abuse and vocational rehabilitation: A survey of policies & procedures. *Journal of Rehabilitation Journal of Rehabilitation, 80*(4), 4–9.

CHAPTER 18

CULTURALLY COMPETENT SERVICE PROVISION: CONSIDERATIONS FOR SUPPORTING VETERANS AND FAMILY REINTEGRATION

KELLIE FORZIAT-PYTEL AND CHRISTINA DILLAHUNT-ASPILLAGA

LEARNING OBJECTIVES

After reading this chapter, you will be able to:

- Understand military culture and experiences of veterans and their families
- Assess the cultural context of relationships, issues, and trends within military populations
- Identify current literature on effective theories, techniques, and interventions that support community reintegration and employment of veterans and their families
- Know community resources that are available to assist military veterans and/or their families within their community

PRE-READING QUESTIONS

1. Do you recognize and understand the key components of military culture?
2. Are you able to describe common military experiences as they relate to mental health and physical health consequences?
3. Can you locate appropriate treatment and resources (e.g., mental health, financial) that specifically support the needs of veterans and their families?

According to the Defense Manpower Data Center (DMDC), current trends indicate there were around 1.3 million ($N = 1,358,761$) active- duty service members in 2022 across Army ($n = 466,897$), Navy ($n = 343,079$), Air Force/Space Force ($n = 332,703$), and Marine Corps ($n = 175,009$) subcomponents (DMDC, 2022). The total number of veterans is even higher; there are over 19 million U.S. veterans, and this population represents 7% of the adult U.S. population (U.S. Department of Veterans Affairs [VA], 2021a). The military is a unique culture that is very different from its civilian counterpart. Military culture has its own values, virtues, beliefs, customs, language, laws, and job titles (Exum et al.,

2011; Goldenberg et al., 2012; Goodale et al., 2012; Hall, 2016), and these elements can impact how individuals think, behave, and live. Service members are held to high standards in this culture that is comprises discipline, order, loyalty, and self-sacrifice and where great importance is given to historic traditions and ceremonies, ethos, the military mission, and group cohesion (Goodale et al., 2012; Hall, 2016; Pryce et al., 2012). Subcultures exist and are dependent on the branch of service (i.e., Air Force, Army, Marines, Navy, Coast Guard, and Space Force) the individual was associated with and their era of service. For example, the war climate for those serving during Operation Enduring Freedom (OEF; Afghanistan in 2001), Operation Iraqi Freedom (OIF; Iraq in 2003), or Operation New Dawn (OND; Iraq in 2010) looked very different than the war climate for those who had served in WWI (started in 1914), WWII (started in 1939), or the Vietnam War (started in 1960). The combat environment for Iraq and Afghanistan wars included artillery fire, roadside bombs, improvised explosive devices, grenades, and sniper attacks (Spelman et al., 2012). These types of weapons and attacks lead to more injuries such as wounds, orthopedic injuries, burns, hearing loss, and traumatic brain injuries (TBIs; Grieger et al., 2006). These outcomes have led to a multitude of mental health problems and psychosocial issues among OEF/OIF/OND veterans. Understanding military culture is paramount to being able to facilitate the counseling process (Hoge, 2011). Military identity may influence one's core sense of self and may impact how one relates to others, one's behaviors, how one dresses, the language(s) one uses, and one's expectations of self (Prosek et al., 2018).

Counseling services may be needed by service members, veterans, and military-connected families and significant others at any stage of military service (e.g., basic training, deployment, after leaving military service). This chapter focuses on (a) the cultural context of relationships, issues, and trends in relation to veteran and family reintegration; (b) current literature on effective theories, techniques, and interventions that can be utilized when working with veterans and their families; and (c) community resources that are available to support military veterans and/or their families as they assimilate into their civilian communities and the civilian workforce.

MILITARY CULTURE: THE CONTEXT OF RELATIONSHIPS, ISSUES, AND TRENDS IN RELATION TO REINTEGRATION

Military culture is composed of a distinct organizational structure and has specific values, beliefs, laws, traditions, language, and experiences (Hall, 2016; Prosek et al., 2018; Redmond et al., 2015). The responsibilities of service members affect all areas of their lives, including how much time service members can spend with their families (Cancio, 2018; Hall, 2016; Meyer et al., 2017). Common positive experiences of veterans and service members include consistent support sources and benefits such as financial incentives, educational funds, and discount programs (Military OneSource, 2022a; National Academies of Sciences, Engineering, and Medicine, 2019). However, the costs of service commitment are considerable. Service also means relocation, frequent separations for a mission, and dangerous and unpredictable work environments (e.g., combat deployments; Booth et al., 2007; Meyer et al., 2017; Sayer et al., 2014). Within the past 20 years of U.S. military overseas contingency operations, 2.77 million troops have been deployed, for a total of over 5.4 million deployments (Wenger et al., 2018). The rate and frequency of deployments are a significant consideration for military mental health professionals, as deployments are associated with challenging mental health outcomes for service members and their loved ones (Cogan et al., 2018; Meadows et al., 2018).

The military population, those currently serving and veterans, can experience a variety of mental health and wellness challenges. Ongoing military mental health issues, rising rates of posttraumatic stress disorder (PTSD), substance misuse, and domestic and community violence among service members have been identified (Hoge et al., 2004, 2006). Deployments are a distinguishing aspect of military service and can contribute to many of the negative consequences of service, including those described. Counselors and other healthcare providers can be an effective support for the military service member, veteran, or any family members who are struggling at any point of the deployment cycle (D'Aroust & Rossiter, 2021; Hall, 2016; Snyder & Monson, 2012). In addition, family readiness groups (FRGs) are available to help create social support systems during deployments. FRGs find ways to improve the flow of information and enhance the resiliency and well-being of service members and their families through the use of practical tools. There are also specific programs (e.g., Families OverComing Under Stress) and organizations (e.g., National Military Family Association [NMFA]) that can assist and support families during times of need.

Deployments

Military deployments can be thought of as forces moving to "active-combat zones and regions identified in multinational partnerships" (Prosek et al., 2018, p. 96). During this time, the service member separates from his or her family for a lengthy period to complete a specific mission (U.S. Department of Defense [DoD], 2012). Missions are categorized as combat (e.g., to uphold peace and security) or noncombat experiences (e.g., search and rescue, development of equipment; Military.com, 2022). Deployments typically occur in phases to encompass the time when official deployment orders are given until the service member returns after the deployment experience (DoD, 2012). Scholars have aligned these phases with "emotional stages" of a deployment (Morse, 2006; Pincus et al., 2001) to depict the common reactions experienced by the service member and their dependents or close others (if applicable). Conceptualizing the stages of a deployment and examining how each one impacts the family members may help mental health professionals as they work with military families.

EMOTIONAL STAGES OF DEPLOYMENT

The emotional stages of deployment include predeployment, deployment, sustainment, redeployment, and postdeployment. (Pincus et al., 2001). Each stage brings challenges for the service member and his or her family members (Cole, 2012). During predeployment, the service member and his or her family members are prophesying about what is to come. This stage often creates anxiety for all of the family members as they prepare for separation (Pincus et al., 2001). Family members may also feel angry, lonely, and rejected by the service member, who is preparing for their mission (Pincus et al., 2001), and arguments could arise or be more prevalent between family members (Pincus et al., 2001; Vogt et al., 2011). The deployment phase is when the physical separation occurs. Increased emotional stress and feelings of sadness, anger, numbness, loneliness, and abandonment are likely to occur for the family members who are left behind (Pincus et al., 2001). The separation may be more or less difficult depending on how much support the stay-behind family members have. The sustainment stage relates to a new normal for the family as the family members begin to restructure processes and find new supports (Pincus et al., 2001). Communication is a critical component during this stage, as the family members left behind are often waiting for the service member to contact them. Depending on the level of communication, feelings of sadness, worry, and frustration may occur (Pincus et al., 2001). In the redeployment stage, the family is anticipating the return (often the month before homecoming) of the service member (Pincus et al., 2001). During this time, family members often experience a mix of emotions such as joy and nervousness as the service member and family must understand what has changed since the deployment and consider how life may be different as a result of the service member being back home (Pincus et al., 2001). The postdeployment stage is when service members and their families reunite. The family must work together to reintegrate (Paley et al., 2013). Following deployment, military families are at their highest risk for dissolution (Negrusa & Negrusa, 2014).

Despite deployments being a time of oscillating feelings for military families, it can also be a time to grow together and strengthen the family unit (Saltzmann et al., 2013). Often individuals are surprised by their resilience.

Active-Duty Status, Experience, and Family Impact

Like all cultures, individuals connected to the military experience positives and negatives in relation to well-being and functioning (e.g., mental health, physical health, social). This section provides a look at the common experiences of the service member; of the immediate family, which is composed of military spouses/partners and children; of the secondary family members (e.g., parents/grandparents of the service member and his or her spouse/partner); and of friends.

SERVICE MEMBER

Service members are dedicated to serving their country. Common reasons service members join the military include family tradition, benefits, the warrior identity, and as an escape from their current lives (Hall, 2016). Service members quickly feel pride in their training and positions. Military life, due to training and demands such as unpredictable work schedules and moving requirements, is not easy, and one of the hardest parts of living the military life is to balance work responsibilities with efforts to form and maintain relationships (Clever & Segal, 2013). Service members in intimate relationships (i.e., have partners) must make challenging decisions regarding commitment and how to maintain a relationship despite physical separation (Clever & Segal, 2013). For service members who have spouses and children, they may feel distress due to conflicting responsibilities to their units and families in times of need (Lester & Flake, 2013). The service member is always balancing his or her unpredictable career and his or her roles at home. For example, service members are likely to miss family gatherings and milestones, since the military comes first (Hall, 2016).

Research that focuses on veterans and service members in the role of a mother is limited. However, service member mothers have been found to experience symptoms of distress, depression, and anxiety throughout the deployment cycle at rates higher than males. They also have high feelings of disengagement from their family during reintegration. Service member mothers also tend to have had greater rates of childhood trauma histories when compared to their male counterparts. In fact, service member mothers who have experienced (a) deployment separation, (b) combat exposure, and (c) adverse childhood experiences, or these things in some combination, are at greater risk for posttraumatic stress and depression symptomatology. This situation can adversely impact the quality and nature of their parent–child relationship and parenting style (Acker et al., 2020; Groer et al., 2016).

Service members see behavior and emotional changes throughout their transitions (e.g., deployment, reunions, retirement; Graf et al., 2011; Pincus et al., 2001; Pryce et al., 2012; Sayers et al., 2009). Research highlights the negative consequences of service and the resulting issues that service members face such as mental health issues (e.g., PTSD, depression), relationship issues (e.g., marriage and parent–child relationship disruptions), and transition issues (e.g., building a new identity and finding new employment after service; Ormeno et al., 2020). Despite the negatives, there are many positive aspects of service, such as a sense of duty, elite training, consistent benefits (e.g., housing allowances, medical care), a sense of community and belonging, and world traveling experiences (Hall, 2016).

SPOUSE

Military spouses are committed to the same serving commitment as their service member. Complex variations in relationship experiences have been found in research for military couples; some relationships experience disorder during deployment and reintegration; however, others flourish

(Bowen et al., 2013). Unique adversities are characteristic of military life that show wide-ranging coping responses (Bakhurst et al., 2017). During military life, spouses often experience challenges with (a) finding and maintaining employment, (b) parenting and child care responsibilities, and (c) platonic and supportive relationships due to continuous relocations and being separated from their service member spouse (DeVoe & Ross, 2012; Drummet et al., 2003; Hall, 2016). When the service member leaves, the spouse functions in a single-parent household (Gladding, 2015); the military spouse is expected to maintain child care responsibilities and routines (DeVoe & Ross, 2012). Marital distress is common throughout the different stages of deployment (Monk et al., 2018; Pincus et al., 2001), and the at-home parent often experiences other strong and fluctuating emotions, such as depression, stress, anxiety, anger, denial, resentment, resilience, and independence (Davis et al., 2012; Monk et al., 2019; Morse, 2006; Pincus et al., 2001; Wilson & Murray, 2016). A spouse's ability to function successfully at home may influence the service member's well-being during deployments (Pincus et al., 2001; Pittman et al., 2004) and affect how well children cope (Huebner et al., 2009). Infidelity is a common concern among the military couple due to tense separations and homecoming adjustments (Snyder et al., 2011). During reintegration, military spouses may be at risk for mental health issues (e.g., depression) when service members return with their own exacerbated mental health concerns (e.g., PTSD symptomatology; Walter et al., 2021). On a positive note, military spouses report the time apart can be time used to appreciate one another (Newby et al., 2005) and to learn how to adapt and be independent (Hall, 2016; Pincus et al., 2001). Spouses also have access to consistent benefits (e.g., medical care, lower- cost shopping and entertainment) and can become part of a strong military community of friendship and support. In addition, laws have been passed that can expedite employment and accreditation for military spouses (e.g., Military Spouse Interstate License Recognition Options, Department of Labor, 2022). There are also a variety of scholarships available for education and career development (Military OneSource, 2022b).

CHILDREN

Military children are regularly adapting to new homes, schools, communities, and family separations (Clever & Segal, 2013). Most of the existing research on children from military families focuses on symptoms of anxiety and depression. The age of the child is a significant factor that relates to his or her ability to cope with the separation and the changes that situation elicits and with the reunion. Developing attachments with the service member may be compromised, so difficulties during reunions could increase (Creech et al., 2014; Creech & Misca, 2017). For example, some children may not understand the circumstances for why a parent leaves, and others may not recognize their returning parent (DeVoe & Ross, 2012). Child maltreatment may become a factor or may increase. These situations could result from the extra stress placed on the parent who is not deployed (Creech et al., 2014).

For young children (3–6 years old), paternal perceived threat during deployment was significantly associated with mother-reported child adjustment and behavior concerns (Hajal et al., 2020). Older children may worry about their deployed parent in terms of safety and well-being (Bello-Utu & DeSocio, 2015), and they typically have more responsibilities than their nonmilitary family peers. This circumstance can be positive, as the youth has opportunities for increased maturity that can lead to positive achievements in social and academic domains (Park, 2011). However, negative reactions are also common. For example, teenagers may be resentful of the service member for being absent in their life (Lester & Flake, 2013) and may experience changes in temperament or interest and performance in school (Chandra et al., 2010; Engel et al., 2010; Lyle, 2006; Pincus et al., 2001). Difficulties in child sleep associated with parent deployment are also noted; researchers suggest that understanding and altering sleep patterns (e.g., helping children fall asleep and stay asleep) could mitigate children's mental health symptoms and increase their emotional well-being (So et al., 2018). Other research has focused on the impact on the health and well-being of children who have injured parents with complex comorbidities (e.g., PTSD, TBI). Rates of preventive care visits for these children often decrease, while rates of visits for injuries, maltreatment, mental health care, and psychiatric medication use increase (Hisle-Gorman et al., 2019). However, military life can also be a positive experience for children. Exposure to different cultures, peoples, and experiences can increase children's self-confidence and ability to accept diversity, can offer a sense of belonging to a community that has a specific culture, and can provide access to educational benefits and lower- cost child care (Hall, 2016).

SIGNIFICANT OTHERS

Research that focuses on the impact military service can have on significant others, such as romantic partners, is limited. Romantic partners of service members are typically not acknowledged or supported via benefits by any DoD organization (NMFA, 2016). Unmarried military partners are viewed as temporary by many individuals in the military (Mewes, 2012); however, these people still experience the trauma and deployment-related stress that accompanies a loved one being in military service just like married partners do (Monk et al., 2018). Married couples report that military service changes the individual family members and the family dynamics, and these changes were noted years after the deployments were over. Though many couples reported continuous struggles with disturbances related to deployment, some couples noted growth in their relationships several years later (Freytes et al., 2017). While limited research is available relating to the effects of military service on parents or friends of service members, stressors for these individuals are also similar. Military partners, parents, and friends of military service members likely face similar challenges regarding the military lifestyle related to moves, separations, and mission- first mindsets as they strive to stay connected (Hall, 2016; Snyder & Monson, 2012). Approximately 50% of active- duty military service members are unmarried but have close relationships with people (i.e., parents, siblings, significant others, and friends) who cannot access the military-provided information and support services (Keyes, 2011). However, today, depending on the military support program, some information and support services may be available (e.g., Military Parent Network) to these individuals.

VETERAN STATUS AND TRANSITION TO CIVILIAN LIFE

A veteran is a person who served in the active military, naval, or air service and who was discharged or released under conditions other than dishonorable (United States Code 38 [38 U.S. Code § 101]). Honorable discharges indicate that the service member met the required elements in their contract and can receive benefits through the VA. Those who do not receive honorable discharges are not eligible for benefits. A service member may choose to retire from the military based on several factors such as contract, age, or years of service (RAND Corporation, 2011). Benefits are granted for those who retire through the VA, and examples of these benefits include the following: medical care, life insurance, disability compensation, housing grants, and education benefits (U.S. Department of Veterans Affairs, 2021b). Many service members' transition to the civilian world includes moving to a more permanent location, obtaining a civilian career, or going back to school. For those who transition to higher education, the Serviceman's Readjustment Act of 1944, commonly known as the GI Bill, will pay for most of the education expenses (e.g., textbooks, tuition; U.S. Department of Veterans Affairs, 2022a).

The decision for someone to separate, or retire, from the military can be difficult and may pose challenges. Appropriate, accessible family support for veterans and their families is critical. Separation from the military impacts the whole family, and many individuals may experience a form of culture shock (U.S. Department of Veterans Affairs, 2022d), as this transition often necessitates an adaptation from a highly regimented lifestyle to a less structured lifestyle and from a culture of teamwork to a more individualistic identity. Veteran community reintegration is a national VA priority, and efforts to support this can be seen at federal, state, and local levels (Elnitsky & Kilmer, 2017).

Common life issues that veterans may need to navigate during retirement and integration into civilian life include (a) relating to civilians who do not understand military service, (b) reconnecting with their families and reestablishing their role in their families, (c) entering the work force (i.e., looking for, applying to, and interviewing for civilian jobs) or returning to an old job position where knowledge and skills may have changed, (d) creating structure since there will no longer be a chain of command that tells the service member what to do, (e) adjusting to a new pace of life and work, and (f) establishing basic necessities (e.g., clothing, housing) and services (e.g., doctor, dentist, counselor; U.S. Department of Veterans Affairs, 2021).

Mental Health and Physical Health Concerns

Individuals who have served in more recent conflicts (e.g., Iraq, Afghanistan) are more likely to endure physical and mental health impairments compared to those who served in earlier eras due to different war contexts (e.g., Epstein et al., 2010; Owens et al., 2007). Approximately 1 in 4 active duty military members show signs of a mental health condition (National Alliance on Mental Health, 2023). Diagnoses of anxiety, depression, and PTSD are seen at higher rates among active- duty and veteran service members compared to the general civilian population (Meadows et al., 2012). Mental health diagnoses of adjustment disorder, alcohol use disorder, anxiety disorders, depressive disorders, insomnia, personality disorders, PTSD, and substance use disorders continue to increase in these two groups (Defense Health Agency, 2022a). About 41% of post-9/11 veterans presented with a need for mental health care (National Academies of Sciences, Engineering, and Medicine, 2018) due to symptoms they experienced while serving that impaired their everyday functioning (e.g., hypervigilance, social impairment, agitation, sleeping issues, guilt). PTSD is often associated with an increased risk for psychiatric comorbidity and decreased psychosocial functioning (Hefner & Rosenheck, 2019; Pietrzak et al., 2010). The prevalence of PTSD in military-connected individuals varies across service eras (Gradus, 2021). For veterans who served in the post-9/11 era, the prevalence of PTSD is estimated to be between 11% and 20% (Gradus, 2021). Veterans are 1.5 times more likely to die by suicide compared to individuals who have never been in the military (U.S. Department of Veterans Affairs, 2019a). Though for many military-connected individuals, PTSD has been linked to increased suicide risk (McKinney et al., 2017) and ideation, research indicates that PTSD, suicidal ideation (SI), and suicide attempts (SAs) may likely be the result of a myriad of comorbid risk factors (e.g., depression) and other trauma-related consequences (e.g., low social support; Lemaire & Graham, 2011). While treatment can be effective in helping to manage PTSD and co-occurring symptoms, service members show low utilization of treatment options and programs and/or are likely to drop out of treatment plans (Hoge et al., 2014).

From 2000 to 2021, approximately 454,000 veterans were diagnosed with a TBI (U.S. Department of Veterans Affairs, 2022e). "The majority of traumatic brain injuries sustained by members of the U.S. Armed Forces are classified as mild TBI, also known as concussion. Most service members who sustain a mild TBI return to full duty within 10 to 14 days through rest and the progressive return to activity process, in which patients gradually return to normal activity using a standardized, staged-approach" (Defense and Veterans Brain Injury Center, 2022, para 1).

TBI-provider resources and clinical and education tools are available to support military and civilian healthcare providers assess and treat service members and veterans with TBIs and their families (Degeneffe, 2021). Resources that address common symptoms such as headache, sleep disturbances, and vision problems are available. In addition, a roadmap that helps healthcare professionals support, counsel, and serve military veterans with disabilities (Frain et al., 2010) and outlines a five-pronged approach that may benefit veterans' outcomes can be found here: https://tacqe.com/rehabilitation-counseling-military-veterans/

Substance use disorders represent a significant risk among military populations. Data shows that about one in three veterans met the criteria for alcohol use disorder, and this is a higher rate than their civilian counterparts (National Institute on Drug Abuse, 2019). Research also confirms there is a strong neurobehavioral basis for alcohol misuse for those who have sustained TBIs. This situation raises a serious treatment concern (Adams et al., 2017; Adams et al., 2020).

In more recent years, scholars have grown to better understand moral injury (i.e., conflict between a service member's action and his or her moral belief system), which can lead to feelings of intense guilt, shame, and social alienation (Griffin et al., 2019; Jinkerson, 2016). This is a unique result of trauma endured as part of service. The cognitive model of PTSD may partially explain the impact of moral injury. A modified cognitive behavioral treatment approach has been designed to address the three principal injurious elements of combat: life-threat trauma, traumatic loss, and moral injury. This approach examined Marines who had been redeployed from the Iraq and Afghanistan wars (Steenkamp et al., 2011).

Sexual assaults have become a serious issue in the military, and reports of sexual assault have increased steadily since 2012 (DoD, 2021). *Military sexual trauma* (MST) is a term that accounts for sexual assault and other activities that occur without consent of both (or all) parties during military service. Researchers have declared that up to 70% of women service members have reported MST, and many of these victims have also experienced disorders such as PTSD, major depressive disorder, suicidality, generalized anxiety disorder, sleep issues, and eating issues (Braun et al., 2021). Counselors should be trained in evidence-based therapies (e.g., prolonged exposure; cognitive processing therapy) that they can use with clients who have experienced MST. In addition, therapists should be aware of and understand other resources (e.g., VA Disability Compensation for Conditions Related to MST, Beyond MST Mobile App for self-help) that could be beneficial for clients to use in conjunction with therapy (U.S. Department of Veterans Affairs, 2022f).

Specifically, among post-9/11–era veterans, there has been an increase in impairments and disability ratings. Forty-one percent (1.8 million) of post-9/11–era veterans have been classified as having a service-connected disability in comparison to 25% (4.7 million) of all other veterans from all other conflicts combined (U.S. Department of Labor, 2020). Almost half of the post-9/11–era veterans had a service-connected disability of 60% or more. In comparison, 41% of veterans from all earlier conflicts had a service-connected disability of 60% or more (U.S. Department of Labor, 2020). As of August 2022, 4.9 million veterans (27% of the total) had a service-connected disability (U.S. Department of Labor, 2023).

> *Disability compensation is a monetary benefit paid to Veterans who are determined by the VA to be disabled by an injury or illness that was incurred or aggravated during active military service. These disabilities are considered to be service connected. To be eligible for compensation, the Veteran must have been separated or discharged under conditions other than dishonorable.* (VA, 2015, p. 1)

For some service members, the psychological wounds of war may be expressed through maladaptive coping, which can include intimate partner violence (IPV; Sayers et al., 2009), drug-related infractions (Baldwin, 2017), and other justice-related concerns. Researchers have determined that 32% of women service members have experienced violence, stalking, or rape during an intimate relationship (Black & Merrick, 2013). In addition, IPV can happen to both male and female service members (Cerulli et al., 2014; Dichter et al., 2011; Iverson et al., 2017). As noted, military relationships undergo unique stressors such as family separations (Burrell et al., 2006) and combat exposure (MacManus et al., 2015), and these stressors may increase the risk of IPV. Finally, parenting stress can be experienced due to separations and need for the service member to prioritize service responsibilities during enlistment (Fischer et al., 2015; Khaylis et al., 2011). For example, the at-home parent must assume all child rearing and household responsibilities both before and during deployments. This situation, then, increases both parents' stress as the home undergoes a primarily solo parenting structure.

Mental Health Treatment Considerations for Veterans and Their Families

Navigation of the transition process alongside a veteran who has significant mental health problems can be daunting and complex. Numerous veteran and family interventions and resources are available to support veterans and military families (see Sherman & Larsen, 2018 for a full list of resources). These interventions and resources target specific areas of support that are needed. For example, one well-known local community group for social support is Team Red, White & Blue (RWB). Team RWB is a veteran-service organization that enriches veterans' lives by connecting them to their communities through physical, social, service, and leadership activities (teamrwb.org). Families are encouraged to join in on events to strengthen relationships within the family and build friendships and support with the other members.

More formal programs have also been created to help military families with various military-life challenges and transitions. Psychoeducational groups that teach conflict management, learning communication, and relapse prevention skills are examples of formal programs that can benefit military families (Snyder & Monson, 2012). Manualized family psychoeducational programs and online and phone-based resources may also be useful to veteran families during transition. According to Sherman and Larsen (2018), "Family psychoeducation is a nonpathologizing, strengths-focused model of care that has documented benefits in the arena of mental illness" (p. 146). A community provider toolkit that explains family psychoeducation is available here: https://www.mentalhealth.va.gov/communityproviders/. Other interventions or supports that are available to military families include different reunification programs (Davis et al., 2012; Fischer et al., 3015; Sherman & Larsen, 2018). Often, these types of programs allow the couple and/or family to communicate and reconnect in either community (e.g., retreats or camps) or home-based interventions. Examples of reunification programs include (1) Project Sanctuary (https://projectsanctuary.us/), which focuses on *reconnecting* family members to each other and to their communities; (2) Gratitude America (http://www.gratitudeamerica.org/), which focuses on preparing service members who have "combat exposure concerns" (e.g., combat stress, TBIs) for the transition to home; and (3) Operation Purple (https://www.militaryfamily.org/programs/operation-purple/family-retreats/), which allows military families the gift of quality time after a transition (e.g., separation) by offering the family getaway retreats.

There are also organizations that create specific resources to help individuals obtain the knowledge they need to competently work with veterans and their families. In 2008, the VA introduced a new mental health handbook, the *Mental Health Treatment Tool Kit*, that offered guidelines for VA hospitals and clinics across the United States (U.S. Department of Veterans Affairs, 2012). Military OneSource is a free service that is provided by the DoD to service members and their families to help with a broad range of concerns, including possible mental health problems (https://www.militaryonesource.mil/). The Psychological Health Center of Excellence provides psychological health research consultation and expertise to leaders, providers, service members, and their families (Defense Health Agency, 2022b). The VA Mental Health Resources provides information about mental health and support services specifically for veterans (U.S. Department of Veterans Affairs, 2022d). The National Resource Directory (NRD) connects wounded warriors, service members, veterans, and their families with national, state, and local support programs. NRD is a partnership among the DoD, the Department of Labor, and the VA (National Resource Directory, 2022).

Veteran Treatment Courts

Veterans who have untreated mental health and substance use disorders may become involved with the criminal justice system. Courts specific to veterans' needs have been designed to respond to the unique experiences that may predispose them to psychosocial mental health problems and challenges, all of which can increase the risk of interaction with the criminal justice system. The veteran treatment court is like other court experiences. It requires regular court appearances, mandatory treatment session attendance, and drug and alcohol use testing (Justice for Vets, 2022). Veterans react well to this structured environment given the structure that they once had in the military. The veteran treatment court can help ensure veterans meet their duties to themselves, the court, and their community (Justice for Vets, 2022). Veterans' justice outreach coordinators are an important part of the veteran problem-solving court.

Traumatic Brain Injury Veteran, Family, and Provider Resources

Common challenges are experienced after one sustains a TBI. Educational information and resources are available to veterans and service members who have TBIs and their families to help them learn about the severity of TBIs, signs and symptoms of TBIs, coping and recovery from TBIs, and prevention of future TBIs (Dillahunt-Aspillaga & Powell-Cope, 2018).

Community providers play an important role in ensuring that veterans receive the care they need. One resource is The Community Provider Toolkit. This resource is designed for healthcare professionals who work with veterans outside of the VA healthcare system (U.S. Department of Veterans Affairs, 2022c).

Vocational Rehabilitation for Veterans

Employment is a critical protective factor against suicide, homelessness, and substance use; it is a social determinant of physical and mental health. Work provides opportunities for social interactions and facilitates community reintegration. Meaningful activity provides a sense of purpose and accomplishment and increases one's self-esteem.

The Veterans Health Administration (VHA) serves veterans who experience employment challenges as a result of mental health, physical, and psychosocial issues. Addressing veterans' employment needs is a critical component of the healthcare system and their services, as employment can work as a protective factor and can promote the overall health and well-being of and community reintegration for veterans. VHA offers vocational services integrated within clinical treatment to promote recovery and community reintegration. These services are provided by rehabilitation counselors and vocational rehabilitation (VR) specialists.

VETERANS HEALTH ADMINISTRATION VOCATIONAL REHABILITATION

In the VHA, VR is a program that assists people with disabilities in obtaining and maintaining employment that is well matched to their skills, abilities, functional limitations, and interests. The VR is housed within the VA healthcare system, and its mission is to provide support to veterans who live with mental illness and/or physical impairment and have barriers to securing and maintaining employment (U.S. Department of Veterans Affairs, 2021c). VR is a clinical service that is integrated within a veteran's overall healthcare. The vision of VHA VR is that all veterans who live with mental illness or physical impairment with barriers to employment who want to work will secure and maintain meaningful, competitive employment that fosters self-esteem, dignity, respect, and independence. It is a recovery program. What makes VHA VR different from other employment programs is the core belief that any veteran who wants to work can successfully do so (U.S. Department of Veterans Affairs, 2021c).

Compensated work therapy (U.S. Department of Veterans Affairs, 2019b) consists of direct hire assistance (community-based employment services and supported employment), provides participants with work restoration services in actual work settings (transitional work), and supports those in school or training and those who desire self-employment. Supported employment and transitional work are provided at every VA medical center.

Vocational and education services can help veterans who have disabilities transition from the military into civilian life by providing skills and incremental exposure to everyday life tasks (Ottomanelli et al., 2019). Veterans often experience long-term challenges that compromise community reintegration (CR; a broad term for return to participation in life roles) and impede their access to community-based services and support (McGarity et al., 2016; Sayer et al., 2014). Therefore, an individually planned and coordinated approach, such as resource facilitation (RF), is needed to address CR barriers (Dillahunt-Aspillaga et al., 2020; Resnik & Allen, 2007; Trexler et al., 2010). RF typically is a statewide telephone or in-person service that is available at no charge for persons who are affected by brain injuries that offers ongoing support to help the individual return to family life, work, school, and the community.

Veteran motivation, caregiver support, and engaged staff at the VA and academic institutions were key drivers for veteran success.

CONCLUSION

Military culture is unique, and counselors who assist veterans need to become competent in understanding this culture. When counselors are culturally competent, they are better able to recognize, implement, and deliver effective and appropriate interventions to service members, veterans, and their families (Prosek et al., 2018). This chapter highlights the unique transition and community reintegration support needs of service members and their families. The case study that follows depicts Greg, a transition service member. Using this case study, practice the application of the information presented in this chapter.

DISCUSSION QUESTIONS

1. Discuss three unique aspects of military culture.

2. Identify three positive consequences of military service.

3. Describe three negative consequences of military service.

   a. How do these consequences vary based on the individual (e.g., service member, dependent, friend)?

4. Examine three support sources that can be used given the negative consequences of military service.

CLASS ACTIVITIES

Case Study: Transition From Active to Veteran Status: Greg's Story

Greg is a 46-year-old male. He served in the U.S. Army for 28 years after enlisting as an infantryman. He spent years living in various locations, having relocated a total of eight times.

Greg was deployed four times to the Middle East. Greg married a civilian wife and has one son who was born during his second deployment. Greg was honorably medically discharged in 2021 due to significant physical and mental health issues that he sustained during his tours. Most notably, Greg was diagnosed with hearing loss, degenerative arthritis, and posttraumatic stress disorder (PTSD). Greg is having a difficult time securing employment since his separation from the military. The family has financial concerns and is struggling to fit into their new civilian community.

Considering Greg's story, please work in small groups to discuss the following:

a. What are the presenting client concerns for counseling and vocational rehabilitation? What do you think is the cause for each of the concerns identified?

b. Which concerns would you address first?

c. What are possible counseling approaches to address these concerns?

d. What community and support resources and services could you offer Greg and his family?

KEY REFERENCES

Only key references appear in the print edition. The full references appear in the digital product on Springer Publishing Connect™: https://connect.springerpub.com/content/book/978-0-8261-5111-7/part/partIV/chapter/ch18

Hall, L. K. (2016). *Counseling military families: What mental health professionals need to know* (2nd ed.). Routledge, Taylor & Francis Group.

Military OneSource. (2022a). *Benefits and resources.* https://www.militaryonesource.mil/benefits-and-resources

National Academies of Sciences, Engineering, and Medicine. (2019). *Strengthening the military family readiness system for a changing American society.* The National Academies Press. https://doi.org/10.17226/25380.

Ottomanelli, L., Bakken, S., Dillahunt-Aspillaga, C., Pastorek, N., & Young, C. (2019). Vocational rehabilitation in the Veterans Health Administration polytrauma system of care: Current practices, unique challenges, and future directions. *The Journal of Head Trauma Rehabilitation, 34*(3), 158–166. https://doi.org/10.1097/HTR.0000000000000493

Prosek, E. A., Burgin, E. E., Atkins, K. M., Wehrman, J. D., Fenell, D. L., Carter, C., & Green, L. (2018). Competencies for counseling military populations. *Journal of Military and Government Counseling, 6,* 87–99. http://acegonline.org/journal/journalof-military-and-government-counseling

Sherman, M. D., & Larsen, J. L. (2018). Family-focused interventions and resources for veterans and their families. *Psychological Services, 15*(2), 146–153. https://doi.org/10.1037/ser0000174

U.S. Department of Defense. (2012). *Military deployment guide.* http://download.militaryonesource.mil/12038/Project%20Documents/MilitaryHOMEFRONT/Troops%20and%20Families/Deployment%20Connections/Pre-Deployment%20Guide.pdf

U.S. Department of Veterans Affairs. (2019). *VHA Directive 1163: Psychosocial rehabilitation and recovery services.* Veterans Health Administration.

U.S. Department of Veterans Affairs. (2021a). *VA benefits for service members.* https://www.va.gov/service-member-benefits/

U.S. Department of Veterans Affairs. (2022c). *Community provider toolkit.* https://www.mentalhealth.va.gov/communityproviders/

CHAPTER 19

RESPONDING WELL TO INDIVIDUALS EXPERIENCING ABUSE AND RELATIONSHIP VIOLENCE

J. RUTH NELSON

LEARNING OBJECTIVES

After reading this chapter, you will be able to:

- Describe which groups are more likely to experience abuse, including intimate partner and relationship violence
- Identify different types of partner violence, including violence toward women with disabilities and toward LGBTQ+ and gender-expansive communities
- Explain how intersectionality plays a significant role and can contribute to an increased risk of partner violence
- Describe how Bronfenbrenner's bioecological theory can help us better understand the context of individuals experiencing partner violence, especially women with disabilities, and inform services and policies to better support survivors

PRE-READING QUESTIONS

1. Which groups and individuals with intersectional identities are at higher risk for intimate partner and relationship violence?

2. In addition to traditional forms of partner violence, what other forms of intimate partner violence may occur for women with disabilities, nonbinary, LGBTQP+, and gender-expansive individuals?

3. How is Bronfenbrenner's bioecological Process–Person–Context–Time (PPCT) model helpful in helping understand how ecological contexts may impact women with disabilities, nonbinary, LGBTQP+ and trans individuals from leaving abusive partners?

4. How does socioeconomic status and housing insecurity play a role in the context of IPV?

5. What are specific recommendations to keep in mind when building a safety plan for a woman with a disability? For an LGBTQP+ individual?

DISPROPORTIONATE RISK OF ABUSE AND NEGLECT FOR PERSONS WITH DISABILITIES

Every day women, men, nonbinary individuals and LGBTQP+, and individuals with disabilities experience abuse, whether it be financial, physical, psychological, sexual, or neglect. Abuse varies widely and includes neglect for basic needs (i.e., food, medical care, hygiene), physical abuse (i.e., resulting in cuts, bruises, burns, broken bones, restraint markings, gunshot wounds), emotional abuse (i.e., verbal or nonverbal behaviors that inflict anguish, mental pain, fear, or distress), and sexual abuse which includes forced or unwanted sexual interaction of any kind (Centers for Disease Control and Prevention [CDC], 2021a; Tracy, 2021a). But these acute or ongoing injuries can also lead to more long-term psychological issues of posttraumatic stress disorder (PTSD), anxiety, suicidal behavior, self-harm, and panic disorder (Tracy, 2021b). Financial abuse—along with emotional, physical, and sexual abuse—includes behaviors to intentionally manipulate, intimidate, and threaten the victim in order to entrap that person in the relationship and is cited as the number one reason survivors do not leave their situations or return to an abusive partner (National Network to End Domestic Violence [NNEDV], 2017). More than 50% of abuse never gets reported and often goes unnoticed even when individuals are seen by emergency department providers due to limited screening tools and assessment (Evans et al., 2017; Morgan & Truman, 2020).

One in seven children are abused, usually by parents/caregivers, and one in ten older adults are abused, usually by a family member (CDC, 2022b; National Council on Aging, 2021). Most abuse occurs at the hands of partners, in the case of adults, although care providers, relatives, and friends can also be perpetrators. Intimate partner violence (IPV) occurs more frequently than every 3 seconds (National Coalition Against Domestic Violence [NCADV], 2020). More than 10 million adults experience IPV each year (NCADV, 2020). Almost one in two women (47.3% or 59 million) in the United States reported any- contact sexual violence, physical violence, and/or stalking victimization by an intimate partner at some point in their lifetime on the most recent National Intimate Partner & Sexual Violence Survey (Leemis et al., 2022). Women with disabilities are at a greater risk than women without disabilities to experience rape, sexual violence other than rape, physical violence, stalking, psychological aggression, and control of reproductive or sexual health by an intimate partner (CDC, 2021b). Men with a disability are more likely to experience stalking and psychological aggression by an intimate partner (CDC, 2021b). Within these prevalence rates, it is important to understand that risk is increased within specific demographic and identity groups. For example, those with disabilities experience abuse at higher rates at all ages than their counterparts without disabilities (Harrell, 2021; Hughes et al., 2012; Khalifeh et al., 2016). It is imperative to understand that the intersectionality of identities can raise the risk of IPV.

CERTAIN GROUPS AND INDIVIDUALS WITH INTERSECTIONAL IDENTITIES AT HIGHER RISK

Women with disabilities (WDs) have a higher risk of being abused by partners as compared to women and men with disabilities, with incidence rates from the literature ranging from 4% to 60% (Breiding & Armour, 2015; Fanslow et al., 2021; Hahn et al., 2014; Slayter et al., 2018). Researchers completed an international meta-analytic review of violence against WDs and found that the frequency and risk of being a victim of IPV were higher in WDs than in those without (Garcia-Cuellar et al., 2022). Financial abuse is the most widespread form of violence in these women, but WDs also experienced emotional, physical, and sexual abuse at alarmingly high rates (Garcia-Cuéllar et al., 2022). Sometimes partners are also personal assistance providers, or other family members may perpetrate abuse (Salwen et al.,

2016). Young adult women (18–21 years) with disabilities have four times the risk as compared to peers without disabilities of experiencing IPV, with a national rate of less than 3% (Slayter et al., 2018).

Men and women with intellectual/developmental disabilities also report high rates of adult abuse. As reported in Platt et al.'s study (2017), 64% of men and 68% of women with a developmental disability experienced abuse at least once. More women than men with developmental disabilities reported adult sexual abuse, but there was no gender difference in the prevalence of any other form of abuse (Platt et al., 2017). A recent meta-analysis suggested a 60% victimization rate of those with intellectual disabilities (Bowen & Swift, 2019).

Ethnic, sexual, and gender identity are additional identities to consider when exploring risk of a client. *Native American women* experience relationship abuse at least 10% more often than women of other ethnicities in two nationally representative surveys (Breiding et al., 2014; Tjaden & Thoennes, 2000), and complexities of jurisdiction of federal, state, and tribal systems fail to effectively charge crimes (Helgesen, 2011; Jock et al., 2022). *LGBTQ+ people* in the United States have also been found to experience higher rates of IPV than the general population, with rates for bisexual cisgender women of approximately two in five and for gender minority people of about one in two (James et al., 2016; Rothman et al., 2012; Walters et al., 2013). However, their stories are usually not studied or examined in the literature (Guadelupe-Diaz, 2019). In particular, bisexual cisgender young adult women and gender minorities face much higher rates of SRV than heterosexual cisgender women (Klein et al., 2022). According to a 2017 report from the National Coalition of Anti-Violence Programs (NCAVP) of Lesbian, Gay, Bisexual, Transgender, Queer and HIV-Affected Hate and Intimate Partner Violence, transgender women who experienced IPV were nearly two and a half times more likely to experience sexual violence and nearly four times more likely to experience financial abuse than survivors who did not identify as transgender women. Additionally, cisgender men surviving hate violence were nearly four times more likely to report experiences of sexual violence than survivors who did not identify as cisgender men. Gay men were more likely to require medical attention, suffer injuries, or die via homicide as a result of IPV and hate crimes (NCAVP, 2018). Nearly half (43%) of LGBTQ+ IPV survivors who sought shelter reported being denied access to shelter and of those, nearly one- third (32%) were turned away because of their gender identity (NCAVP, 2017).

Transgender individuals may be as much as 2.2 times more likely to experience physical IPV and 2.5 times more likely to experience sexual IPV compared to cisgender individuals (Kattari et al., 2022; Peitzmeier et al., 2020). Within trans populations, the 2015 U.S. Transgender Survey of 27,715 participants reported that 54% experienced some form of IPV throughout their lives. Specific subpopulations within the transgender community may be at even higher risk for psychological, physical, transrelated IPV and stalking by an intimate partner, such as those with disabilities, those who are homeless, those who engage in sex work, or those who are undocumented (James et al., 2016; King et al., 2021). In a secondary analysis of the National Transgender Discrimination Survey (Seelman, 2015), transgender people of color, those with disabilities, and those more frequently perceived to be transgender by others are more likely to experience unequal treatment in domestic violence centers.

Although women experience IPV at higher rates in general and suffer more physical harm, *men* tend to be underserved, with few screening protocols validated for nonfemale clients, as medical providers aren't routinely asking men these questions (Velonis et al., 2021), and limited safe places to go, as many shelters are women-only facilities and because men are less likely to report (Machado et al., 2017). A significant number of males—between 14% and 20%—experience IPV (Bazargan-Hejazi et al., 2014, Black et al., 2011). A U.S. surveillance study found 14% of men reported ever experiencing severe nonsexual physical violence from a partner (Black et al., 2011). A probability cross-age sample of California residents found gay men had 2.5 odds of both lifetime and 1-year IPV compared to heterosexual men (Goldberg & Meyer, 2013).

INTIMATE PARTNER ABUSE

IPV can take many different forms, especially in minority populations such as those with disabilities and those from LGBTQ+, nonbinary and trans communities. IPV includes physical violence, sexual violence, stalking and psychological aggression (CDC, 2022b). *Physical violence* is the use of physical force against someone (CDC, 2022b). It can take the form of slapping, pushing, kicking, biting, inflicting burns, bed sores from not being appropriately and regularly moved, to injury with a gun and knife and/or nonfatal strangulation (NFS), which is now seen as a high-risk factor for a lethal attempt and subsequently is a felony in several states (Breiding et al., 2015; Monahan et al., 2022).

Sexual violence is "forcing or attempting to force a partner to take part in a sex act, sexual touching, or a non-physical sexual event (e.g., sexting) when the partner does not or cannot consent" (CDC, 2022b, p. 1). *Stalking* is a pattern of repeated, unwanted attention and contact by a partner that causes fear or concern for one's own safety or the safety of someone close to the victim (CDC, 2022b, p. 1). *Psychological aggression* is the use of verbal and nonverbal communication with the intent to harm another partner mentally or emotionally and/or to exert control over another partner (Breiding et al., 2015; CDC, 2022b). It can include yelling, demeaning someone with name calling, threatening violence and abandonment, and gaslighting or playing "mind games where the perpetrator gives false information to the victim, making them doubt their memory and perception, and destroying property" (Breiding et al., 2015, p. 11).

Individuals with disabilities tend to experience more severe forms of physical abuse and may stay within such relationships longer than others (Brownridge, 2006). The American Psychological Association (2022) delineates forms of disability-related abuse as follows: removing or destroying a person's mobility devices (e.g., wheelchairs, scooters, walkers), denying access to or taking prescribed medication from someone, forcing someone to take medication against their will, forcing someone to lie in soiled undergarments, preventing access to food, inappropriately touching a person while assisting with bathing or dressing, and denying access to disability-related resources in the community or healthcare appointments. Those with more severe physical disabilities are at a heightened risk of IPV due to their increased dependence on partners or personal assistants for care. Abusive actions may also include withholding mobility supplies or threatening partners with institutionalization (Lund, 2011; Plummer & Findley, 2012). Uniquely, the "whittling away of self-esteem associated with having a disability as a precursor to abuse" may also exacerbate WDs' potential for experiencing or remaining in a violent relationship and/or seeking help in such a situation (Nosek et al., 2001, p. 124).

LGBTQ+, nonbinary, and trans community members face additional types of abuse that are unique to their contexts. For the LGBTQ+ community and nonbinary and transgender individuals, their IPV can look different and not follow the formulaic story of the cisgender heterosexual male abusing the cisgender heterosexual female. These individuals may experience heterosexist or cis-sexist language by partners. This refers to positioning heterosexuality as superior to LGBTQ+ relationships (Family Justice Center Alliance & Family Service of Piedmont [FJCA/FSP], 2022). An example could be "You always wanted to be with girls" could be an abusive statement made toward a bisexual cisgender female or belittlement of their gender (Kattari et al., 2022). Another abusive statement would be, "I'm going to out you to your family or work colleagues." If LGBTQ+ individuals come out about their sexual orientation, they could be fired from a job, kicked out of a home, or physical or verbally victimized (James et al., 2016). In 30 states it is illegal to kick someone out of housing due to their sexual orientation, but it still occurs (FJCA/FSP, 2022). In addition to the IPV, LGBTQ+ students also experienced discrimination when seeking support and experienced institutional betrayal and internalized homonegativity (Klein et al., 2022). Trans community members may also face abuse, as a partner may take abusive control of medical supplies needed (FJCA/FSP, 2022).

ECOLOGICAL CONTEXT MATTERS: WHY SURVIVORS MAY CHOOSE NOT TO REPORT

When trying to understand the intersectionality of an individual and their contextual lives and how better to support individuals experiencing abuse, particularly women, nonbinary LGBTQP+ and trans individuals with disabilities, Bronfenbrenner's bioecological Process–Person–Context–Time (PPCT) model (1979, 2005) can be helpful in thinking about layers of bidirectional influences on the individual. This model helps us better understand the multiple contexts of how women are influenced and helps explain growth and change over time through bidirectional influences. Bronfenbrenner's model (2005) includes four key components: (a) the developmental *process* of interactions between the person and their environment; (b) the *person*, with her or his individual biological, cognitive, behavioral, and emotional characteristics; (c) a *context* of multiple nested levels or systems influencing development; and (d) various types of *time*, such as historical time and its influences. The following sections will highlight the various ecological contexts that impact an individual's experience when encountering relationship violence and how they may discourage disclosure of IPV.

Historical Influences

Bronfenbrenner's theory wisely includes the effects of historical and current events and how they impact individual circumstances. The COVID-19 pandemic increased IPV, with increased severity for those already experiencing IPV and instigated novel cases (Peitzmeier et al., 2022; Piquero et al., 2021). New IVP or increased severity of IVP was more likely to occur in essential workers, people who are pregnant, those unable to afford rent, those who are unemployed/underemployed or had recent changes to their job, those who had partners with recent changes to employment, and those who had gotten tested or tested positive for COVID-19 (Peitzmeier et al., 2021). COVID-19 brought about job losses, and the United States is currently experiencing high economic inflation, largely due to the impact of COVID-19 and disruption of global supply chains. These contexts play a role in whether or how an individual is impacted when experiencing violence. These factors are likely to further encourage a WD or nonbinary individual with a disability or a transgender individual with a disability to stay with partners whom they may depend on for financial support.

Socioeconomic Status

Socioeconomic status (SES) refers to one's income, occupation, and education or their family income, occupational, and educational status (American Psychological Association, n.d.). People with disabilities tend to experience lower SES than people without disabilities (Department of Labor [DOL], 2021). This may occur in terms of education, income, or both. In a recent U.S. government report, the proportion of WDs living below the federal poverty level is 1.4 times higher than for men with disabilities and 2.2 times higher than for women without disabilities (these differences are all statistically significant). Additionally, one-quarter of WDs between the ages of 25 and 54 (prime working age) and nearly 10% of employed WDs were living in poverty in 2020 (DOL, 2021). Of working women ages 16 to 64, only 33.7% of WDs were working as compared to 76% of women without disabilities, but this rate has increased from prior years with the advent of COVID-19 and flexibility in working from home (DOL, 2021). The COVID-19 pandemic multiplied the effects on WDs as their unemployment rates jumped 8 percentage points higher than the previous year (DOL, 2021).

Another key contextual variable is the type of work WDs participate in. Women are more likely than men to work in management, professional, and related occupations; service occupations; and sales and office occupations (DOL, 2021). The authors of this study suggest it could be related to academic attainment, and that could be partially true, but further analyses found that lower salaries held true for WDs even with higher education such as holding bachelor and graduate degrees (DOL, 2021). WDs are less likely to work in management, professional, and related occupations and more likely to work in service or sales and office occupations compared to women without disabilities, which likely contributes to reduced income, and are also more likely to need public health insurance (DOL, 2021). The United States is not alone in this divide. In the 2009 to 2014 Life Opportunities Survey in the UK (N + 32,355 observations; Kim et al., 2020), disabled women were significantly less likely to be employed, least likely to work full-time, and least likely to be supervisors and felt more limited in the type and amount of paid work.

After the Americans with Disabilities Act (ADA) was passed, employment of people with disabilities actually decreased due to people's perceived and inaccurate assumptions of costly and "difficult" accommodations that would need to be provided (Hoffman, 2008). Further, if mothers with disabilities are triply marginalized: for being a woman, for having a disability, and for having a child (Buonocore Porter, 2018). Buonocore Porter talks about the maternal or caregiver wall, where employers can be discriminatory and inflexible, leading to a lack of time, lack of money, and prejudicial stereotypes against mothers and their work productivity. Mothers need time for their children's medical appointments, school conferences, and to care for children when sick, and employers are not willing to work around this. Mothers may also lack money due to their lower-paying positions.

Housing Insecurity

Housing insecurity caused by underemployment or lack of employment or lack of shelter space may also lead women with and without disabilities to remain in unsafe situations. In a large sample of mothers from domestic violence shelters in an urban area, one-third (36%) reported housing instability over the subsequent 2 years, with 11% experiencing homelessness (Gilroy et al., 2016). Pregnant participants experiencing IPV conveyed to researchers that they had no choice but to deal with the abuse, and the authors suggest that one of the many reasons they may not have felt they could end the relationship was housing, as IPV survivors are at a heightened risk for housing instability (Herbell et al., 2020). Housing is a top priority for survivors (Dichter et al., 2017; Sullivan et al., 2019), as housing is the first step in healing from the trauma of abuse (Clough et al., 2014). Permanent housing also allows children to feel less stressed and more stable and establish a routine during a transition (Bomsta & Sullivan, 2018). Herbell et al. also found that a number of additional barriers to housing include a lack of housing in rural areas, lack of fair rent in urban areas, and landlord discrimination. Marçal et al. (2022) also found that IPV exposure at age 5 was associated with increased housing insecurity at age 9, which was associated with increased adolescent depression and anxiety at age 15. Housing insecurity mediated the link from IPV exposure to adolescent depression (Marçal et al., 2022). Housing instability creates additional stress on the parent and child and at a time when children need security and stability to build healthy Erikson psychosocial stages of trust/distrust and autonomy.

Geographical Location

WDs may have particular concerns regarding the lack of anonymity in many small, rural communities (Sandberg, 2013) and the likelihood of them or their perpetrator of abuse having personal relationships with individuals in positions of power (e.g., police, judges). Women in rural areas were less likely than those in urban areas to find the police or physicians to be helpful in addressing IPV due to the perceived lack of anonymity (McCall-Hosenfeld et al., 2014; Shannon et al., 2016). Rural survivors are also less likely to reach out for services. WDs may not disclose they have a disability for fear that their children could be removed or perceived to be less competent, and if involved in court proceedings, many will self-medicate rather than disclose their disability (Douglas, 2018).

Gender Identity

James et al. (2016) found that 48% of transgender individuals in their study experienced discrimination, harassment, or violence based on their gender identity and therefore are not likely to want to disclose their IPV. Trans survivors may feel their experiences aren't severe enough to be abuse or aren't worthy of help or attention (Guadalupe-Diaz, 2019). Researchers found that transgender males and nonbinary participants were less likely to report their abuse to friends and family and formal resources, especially police, due to perceptions that law enforcement has been unsafe in the past (e.g., criminalizing their behavior or illegally arresting them for sex work; Guadalupe-Diaz, 2019; James et al., 2016; Kurdyla et al., 2021; Messinger, 2017). Reporting IPV posed a double threat to their gender identity: a threat to their masculinity and feeling inadequate due to their trans status (Kurdyla et al., 2021). When individuals did disclose, there was a sense of urgency from threats to their physical life and safety, as well as increasing mental health concerns, and they carefully managed who they disclosed to (usually friends supportive of their gender identity) because it meant usually disclosing their gender identity and/or sexual orientation, which could have ripple effects to their jobs, living situations, and housing (Kurdyla et al., 2021).

Bidirectional Effects

WDs may have children with their abusers, and children and teens observing severe violence are impacted socioemotionally and behaviorally (Anderson & van Ee, 2018; Fong et al., 2019; Peterson et al., 2018; Vu et al., 2016). Ballan et al. (2014) reported from their study of WDs from the specialty domestic violence center that 43% of individuals experiencing IPV were married and 82% of them had children with their abusers. Many may not report abuse for fear they may lose their children, being doubly marginalized as a woman with a disability and experiencing IPV. Nearly a third (28%) of children in the United States witness IPV against their mothers (Finkelhor et al., 2013). IPV can cause adverse parenting practices, emotional dysregulation, and maternal PTSD, all supported as mechanisms that can lead to negative mental health outcomes in the children (Greene et al., 2018; Harding et al., 2013). Although neither physical nor psychological IPV was directly associated with child internalizing or externalizing problems, mothers' PTSD symptoms and parenting practices both mediated the link from IPV to child behavior problems (Greene et al., 2018). Survivor parents may also be overprotective and further isolated, hesitating to engage in even common activities such as taking the children to a park (Herbell et al., 2020). There may also be longer- term consequences, as Slayter et al. (2018) found a significant association between 18- and 21-year-old individuals with disabilities experiencing IPV who had observed parental IPV as a child and also experienced child abuse themselves.

Children and teens can also be resilient and can play an agentic role in providing supportive actions to their survivor parent (Johansen & Sundet, 2021; Overlien & Hyden, 2009). Some parents increase their authoritative positive parenting strategies (e.g., affection, strong communication) with positive outcomes in children, and others may increase authoritarian parenting (e.g., little nurturance, little communication), which can lead to negative sequelae (Ehrensaft et al., 2017; Greeson et al., 2014). Research has found that even having one adult (inside or outside the family) a child can trust consistently can be protective against poor mental health outcomes and self-harming behaviors in those affected by IPV during childhood (Bellis et al., 2017). Other positive coping strategies from a meta-analysis of children experiencing violence that fared better included informational or emotional support and problem- solving, distancing from the conflict, cognitive redefinition, and emotional self-regulation strategies (Hines, 2015).

Many contextual barriers—historical influence, SES, housing insecurity, geographical location, gender identity, and bidirectional effects with children—can interfere with leaving an abusive partner, but additional ecological contexts may also bring support to victims such as support groups, community groups, and faith- based groups.

RESPONDING WELL

Safety Procedures

In responding well to WDs, nonbinary individuals, and LGBTQ+ and gender- expansive individuals experiencing abuse and IPV, providers must always provide safe, person-centered, nonjudgmental, and helpful responses that are culturally competent. Providers must acknowledge the lethality of relationship violence and ascertain if the person is safe or not and build safety plans if the individual does not feel able to leave the situation at that time. Assessing for abuse should always occur in private and be kept confidential, except when contraindicated by mandatory reporting laws (Salwen et al., 2016). This may need to be done online, where they can directly speak or enter information in case the abuser is also providing direct care or is an intimate partner.

Disability-Related and Gender-Expansive Accommodations

For those with disabilities, service providers will need to have an assessment separate from an intimate partner who may accompany clients to appointments (Ballan & Freyer, 2017). It is also important to determine if the abusive partner is responsible for assisting with activities of daily living (ADLs). If the survivor is dependent on the abusive partner for ADL assistance, reporting abuse could result in the loss of the individual responsible for helping to meet most basic needs. In addition, fear that leaving the relationship will lead to further isolation is an obstacle to successful separation and safety planning (Ballan & Freyer, 2017). A social worker may need to connect survivors to community resources that can help with backup care, provide guidance on hiring and managing those who assist them, or facilitate achievement of new skills or skills that will decrease their need for support from others (Ballan & Freyer, 2017; Saxton et al., 2001). Mandatory reporting laws may dictate what may need to be reported, but it is important to know that individuals with disabilities distrust adult protective aervices (APS), as it may lead to a loss of independent functioning, especially those with more severe disabilities who need daily ADL support (Douglas, 2018).

Responders should always listen empathically and nonjudgmentally as to what the survivor wants to do, and if they are not wanting to leave at this point in time, ask about if they would like further resources to have on hand (Salwen et al., 2016). If the survivor is trans or LGBTQP+, one will need to also consider the consequences of disclosing abuse (e.g., outing, loss of job, housing) and really listen to the survivor as to how they would like to proceed.

Responders should also address disability-related needs and whether that involves helping them get connected with mental health or other needed services (e.g., medical appointments, physical therapy, counseling). Ballan and Freyer (2017) discovered that few medical providers recognized IPV and even when they did, only a small percentage then connected WDs with IPV resources and organizations of support. It is important that providers seek out and build intercultural awareness of these communities, if not already a member, so that they can connect individuals with disabilities to these disability communities as well as other supportive communities. Building intercultural competence begins with understanding the vibrant disability culture and the LGBTQ+, nonbinary, and transgender cultures (Boroughs et al., 2015, FJCA/FSP, 2022; Forber-Pratt, 2019). It is also important to gain training on microaggressions against those communities, such as learning more about disability etiquette (Diamond, 2012; Olkin et al., 2019). Building networks with domestic violence advocates and referring survivors to them with their specialized backgrounds remain critical. Consider the following awareness exercises:

- Immerse yourself in narratives and listen well to each individuals' experiences.
- Recognize your own intersectionality and how that may impact your behavior toward those experiencing IPV.
- Think complexly about the increased risks of multiple identities.
- Understand there are multiple models of disability (see Nelson et al., 2017) and realize how the social model tends to better empower survivors with disabilities.
- Recognize the change that can happen within the environment—programs, attitudes, architectural access—so that individuals with disabilities have more access to domestic violence shelters, programming within such shelters, employment, and psychological services to support survivors.

However, since less than half of all safe homes, shelters, and transitional housing services provide mental health services to survivors of IPV (Hines & Douglas, 2011), agencies addressing IPV, including WDs, must offer accessible comprehensive mental health services, and service providers need to be prepared to ask these questions of local resources. Since many domestic violence shelters are for women only, providers need to have a list of safe shelters that also will serve LGBTQP+, nonbinary, gender-expansive, and trans communities that may not identify as a woman. Shelters should also provide LGBTQP+ supplies and needs such as hormone therapy, binders, gap makeup, and clothing. Shelters should also be aware that perpetrators may go there if they are the same gender and protect against that. This community is also quite small, so be aware of that and connect them to the Trans Life Line, PFLAG, and other supportive local organizations that provide specialist positions for trans individuals (FJCA/FSP, 2022).

Intervening well also means building individual competencies in those experiencing abuse. Building direct skills through curriculums such as the ESCAPE-NOW (Khemka & Hickson, 2015) curriculum to increase self-efficacy, empowerment, and self-determination for those with intellectual disabilities is one example. Connecting individuals to accessible job training and education so that they can pursue economic self-sufficiency is also essential. Building community and social support is critical, thus helping to build peer and social networks and repair or identify healthy family/caregiver relationships, service systems, and community partners that can collaborate and support WDs (e.g., disability-specific organizations and advocate resources like the Abused Deaf Women's Advocacy Services). To intervene well with children and teens exposed to IPV violence, Berg et al. (2020) suggest building general education and awareness of the effects of violence exposure on children for providers, provide trauma-informed care, emulate cultural humility, and improve collaboration across service domains (e.g., social services, legal systems, healthcare providers) for individuals and their families impacted by partner violence.

Kulkarni (2019) put forth four culturally competent principles to keep in mind when responding to survivors of IPV: (a) power sharing, (b) authenticity, (c) individualized services, and (d) systems advocacy. Power has been taken away from survivors, and empowering survivors to identify their needs and make their own decisions is first and foremost. When providers are culturally sensitive, avoid judgment and microaggressions, and have training in various minority cultures, they can be more authentic in their relationship with the client and develop better individualized plans. Individualized services are needed even more so for WDs, LGBTQP+, trans, and gender-expansive clients with multiple intersectionalities and safety considerations.

CONCLUSION

The experience of intimate partner and relationship violence is more common within particular populations, including women with and without disabilities, men and women with intellectual disabilities, Native American women, elderly women, LGBTQP+, and gender- expansive individuals. Women with and without disabilities are most likely to experience relationship violence. While traditionally less focused on, male victims comprise 14% to 20% of those who are victimized, and many do not report because of the stigma associated with gender and masculinity social norms. Partner violence includes physical and sexual violence, stalking, and psychological aggression with the purpose of trying to control partners. Disability-related violence can look different: destroying assistive technology, preventing access to basic needs such as food and medications, inappropriately touching a person while assisting with bathing or dressing, and demeaning them for their disability status. LGBTQP+ and gender- expansive communities may experience violence in the form of belittling of their gender and outing them without consent. Intersectionality of multiple identities can raise the risk of IPV, and providers need to consider each of these social locations so as to better develop individualized safety plans. Bronfenbrenner's bioecological theory provides a model of nested systems and influences that impact how an individual may respond to IPV, including barriers in historical context, SES, housing insecurity, geographical location, gender identity, and bidirectional effects with children. Responding well to WDs and LGBTQP+ and gender-expansive communities begins with understanding these cultures better, listening carefully, and being knowledgeable about the safety concerns of leaving the relationship, providing culturally sensitive and disability-related accommodations in safety planning and next steps forward.

DISCUSSION QUESTIONS

Brainstorm the following questions in small groups.

1. How may a woman with a disability and of a faith background experiencing intimate partner violence be impacted by contextual systems of Bronfenbrenner's ecological model?

2. How may it lead to her not leaving the situation? How may the following systems impact her actions?

CLASS ACTIVITIES

Case Study: Experiencing Abuse as a Woman With Multiple Disabilities

Background

Avery is a 28-year-old cisgender, bisexual woman with periodic depression and anxiety with rheumatoid arthritis in her joints, primarily her knees. At times she has used a cane and/ or walker as she experiences more severe flare-ups. She has a long-term partner of 6 years,

Shannon, a 33-year-old cisgender, lesbian female who has recently been more controlling of her partner's activities and having angry outbursts over small things (e.g., standing in front of the TV, not completing all the laundry). She is very suspicious and has started accusing Avery of having an affair with their next- door neighbor, Paul. Shannon has even gone so far as to start tracking Avery with her phone when she leaves for doctor appointments or to get groceries and will send menacing texts if not home within a certain amount of time. Her partner has also told Avery that "You are damaged goods. No one else will want to be with you." Avery isn't involved with another person romantically or sexually and doesn't understand why Shannon thinks this is the case. Shannon has started using this premise to slap her and force her into sexual activities even when she does not want to. She has also been taking away Avery's medication for her mental health disabilities and arthritis and refusing to help her when she's struggling to get up or move. Avery feels like she's becoming more and more isolated, other than online Zoom meetings with work colleagues, as she works remotely since COVID-19. Shannon is very careful not to abuse her while she's on work calls. Shannon, however, is currently unemployed and takes much of Avery's earned money and controls the finances. Avery's family lives in another city 3 hours away, so she doesn't have much in the way of family support. A couple of friends have reached out, but Avery hasn't shared what's going on at home. She's ashamed and can't believe that this is happening to her and she would have to share her sexual orientation. Shannon used to be a good partner until COVID-19 hit and she lost her job.

Guided Analysis

This case study is not unusual in that 40% to 50% of women experiencing IPV will be married or in a long-term relationship, and women with both physical and mental health disabilities are much more likely to be targeted (Hahn et al., 2014). Avery's abuser uses physical abuse (slapping), sexual abuse (forced to have sex, which is rape), emotional abuse (demeaning statements, menacing texts, yelling, controlling her activities), financial abuse (controlling the finances and taking most of the monies), disability-related abuse (taking away medications, refusing to help her with mobility), and technology-related abuse (tracking her via her phone and sending abusive texts). She is also not currently working, which can increase the severity of abuse and is a correlate of financial abuse. Some research (Peitzmeier et al., 2021; Piquero et al., 2021) noted that novel cases of abuse appeared with the advent of the stay-at-home orders with COVID-19 and the loss of jobs and economic downturn. This appears to be the case with this couple.

Avery is isolated with her family farther away. Sometimes people are estranged from family because the family doesn't approve of the partner, their sexual orientation or gender identity, or how they are being treated. Women with disabilities may also be more isolated from communities due to their disability and dependence on their partner for ADLs (Copel, 2006). A couple of friends have reached out, but Avery is too ashamed to admit what is happening and it's hard for her to believe. She is in shock due to the trauma of what she's been experiencing, likely first denying and minimizing her partner's behaviors. Avery also doesn't have the energy or motivation with her depressive symptoms to seek out help, but this has increased both her depression and anxiety symptoms tremendously. Safe person-centered care would encourage counseling for her mental health symptoms and address the violence at the same time. A suicide threat assessment should be done with a history of depression. It would be important to listen to Avery carefully as to what she wants to do, encouraging her to leave and realizing that if she chooses to leave and where to go, that is the most dangerous time for her personally. Her phone location should be turned off (e.g., turn off Find My iPhone) if she leaves. If she doesn't want to leave the situation immediately, then provide information about local domestic violence centers and local/national hotlines for IPV and suicide (#988), and have a stash of her medicines and doctors' information and prescription information with a friend or family so that she will be medically safe when she leaves. Encourage her to get all account/passcode information for her financial accounts. If she does desire to leave and is thinking of staying with a friend or family, encourage staying at a shelter where Shannon is unaware of where she will be. Shannon likely knows addresses of family and friends or could get that information. If Avery is using a walker or cane, depending on the severity of her rheumatoid arthritis, one should check out the physical accessibility (e.g., entry, one level, shower supports, one level bedroom/bed) of the domestic violence shelter.

KEY REFERENCES

Only key references appear in the print edition. The full references appear in the digital product on Springer Publishing Connect™: https://connect.springerpub.com/content/book/978-0-8261-5111-7/part/partIV/chapter/ch19

Ballan, M. S., & Freyer, M. B. (2017). Supporting female survivors of intimate partner violence with disabilities: Recommendations for social workers in the emergency department. *Social Work in Health Care, 56*(10), 950–963. https://doi.org/10.1080/00981389.2017.1371099

Bowen, E., & Swift, C. (2019). The Prevalence and correlates of partner violence used and experienced by adults with intellectual disabilities: A systematic review and call to action. *Trauma, Violence & Abuse, 20*(5), 693–705. https://doi.org/10.1177/1524838017728707

Breiding, M. J., & Armour, B. S. (2015). The association between disability and intimate partner violence in the United States. *Annals of Epidemiology, 25*(6), 455–457. https://doi.org/10.1016/j.annepidem.2015.03.017

Copel, L. C. (2006). Partner abuse in physically disabled women: A proposed model for understanding intimate partner violence. *Perspectives in Psychiatric Care, 42*(2), 114–129. https://doi-org.ezproxy.bethel.edu/10.1111/j.1744-6163.2006.00059.x

García-Cuéllar, M. M., Pastor-Moreno, G., RuizPérez, I., & Henares-Montiel, J. (2022). The prevalence of intimate partner violence against women with disabilities: A systematic review of the literature. *Disability and Rehabilitation, 45*(1), 1–8. https://doi.org/10.1080/09638288.2022.2025927

Jock, B. W., Dana-Sacco, G., Arscott, J., Bagwell-Gray, M. E., Loerzel, E., Brockie, T., Packard, G., O'Keefe, V. M., McKinley, C. E., & Campbell, J. (2022). "We've already endured the trauma, who is going to either end that cycle or continue to feed it?": The influence of family and legal systems on Native American women's intimate partner violence experiences. *Journal of Interpersonal Violence, 37*(21-22), NP20602–NP20629. https://doi.org/10.1177/08862605211063200

Kulkarni, S. (2019). Intersectional trauma-informed intimate partner violence (IPV) services: Narrowing the gap between IPV service delivery and survivor needs. *Journal of Family Violence, 34*(1), 55–64. https://doi.org/10.1007/s10896-018-0001-5

Lund, E. M. (2011). Community-based services and interventions for adults with disabilities who have experienced interpersonal violence: A review of the literature. *Trauma, Violence, & Abuse, 12*, 171–182. https://doi.org/10.1177/1524838011416377

Platt, L., Powers, L., Leotti, S., Hughes, R. B., Robinson-Whelen, S., Osburn, S., Ashkenazy, E., Beers, L., Lund, E. M., Nicolaidis, C., & The Partnering With People With Disabilities to Address Violence Consortium. (2017). The role of gender in violence experienced by adults with developmental disabilities. *Journal of Interpersonal Violence, 32*(1), 101–129. https://doi.org/10.1177/0886260515585534

Salwen, J. K., Gray, A., & Mona, L. R. (2016). Personal assistance, disability, and intimate partner violence: A guide for healthcare providers. *Rehabilitation Psychology, 61*(4), 417–429. https://doi.org/10.1037/rep000011

CHAPTER 20

IMMIGRANTS, REFUGEES, AND ASYLUM SEEKERS: THE PSYCHOSOCIAL COST OF WAR ON CIVILIANS

MARK A. STEBNICKI

LEARNING OBJECTIVES

After reading this chapter, you will be able to:

- Identify and recognize the unique aspects of trauma and the clinically significant mental health symptoms experienced by immigrants, refugees, and asylum seekers from poor and war-torn countries

- Analyze specific issues in premigration, migration, and postmigration resettlement efforts and the unique medical, physical, psychosocial, and psychological stressors associated with successful transition

- Differentiate Western-based medical and psychological assessment, diagnosis, and treatment efforts from that of culturally based approaches that enhance optimal wellness during transition to postmigration resettlement

- Examine the mandatory humanitarian medical, physical, and psychological triage, assessment, and treatment efforts that occur during postmigration resettlement

PRE-READING QUESTIONS

1. What are the unique medical, physical, psychosocial, and psychological stressors and conditions associated with immigrants, refugees, and asylum seekers transitioning from war-torn countries to the United States?

2. How would you differentiate the trauma experiences of immigrants, refugees, and asylum seekers from that of the general population of Americans?

3. Describe the culturally based psychosocial stressors and unique losses experienced in the lives of immigrants, refugees, and asylum seekers from war-torn countries.

The world has been at war since the beginning of time. The majority of deaths that occur during times of war do not involve military personnel (Stebnicki, 2021a). Rather, 90% are composed of civilian casualties (Wiist et al., 2014). Since the Russian Federations' armed attack on Ukraine (February 24, 2022) and ongoing as of summer 2022, the Office of the United Nations High Commissioner for Human Rights (UNHCR) reported 4,889 civilians killed and 6,263 injured (UNHCR, 2022a). Now into its second year war with Russia, over 6.7 million refugees have left Ukraine. The concerns with civilian casualties and refugees globally is the long-term medical, physical, and psychological trauma that is complicated by a world at war with no predictable end in sight. Since World War II, 127 different wars have been fought globally with more than 40 million civilian deaths (Hanson & Vogel, 2012). World War II alone was responsible for more than 27.3 million civilian casualties (War Chronicle, 2016). Other examples since the mid-20th century include over 5.4 million civilian deaths in the Democratic Republic of Congo; 2 million civilian deaths related to the Khmer Rouge killing fields; 2 million civilian deaths in Rwanda; and 200,000 civilian deaths from the Bosnian civil war in the Balkins (Genocide Intervention Network, 2016). During more recent 21st-century conflicts, the Global War on Terrorism, which includes Operation Iraqi Freedom, Operation Enduring Freedom, Operation New Dawn, and Operation Inherent Resolve, has resulted in more than 900,000 casualties that include U.S. military members, allied and opposition fighters, civilians, journalists, and humanitarian aid workers (Watson Institute for International and Public Affairs, 2021). Besides civilian and military casualties, the Global War on Terrorism that began post-9/11 was estimated to have cost $8 trillion in direct cost of war based on the Department of Defense Overseas Contingency Operations Budget. Civilian causalities (direct and indirect) owing to enemy combatants are difficult to obtain because there are no standardized reporting procedures for these (Physicians for Social Responsibility [PSR], 2016). PSR suggests that the U.S. military and the Department of Defense do not provide an accurate accounting of civilian causalities during war time.

Global security is reportedly in one of its most capricious states in modern times. Some would say that we are in the midst of World War III as a result of the Islamic State of Iraq; al Qaeda; the Taliban; and newer global threats by Russia, China, North Korea, and other hostile insurgencies where civilians are at the epicenter of armed conflict and the quest for power and control of land and resources. Geographic relocation to the United States and other countries is no longer just for immigrant job seekers or a quest to improve one's quality of life. Rather, the journey is long, perilous, and primarily for the purpose of basic survival, just to be able to stay alive and have basic food, water, shelter, and a safe environment to exist.

What is at stake is the safety and security of U.S. citizens' and other global civilian populations' mental and physical well-being (Hocking, 2018; Oppedal & Idsoe, 2015; Pluck et al., 2022). We are confronted by simultaneous technological, person-made, and biological threats in our homeland perpetrated by antigovernment groups, terrorist networks, and other dark entities that have flown under the radar for decades (Joint Chiefs of Staff et al., 2016).

The United States has been blessed with a democracy that respects and upholds civil liberties for the most part. It has a strong humanitarian base of nonprofit organizations and faith-based groups to help those in need of food, clean water, shelter, clothing, and mental and physical healthcare. However, the same opportunities are not afforded to civilians in war-torn countries where torture, rape, imprisonment, and execution are daily threats to minority and disempowered indigenous groups (Goodman et al., 2017; Spaas et al., 2022; Stebnicki, 2016, 2018, 2021a). As a consequence, millions of immigrants, refugees, internally displaced persons, and asylum seekers from war-torn countries seek to find safe havens in the United States and other nations that value human life and civil liberties.

DEFINITIONS

The U.S. Citizenship and Immigration Services (USCIS, 2022) under the U.S. Department of Homeland Security delineates the complex law and path to citizenship as it relates to immigrants, refugees, and asylum seekers. The USCIS (2022) makes decisions based on policies and laws that were first introduced in the Immigration and Nationality Act (INA). The INA was shaped by the McCarren–Walter bill in 1952, which created Public Law 82–414. An extensive policy manual exists (USCIS, 2016b), which provides full disclosure of all policies related to rights, responsibilities, and processes of naturalization, continuous residence, individuals and groups under temporary protected status (TPS), and overall policies related to immigration. The intent of the policy manual is to provide transparency to all public, private, and governmental entities concerning global populations of persons and groups that want to enter the United States each year. The law itself is quite complex and is beyond the scope of this chapter to be discussed comprehensively. The interested helping practitioner and students may want to consult the USCIS updated policy manual, as federal regulations, definitions, and specific issues relating to immigrants, refugees, and asylum seekers change frequently, particularly as new administrations are elected to office (USCIS, 2022). Definitions are described in the following sections so as to clarify the individuals who comprise the populations and cultures we refer to as immigrants, refugees, and asylum seekers.

Immigrant

Generally, the term *immigrant* is defined as a person who is a migrant from another country, either lawfully or unlawfully, with the intent to take up permanent residence in the United States (Department of Homeland Security, 2016). Under the *immigrant class of admission* category (Department of Homeland Security, 2022), a lawful permanent resident (LPR), or "green card" recipient, may live and work anywhere in the United States if they apply to become a permanent U.S. citizen and if they meet all the eligibility criteria. The Immigration and Nationality Act provides several broad categories of admission for foreign nationals to gain LPR status with the intent of family reunification, economic sustainability, and humanitarian outreach. The secretary of Homeland Security has the power to designate individuals and groups from foreign countries under TPS, which grants foreign nationals temporary and lawful permanent residence in the United States. This would typically be done in cases in which returning to his or her country of origin would likely result in imprisonment and/or harm would come to him or her; in many circumstances, the individual's return would result in death, such as Afghanis and Iraqis returning to their country of origin.

The uninformed and culturally insensitive often use the term *illegal aliens* for immigrants who have entered the United States lawfully and unlawfully. There is a certain degree of stigma and stereotype associated with the term *alien* because of its dehumanizing aspects. Thus, it becomes more humanistic and culturally appropriate to use the terms *LPR* and *U.S. citizen* when referring to those who immigrated lawfully to the United States and have been granted residency or citizenship status.

Refugee

The USCIS (2022) defines a *refugee* as someone who (a) is located outside the United States and is in need of humanitarian assistance; (b) demonstrates he or she has been persecuted owing to race, religion, nationality, political opinion, or membership within a particular social group and is not firmly resettled in another country; and (c) meets all the requirements for admission contingent on background screenings (i.e., mental, physical, criminal). Additionally, the United States provides *refugees* who have been persecuted or have a rationally based fear of being persecuted two programs: a *refugee* program outside the United States for their immediate relatives and an asylum program for *asylees* and their immediate relatives living in the United States (Department of Homeland Security, 2022).

Asylum Seeker

Each year people come to the United States seeking asylum because of threats to their safety and fear of persecution. Generally, the USCIS defines an *asylum seeker* as a person who, because of race, religion, nationality, membership in a particular social group, or political opinion, has been threatened with violence, persecution, and fear that he or she will suffer persecution. Asylum seekers are a new phenomenon to the United States and European nations for the 21st century because of the immense volume of populations seeking safety and security from war-torn countries. This sociopolitical phenomenon requires governments to seriously consider the human, moral, and ethical issues related to accepting and not accepting, screening, and adjudicating such populations of individuals. Issues related to terrorism, criminality, pandemic viruses, and other consequences are quite challenging for the mental and physical health and welfare of the civilized world today. As a result of case law in the United States, as well as changes in new political administrations, applicant asylees' futures are based on changing rules, policies, and procedures for temporary and permanent admission to the United States.

PREVALENCE, INCIDENCE, AND ETIOLOGY

Worldwide there are more than 89.3 million refugees, asylum seekers, and internally displaced persons from war-torn countries forced to flee their homelands (UNHCR, 2022b). The UNHCR's global trend report, compiled by governments and nongovernmental-partnering organizations, shows an enormous increase in these indigenous populations because of war and threats of safety and security. The Migration Policy Institute (MPI, 2022), a nonpartisan research and statistical analysis institute that collects data from the U.S. State Department's Worldwide Refugee Admissions Processing System (WRAPS) and Department of Homeland Security's Yearbook of Immigration Statistics, reports that 11,411 authorized refugees legally resettled in the United States during the first 6 months of 2022. This figure represents the lowest number of refugees admitted to the United States on record, with 1980 being the highest on record at 207,116. The U.S. State Department (2022) reports that 11,814 refugees were admitted to the United States during 2021. The following sample countries of origin, from the highest to lowest admissions during 2021, include Democratic Republic of Congo ($n = 2,868$), Burma ($n = 2,115$), Ukraine ($n = 1,927$), Afghanistan ($n = 604$), Iraq ($n = 537$), Syria ($n = 481$), Eritrea ($n = 475$), El Salvador ($n = 365$), Moldova ($n = 364$), Sudan ($n = 254$), Guatemala ($n = 247$), and Columbia ($n = 215$). All other countries of origin admitted to the United States for 2021 were under 200 persons. The majority of these indigenous populations have been forced out of their homelands and have resettled across about 41 states in the United States.

Astonishingly, there are more than 6.8 million refugees across the African continent with another 5.2 million requiring humanitarian assistance due to intensified conflicts; extreme climate change weather conditions; and severe deficits in housing, nutrition, healthcare, and economic stability (U.S. State Department, 2022). The United States anticipates being a key partner with UNHCR in the re-settlement of refugee minors to other countries, including the United States, in the coming years. Additionally, another global hotspot requiring humanitarian support for immigrants, refugees, asylum seekers, stateless persons, and those forcibly displaced are populations that come from Latin American countries and the Caribbean. At least 50% are children and adolescents. The United States has addressed this need through the Deferred Action for Childhood Arrivals (DACA) program. Launched in 2012, the program estimates for 2021 there were 611,470 active DACA recipients, with approximately 1.2 million currently navigating through the complex process of citizenship in the United States. A number of persons under DACA could potentially become permanent U.S. citizens under the DREAM Act of 2021.

Despite the hysteria among some Americans, the majority of applications for asylum and resettlement are being handled by multiple other countries worldwide, with Germany and other Eastern and Western European nations providing a majority of humanitarian support, not the United States. Multiple governmental and nongovernmental organizations in all 50 states have provided basic needs for these indigenous groups. The USCIS (2020) has completed more than 7.6 million applications, petitions, and requests for U.S. citizenship during fiscal year (FY) 2020, which was the lowest in the last 5 years and was driven primarily by the COVID-19 pandemic. Currently, it would appear that the immigration processing system is significantly behind due to the pandemic, is overworked and understaffed, and at times lacks the much-needed political support to lift caps on indigenous peoples who flee their country of origin to the United States to escape political persecution, torture, genocide, and being forced into military service for ongoing tribal wars.

The etiology of indigenous populations seeking asylum to other countries appears to be driven by a number of factors. Indeed, war is at the epicenter of this human suffering as millions are forced to relocate geographically. This person-made disaster points to the overall lack of respect, empathy, and protection for human life perpetrated by brutal governments, religious zealots, and other indigenous tribal warring groups. The known causes are also exemplified by civil and religious armed conflicts; continuous bombing of villages and towns; violence perpetrated by drug warlords; forced sexual prostitution and slavery; human trafficking; imprisonment by the government for possessing the "wrong" sociopolitical or religious beliefs; racism; discrimination; forced isolation/internal displacement; detention camps; deprived access to adequate mental and physical healthcare; and withholding of basic food, water, shelter, and clothing for warmth (Cigrand et al., 2022; Schick et al., 2018; Stebnicki, 2016, 2018). Overall, it is an incomprehensible task for any one government, organization, or agency to provide assistance for all those in critical need.

SOCIOCULTURAL FAMILIAL IMPACT OF WAR

Acts of genocide, ethnic cleansing, political persecution, and other atrocities have wounded the soul of indigenous populations. Although this chapter focuses on civilians that forcibly must leave their country of origin, we should also be mindful of the psychological cost of war on U.S. military personnel who are at the epicenter of peacekeeping, humanitarian efforts, or fighting enemy combatants (Stebnicki, 2021a). The mission creep, operation tempo, and frequent deployments for service members can be relentless, creating a type of moral injury, operational stress, and complex posttraumatic stress disorder (Tick, 2014), all of which have clinically significant medical, physical, psychosocial, and psychological conditions requiring immediate attention. The men and women who serve with U.S. Customs and Border Protection also have unique occupational stressors. They are at the epicenter of severe illnesses and death of immigrant and refugee family members who spent months waiting in detention centers to be processed through the U.S. Immigration and Citizenship Services. Thus, the mental health and related fields are only beginning to understand the impact that war has on cultures, civilians, active-duty service personnel, veterans, and military family members, as well as the men and women tasked with border protection.

Immigrant and refugee women are a particularly vulnerable population and comprise about 51% of foreign-born nationals who enter the United States each year (Goodman et al., 2017). Some immigrant and refugee women may frequently experience rape, torture, and human trafficking. Oftentimes, this results in complex trauma that is difficult to treat given the stark cultural differences in traditional Western psychotherapy evidence-based practices (e.g., cognitive behavioral therapy [CBT], eye movement desensitization and reprocessing [EMDR], talk therapies) versus other indigenous healing modalities that are culturally contextualized because they are focused on language, meaning, and sacred rituals (Every et al., 2017; Stebnicki, 2016).

There are significant adjustment issues for immigrant and refugee women that are different from those for men acculturating to the United States. Although, there are similarities because they both may have to learn a new language; seek appropriate healthcare, support services, and transportation; and deal with mental health and other psychosocial adjustment and acculturation issues, compared to immigrant and refugee women, men have increased work opportunities, reduced childcare responsibilities, and reduced traditional household duties that are typically relegated to women (Women for Women International, 2022).

Employment is commonly identified as a vital indicator of cultural adjustment. However, studies report obstacles for women in the work environment relating to discrimination and social injustices. For instance, Afsharian et al. (2021) report that many immigrants, particularly women, are subjected to physically and psychologically unsafe work environments where there is a higher incidence of job harassment and discrimination. Other challenges for immigrant and refugee women are the high incidence of sexual trauma, physical abuse, maternal and infant mortality, and multiple other cultural adjustment issues creating psychological distress. Studies suggest that many immigrant women are devaluated and disregarded by Western medical practices. This creates health disparities among an already vulnerable population of immigrants, refugees, and asylum seekers in the United States (Rogers et al., 2020).

Immigrant, refugee, and asylum seeker children and adolescents are especially vulnerable and profoundly affected medically, physically, and psychologically by war. There is long-term exposure to political, cultural, and sexual violence, as well as other traumatic experiences that create cultural adjustment issues (Costa et al., 2021; Elkon-Tamir et al., 2021; Spaas et al., 2022). In the United States, it is estimated that approximately 43% to 50% of all refugees are children and adolescents (American Psychological Association, 2010; U.S. State Department, 2022). In fact, many families are often forcibly separated or relocated or detained in detention facilities, creating a family crisis accompanied by the loss of family rituals and identity (Oppedal & Idsoe, 2015; Steel et al., 2011).

Another highly vulnerable population are unaccompanied minors, primarily because they are exposed to more frequent and intense traumatic incidents than accompanied immigrant and refugee children. During 2021 there were over 4,200 migrant children being held in detention centers on the U.S. border (Ordonez, 2021). The MPI (2022) reports that during 2019 approximately 11,500 unaccompanied children were detained at the U.S.–Mexico border where they were housed in Border Patrol facilities. In the first 6 months of 2022 tmore than 290 migrant families died attempting to cross over from the Mexico–U.S. border.

Indeed, the cascade of medical, physical, psychosocial, and psychological conditions are far-reaching for immigrant and refugee minors. Complicating issues related to unaccompanied minor asylum seekers include their stage of social–emotional development where many are trying to adapt, process, and navigate through normative child and adolescent social–emotional growth patterns while resettling in the United States. There are also issues related to acculturation to other foreign cultures and surrogate families, chronic and persistent posttraumatic stress symptoms, major depressive disorders, lack of knowledge about psychosocial resources, and the ability to sustain post-resettlement psychological adjustment (Fuhrer et al., 2020; Schick et al., 2018).

The significant loss of parents, family, friends, homes, schools, and other familiar daily routines for immigrant children and adolescents creates deficits in appropriate medical, physical, psychosocial, and psychological healthcare (Gargano et al., 2022; Lies et al., 2019), many of which may go underreported, undiagnosed, or undertreated. Overall, immigrant and refugee children and adolescents have been one of the most vulnerable populations with significant challenges for resettlement outside their country of origin. For instance, since the 1990s, twell over 2 million children have been killed, 6 million disabled, and 20 million left homeless as the result of war (Stichick & Bruderlein, 2001). The United Nations (2016) reports that between January 2011 and June 2015, about 1,400 boys and girls have been abducted in Iraq by al Qaeda and ISIS. In addition, more than 3,000 children have died as the result of improvised explosive device (IED) explosions.

There are severe mental, physical, social, emotional, psychological, and spiritual consequences to these cultures, which have created a historical trauma that is passed down to many future generations (Stebnicki, 2016). This humanitarian crisis requires a long-term plan to bridge the gap between Western mental health treatment strategies and adapting culturally relevant approaches for indigenous groups exposed to war (Every et al., 2017; Hanson & Vogel, 2012; Miller & Rasmussen, 2010; Nose et al., 2017; Steel et al., 2011). The complex trauma acquired by armed conflict, poverty, malnutrition, and displacement into overcrowded and impoverished refugee camps and detention centers has created mental and physical trauma, anxiety and major depressive disorders, and sleep disturbances resulting in permanent mental and physical disabilities (Lies et al., 2019; Stebnicki, 2016). The destruction of social networks and those who are survivors of forced child military service, sexual assault, and the loss of social and material support, as well as widows and orphans, has created a complex trauma that cannot be addressed purely from Western models of mental health treatment. Rather, exposure to war on civilians requires integrative, culturally sensitive approaches to heal the symptoms of posttraumatic stress and the daily stressors of survival on war-affected indigenous populations.

A humanitarian crisis of epic proportions exists on a global basis for immigrants, refugees, internally displaced persons, and asylum seekers from war-torn countries (Homeland Security, 2022). The complex global security both at home and abroad has far-reaching implications for the sociocultural and psychosocial health, safety, and welfare of all the planet's populations. The complex trauma experienced by immigrants, refugees, and asylum seekers appears to be a silent epidemic for most Americans (Stebnicki, 2016, 2018). The critical challenges for these indigenous/ethnic groups rarely come into the consciousness of "things to worry about" for most Americans, unless, of course, one or more of these groups lives in your community or you read these on social media and misinformed news reporting. It certainly becomes an issue for Americans who identify with or belong to the ethnic heritage of these groups. The reality is that no amount of money or donations can heal the suffering of foreign nationals, which can be viewed on the nightly news and other 24-hour electronic media news outlets.

Fear and ignorance are easily spread by some U.S. politicians who misuse language (i.e., illegal aliens, Muslim terrorists), which ultimately stigmatize ethnic minority groups. Truly, language has the potential to harm or heal. The 2020 COVID-19 pandemic and derogatory former president's disparaging comments about its Asian origins saw a dramatic rise in Asian American violence in the United States that continues today. Stigmatizing language communicated about different minority groups has the potential to perpetrate overt acts of prejudice, discrimination, and intentional/unintentional racism. Misuse of language by well-intentioned U.S. lawmakers who have created legal terms, such as *Hispanic*, also has the potential to stigmatize minorities because it does not consider cultural identity (i.e., Latinx, Columbian, Mexican American) and within-group differences. The various terms we use to describe other cultures tend to seep into the unconsciousness of many Americans. Consequently, we normalize the stigmatizing language used to describe different minorities and can easily become intolerant of others, which hinders our ability for compassion and empathy.

As mental health and psychosocial rehabilitation professionals, we must deflect the negative attitudes and overt prejudices that are sustained in the larger society. We are held to a much higher standard due to our ethical obligations and interest in serving others in a humanistic manner. The groups most affected have sustained enough harsh treatment for one lifetime. Thus, we have an ethical obligation to build cultural awareness, knowledge, and skills to work with others who are culturally different. Unfortunately, the majority of practitioners do not have training to work with the complex trauma experienced by immigrants from war-torn countries (Stebnicki, 2015). Despite training in multicultural counseling, most practitioners do not have the language skills and cultural knowledge to work with these indigenous populations. This should not prevent mental health professionals from responding to the humanitarian need in an empathic way of being. Accordingly, special training is required to work competently and ethically with immigrants from places in the far reaches of the globe, which is discussed later in this chapter.

GOVERNMENT-DRIVEN DISASTER RESPONSE AND STRATEGIC INITIATIVES

There is a human cost to living in an unpredictable world that has experienced person-made disasters perpetrated on defenseless and disempowered civilians who are exposed to war. Yet there is a fundamental human right recognized by the United Nations that every person has a right to leave their country and seek asylum to avoid persecution and to change their nationality. It is a concept as old as biblical times. There are no peaceful political resolutions for some immigrants, refugees, and asylum seekers in many scenarios. As a consequence, there are always civilian casualties as a result of war. Historically, there has always been a humanitarian response in times of large-scale disasters. Therefore, having some faith there will always be humanitarian efforts, as well as compassion for others, requires a determined, hopeful, positive, and optimistic view of the world.

Humanitarian efforts are seen in many corners of the Earth where agencies and organizations have mobilized to cobble together basic services for food, clean water, shelter, clothing, and medical healthcare (e.g., American Red Cross, Doctors Without Borders, International Federation of Red Cross and Red Crescent Societies, Mercy Corps). Every nonprofit agency, faith-based organization, or government entity has its own conceptual and philosophical approach to assisting with food, clean water, shelter, clothing, healthcare, financial supportment, and spiritual care. However, it is critical that some organizations take charge of planning, coordinating, organizing, and leading a unified coalition of care providers and volunteers to be effective in large-scale disaster response, such as the masses of immigrants, refugees, and asylum seekers fleeing their homelands and geographically relocating all over the world.

The Strategic Foresight Initiative (SFI) action plan developed by the Federal Emergency Management Agency (FEMA, 2012) is one example of an agency that has stepped up to the challenge of addressing the needs of immigrants, refugees, and asylum seekers in the United States and has projected and anticipated potential crisis outcomes up to the year 2030. Although FEMA's mission is not humanitarian in nature, the SFI action plan provides a comprehensive crisis response plan for handling the influx of indigenous/ethnic populations. This transformative crisis response and disaster plan is intended to advance strategic planning at the local, county, state, and federal government levels to be prepared for potential associated risks of epidemics, pandemic health, illness and disease concerns, biological risks, and other crises that might erupt as a result of populations from war-torn countries arriving to the United States.

The guideposts presented in FEMA's SFI report explore and highlight other critical areas of epidemic and pandemic concerns such as the (a) increasing complexity and decreasing predictability of living in a secure homeland environment; (b) evolving mental, medical, and physical healthcare needs of all Americans and at-risk populations; and (c) future resource constraints of fiscal, technological, and highly trained personnel to work at the epicenter of disaster. An abbreviated list of SFI scenarios includes understanding the preparation, prevention, protection, and disaster response in dealing with the healthcare of older aging adult populations, persons with chronic illnesses and disabilities, technology, terrorism in the homeland, pandemics, drought, and multiple other critical incidents that deal with the strain of economic resources, the deteriorating infrastructure, and other major threats that are both person-made and biological in nature.

The United States is the world's strongest nation enjoying the advantages of civil rights for all cultural minority groups (e.g., persons of racial/ethnic diversity; persons with disabilities; persons who identify as lesbian, gay, bisexual, and transgender [LGBT]), state–federal programs for disability benefits (e.g., workers compensation, supplemental security income [SSI], Social Security disability insurance [SSDI]), technology, energy, and alliances and partnerships with other countries to decrease security threats on multiple levels. Despite these strengths, there are countries, governments, and other dark entities outside and within the United States that would like to undo the benefits, civil rights, and social justice progress afforded to Americans.

For example, the 2015 report of the military's contribution to national security (Joint Chiefs of Staff et al., 2016) identifies threats to our national security. These include but are not limited to (a) Russia, which has repeatedly demonstrated a lack of respect for the sovereignty of its neighboring countries and other actions that violate multiple human rights agreements; (b) Iran, which also has interest in pursuing nuclear and missile delivery technologies and state-sponsored terrorism and has undermined stability in Middle Eastern countries such as Israel, Lebanon, Iraq, Syria, and Yemen; (c) North Korea, which is also very active in the pursuit of nuclear weapons, ballistic missile testing, and cyber-attacks and has repeatedly and contentiously confronted and bullied Korea and Japan with harm; and (d) China, which has added much anxiety and tension to the Asia-Pacific region not only militarily but by claiming its territories that include nearly the entire South China Sea.

Indeed, this 2015 report has been spot-on, particularly with the Russian invasion of Ukraine that began February 2022. All security risks and potential critical incidents listed earlier have the potential to destabilize countries in a wide range of areas. This ultimately results in creating a global environment of immigrants, refugees, and asylum seekers that could potentially overwhelm a country's infrastructure, economy, healthcare systems, and overall quality of life. Countries that do not advocate and codify into law basic human rights and protections for racial/ethnic minority groups, gender equality, persons with disabilities, and other vulnerable populations cannot provide a safe haven for humanitarian needs and the compassion required to assist in resettlement efforts. Indeed, countries that have security threats to their democracy and ongoing internal sociopolitical crises with the intention to destabilize systems of social justice and create civil war all have the potential to be vulnerable to chaos and instability. The key point is that the government and antigovernment factions that make up these suppressive groups have unpredictable behaviors that threaten the health, safety, and welfare of Americans and all other allied countries' around the world. Regardless of one's political, moral, and philosophical beliefs regarding the engagement in war, the presence and actions of the U.S. military, its allies, and its partners are critical to deter aggression and defeat extremist groups in key global hot spots and in our own homeland. History has shown that the real victims of war are defenseless and disempowered citizens.

Presently, we have incurred multiple limitations that exceed our resources in response to complex critical incidents occurring simultaneously (e.g., pandemic viruses, terrorism, conflict/war, cyber-security, natural disaster increasing climate refugees, and biological threats). From a sociopolitical perspective, issues related to immigrants, refugees, and asylum seekers cannot become a low priority for government agencies. Thus, it is critical that the United States set an example of service and compassion to respond to the humanitarian needs of other global populations.

GUIDELINES FOR MEDICAL AND MENTAL HEALTH SCREENINGS FOR NEWLY ARRIVED IMMIGRANTS, REFUGEES, AND ASYLUM SEEKERS

The Centers for Disease Control and Prevention (CDC, 2022) and the Division of Immigrant, Refugee, and Migrant Health offer technical instructions to medical providers in several categories such as

(a) health education and communication tools for guidance to state, regional, and county health departments; (b) profiles on refugee health; (c) international adoption guidelines; (d) current status of migration border health; and (e) laws and regulations related to immigrant, refugees, and migrant health. The intention of this division of the CDC is to promote healthy resettlement, offer technical guidelines and support to physicians and other healthcare providers, alert the public of the status of overseas travel, and provide other guidance for the overall public health in the United States. The interested reader is encouraged to view updates on the CDC website for current rules, regulations, and provider guidance given the changing sociopolitical climate and viral pandemics, which require other layers of health screenings, prevention, and programs to deter a public health crisis.

The long journey of immigrants, refugees, and asylum seekers is a testament to their psychological, emotional, and physical resiliency. However, many die along this perilous journey. In fact, during the first 6 months of 2022, 290 migrant families died on the U.S.–Mexico border (MPI, 2022). Hundreds and thousands of other migrants over the years have died traveling through Central American countries torm by civil war due to hostile environments; disease; and lack of food, water, and shelter. The dying and death experiences of migrant family members on their journey through the Americas have created a unique type of complex trauma, bereavement, and prolonged grief experience (Stebnicki, 2016, 2021b). Exposure to profound stressors and traumatic events predisposes immigrants, refugees, and asylum seekers to a life of chronic and persistent mental and physical health conditions, causing permanent disability. More specific, the chronic and persistent risk factors that predispose immigrants, refugees, and asylum seekers to a lifetime of disabilities include depression, posttraumatic stress symptoms, anxiety, prolonged grief disorders, panic attacks, substance use disorders, somatization, and traumatic brain injuries (Fuhrer et al., 2020; Nosé et al., 2017; Pluck et al., 2022; Stebnicki, 2018; Tribe et al., 2019).

The etiology and underlying cause of immigrants', refugees', and asylum seekers' poor mental and physical health conditions are well documented in the literature (CDC, 2022; Fazel et al., 2005; Hanson & Vogel, 2012; Higson-Smith, 2013; Lies et al., 2019; Miller & Rasmussen, 2010; Pells & Treisman, 2012; Spaas et al., 2022). It is unimaginable for most Americans to understand the horrific life that some have endured. This includes but is not limited to exposure to war and combat at an early age, state-sponsored violence and oppression, torture, internment camps, human trafficking, displacement from one's home and country, loss of family members and prolonged separation, the stress of adapting to a new culture, and living in poverty and unemployment. Indeed, the process of resettlement and psychosocial adjustment to living in a new country does in fact require medical and mental health interventions.

Arredondo et al. (1996) suggest that it is essential for counselors to first understand three stages of migration that impact the medical, physical, and psychological health of migrants: premigration, the journey (migration), and postmigration. Each phase has unique characteristics that help define the unique losses and traumas that immigrants, refugees, and asylum seekers experienced to support their goals in postmigration resettlement. For instance, some populations were stolen from Africa and forced into slavery while others were forced into sexual servitude. Many were subjected to war and political violence and separated from their families. Losing one's identity within their culture or homeland can be disempowering but oftentimes coexists with traumatic experiences. In another study using a phenomenological research design, Cigrand et al. (2022) conducted and analyzed interviews of 15 Latinx and Asian immigrants and refugees who shared their stories of premigration, migration, and postmigration experiences. As they described their experiences, four themes emerged that helped counselors better understand their journey into postmigration resettlement. Themes that were identified include (a) the dire decisions they had to make (e.g., sociopolitical forces influencing their departure, war, impact on their mental and physical well-being); (b) resilience and perseverance to make the arduous journey (e.g., oppression in their country, motivation for a better quality of life); (c) trauma and losses (e.g., physical injury and violence, civil wars, loss of family members); and (d) human rights violations they experienced (e.g., exploitation, discrimination, criminalization).

Indeed, counseling professionals are trained in multicultural counseling approaches, yet few have the opportunities to work with global populations of immigrants, refugees, and asylum seekers. Professional counselors are encouraged to seek additional training in working with specific cultural groups in postmigration resettlement. There may be multiple opportunities for counselors to advocate for and serve global populations of individuals in their region of the country either in faith-based organizations, private practices, or through the federal government. Facilitating counseling approaches that secure cultural pride is at the foundation of culturally competent counseling. The section that follows, derived from federal government guidelines and research-based entities, offers guidelines to professionals that assist in the diagnosis and treatment of mental health conditions and psychosocial approaches that enhance optimal medical, physical, psychosocial, and psychological well-being of immigrants, refuges, and asylum seekers to enhance successful postmigration resettlement.

Triage of Immigrants, Refugees, and Asylum Seekers

Under the authority of the Public Health Service Act, the U.S. Department of Health and Human Services (DHHS, 2022) and the CDC's Division of Immigrant, Refugee, and Migrant Health (CDC, 2022) outline regulations for medical and mental health screenings of immigrants, refugees, and asylum seekers pursuing lawful permanent residency in the United States. The process and regulations are quite complex. Thus, for a more comprehensive review, readers should consult the References for the various U.S. government websites for updated policies, regulations, and federal guidelines to healthcare providers.

One of the first steps in this process is developing health clinics in the homeland and overseas for the purpose of triaging refugees and asylum seekers. Clinicians perform a variety of medical and mental health evaluations using medically trained American-born interpreters and bicultural interpreters. Based on the severity of symptoms presented by the refugee patient and his or her ability to function in daily life, the medical evaluations are triaged into three separate groups. Group I includes those refugees with chronic, serious, and acute health conditions that require immediate follow-up. Group II includes refugees with less acute mental health or psychiatric symptoms that only require routine follow-up care. Group III involves refugees without any identified mental or physical symptoms that require routine or immediate care.

Refugees' Mental and Physical Assessment

Medical, physical, psychosocial, and psychological complaints are quite common among immigrants, refugees, and asylum seekers from many countries. Yet only a small portion of these groups receives the appropriate diagnosis and culturally focused treatment to enhance optimal wellness (Fuhrer et al., 2020; Hocking, 2018; Pluck et al., 2022). In the United States, guidelines and procedures for the mental and physical assessment are comprehensive and mandatory for all immigrants, refugees, and asylum seekers pursuing permanent citizenship. The goal is to prevent, detect, and intervene in mental or physical health conditions that require urgent or immediate attention and to generally assess those refugees who require referral and follow-up care with other providers. For instance, there are strict guidelines to prevent the spread of COVID-19 and its mutant variants as well as other viruses that could cause a global pandemic. There are also intestinal parasites that have been identified in other countries whereby the refugee may require social isolation, treatment, and/or vaccination if available. The following are a sample of mandatory guidelines for medical and mental health professionals to implement in terms of screenings and evaluations:

- Review of any available premigration medical and mental health records from the refugees' country of origin

- Current medical history, physical exam, use of prescription medications, allergies, and particularly screening for such neurological conditions as traumatic brain injury

- Exposure to any occupational hazards, as many indigenous minority groups have worked in agriculture, mining, and factory occupations that have a high-risk exposure to toxins

- The level of exposure to combat and other traumatic events, particularly screening for symptoms of posttraumatic stress

- Screening for other mental health conditions such as depression, anxiety, and substance use disorders; screenings for drug and alcohol use also include any use of traditional herbal indigenous substances such as khat

- Specialized child screenings that include childhood immunizations, vaccinations, allergies, any malnutrition, maltreatment, scars, physical deformities, the child's patterns of normal development, level of education, and any somatic complaints

- Social–familial–cultural history, as well as educational, occupational, or literacy levels

If significant positive findings emerge from any of these assessments, it is quite typical that follow-up clinical observations and assessments are warranted. All critical information is provided to resettlement agencies so that individual needs can be met. It is particularly important that on initial assessment vulnerable populations are identified because of some unique needs requiring follow-up care. Some vulnerable populations include the following individuals: (a) pregnant women and infants; (b) severely disabled individuals and those who have chronic illnesses; (c) those who exhibit chronic and persistent psychiatric symptoms; (d) those who are developmentally disabled and those who possess other neurocognitive conditions; and (e) those who are aged, elderly, or frail.

CULTIVATING A WORKING ALLIANCE WITH REFUGEES: CONSIDERATIONS FOR MENTAL HEALTH AND PSYCHOSOCIAL REHABILITATION PROFESSIONALS

It is of paramount importance that mental health and psychosocial rehabilitation professionals use culturally sensitive approaches when interacting with immigrants, refugees, and asylum seekers, many of whom are significantly culturally different from the professional's background. Rapport building and earning the circle of trust is paramount for forming a strong working alliance. The use of culturally appropriate empathy and other therapeutic techniques (e.g., eye contact, social distancing, body language) are critical elements during therapeutic interactions. Mental health and psychosocial rehabilitation professionals should anticipate some level of difficulty during rapport building, which is a natural artifact of working with immigrants, refugees, and asylum seekers. Some examples of these difficulties exist because:

- Many cultural groups distrust Americans because they were taught to fear them by their country of origin.

- The U.S. military may have invaded their country, which destabilized their government and destroyed their homeland.

- Americans are many times viewed as violent people as portrayed in movies and other electronic media.

- Some indigenous groups may view mental health professionals as an extension of their previous punitive government.

- Some indigenous groups may not understand the American lifestyle behaviors as portrayed in the electronic and social media.

- Most indigenous groups do not have a mental health provider system such as the United States, and many do not endorse mental health counseling because they were taught not to disclose personal problems and issues to strangers.

Facilitating culturally sensitive approaches with immigrants, refugees, and asylum seekers also requires some knowledge, awareness, and skills in the following areas:

- Knowledge of the geographic location and salient aspects of the refugee's culture (i.e., religious and spiritual beliefs, occupations, daily lifestyle habits, form of government, system of healthcare and education)

- Competencies in the use of cultural empathy (i.e., use of eye contact, nonverbal language, spatial distance, time orientation)

- Administration and use of all assessments (standardized and nonstandardized) and an understanding that most assessments were not culturally normed on the population being served

- The mental health professional's overreliance on Western mental health counseling theories and techniques ignoring culturally focused approaches

- The mental health counselor's use and overuse of diagnosing and treating mental health disorders as they relate to the *Diagnostic and Statistical Manual of Mental Disorders, Fifth Edition (DSM-5) and DSM-5-TR* criteria (American Psychiatric Association, 2013, 2022)

First Steps in Cultivating a Working Alliance

Many immigrants, refugees, and asylum seekers want to escape their countries of origin because of mental and physical torture, mass violence and genocide, witnessing the killings of family members and friends, sexual abuse, kidnapping of children and women to be used in forced sexual prostitution, looting of personal possessions by the government/military, starvation, and deprivation of food, shelter, and clothing. The acts of brutality perpetrated on these indigenous groups have created distrust among almost everyone except the friends and family whom they journeyed with to find safe haven. Accordingly, mental health professionals can cultivate a working alliance possessing awareness, knowledge, and skills in the following areas:

- Use language interpreters when necessary for communicating, and always attend to the person you are speaking to, not the interpreter. It is preferable to use an interpreter from the indigenous group you are serving.

- Find a tribal leader, elder, or some other member of the refugee group who has knowledge of the specific culture and the needs of his or her own people.

- Collaborate, support, and coordinate services, working through one or two persons who are indigenous to the culture, which can help build trust among others in the group.

- Understand that "silence" does not imply resistance. Rather, many refugees have a natural reluctance toward Americans or engaging in Western models of therapeutic services from someone outside their culture.

- Understand how to interpret the emotions and cognitions of refugees, which is critical to engaging in therapeutic alliances. For instance, many refugees may exhibit feelings of rage and anger. This should not be anthologized. Rather, anger and rage are many times experienced as inconceivable betrayal by the government they once trusted. There are many other emotions that require other interpretations.

■ Use natural spaces or the natural environment to build a rapport and working alliance with someone. An office space or building can potentially intimidate many indigenous populations and may retraumatize these individuals as a representation of the brutal government from which they fled.

Second Steps in Cultivating a Working Alliance

There are no words to describe the horrific trauma that many refugees have experienced. A seasoned humanitarian mental health professional understands the refugee's risk factors and long-term mental health problems and knows how to reduce further traumatic exposure by creating a *circle of trust*. This trust can potentially be developed by the strategies offered in the section "First Steps in Cultivating a Working Alliance" and can be strengthened by the following therapeutic culturally endorsed interventions:

■ Mental health professionals should view refugees as "survivors" rather than "victims." There are extraordinary stories of survival that can help build resiliency among others in the refugee groups. Shared storytelling among group members that are matched appropriately (men to men; women to women) is critical. Individual therapeutic interaction for many indigenous groups is not a natural way of healing. Thus, the group is only as strong and resilient as those that comprise the group. Refugee groups can draw to one another because they have earned the circle of trust.

■ The numbness and shock of being a survivor of the horrific extraordinary stressful and traumatic events experienced by the refugee may linger much longer than anticipated. Everyone heals at his or her own rate and pace; however, the level of intensity and posttraumatic stress symptoms may endure for months after an arrival to a safe-haven country.

■ It is essential to listen to and elicit immigrants', refugees', and asylum seekers' stories regarding their premigration, journey (migration), and postmigration experiences. Each phase has unique characteristics that can help define the unique losses and traumas they have experienced. Culturally competent professionals understand how they can use this information for strengthening the therapeutic bond.

CONCLUSION

The etiology of the worldwide pandemic of immigrants, refugees, and asylum seekers is clear. It is war that is at the foundation of all human suffering as millions are forced to relocate geographically. This epidemic of person-made disaster points to the overall lack of respect and empathy for human life perpetrated by brutal governments, religious zealots, and other indigenous tribal warring groups. The known causes are also exemplified by civil and religious armed conflicts; continuous bombing of villages and towns; violence perpetrated by drug warlords; forced sexual prostitution and slavery; imprisonment by the government for possessing the "wrong" sociopolitical or religious beliefs; racism; discrimination; forced isolation/internal displacement and detention camps; deprived access to adequate mental and physical healthcare; and the withholding of basic food, water, shelter, and clothing for warmth. Counseling professionals have had few opportunities to work with global populations of immigrants, refugees, and asylum seekers. Given the changing demographics in the United States, professional counselors are encouraged to seek additional training in working with specific cultural groups in postmigration resettlements. Facilitating counseling approaches that secure cultural pride is at the foundation of culturally competent counseling.

CLASS ACTIVITIES

1. Have students imagine and discuss the psychosocial issues faced by immigrants and refugees attempting to come to America for a better life. Specifically, how will they obtain food in overcrowded camps? How will mothers take care of their infant children? How will they be able to access adequate medical care if a member gets sick? What are the societal attitudes they are likely to encounter?

2. Other than war, fear of gangs, and the poor available job economy in these countries that are being fled, what is another growing significant global issue facing many countries that has gradually occurred over the past 20 years? Discuss.

KEY REFERENCES

Only key references appear in the print edition. The full references appear in the digital product on Springer Publishing Connect™: https://connect.springerpub.com/content/book/978-0-8261-5111-7/part/partIV/chapter/ch20

Costa, D., Biddle, L., & Bozorgmehr, K. (2021). Association between psychosocial functioning, health status and healthcare access of asylum seekers and refugee children: A population-based cross-sectional study in a German federal state. *Child and Adolescent Psychiatry and Mental Health, 15*(59), 1–15. doi.org/10.1186/s13034-021-00411-4

Fuhrer, A., Niedermaier, A., Kalfa, V., & Mikolajczyk, R. (2020). Serious shortcomings in assessment and treatment of asylum seekers' mental health needs. *PLoS ONE, 15*(10), 1–13. doi.org/10.1371/journal.pone.0239211

Goodman, R. D., Vesely, C. K., Letiecq, B., & Cleaveland, C. L. (2017). Trauma and resiliency among refugee and undocumented immigrant women. *Journal of Counseling and Development, 95*, 309–321. https://doi.org/10.1002/jcad.12145

Hanson, E., & Vogel, G. (2012). The impact of war on civilians. In L. L. Levers (Ed.), *Trauma counseling: Theories and interventions* (pp. 412–433). Springer Publishing Company.

Oppedal, B., & Idsoe, T. (2015). The role of social support in the acculturation and mental health of unaccompanied minor asylum seekers. *Scandinavian Journal of Psychology, 56*, 203–211. https://doi.org/10.1111/sjop.12194

Spaas, C., Verelst, A., Devlieger, I., Aalto, S., Andersen, A. J., Durbeej, N., Hilden, P. K., Kankaanpaa, R., Primdahl, N. L., Opaas, M., Osman, F., Peltonen, K., Sarkadi, A., Skovdal, M., Jervelund, S. S., Soye, E., Watters, C., Derluyn, I., Colpin, H., & De Haene, L. (2022). Mental health of refugee and non-refugee migrant young people in European secondary education: The role of family separation, daily material stress and perceived discrimination in resettlement. *Journal of Youth and Adolescence, 51*, 848–870. doi.org/10.1007/s10964-021-01515-y

Stebnicki, M. A. (2015, October). The psychosocial cost of war on non-military civilian populations: A global perspective. Presentation made at the Annual Conference of the Licensed Professional Counseling Association of North Carolina, Raleigh, NC.

Stebnicki, M. A. (2021a). *Clinical military counseling: Guidelines for practice.* American Counseling Association.

CHAPTER 21

KEY CONCEPTS AND TECHNIQUES FOR AN AGING POPULATION OF PERSONS WITH DISABILITIES

EVA MILLER AND SUSANNE M. BRUYÈRE

LEARNING OBJECTIVES

After reading this chapter you should be able to:

- Understand the importance of addressing the vocational and employment goals of older individuals in the clinical process
- Identify how employment discrimination may occur for older individuals
- Become familiar with the developmental and sociological models for aging and how they inform clinical intervention around work and employment for older individuals
- Discuss with both individuals and employers ways in which workplace policies and practices can enhance the productivity, retention, and job satisfaction for older workers

PRE-READING QUESTIONS

1. Why might it be important for rehabilitation and other counseling professionals to focus on the vocational interests and employment outcomes for older clients?

2. What might be some of the barriers to equitable access to employment for older workers that counselors might want to address and prepare them for?

3. How might counselors assess the vocational/career/employment interests of older individuals?

4. How might employers create a more inclusive workplace for older employees?

5. How can counselors serve as consultants to employers on older worker issues?

Older workers are one of the fastest-growing subsets of the American workforce; many more people are working into their later years, a trend that is expected to continue. A number of factors are driving this trend. Many older Americans are now healthier later in life, they have a longer life expectancy, and they are better educated than previous generations, which increases their likelihood of staying in the labor force and retaining their autonomy and dignity. According to the Social Security Administration (2021), the number of Americans 65 and over will increase from 57 million in 2021 to about 76 million in 2035. Many of these older Americans are now continuing to work beyond the previously anticipated retirement age of 65, as their life expectancy during their retirement age is longer. In 1940, the life expectancy of a 65-year-old was almost 14 years, whereas today it is estimated at over 20 years (Social Security Administration, 2021). Many older workers therefore anticipate needing more resources to support a longer retirement tenure; this is one factor in older workers remaining employed.

People are working later in life for a number of reasons besides increasing longevity into the retirement years and the need for additional economic support. Changes in Social Security and retirement public policy as well as economic necessity have been motivators for some, but for others a desire for continuing professional and workplace social community engagement is a key factor (Kita, 2019). Personal fulfillment and the social benefits of work are additional factors why older workers, as well as the general workforce across all ages, find work fulfilling and want to stay engaged in vocational pursuits. Recognizing this in the larger social American policy and community context, there are increasing efforts to promote financial independence, emotional health, and physical wellness among the growing population of older individuals (Gonzales et al., 2015).

With more aging workers deciding to stay in the workforce, it is imperative that workplaces adjust their policies and practices to accommodate their retention and build more age-inclusive workplace cultures. Older people have often historically been devalued by society, discriminated against with regard to employment, discouraged from making their own decisions about a variety of aspects of their lives, and forced to make residential relocations into institutions that may not encourage or allow dependence of thought or action (Kampfe, 2015). The growing numbers of people staying in the workforce longer is forcing needed changes to this scenario.

As the baby boom generation continues to age, the number of 65- to 74-year-olds in the labor force is projected to increase more than workers in other age groups (U.S. Bureau of Labor Statistics, 2021). The percentage of workers aged 75 years and older in the labor force is expected to grow by 96.5% over the next decade, from 8.9% in 2020 to 11.7% in 2030 (U.S. Bureau of Labor Statistics, 2021). In contrast, participation rates for most other age groups in the labor force are not projected to change much over the 2014 to 2024 decade (Toossi & Torpey, 2017).

The aging population is also likely to result in an increasing number of people with disabilities in the workforce who may have difficulty with work performance and staying employed, especially in positions with higher physical demands in the job (Converso et al., 2018). Workplaces and workers must be equipped to take advantages of workplace policies and practices that heighten the likelihood that older workers are able to stay in the workforce, retain their productivity, and experience the significant job and life satisfaction that they deserve. Yet a 2013 study conducted by Cornell University and the Disability Management Employer Coalition (DMEC) revealed although 86% of employers polled were concerned about the impacts of an aging workforce, only 36% addressed aging in absence and disability management (ADM) program design (Bruyère et al., 2019; Switzer et al., 2014).

Rehabilitation and other counseling service providers can assist in raising awareness both with employers and with aging workers about effective policies and practices that can minimize the negative impact on work productivity that they might experience and maximize longevity in the workforce. To do so, effective counseling practices should increasingly include attention to preparing both individuals and their workplaces for the impact of the aging process. Proactive education on ways to maximize the productivity of an aging workforce, effective case management, and workplace accommodations can significantly contribute to maximizing aging-worker retention.

DEVELOPMENTAL MODELS OF AGING

Addressing the needs of our aging workforce involves understanding human development. All people age, but how we age varies considerably from person to person. Most would agree the aging process involves a natural decline in physical, social, and biological processes, but what about the fact that older adults have limited time to pursue their dreams and resolve regrets they may harbor? What about the older person who is forced to work well past her ideal age of retirement due to financial needs? What constitutes "healthy" aging? In order to understand how people function in their later years, it is important to understand a person's development across the life span. There are a number of models that explain human development, including Freud's psychosexual theory of development (1905), which focuses on childhood conflict to explain personality development, and learning theory, which emphasizes rewards, punishments, and imitating others as part of the learning process. We also have Vygotsky's sociocultural theory of development (1929), which maintains learning is influenced by the sociological context in which we are raised.

While each of these models contributes to our understanding of development, one of the most influential models of human development germane to counseling and public healthcare is Erikson's model of psychosocial development (1950). Erikson's theory is based on the *epigenetic principle,* which means a person passes through predetermined developmental stages over a lifetime and each of these stages builds upon a previous stage. At each stage, we face a developmental "crisis" or a life challenge we must overcome in order to move successfully to the next stage of development. Erikson underscored the role of social interaction and relationships in human development and believed the ability to overcome age-related struggles leads to the development of personality traits that facilitate confidence, resilience, and well-being. Erikson maintained old age, the last of eight stages of development, is characterized by *integrity* versus *despair,* which begins at age 65 and ends at the time of death. In this stage, conflict centers around existential uncertainties that involves questioning whether we have led a rewarding and meaningful life. Integrity, or the ability to look back on one's life with feelings of pride and accomplishment, involves self-acceptance, feeling a sense of connectedness with others, having few regrets, and coming to terms with our mortality. Despair involves feelings of bitterness, discontentment, guilt, depression, and hopelessness. Erikson (1950) believed most people do not experience complete integrity or total despair, but instead strike a healthy balance between the two while examining and trying to make sense of their lives. For older people, this entails reconciliation of the past as well as dealing with current life issues such as being forced to work past one's planned age of retirement due to economic hardship, developing a chronic illness, caring for an aging life partner or parent, and the passing of family and friends. As such, having a solid understanding of the developmental process can improve counselors' and case managers' ability to help older adults navigate this last stage of development.

SOCIOECOLOGICAL MODELS OF AGING

Bronfenbrenner's theory of socioecological development (1977) provides one of the most widely accepted explanations of the influence a person's environment has on their development. According to Bronfenbrenner, a person is viewed as inseparable from their environment and all aspects of development are interwoven. People are embedded in a series of four interactive systems that determine how we think and feel. To illustrate Bronfenbrenner's model from an aging perspective, an example would be an older person at the center of their socioecological system where they are surrounded by family, friends, coworkers, and those most important to them who comprise his or her *microsystem.* Next, we have the older person's *mesosystem,* which involves interconnections among the major settings in which they come into contact (e.g., family interactions, spiritual affiliations, and work). This is followed by the *exosystem,* which includes social settings surrounding older individuals such as their neighborhood and political institutions. The final system is the *macrosystem,* which involves the social, legal, economic, and political systems that surround such individuals. It is this final system where they are either encouraged or excluded and where ageism becomes a factor for some. According to Braimah and Rosenberg (2021), the complexities of aging require careful consideration of the interconnected influences of one's environment. For example, if an older person lives in a neighborhood where they feel afraid or they experience discrimination, the impact is likely to be toxic to their well-being.

THEORETICAL AND CLINICAL IMPLICATIONS

Historically, old age was viewed as a time fraught with disease and disability. Cumming and Henry (1961) introduced their *disengagement theory* to describe old age as a period of withdrawal or disengagement from social interactions and activities. According to disengagement theory, older individuals relinquish their roles in society to make way for younger generations. We see this happen regularly, with older workers getting pushed out of the labor force and being replaced by younger employees. Another prominent psychological theory that views old age in a broader sense is Havighurst's (1961) *activity theory,* which maintains old age is a time to modify or substitute one's roles and activities to maintain a positive sense of self. For example, an older person might change their role of employee to volunteer when they retire. Another well-known theory, the *continuity theory of aging* (Atchley, 1989), maintains that as people grow older, their personality and level of activity continue just as when they were younger and past coping strategies are used to deal with physical, financial, and social problems. This theory aligns with a solution-focused psychotherapeutic approach that encourages the use of problem-solving as opposed to getting "stuck" and feeling helpless. Indeed, aging necessitates major life changes for many, and aging theories can guide practitioners in their efforts to help older adults traverse these crucial adjustments.

There are myriad clinical considerations that affect older adults; however, for the purposes of this chapter, we will address the primary issues associated with an aging workforce. To begin, it is important to examine some pertinent aging demographics. According to the Administration on Aging (AoA, 2021), 9.8 million (18%) Americans ages 65 and older were working or were actively seeking employment in 2020; however, the unemployment rate for older adults more than quadrupled following the COVID-19 pandemic. In addition, 4.9 million Americans (almost 10%) age 65 and over lived below the poverty level in 2019, and the highest poverty rates were experienced among older Hispanic and African American women who lived alone. Indeed, many older adults, especially women of color, are facing heavy economic burden but are unable to retire. The inability to retire as planned is unfortunate, as approximately 20% of adults ages 65 and over have reported they could not function at all or had considerable difficulty with at least one of six functional domains (i.e., trouble seeing and hearing, problems with mobility, communication problems, cognitive issues, and problems with self-care (AoA, 2021). With regard to their health, most older Americans have at least one chronic condition, and many have multiple conditions. In fact, aging is associated with the increased risk of many diseases, including heart disease, diabetes, arthritis, Alzheimer disease, and cancer (Centers for Disease Control and Prevention [CDC], 2022), yet many people with these chronic conditions are working well past their preferred age of retirement. Other issues that impact an older person's well-being include social isolation, inadequate technological supports (e.g., poor Internet service and outdated computers), being a primary caregiver for a life partner or a grandchild, and the need for in-home or skilled nursing care (Cox, 2020). As such, counselors, case managers, and those in healthcare should be cognizant of these and related issues when addressing the needs of our aging workforce.

For individuals with serious mental illness (SMI), the aging process may be accelerated and is associated with reduced life expectancy as compared to the general population (SAMSHA, 2021). According to the World Health Organization (WHO) (2021), approximately 13% of adults ages 70 years and over had a mental disorder in 2019 (namely anxiety and depressive disorders), yet most mental health service dollars are usually targeted for young adults, adolescents, and children. WHO (2021) also reported the rate of mental disorders is higher among older adults living in poverty, and while older women tend to have higher rates of mental disorders than men, this gap fades with increased age (e.g., 80s and over). Other factors that contribute to the reduced life expectancy of people with SMI include inadequate access to preventive healthcare, greater exposure to chronic stress and trauma, increased risk of suicide, and factors associated with low socioeconomic status (Substance Abuse and Mental Health Services Administration [SAMHSA], 2021). In addition, some studies suggest psychological distress is higher among marginalized groups of older individuals, including persons of color and LGBTQ+ groups (Carpenter et al., 2022). With regard to suicide, the rate for males aged 75 and over was the highest of all age groups in 2020 (CDC, 2022). In addition, according to the CDC (2022), 6.2 million Americans have Alzheimer disease, the most common type of neurocognitive disorder and the fifth leading cause of death among people ages 65 and over. As such, facilitating access to health and mental health services and supports for older workers is imperative.

While substance use tends to decline after young adulthood, nearly 1 million adults aged 65 and older have a substance use disorder ([SUD], SAMHSA, 2019). Alcohol is the most widely used drug among older individuals, with approximately 65% of those age 65 and older reporting high-risk drinking, defined as exceeding daily guidelines (two drinks for men and one for women) at least weekly (National Institute on Drug Abuse [NIDA], 2020). In addition, older adults are often prescribed more medications than other age groups, leading to a higher rate of exposure to potentially addictive medications. For example, chronic pain may be more complicated in older adults experiencing other health conditions, often leading to increased use of prescription opioid medications for pain relief. According to NIDA (2020), the primary takeaways regarding substance use among older adults include the following: substance use among older adults is increasing; older adults are more highly susceptible to drugs and alcohol effects than younger adults; they are more likely to unintentionally misuse medications by forgetting to take them or taking too many; and they may use substances to cope with life changes such as retirement, declining health, a change in living situation, and issues related to grief and loss. Recognizing the value of older workers and facilitating their ability to overcome substance use issues can have a profound impact on their employment success as well as their overall life satisfaction.

ASSESSMENT OF OLDER ADULTS

As with other age groups, treatment for older individuals begins with proper assessment; however, there are a number of noteworthy considerations to keep in mind when examining older adults. One of the first things to address is why the person is being referred for testing, as this will guide clinicians in choosing the most relevant test instruments. Ask yourself, "What is the presenting problem(s)?" If the older person is unable to tell you why they have been referred for assessment, after obtaining the person's written permission, you may wish to consult with family members or friends who know the person well. The referring party is usually a good source as well. It is also important to note that many older adults do not have experience in the standardized testing process and may feel threatened or intimated when informed they are going to be tested. As such, older adults may benefit from additional explanation to clarify what the test measures, its relevance to their current issues, and the benefits of the test results as they relate to them (Kampfe, 2015). Providing reassurance may also be helpful. For example, the counselor or case manager can inform the person that the questions that will be asked are standard questions asked of all clients who come in for testing. This strategy may be especially helpful for individuals referred for cognitive problems (e.g., memory impairment), as they may become suspicious about why they are being assessed and exhibit increased anxiety, which can render their test results invalid.

Respecting one's culture is another important factor to consider when assessing older individuals. One way to do so is to use the method that entails a person's level of *education*, their *culture* and level of acculturation, *language* proficiency, *economic* issues, *communication* style, *testing* situation and one's *comfort* and level of motivation, intelligence, and the context of one's immigration (Fujii, 2018). Another helpful strategy that can be used when assessing older adults is to carefully observe their behavior (also called *subjective assessment*). This is true of all types of assessments, whether it be a vocational assessment or a depression inventory. Practitioners will want to note behaviors indicative of anxiety, boredom, and confusion, among others, as these behaviors can influence assessment outcomes. For example, the detection of anxiety in older individuals may be complicated and can be easily confused with normal aspects of aging such as age-related cognitive decline (Balsamo et al., 2018).

Functional assessments are critical for older workers, given their increased likelihood for chronic illness and disability. There are many instruments from which to choose, and the types of functional assessments selected will vary depending on individual need (e.g., the functioning of 60-year-old may vary widely from that of someone who is much older). However, important areas to assess are the person's ability to carry out essential responsibilities (e.g., manage household and work) and their physical, psychological, and social limitations. Goldman (2020) noted it is prudent to examine physical movements such as lifting and walking and integrating these activities into one's ability to fulfill occupational and social roles when completing a geriatric assessment. According to Goldman, impairment of functional status can be triggered by the onset of deconditioning, disease, changes in social support or environment, and advanced age, all of which can impede an older worker's job performance. Variables such as lifestyle, coping abilities, activity accommodations, medical care, external supports, physical and social environments, therapeutic regimens, and rehabilitation can mediate the severity of functional limitations and subsequent development of disabilities (Ng & Law, 2014).

Research shows people's goals and strategies for participating in the workforce and accomplishing work goals change over time due to age-related losses, gains, and shifts in priorities (Heckhausen et al., 2019). Career assessment plays a vital role in the conceptualization of older workers' employment goals. Some of the most widely used career-related inventories are Holland's (1997) *Theory of Career Choice*, the *Strong Interest Inventory* (Hansen, 2000), and the *Myers Briggs* (Myers, 1962). For older workers with significant disabilities, a referral for a comprehensive vocational evaluation may be indicated. Vocational rehabilitation counselors specialize in vocational assessment and helping people with physical, mental, developmental, and emotional disabilities find employment and live independently. The increased number of older adults in the workforce also entails an increased number of older individuals with disabilities in the workforce, who will likely qualify for protection under Title I of the Americans with Disabilities Act, including protection against employment discrimination and the receipt of reasonable accommodations. However, due to fear of ageist attitudes and a host of reasons, older persons may be reluctant to request accommodations, or they may be unaware of their protection rights (Dong, 2018), and rehabilitation counselors who are trained to assist workers in overcoming employment barriers are in a great position to advocate on behalf of older workers.

A general mental health assessment for older adults typically includes a comprehensive social history (e.g., living situation, family, support systems, employment status, and quality of work setting), a developmental history, a psychological history that includes current mental health issues (e.g., presenting problem and previous counseling), substance abuse history, documentation of physical issues and current medications, behavioral observations, formal testing (if indicated), and any other relevant information that guides treatment planning. Older adults with SMI are especially at risk for missed or inaccurate diagnoses of mental health issues, as psychiatric symptoms may overlap with multiple co-occurring illnesses, making it difficult for practitioners to form an accurate diagnosis. For example, psychosis (e.g., delusions and/or hallucinations) in older adults is often a symptom of another primary disorder, including a neurological disorder, illicit substance use, prescribed medications, or delirium (disturbance in attention and awareness that develops quickly and tends to fluctuate in intensity during the course of a day), rather than a primary psychotic disorder or SMI (SAMHSA, 2021). Therefore, a thorough evaluation of an individual's physical and mental health and their medical history is vital to understanding the underlying cause of a symptom and arriving at an accurate diagnosis, and counselors and case managers who work with older persons will want to receive training specific to this population. It should be noted, however, that because of the complexities often found in older adults (e.g., cognitive issues, chronic health issues), a referral for thorough psychological or neuropsychological assessment may be indicated.

Some of the most common mental health instruments used by counselors, case managers, social workers, and those in public healthcare are relatively easy to administer and score; however, training and supervision are needed to ensure proper use for novice practitioners. Examples of instruments commonly used to assess for depression and anxiety among older adults include the *Geriatric Depression Scale* (Yesavage et al., 1983) and the *Geriatric Anxiety Scale* (Mueller et al., 2015). The *Patient Health Questionnaire* [(PHQ-9); Kroenke & Spitzer, 2002) is another good depression inventory many practitioners use to monitor the severity of depression and response to treatment. In addition, the *Mini Mental State Exam-II* (Folstein et al., 2010) is one of the most frequently used brief assessments of cognitive impairment. Life satisfaction, hope, resilience, and social supports are also factors to consider when evaluating older adults, and there are many questionnaires designed to assess these traits.

With regard to substance abuse and assessment, older adults are less likely to receive screening and assessment than younger adults, which can be dangerous, as they are more likely to feel the negative effects of alcohol and drugs and are more likely to take multiple medications, which can lead to fatal drug interactions (SAMHSA, 2020). In addition, approximately 36.8% of older adults with SUDs also have co-occurring mental health issues, and 10.7% of adolescents had a SUD co-occurring with mental illness (SAMSHA, 2020). A wide variety of instruments can be used to detect SUDs among older adults. The *Alcohol Use Disorders Identification Test* (AUDIT; Aalto et al., 2011) was developed to screen for heavy alcohol use and can readily identify alcohol misuse in people ages 65 and older. The *Senior Alcohol Misuse Indicator* (Purcell & Olmstead, 2014) is another reliable, five-item questionnaire that identifies older adults who may engage in risky alcohol use. The *Alcohol, Smoking and Substance Involvement Screening Test* (ASSIST) is another widely used questionnaire developed by WHO (2010) to assess for substance misuse, including alcohol and tobacco use. According to SAMHSA (2020) SUD assessment should include mental health, medical, family, vocational, social, sexual, financial, legal, substance use, and SUD treatment histories. A physical exam is also recommended to assess for co-occurring physical issues that can impact an older person's mental health as well as to assess for problems secondary to the substance abuse (e.g., sleep problems, chronic pain). The assessment should also include biological screening measures, such as urine screens for benzodiazepines and opiates, breath alcohol testing (i.e., Breathalyzer), and lab work.

The testing site is another area to consider when assessing older adults. For example, older adults should be informed in advance of the upcoming assessment(s), and, to ensure optimal performance, they should be asked to bring all assistive devices to the testing site (Kampfe, 2015). There are many assessment instruments designed specifically for older individuals, and the appropriate test battery will depend on the reason the person is being referred for assessment. However, it is important to note that not all assessments for older individuals were normed for older adults and these test results should be interpreted with caution and, whenever possible, a different instrument should be selected. In addition, due to their age, older individuals often benefit from a thorough geriatric assessment that includes a functional assessment, a medical exam, cognitive assessment, home safety assessment, neurologic assessment, pain assessment, a nutritional assessment, and for some, hospice and end-of-life assessment.

Testing considerations and accommodations for older workers are other important areas to address. For example, people with sensory impairments and those with reduced energy levels or disabling physical conditions may show signs of fatigue and can benefit from accommodations during testing. Many older adults also report restrictions in their ability to carry out meaningful activities of daily living and should be assessed for this as well. In addition, according to Kampfe (2015), reflex speed tends to decrease and sensory loss increases with age, so power or practical tests may be more meaningful than speed tests. Other practices to consider when assessing older workers include using situational or ecological evaluations (i.e., assessment using actual employment and community settings) and implementing job trials, which can provide a more accurate representation of an older worker's job skills than paper-and-pencil or computer-generated tests.

Given the increased likelihood of chronic illness, disability, and sensory impairments among older adults, it also is important to ensure there is adequate lighting and that the older person can hear, and you will want to test the person in the language of their choice. If you suspect the older person is experiencing hearing problems, you might administer the *Hearing Handicap Inventory for the Elderly – Screening Version* (Weinstein, 1986), a 10-item, self-administered questionnaire developed to measure social and emotional problems secondary to hearing impairment. Using large fonts is one way to address this issue. A quick way to test if a person can see is to simply ask them to read a brief statement placed in front of them. If a person is unable to read at the level required for the testing instrument you have chosen, it will be necessary to select another instrument or to test the person verbally. Ascertaining a person's preferred language for testing can be accomplished by asking the person prior to the time the assessment is scheduled to make sure you can access the testing instruments in their language. If you need to assess an older person in a language other than their preferred language (e.g., the instrument is not available in their preferred language), an interpreter may be used, but caution must be taken when interpreting the test results.

INTEGRATION OF LIFE EXPERIENCES

An individual who is aging successfully has a more integrative experience that includes acceptance of the past, resolution of conflicts, and reconciliation of reality with the ideal self than a person who utilizes escape and obsessive reminiscence of the past. Life reviews may allow clients to integrate life experiences and create new meaning to promote the resolution of conflicts and reconciliation with others in preparation for life transitions and the termination of life. Life planning may assist older persons in clarifying transferable vocational or leisure skills, planning for age-related change, and setting goals. Personal control is vital in maintaining mental health and life satisfaction (Kampfe, 2015). The ability to make decisions, self- regulate behavior, and control the environment is positively associated with psychological well-being. Paid work is recognized as an important source of well-being for older men and women because work provides a sense of independence and competence outside of immediate family networks. Counseling interventions that encourage personal control rather than focus on diagnosis and pathology may be more effective in promoting the well- being of older persons.

COUNSELING AND CASE MANAGEMENT

The aging population requires multiple services from a number of professionals, including case managers, counselors, healthcare providers, and human resource employees. To facilitate positive outcomes for aging populations, interagency collaboration offers an opportunity for enhanced employment outcomes. Casework is the common denominator that cuts across various service professionals and is relevant to deconstructing disincentives for either maintaining or returning to work. In addition, given the myriad factors associated with aging, counselors and case managers will want to conduct a thorough intake to ensure their ability to develop a complete clinical picture of their older clients. It is also prudent to ensure accurate understanding of the older person's goals, including both personal and work-related goals, to maximize treatment outcomes. Helping clients identify barriers and assisting them in overcoming these barriers can also abet the treatment process. For example, Miller et al. (2016) analyzed Rehabilitation Services Administration data for vocational rehabilitation clients age 55 and over with diabetes and found successful employment was most highly correlated with access to rehabilitation technology (e.g., mobility devices), the ability to live independently, and having good job support services (e.g., job retention support). Case managers and counselors who work with older workers should also be familiar with services for older adults in order to make appropriate referrals. Common social assistance programs used by older adults include healthcare, food and shelter, access to medicine, assistance with language and physical barriers, community integration programs, vocational services, and other services offered through government and nonprofit agencies. In addition, older adults may not know what to expect if they are attending counseling or seeing a case manager for the first time and will likely benefit from additional explanation of the process (Kampfe, 2015). It is also advisable for mental health and medical professionals to engage older adults by using promotional materials that highlight the benefits of counseling and related services for older adults. This can be accomplished by increasing mental health literacy among older adults by using terminology they can understand, adapting to meet the needs of older adults (e.g., allowing for extra time for sessions and providing accommodations for sensory problems), and providing training on aging for mental health professionals (O'Donnell et al., 2021). In addition, it is important to recognize potential biases and to keep an open mind when working with older adults, as agism is an ongoing issue among counselors (e.g., Wagner et al., 2019).

Older adults experience similar rates of mental health problems to the general population, yet they are more likely to encounter mental health care inequalities due to limited access to mental health services, underidentification of mental health issues, and overreliance on pharmacological interventions (Cremers et al., 2022). According to Cremers et al., mental health inequalities result from a number of issues, including a lack of transportation and financial constraints, family members and other care providers' difficulty identifying mental health problems in older adults, stigma about the mental health needs of older adults, and poor mental health literacy among older adults. In addition, SAMHSA (2021) noted clinical case management and counseling for older adults with mental illness tend to be complex and require consideration of the impact of aging as well as current physical and mental symptoms because older individuals often experience greater barriers than younger and middle-aged adults. Examples of some of the most prevalent barriers include inadequate insurance coverage for treatment of mental disorders; a shortage of trained geriatric mental health clinicians; lack of culturally and linguistically appropriate care; limited physical mobility and access to transportation; limited coordination among primary care, mental health, and aging service providers; and stigma surrounding mental health disorders and treatment (SAMHSA, 2021). As such, proper referrals, ongoing coordination of services, and education about aging services can significantly contribute to the well-being of many older adults by promoting their autonomy, competence, and increased motivation to actively participate in mental health–related services.

Effective counseling also entails proper treatment planning, as life span developmental research shows motivational goals in older age differ from goals of younger people, and dealing with loss often becomes more salient than in previous years (Sittler et al., 2022). For example, when a person's resources are insufficient to pursue all or most of one's goals, people are likely to focus on their most urgent goals. Sittler et al. found older adults age 70 and over were most concerned with their health, cognitive functioning, and the well-being of family members and friends and occupational activities and sexuality were least important. Conversely, older adults who are still working may have counseling goals relating to employment as well as managing financial, medical, family, and other salient life issues. Regardless of the chosen psychotherapeutic approach, it is important to remember that older adults' definition of aging is multidimensional, and while physical health is a frequently reported issue among older adults, other commonly reported counseling concerns are social support, financial resources, lifelong learning/stimulation, a sense of engagement, and maintaining one's purpose in life (Fullen et al., 2018). Fullen et al. recommend using *a whole person wellness paradigm* when working with older adults to decrease internalized ageism (e.g., negative attitudes toward one's own aging) and to promote positive perceptions of aging. Specifically, they recommended a multidimensional wellness model for working with older adults that includes the following domains: (a) developmental, (b) cognitive, (c) physical, (c) emotional, (d) spiritual, (e) relational, (f) vocational, and (g) contextual. As such, by emphasizing wellness, there is potential for counselors and case managers to broaden their clients' perspectives on aging by encouraging them to consider aspects of aging well that are not exclusively based on physiological or functional domains. To illustrate, Färber and Rosendahl (2020) conducted a meta-analysis of existing research on the correlation between resilience and mental health in older adults and found resilience was clearly associated with better mental health.

While many older adults may choose to obtain counseling at a counselor's office, counseling older adults in their homes is also highly effective (e.g., eliminates mobility and transportation concerns). According to Boyd-Franklin and Bry (2019), in-home counseling entails a problem-solving approach that combines structural and behavioral family systems theory to assist older adults with multiple problems focus and prioritize their issues. Older adults may also benefit from the use of telehealth but may be reluctant to use technology-facilitated mental health and physical care. Wilson et al. (2021) examined how and why older adults choose to use e-health and noted the most prevalent barriers to e-health use were a lack of self-efficacy, knowledge, support, functionality, and information provision about the benefits of e-health. As such, it behooves counselors and case managers to encourage older adults to learn to use telehealth, as this is a viable solution for overcoming the barriers to timely access and effective healthcare. Tyler et al. (2018) maintain that if older people are to continue to contribute to society as capable and confident individuals, internet participation should be available as a viable option for them to articulate their goals, needs, and aspirations. In addition, internet use affords opportunities for older adults to enhance social participation and inclusion (e.g., online support groups), which can improve their quality of life.

Older adults benefit from a variety of counseling modalities. One highly effective approach for addressing developmental issues among older adults is life review therapy (LRT), which was designed for older adults to help them attribute meaning to positive and negative memories across the life span (Butler, 1963). According to Butler, reminiscing about one's past is not a sign of cognitive decline, but rather a naturally occurring progression given the closeness to life's end. LRT entails a structed variation of reminiscence therapy that addresses specific lifetime periods (e.g., childhood, adolescence, adulthood, and life summary) and has been shown to be effective for addressing end-of-life issues and related mental health problems among older adults and individuals with chronic illness (Kleijn et al., 2021; Westerhof & Slatman, 2019).

Berry and Berry (2018) examined the lived experiences of older adults participating in wellness counseling groups to increase understanding of the most salient challenges they face. The results showed the most significant issues identified were the desire to preserve family traditions and cultural identity, feelings of loneliness and isolation, the ability to control self-care, and death and dying concerns. Participants also identified spirituality and humor as useful coping mechanisms. Due to participant concerns regarding loss of control and their desire to make personal choices about their healthcare needs, Berry and Berry underscored the merits of psychoeducation as an important part of healthcare, social work, and counseling services. Indeed, education is an excellent means for empowering aging adults to attend to their self-care and learn new skills associated with health and well-being. The authors also noted humor (when employed in a sensitive manner) can be helpful to establish rapport and to facilitate reframing negative experiences.

Other counseling approaches that can be effective for working with older adults include solution-focused approaches designed to address current and specific issues; person-centered therapy, which encourages a supportive counseling environment; and positive approaches designed to instill hope and an optimistic life view. When addressing work-related case management and counseling issues, it is important to note fulfilling work comprises job satisfaction, meaningful work, positive work engagement, and a workplace that entails positive emotions (Allan et al., 2019). A strengths-based model that entails positive psychological interventions (hope, strengths, adaptability, and empowerment interventions) instilled within career and work counseling has also been shown to be effective (Owens et al., 2019).

PROACTIVE EMPLOYER RESPONSE

A major issue for aging workers and their employers is the work environment and whether it might be unfriendly and perhaps even discriminatory toward older workers. A significant factor influencing the decision to retain or eject older workers is no doubt the culture of the workplace itself (Chiesa et al., 2019). Another factor is the misperception that older workers are more costly in terms of health insurance, low productivity, and missed days of work (American Association of Retired Persons [AARP], 2015).

Research suggests employers discriminate against older workers in the job application process (AARP, 2018; Perry et al., 2016; von Schrader & Nazarov, 2016). In addition, the stereotypes that younger workers have of their older peers can greatly influence workplace dynamics. Traditional stereotypes of older workers (e.g., being inflexible, sick, and unwilling to learn new technology) continue to persist at many levels (Chiesa et al., 2019; Ng & Feldman, 2012; Posthuma & Campion, 2009). Such stereotypes clearly have had an influence on older workers' labor force participation in the past. Workers who experience age discrimination are more likely to leave their current employment setting and less likely to remain employed. Age-based stereotyping perpetuates discriminatory practices and discourages elderly workers from remaining in or returning to the workplace (Kampfe et al., 2007).

Around 30,000 charges are filed annually in the United States under the Age in Employment Act of 1967 (ADEA), a law that protects workers 40 and over from discrimination in employment on the basis of age. Although the majority of ADEA charges cite termination-related issues (63%), a growing number over the last 20 years cite issues of employment relations (including harassment and discipline). The age group with the highest charge rate (number of charges per 10,000 in the labor force) is those approaching full retirement age (62- to 64-year-olds), indicating that these workers are perhaps feeling pushed out of the workforce prematurely (von Schrader & Nazarov, 2016). Age discrimination in the workplace is often difficult to detect and can be hidden within management practices that target older workers, such as incentivized layoffs, restriction of training to new hires, and internal ranking systems (Woolever, 2013). Age discrimination may also manifest as disability discrimination: Nearly 60% of disability discrimination claims filed under the Americans with Disabilities Act (ADA) come from people over age 40 (Bjelland et al., 2010), and 16% are filed by people older than 55 years (Bruyère et al., 2010).

Keeping the senior worker not only preserves valuable institutional knowledge and memory but also creates beneficial diversity in the workplace. Incentives and workplace support will be needed to encourage employers to retain older workers and to encourage older workers to remain in the workforce. In a review of studies related to healthy aging and workplace productivity conducted by Barakovic-Husic et al. (2020), the most prominent works identified suggest policies that encourage lifelong learning and a workforce that comprises both younger and older workers, as well as gradual retirement. Employers must create workplace policies and practices and effective intergenerational inclusion initiatives that support worker retention. This process may include adopting new management styles and work- setting protocols that focus on an age-diverse workforce. Human resource policies and practices should reflect alternatives that will respond to the older workers' desire for flexible working hours, part-time positions, and the ability to choose what part of the day they work. Increasingly cited as a workplace accommodation among older workers is the desire for flexible work arrangements (e.g., alternative schedules, reduced working hours, nonmonetary benefits; Tishman et al., 2012). Flexible workplace, telecommuting options, and flex-time agreements can help fill this need (Kampfe, 2015; von Schrader et al., 2013).

Benefit plans may also create disincentives for retaining older workers. Many plans can send mixed messages to older workers; some create incentives to retire, while others encourage continued labor force activity. Some employers are creating healthcare and retirement policies that offer incentives to older workers to stay engaged in the workforce, such as phased retirement, "in demand" workforce for specialized consulting, senior staff mentors for new workers, casual/part- time workers' programs, discounts on pharmaceuticals, specialized health screenings, long-term care insurance, preretirement planning, and prorated benefits for employees on flexible work schedules (Society for Human Resources Management/Sloan Foundation, 2015; Tishman et al., 2012; von Schrader et al., 2013).

Managers play an important role in retaining older workers. Managers may perpetuate stigma about aging or disability and fail to recognize workplace issues as they arise—or they avoid performance discussions and encourage the use of disability leave rather than addressing issues in the work environment (Coduti et al., 2015). Managers also have a strong impact on the workplace culture, and employees who report to managers who are aware of their organization's policies about disability and diversity are less likely to experience bias or discrimination (Nishii & Bruyère, 2014). The second most common basis for disability discrimination charges is "retaliation," which includes harassment and discipline issues. These are areas in workplace culture where supervisory influence can make a great deal of difference (Bruyère et al., 2010). When managers and the organization foster a culture of flexibility and accommodation, all employees see requests for accommodations as less unusual and are more likely to accept accommodations as supports that improve productivity (Nishii & Bruyère, 2016). Employers may find that some human resources (HR) practices considered "universal" are, in practice, less fit for the needs of older workers and may wish to examine their current HR management in terms of sets of practices centered around developing existing skills, maintaining current levels of functioning, using existing resources, and accommodating new issues (Kooij et al., 2014). These categories of practice parallel and support the standard of care (SOC) framework of aging.

Finally, it is important to address intergenerational conflict and concerns. Positive exposures to team members of different ages through selective work group composition or focused interventions may support a positive organizational climate for aging (Truxillo et al., 2015). For example, some manufacturing companies are concertedly using intergenerational teams to enhance innovation and creativity and improve productivity. In a survey of manufacturers and a series of interviews with manufacturing industry leaders conducted by the Manufacturing Institute of the National Association of Manufacturers in 2021 and funded by the AARP, results show that those firms who successfully manage multigenerational teams target knowledge transfer, recruitment, and staff feedback to mitigate staff turnover, enhance innovation, and boost company morale and motivation (AARP/Manufacturing Institute, 2021). More research and innovative practices are needed to continue to confirm the value of these approaches to maximizing productivity and job satisfaction for workers of all ages.

COUNSELOR PRACTICE, TRAINING, AND RESEARCH IMPLICATIONS

Practice Implications

The purpose of this chapter is to highlight the importance of the role of counselors who work with individuals with chronic illness and disability to be able to support the continuing vocational interests and longer-term employment success of these service recipients who are also older. As documented earlier, the workforce is aging, and yet many individuals want to maintain employment, both for economic reasons but also life satisfaction and the ability to meaningful contribute to the communities in which they live. These individuals may be needlessly kept from the workforce or from realizing their full potential to contribute to the workforce due to discriminatory attitudes and workplace practices that do not facilitate their retention. It is therefore imperative that counselors become aware of the unique interests of older workers in employment retention and how they can better empower them to be self-advocates in this process. In addition, counselors can serve a consulting role in informing employers about good practices in workplace accommodation, inclusive workplace culture, and workplace policies and practices for retention and continuing engagement of older workers.

Education and Training Implications

Employers and their aging employees will need further information to support an expanding older cohort in the workforce, who very much want to continue working and yet may incur disabilities. Counselors can provide individual supports to older clients who are experiencing disabilities that may impact work performance, and they can also offer consultation to employers about the accommodation process. To be able to confront myths and stereotypes, counselors will need to have knowledge of the intellectual, social, and emotional well-being of older adults, as well as accommodations that can mitigate the limitations that may naturally occur in the aging process. Counselor educators can better prepare counselors-in-training for this task by including aging issues throughout the counselor education curriculum.

Personal experiences with various groups of people and social learning experiences shape one's viewpoint toward a group. Counselors-in-training may have had prior exposure to negative stereotypes about persons with disabilities, have been repeatedly exposed to negative stereotypes about aging (ageism), have a prejudice against older persons (gerontophobia), have a fear of aging or of associating with older persons, or have other attitudinal barriers or misconceptions (Kampfe, 2015). Both personal and societal attitudes toward the aging process and older populations are appropriate to explore in specific courses such as psychosocial, cultural diversity, counseling theories, career development, and human growth and development coursework. The ultimate goal is for issues on aging to be infused throughout the curriculum. Inclusion of material on multicultural aspects of human relationships is intended to increase trainees' multicultural awareness, knowledge, and skills through developing an understanding of one's personal values, attitudes, motivations, and behaviors. Retraining, adaptive devices, physical therapy, and occupational therapies can assist workers injured on the job, regardless of their ages. However, counselors should be aware that age-related changes in stamina and healing may require that older employees who do receive on-the-job injuries may need to be afforded additional time and extended therapy to fully restore optimal functioning.

Infusion of information regarding this population into existing counselor accreditation–approved curricula is vital if the counseling profession is to become a resource for the development of strategies to maintain the economic independence of older citizens. Such courses can also expose counselors-in-training to the issues and attitudes that impact the employment of older workers, particularly those with disabilities. Select rehabilitation scholars have been promoting such inclusion for years (Kampfe et al., 2005; Kampfe et al., 2007), but this continues to be a needed but largely unrealized inclusion in rehabilitation curriculums.

Research Implications

Research is needed on the issues of aging workers, such as training needs, career transition issues, and retirement planning. Continued research is also needed on which accommodations, workplace modifications, and changes to policies and practices positively impact the retention and continued productivity of an aging workforce. As even yet older workers are staying in the workplace and as workplaces change in response to contemporary economics and environmental demands, continued attention to what will be useful to maintain the productivity and job satisfaction of older workers will be a continuously evolving agenda. Counselor practitioners are in a unique position to contribute to needed research design conceptualization, metrics, and analyses to test the multiplicity of interventions we will be exploring in the coming years to keep our aging workforce healthy and intellectually engaged in the employment environment. Counselors are experientially qualified to provide the needed services to keep this population productive and more fully engaged in their communities and continuing employment.

CONCLUSION

The purpose of this chapter was to highlight the importance of the role of counselors who work with individuals with chronic illness and disability to be able to support the continuing vocational interests and longer-term employment success of older service recipients. Older adults have historically been devalued by society, but the growing number of older people staying in the workforce longer is forcing needed changes to this scenario. Rehabilitation and other counseling service providers are in an excellent position to raise awareness, both with employers and with aging workers, about effective policies and practices that can minimize the negative impact on work productivity they might experience and maximize longevity in the workforce. Counselors are also in a unique position to contribute to much-needed research design conceptualization, metrics, and analyses to test the multiplicity of interventions we will be exploring in the coming years to keep our aging workforce healthy and intellectually engaged in the employment environment. Recognizing that older workers can bring significant value to the workplace, especially when they are able to leverage their extant knowledge, skills, and abilities through skill updating, work experience enhancements, and work accommodations may improve outcomes not just for older workers but for work environments and society as a whole.

CLASS ACTIVITIES

1. Review information on two to three age and employment discrimination claims cases and write a two- to three-page paper on the key issues in age discrimination and workplace barriers for older workers presented in these cases.

2. Interview an older worker and find out about what their own experience has been in their later years. Do they feel that they have been treated differently? If so, how?

3. Interview an employer around their workplace policies and practices for older workers. Do they have targeted policies/practices for affirmative recruitment and retention? If so, what are these targeted policies/practices?

4. Write a paper that details the legislative and public regulatory frameworks that can impact older workers and how they may have both positive and negative impacts.

5. Design a counseling protocol (list of interview questions, battery of related assessment tools) that will assist you as a counselor to address the unique employment/vocational interests/considerations of older clients.

KEY REFERENCES

Only key references appear in the print edition. The full references appear in the digital product on Springer Publishing Connect™: https://connect.springerpub.com/content/book/978-0-8261-5111-7/part/partIV/chapter/ch21

Age Discrimination in Employment Act of 1967, Pub L. No. 90–202, 29 USC 621.

American Association of Retired Persons (AARP) (2015). *The surprising truth about older workers*. AARP The Magazine. https://www.aarp.org/work/age-discrimination/older-workers-more-valuable/

Barakovic-Husic, J., Malero, F. J., Barakovic, S., Lamesky, P., Zdravevski, E., Marevsova, P., Krejcar, O., Chorbev, I., Garcia, N., & Trajkovik, V. (2020). Aging at work: A review of recent trends and future directions. *International Journal of Environmental Research and Public Health, 17,* 7659. https://doi.org/10.3390/ijerph17207659

Bruyère, S., von Schrader, S. & VanLooy, S. (2019). Chapter 16: Employment strategies for older adults. In I. Schultz & R. Gatchel (Eds.), *Handbook of rehabilitation of older adults*. Springer International Publishing.

Goldman, L. G. (2020). *Geriatric assessment*. https://www.sciencedirect.com/topics/pharmacology-toxicology-and-pharmaceutical-science/functional-status

Miller, E., Gonzalez, R., & Kim, J. H. (2016). Vocational rehabilitation outcomes among older adults with diabetes. *Journal of Vocational Rehabilitation, 44*(1), 109–121. https://doi.org/10.3233/JVR-150784

Society for Human Resource Management/Sloan Foundation. (2015). *SHRM survey findings: The Aging Workforce – Recruitment and retention*. https://www.shrm.org/resourcesandtools/hr-topics/talent-acquisition/documents/2015%20gap%20analysis.pdf

V

NEW DIRECTIONS, ISSUES, AND PERSPECTIVES

The final section of this text addresses several other contemporary issues faced by persons with chronic illness and disabilities (CIDs) that are relevant to counselors and practice. In addition to psychosocial adjustment, multiple other variables affect adaptation and overall well-being of persons with CID. The authors in Part V discuss various topics including positive psychology and current well-being interventions regarding quality of life, the human aspect of ongoing advances in assistive technology and accessibility, discussing religion in counseling and various religious and beliefs, the growing injustices in America and abroad with the resulting negative impact on those who are oppressed and discriminated against, and the alarming impact increase of mental health issues as a result of overuse of social media. Finally, the coeditors discuss reflect on how persons with disabilities have been perceived and treated by society over the centuries, where we are currently regarding global changes and diminishing resources, and considerations for counselors in the future as they learn to adapt to the needs of persons with CID.

MAJOR HIGHLIGHTS IN PART V

- Chapter 22 provides an overview of rehabilitation interventions designed to positively influence quality of life (QOL) and well-being. The authors define subjective well-being and quality of life and review literature outlining facilitators and barriers to well-being. The chapter contains a review of intervention research in well-being and QOL, including interventions that address disability-related impediments, positive psychology and strengths-based approaches, and macro-level interventions designed to address systemic barriers to well-being for disabled people. The authors conclude with guidance for counselors working with clients on how to understand well-being needs and identify person-centered intervention targets.

- The World Health Organization (WHO) estimates that about a third of the population has a need for some kind of assistive technology (AT). Chapter 23 provides an overview of AT, as a wide range of devices and technologies that promote quality of life among individuals with disabilities. The range of potential impacts includes facilitating education, employment, leisure, and community involvement. In this chapter, the authors provide a discussion of barriers to AT access and use, and effective models for guiding AT selection and maintenance. The authors propose a team approach, citing the important distinction that the necessarily knowledge and skills for comprehensive AT service provision are not germane to one profession or discipline. The chapter concludes with ethical consideration for AT services.

- The authors of Chapter 24 define the major religions in the US, how they are distinguished from one another, and how they view persons with CID as well as the importance of religion and spirituality are for persons with CID. They also discuss how our religious and belief systems are impacted psychologically in terms of adaptation or adjustment to disability following a CID. Finally, the authors discuss counseling strategies and various approaches to therapy for this population since the majority of Americans and other countries largely believe in an omnipotent entity or faith in spirituality and religion.

- The authors of Chapter 25 explore centuries old social justice inequities, oppression, discrimination, and resulting poverty of social injustice toward persons with CID and those of minority. This has been an ongoing global phenomenon that has detrimental effects on those individuals and their families affected by it in terms of quality of life, health care, employment, life satisfaction, internalized oppression, and personal growth. In counseling this most disenfranchised population, the authors address the social justice counselor who not only is equipped to provide counseling and guidance to this population, but also trained in advocacy, both for and with one's clients may be unjustly denied services. The social injustice counselor aims to improve the system by making sure the playing field is fair and just for this vulnerable population.

- The authors of Chapter 26 explore another contemporary and increasingly alarming negative impact on one's mental health due to using or overusing social media. Growing research over the past decade demonstrates that young women in particular use social media sites (SMS) to look for social rewards and capital from posting photographs, outings, and movie reels for likes and flattering comments from their followers for external validation. When this doesn't occur, or conversely the user is bullied or humiliated by follower comments, the negative impact on mental health and the devastating. There is growing empirical evidence that some adolescents and young adults may experience eating disorders, or body image, lowered self-worth and confidence, or suicide. The authors discuss various intervention and treatment approaches for this growing mental health crisis.

- Finally, Drs. Marini, Fleming, and Bishop discuss their career observations and knowledge regarding the psychosocial aspects of chronic illness and disability. They each proffer their own distinct opinions of where society has been regarding the attitudes and treatment of persons with disabilities, the current global issues facing humanity and its trickle-down impact on those with CID, and where, as students, counselors and rehabilitation educators need to go moving forward. Marini's Part A conveys how the have-nots have historically been treated unjustly and reflects upon the recent global and U.S. responses to the pandemic, increasing war, violence, and climate refugees, racial unrest contributed in part by political turmoil, and rapid population growth with countries vying for diminishing resources. He indicates that although America is a wealthy nation that will be one of the last countries to experience the ramifications of these converging humanity issues, they will eventually arrive at our front door. Although those living in poverty with or without disabilities at a higher mortality rate at much lower ages than those with wealth, there is little effort at this time to alter this trajectory. The result for persons with CID living off a meager income, will only exacerbate the mortality rates. Dr. Fleming, in Part B, reflects on how the field must adapt and reconsider the role of the rehabilitation counselor in more effectively responding to social and economic inequity as described in Part A. She challenges those working in counseling and social services to shift our mindset of how to improve quality of life and affect change from solely focusing on individuals to also highlight and work to remove systemic barriers for marginalized people, including those with disabilities. Both are important. This shift will require an acknowledgement of the assumptions engrained in our policies, and for us to look to the disability community for guidance and leadership on meaningful changes that need to be made. Another area of focus is increasing representation of disabled counselors and scholars, requiring us to acknowledge and address inaccessibility within our educational and professional spaces. The disability community has always been their own best and most effective advocates. Our role as professionals is to be ready to provide the kinds of supports and research that are needed to respond to individual and social barriers as identified by those directly impacted. Bishop reflects on the text itself, in the context of its several editions. He discusses the current edition and the contributions of its authors and reflects on the changes in disability and rehabilitation since Marini and Dell Orto published the first edition.

CHAPTER 22

INTERVENTIONS TO IMPROVE THE WELL-BEING OF PEOPLE WITH DISABILITIES AND CHRONIC ILLNESS

ALLISON R. FLEMING, EMRE UMUCU, AND BRIAN N. PHILLIPS

LEARNING OBJECTIVES

After reading this chapter, you will be able to:

- Define subjective well-being and quality of life
- Consider well-being within the context of disability
- Understand models and approaches for improving well-being in disabled populations
- Analyze the purpose, application, and evidence for interventions to promote well-being within and across categories
- Evaluate approaches for understanding barriers to well-being in clients, and how to select well-being interventions to support clients that match their needs and circumstances.

PRE-READING QUESTIONS

1. What does well-being mean? What aspects of life are considered when we think about our own well-being?
2. What is the role of a rehabilitation counselor or related professional in improving well-being?

WHAT IS WELL-BEING?

Understanding and improving well-being is the primary goal of all rehabilitation interventions (Crewe, 1980). Integrative conceptualizations of well-being include attention to both objective and subjective indicators of "living a good life" (Costanza et al., 2007). Rehabilitation counselors have the abilities and resources to help individuals address their well-being through a variety of counseling and rehabilitation interventions. We will start this chapter with a brief definition of well-being, and the related concept of quality of life (QOL). Definitions for subjective well-being and QOL are available from several highly esteemed sources, and these terms are often used interchangeably (Roessler, 1990) as we do in this chapter. Ed Deiner, arguably one of the leading well-being researcher in social psychology and related fields provides this definition for subjective well-being: "that a person thinks [their] life is desirable regardless of how others see it", and "pleasant and good" (Deiner, 2009, p. 1). Deiner's definition is consistent with several others that use similar terms. For example, the World Health Organization (WHO, 1998) defines QOL in a similar fashion, "individuals' perceptions of their position in life in the context of culture and value systems in which they live and in relation to their goals, expectations, standards, and concerns" (p. 2). Notedly absent from this definition are objective indicators of well-being, including health, comfort, status, or wealth (Deiner, 2009). However, we know that the experience of health problems, inability to meet basic needs, or not being able to access opportunities in desired social, economic, and educational contexts are threats to well-being. In fact, empirical studies support the connection between material living conditions and life satisfaction (Vladisavljevíc & Mentus, 2019).

QOL can be understood as how satisfied a person is with life in general and with particular aspects of life and is often expressed as a result of the person's internal assessment and subjective perception of a set of personally meaningful standards (Bishop & Feist-Price, 2002; Terry & Huebner, 1995; WHO, 1998). Evidence has been found that this multi-factor definition of QOL encompassing several features of life in QOL perception applies to children as young as third grade (Terry & Huebner, 1995) and these perceptions are variable over time (Bishop et al., 2008). Two more specific aspects of well-being have emerged: health-related quality of life, and psychological well-being. Health-related QOL is often used as a patient reported health outcome, and refers to individual perceptions of functioning (Centers for Disease Control and Prevention, 2018). Psychological well-being is a term more often used by those concerned with mental health, and refers to psychological functioning and personal growth within the context of the person and environment interaction (Ryff, 1989). The Ryff (1989) model of psychological well-being, the most widely accepted model (Villieux et al., 2016), includes six dimensions: self-acceptance, positive relations with others, autonomy, environmental mastery, purpose in life, and personal growth. QOL and well-being research is an evolving science, crossing many disciplines (Centers for Disease Control, 2018). More recently, new theories on well-being such as Seligman's PERMA (i.e., positive emotion, engagement, relationships, meaning, accomplishment) covers both subjective and psychological well-being (Seligman, 2011).

Over years of research, one area of agreement is that well-being and quality of life are multidimensional constructs. Consistent with this idea, researchers have proposed that in order to gain a better understanding, we must consider several aspects of how we think about our well-being (Deiner, 1984). Over time, researchers have organized findings on how we consider our QOL and well-being into what are known as life domains, understood as aspects of our life and experience. Common life domains considered include: (a) physical health; (b) mental health; (c) social support and social relationships; (d) level of independence and ability to direct one's life and choices; (e) employment and productive activity (i.e., pursuing education, volunteering, caring for family); (f) environmental influences; (g) material and economic well-being; (h) and spirituality, religion, and personal beliefs (Bishop, 2005; WHO, 1998). Within this set of core areas, we likely place different importance or value on these life domains and how we consider them as they contribute to our QOL and well-being (Bishop, 2005). It is also likely that the importance we give to each of these domains may shift over time, either because of typical growth and maturation with age or an event or development in our life that prompts a shift. For example, physical health may not be something we consider strongly in our QOL valuation until we incur a chronic health condition that impacts our health and functioning in significant ways.

INTERNAL AND EXTERNAL CONTRIBUTORS TO WELL-BEING AMONG DISABLED POPULATIONS

Rehabilitation researchers have undertaken important studies of how incurring a disability, undergoing treatment, managing disability related symptoms, and experiencing resulting changes in roles and activities impacts QOL of persons with disabilities. Researchers have also sought to compare how people with disabilities report their QOL as compared with nondisabled people. Findings have indicated that, as a group, people with disabilities report lower levels of life satisfaction than those without disabilities, although disability severity is not directly related (Fuhrer, 1994; Fuhrer et al., 1992). Individuals place greater importance on community and contextual factors, such as employment, leisure, social relationships, income, self-assessed health, contact with friends and acquaintances, safety, and opportunity to take part in activities that are customary based on age, gender, and culture (Clayton & Chubon, 1994; Crewe, 1980; Fuhrer, 1994; Fuhrer et al., 1992; Kinney & Coyle, 1992; Whiteneck et al., 2004).

Foundational studies in disability samples can help us understand what areas disabled people report as most important to them when they think of their well-being. While terminology was often slightly different, common features emerged: emotional well-being, health, social and family involvement, material well-being, work or productive activity, self-determination, autonomy and personal choice; personal competence, community adjustment, and IL skills; community integration; social acceptance, social status, and ecological fit; personal development and fulfillment; residential environment; recreation and leisure; normalization; individual and social demographic indicators; civic responsibility; and support services received (Cummins, 1996; Davis et al., 2017; Hughes et al., 1995; Kinney & Coyle, 1992). While most of these domains are the same for individuals who do not have disabilities, the differences are likely related to the disability experience and specific barriers or concerns that disproportionately impact disabled people. Considerations of autonomy and personal choice, competence, community integration, normalization, and accessibility take on additional meaning within the context of disability, and the realities of living in a world where your choices and activities are often limited by the social and architectural environment and how others view your capacity.

Disabled activists argue that devaluation of disabled lives is connected to non-disabled people's perception of quality of life, and their assumption that a person who has a disability cannot contribute to society, have a good life, or be content (Longmore, 1995). Tamara Dembo, a foundational scholar in disability literature, explains this in her conception of the insider-outsider dynamic. Dembo explained that nondisabled people (outsiders), only think about the difficulty or complications associated with a disability experience and thus have a negative impression of what QOL must be. The disabled person (insider), considers their QOL more broadly, encompassing positive aspects of their experience and how their disability may shape or define their identity. Individuals who are close to a disabled person are also more likely to consider a balanced view and have a more favorable impression of QOL (Dunn et al., 2016; Wright, 1988). Recalling that our perception of well-being is shaped by our feelings of how desirable our life is, it is reasonable to suggest that societal views and messages about disabled people likely influence how individuals view their life quality. Ableism and disproportionate impact of unemployment, poverty, and health burdens experienced by disabled people cannot be separated from our discussion of well-being and serve as potential intervention target areas.

INTERVENTION RESEARCH IN WELL-BEING AND QUALITY OF LIFE

With an understanding of the varied aspects of individual consideration in well-being and QOL, we can move on to identifying examples of interventions targeted to the disability community designed to enhance well-being. As a field, we are still building our capacity to identify evidence-based practices within well-being therapy or other positive psychological approaches that will increase QOL. A range of interventions are available that appear to increase well-being by targeting important life domains, increased function, or enhancing personal strengths to alter how individuals respond to their circumstances. Disabled people continue to be marginalized in the United States and around the world, and are overrepresented in racialized communities and among individuals experiencing poverty, introducing additional oppression (Nerlich et al., 2021). While efforts to increase well-being at the individual level are needed and wanted, we must also consider the macro-level as well-being is negatively impacted by oppression, marginalization, and lack of opportunity experienced by disabled individuals (Melton, 2018). The following is a review of intervention research in well-being and QOL, including those that address disability-related impediments, positive psychology and strengths-based approaches, and macro-level interventions designed to address systemic barriers to well-being for disabled people.

Individual Functioning

Researchers have integrated quality of life and well-being as outcome variables in intervention studies (McKay et al., 2018; Phillips et al., 2021), and findings provide us with understanding of how promoting function or opportunity in valued life domains may positively influence well-being. Examples of areas considered when we assess our well-being include social inclusion and support, having valued social roles including work, autonomy and personal choice, and physical and mental health. Observational research has helped us to understand that disabled and nondisabled people have similar thoughts on the importance of life domains, but barriers caused by marginalization, exclusion, and inaccessibility disproportionately impact satisfaction in these domains for disabled people. While our review was not exhaustive, we found several examples of intervention studies in rehabilitation settings with disabled populations that measured QOL or well-being impact. These are just a few targeted examples, and it is highly likely that other similar interventions may have had the same impact but did not measure QOL outcomes. Only a sub-set of studies in recent reviews collected data on quality of life or well-being (McKay et al., 2018; Phillips et al., 2021).

SOCIAL CONNECTIONS AND SUPPORT

Social connectedness, belonging, and social support are considered by some to be a human need, and strongly influence our well-being (Baumeister & Leary, 1995; Deci & Ryan, 2000). While disability in and of itself does not necessarily impact the ability to engage in meaningful relationships, individuals with disabilities are more likely to report social isolation and loneliness. Some disabilities manifest themselves cognitively or emotionally and directly impact the way that an individual relates with others, interfering with relationship building. External influences also impact socialization, for example the social stigma that surrounds disability. Stigma may cause others to avoid people they know to be disabled, or view people with disabilities as objects of pity or in need of assistance and not as person with whom a genuine relationship is desired. Some medical conditions that require significant management or fatigue that result in reduced social participation or are commonly experienced with secondary depression that reduces one's interest in social interactions.

Interventions can help individuals secure or maintain social connections and supports and may ultimately result in improved well-being. An example of a relevant intervention is encouraging individuals to reach out and increase connectedness or supporting individuals through stigma reducing intervention to help them feel more comfortable engaging with others (Sibitz et al., 2013). Another approach may be to address barriers that interfere with social interactions, for example, a promising intervention for people with hearing loss that included support for implementing communication devices in real-world settings to facilitate improved communication (Deal et al., 2017). Alternatively, interventions may be targeted at the environment, creating a scenario where people can find belonging and be accepted and appreciated for who they are without any need for them to change. In the psychiatric rehabilitation sphere, Clubhouse is a good example of this type of environmental facilitator where the Clubhouse itself is a community where people are always welcome as "members for life" and members reach out to each other for check ins and organize group events (Clubhouse International, 2022). Several studies of Clubhouse members have shown increased well-being after joining (Gold et al., 2016; Mowbray et al., 2009; Tsang et al., 2010). Considering the high level of stigma associated with mental illness, the Clubhouse approach is a powerful way to help people feel accepted and valued in a world where they are often not and shows promise in its potential to increase well-being.

VALUED SOCIAL ROLES

Another life area that commonly contributes to our well-being perceptions is the degree to which we have the opportunity to engage in valued social roles. In the United States, work is particularly defining. Disability may interfere with ability to work for a number of reasons, either because of increased supports or accommodations needed to complete job tasks, a gap in training or education necessary to meet job requirements, or lack of opportunity because of ableist assumptions that disabled people are not qualified. Interventions may support disabled people in returning to work or other activities that they did prior to disability onset, or engage in activities typically expected for someone their age. A powerful example comes from Agrability, a program that addresses accommodation and accessibility needs on farms and ranches (Fetsch et al., 2018; Fetsch & Turk, 2018), showing that participants experienced increased well-being after regaining access to farming and ranching activities. Similarly, an on-site return to work intervention that included assessments and accommodations for individuals after a stroke resulted in increased well-being among participants (Ntsiea et al., 2015). Another work-related intervention was demonstrated by Katz and colleagues (2013) showing well-being gains among individuals in a mental health recovery program after engaging in a small business opportunity as part of their recovery program.

AUTONOMY AND PERSONAL CHOICE

Autonomy, like belonging and social connectedness, is considered a human need that influences well-being (Deci & Ryan, 2000). Disability in and of itself does not reduce autonomy automatically, but some disabled people may experience socioecological and cultural threats (e.g., environmental barriers or attitudinal barriers) to autonomy because of assistance needs, or experience overprotection and are not permitted to make their own decisions and manage their own life. For example, individuals with intellectual and developmental disabilities and those with significant and persistent mental illness are more likely than others to need assistance with decision making and independent living, and as a result have higher rates of guardianship or other care taking situations that limit their ability to control their own lives and situations (Kohn et al., 2012). However, studies have repeatedly shown a relationship between self-determination, control over one's life, and independence and quality of life (Jameson et al., 2015). Interventions that increase self-determination and empowerment may increase well-being, as shown in an example program that included coaching and mentoring for youth with disabilities in foster care (Powers et al., 2012).

PHYSICAL AND MENTAL HEALTH

Individuals with disabilities are disproportionately likely to experience poor health as compared to nondisabled people. Studies consistently show that disabled people experience higher rates of early death, preventable illness, severe medical complications and hospitalizations. Individuals with disabilities are also more likely than nondisabled peers to smoke, live sedentary lives, be obese, and incur diabetes and heart disease (Froehlich-Grobe et al., 2021). Interventions to support physical and mental health are another way to increase well-being, by way of supporting continued health and wellness or reducing the negative impact of a disability condition. For example, an intervention focused on increasing physical activity for older adults at risk for mobility related disability slowed the decline of QOL that is expected in this population (Groessl et al., 2019). Other studies supporting individuals with disabilities in self-management of healthy behaviors have also shown increased well-being outcomes (Ravesloot et al., 2016).

Positive Psychology and Wellness Interventions

Central to positive psychology is the belief that strengths, virtues and positive dispositions can be used to improve health and well-being and support people to reach potentials beyond what can be accomplished from remediation of pathology or impairment alone (Seligman & Csikszentmihalyi, 2000). The philosophy of rehabilitation counseling is infused with the tenets of positive psychology (McMahon & Kim, 2016). McCarthy (2014) stated positive psychology to be part of our disciplines' DNA. Beatrice Wright, a pioneer of positive psychology and leader in rehabilitation counseling, emphasized the importance of a strength-based approach to service provision for people with disabilities (Wright, 1960, 1983). The renewed interest in positive psychology has brought a multitude of empirical studies validating the framework (Chou et al., 2013; McMahon & Kim, 2016). Positive traits such as hope, mindfulness, spirituality, and forgiveness have consistently been shown to correlate with positive outcomes (Leclaire et al., 2018; Müller et al., 2016; Phillips et al., 2022).

Wellness interventions may focus on achieving wellness in physical, psychological, or spiritual domains, and have been demonstrated to make a positive impact on people with disabilities and chronic illnesses, such as maintaining and increasing quality of life (Ng et al., 2013; Stuifbergen, Morris, et al., 2010). Strategies that can promote wellness may include helping people with disabilities develop coping strategies, participate in health promoting behaviors, and set goals (Putnam et al., 2003). Interventions that incorporate mindfulness, gratitude, service to others, and strategies to enhance social connections have also demonstrated promising results to increase well-being across disability populations (Leclaire et al., 2018; Myers et al., 2018; Müller et al., 2016; Müller et al., 2020; Stuifbergen et al., 2010; Zemper et al., 2003).

Researchers have also developed positive psychology interventions (PPIs) and positive psychotherapy (PPT; Rashid & Seligman, 2018) to focus on not just "pathology and mental illness" but also "mental health and well-being" in psychotherapeutic interventions. PPT, an emerging psychotherapy approach, "is an incremental change to balance therapeutic focus on weakness" (Rashid & Seligman, 2018, p.3). PPT is an important development in the mental health field because it aims to (a) expand the scope of psychotherapy, (b) broaden beyond the medical model, (c) expand the outcome of psychotherapy, and (d) attenuate the impact on the clinician (Rashid & Seligman, 2018). PPT is primarily based on two major theories (Rashid & Seligman, 2018):

1. PERMA Theory of Well-Being (Seligman, 2011): PERMA is Seligman's well-being theory which P stands for positive emotion (e.g., joy); E stands for engagement (e.g., flow); R stands for relationships (e.g., secure relationships); M stands for meaning (e.g., sense of purpose in life); and A stands for accomplishment (e.g., pursuing success).

2. Character Strengths (Peterson & Seligman, 2004): Character strengths are "the psychological ingredients – processes or mechanisms– that define the virtues" (Peterson & Seligman, 2004, p.13). There is a total of 24 Character Strengths under the umbrella of six virtues (i.e., wisdom, courage, humanity, justice, temperance, transcendence).

Both PERMA and character strengths are malleable, meaning that they can be measurable, teachable, and learnable (Rashid & Seligman, 2018; Seligman, 2011). PPIs and PPT both focus on cultivating PERMA and character strengths. PPT integrates symptoms with strengths, weaknesses with values, resources with risks, and hopes with regrets to find a balance in understanding human behaviors (Rashid, 2015); therefore, we believe that PPT can be used as one of the standalone intervention or in conjunction with other traditional psychotherapy approaches (e.g., Cognitive Behavioral Therapy [CBT]).

EMPIRICAL SUPPORT FOR POSITIVE PSYCHOLOGY INTERVENTIONS

Growing research has examined the effectiveness of positive psychology interventions in people with disabilities. Results have been promising, with a variety of approaches showing positive impact on health and well-being across disability samples. Müller and colleagues (2016, 2020) engaged two samples comprised of community-dwelling people with chronic pain and a physical disabilities in tailored positive psychology interventions. They found that participants in both studies experienced improved pain-related outcomes, life satisfaction, positive affect, and reduced depression (Müller et al., 2016; Müller et al., 2020). The exercises included topics such as kindness, gratitude, relationships, and spirituality. For example, the kindness exercise in the initial study consisted of asking participants to perform good actions for others (Müller et al., 2016). In the follow up study, the exercises included topics such as flow, relationships, and optimism (Müller et al., 2020). More specifically, the relationships exercises comprised of topics focused on helping individuals strengthen and prioritize their enjoyment in relationships (Müller et al., 2020).

In two studies of participants with Multiple Sclerosis (MS), researchers found that positive psychology interventions resulted in improved well-being outcomes. In a pilot study testing a 5-week group positive psychology intervention, researchers found that participants with multiple sclerosis had reduced depression and fatigue post-intervention (Leclaire et al., 2018). The intervention included five positive psychology exercises, which are gratitude for positive events, personal strengths, gratitude letter, enjoyable and meaningful activities, and remember past successes (Leclaire et al., 2018). As an example, the gratitude for positive events exercise entailed asking participants to recall three positive events that happened in the last week and to write about them and their feelings associated (Leclaire et al., 2018). In another study, people with multiple sclerosis who participated in a multi-day educational wellness program had improved self-efficacy and health-related quality of life (Ng et al., 2013). The educational wellness program encompassed components such as self-management and stress reduction (Ng et al., 2013).

Positive psychology interventions focused on wellness have also shown notable improvements in health-related quality of life, with promising results noted in several disability populations. Zemper and colleagues (2003) engaged a sample of people with spinal cord injuries in a wellness program comprised of topics on lifestyle management, physical activity, nutrition, and secondary conditions preventions. After participating, participants reported having fewer and less severe secondary conditions, and improved health-related self-efficacy and health behaviors (Zemper et al., 2003). Hutson and colleagues (2022) engaged individuals with rheumatoid arthritis, in a 30-day wellness intervention, completers showed reduced pain, functional impairment, cognitive/physical impairment, depressive symptoms, anxiety, and insomnia. The intervention focuses on five wellness strategies, including exercise, mindfulness, sleep, social connectedness, and nutrition (Hutson et al., 2022). In another study, women with fibromyalgia syndrome who participated in a wellness intervention demonstrated improved health-promoting behaviors and quality of life (Stuifbergen, Blozis, et al., 2010). The intervention addressed topics such as maximizing health, adjusting lifestyle, exercising and physical activity, eating healthy, and managing stress over a 30-month period (Stuifbergen, Blozis, et al., 2010).

People with intellectual and developmental disabilities who participated in a telehealth mindfulness-based health wellness intervention helped them improve physical wellness via mindfulness strategies and knowledge of healthy diet (Myers et al., 2018). The mindfulness-based health wellness program includes five components, including physical exercise, healthy eating and nutrition, mindful eating, visualizing/labeling/responding to hunger, and meditation (Myers et al., 2018). For people with chronic severe mental illness, participating in a wellness education group intervention helped them with socialization, education, and motivation to change (Van Metre et al., 2011). The intervention included an eight-week curriculum addressing topics including diet, stress and anxiety, recovery, depression, doctor's visit, oral health, sleep, and financial health (Van Metre et al., 2011). A 90-day self-management mental wellness intervention demonstrated reduced depressive symptoms, anxiety symptoms, functional disability as well as increased sleep quality, happiness, resilience, enthusiasm, and optimism for individuals with psychiatric disorders (Rolin et al., 2020). The intervention focused on mindfulness, sleep, social connectedness, nutrition, and positive psychology-focused exercises (Rolin et al., 2020).

Positive psychology interventions and therapeutic approaches provide us with promising avenues to support individuals with disabilities to increase their well-being in multiple life domains. Research supports the application of these interventions across disability populations, with a variety of different strategies, exercises, and intensiveness of intervention protocols. Counselors can learn much from adopting these approaches, designed to increase strengths rather than "fixing" problems. Finally, these interventions are consistent with rehabilitation philosophy and tradition, with a strong history of application by foundational scholars (McCarthy, 2014; Wright, 1960, 1983).

SOCIAL DETERMINANTS OF HEALTH AND THEIR INFLUENCE ON WELL-BEING

The World Health Organization (WHO) identified Social Determinants of Health as an alternative view on quality of life and well-being. The Office of Disease Prevention and Health Promotion defines the term, "Social determinants of health are conditions in the environments in which people are born, live, learn, work, play, worship, and age that affect a wide range of health, functioning, and quality-of-life outcomes and risks" (WHO, 2022, p. 1). The Social Determinants of Health model acknowledges the entrenched connection between well-being and access to resources (Froehlich-Grobe et al., 2021). Resources commonly refer to finances, but also extend to social capital and connectedness. The context of where we live, work, and spend our time influences whether we can make choices that will improve our health and well-being, and how we might do so (Braveman et al., 2011). Mounting evidence demonstrates that people who live in socially disadvantaged areas are prone to experience more difficulty finding appropriate housing, are more likely to be victims of crime, and are less likely to have access to needed social services, space for physical activity, or healthy food (Drake & Rudowitz, 2022). Discrimination, exclusion, and chronic stress have also been identified as threats to health and well-being (Deiner & Seligman, 2009; Froehlich-Grobe et al., 2021).

Historically, application of the medical model of disability and ableist views have created a social context where the terms disabled and "healthy" and "happy" may seem incompatible, and where disabled people who have satisfying lives with fulfilling relationships, careers, and hobbies are seen as "inspirational" or having "overcome their disability." This view lacks appreciation for evidence that people born with or incurring disability adapt, but often live in environments that are not conducive to the strategies they have developed to be able to pursue the activities they want, with people they choose, in spaces they find most desirable (Andrews et al., 2019). Supportive environments for disabled people are accessible, socially affirming, and include available technology, services, and resources. What if instead of focusing on the person and what they can do to increase well-being, we turned our attention to the environment to promote equitable access as a way to influence well-being? In favor of broadening our view on the role of rehabilitation professionals in addressing well-being from the micro to the macro through an equity lens (Bhattarai et al., 2020), we will present a discussion of macro interventions and their potential to increase well-being in disability communities.

What Are Macro Interventions and How Do They Address Well-Being?

Macro interventions are best understood as those leveraging community organizing, community partnerships, participatory action research, social action, or legislative action and policy change to increase the well-being of individuals in communities (Ferguson et al., 2018). Examples of the impact of macro interventions include improving economic conditions, changing unfair policies, reforming human services, and expanding equity and human rights (Ferguson et al., 2018). The impact of macro-interventions are measured at the community level (Thyer, 2008). For example, do people with access to home and community-based services report higher quality of life than those without access? Do disabled children who live in communities with adaptive sports programs report greater well-being than children who live in communities without these programs?

Bearing in mind the significant marginalization of disabled people in the U.S. and globally, and the threats associated with well-being related to poverty, social isolation, and poor health- macro interventions appear a promising avenue for improving well-being and quality of life for disabled people and serve as a compliment to individualized interventions. The macro view on interventions is also consistent with the need to consider intersectionality, as disability status alone is not sufficient to understand context. Disabled people of color, LGBTQA disabled people, and those otherwise marginalized will experience different kinds of oppression and have different considerations for well-being (Withers et al., 2019). As a method for identifying appropriate example of macro-interventions, we considered three areas identified among disability advocates (National Disability Rights Network, 2022): economic, vocational, and political accessibility.

ECONOMIC RESOURCE GAPS

Individuals with disabilities are much more likely to experience poverty than people without disabilities (Erickson et al., 2019). Common explanations for this relationship between poverty and disability include the increased costs brought on by disability (e.g., medical bills, medications, assistive devices) and the potential reduction in wages due to medical absences, unemployment, or underemployment (Coleman-Jensen & Nord, 2013). The poverty–disability connection has been described in the literature as "a trap" (Stapleton et al., 2006, p. 701), "intractable" (Sylvestre et al., 2018, p. 153), and the "elephant in the room" (Hughes & Avoke, 2010, p. 5). More concerning, the relationship between disability, poor health, poverty, and unemployment appears cyclical (Lustig & Strauser, 2007).

Food insecurity serves as a specific and tangible consequence of insufficient economic resources and is disproportionately experienced by households with at least one disabled member (Brucker & Coleman-Jensen, 2017). People experiencing food insecurity have regular concerns over amounts and quality of available food and may decrease portions or skip meals to adjust (USDA, Economic Research Service, 2018). Of particular relevance to the disability community, food insecurity is associated with higher rates of cognitive impairments, mental health conditions, diabetes, heart disease, and cancers, among other health concerns (Harvey et al., 2022). Huang et al. (2010) found that both resource limitations and competing expenditure demands contribute to food insecurity in households impacted by disability and that "protective effects of economic resources against food insecurity may differ for people with and without disabilities" (p. 118).

The United States Department of Agriculture (USDA) runs several programs to combat food insecurity, including experimental interventions designed to increase autonomy and ability to make healthy food choices. One example of a macro-intervention, Fair Food Network Double Up Food Bucks (DUFB), was implemented in Kansas and Missouri with funding from the USDA food insecurity incentive program (Harvey et al., 2022). Program participants were incentivized to purchase fresh fruits and vegetables from participating farmers markets and local merchants by receiving an extra dollar in benefits (a "food buck") for every dollar spent on fresh produce. Participants could use these "food bucks" to purchase additional fruits and vegetables once their benefits ran out. Benefit recipients in the targeted communities reported increased intake of fresh produce, and credited the incentive program. Gains in QOL were reported by participants who were experiencing food insecurity (Harvey et al., 2022).

UNEMPLOYMENT AND UNDEREMPLOYMENT

Unemployment and underemployment are consistently identified as issues that disproportionately impact disabled people. Long-standing trends are evident, showing significant gaps in employment rates and wages of working-age adults with disabilities compared to nondisabled peers (Sevak et al., 2015). From a well-being perspective, researchers have provided causal links between unemployment and reduced physical and mental health, social isolation and loneliness, unhealthy behaviors, and even increased risk of mortality (Puig-Barrachina et al., 2011). In the employment arena, macro-interventions may take different forms, such as examining laws and policies preventing employment discrimination, educational programs preparing individuals for the labor market, and benefits and systems extended to people who experience temporary or long-term unemployment due to illness or disability. An example of a study of macro-interventions to influence employment rates is found in an analysis of different policies of employment protection laws and public welfare benefits in different countries. Researchers analyzed employment trends in five countries (United Kingdom, Canada, Norway, Denmark, and Sweden) with a range of legal protections for firing workers for reasons related to chronic health conditions, and generosity of public benefits for individuals unable to work (Holland et al., 2011). Findings revealed that generous social welfare benefits were not correlated to lower levels of employment among individuals with work-limiting disabilities. Additionally, it appeared that countries with greater financial and policy emphasis on employment protections had higher rates of employment among disabled workers than countries that did not (Holland et al., 2011). These findings illustrate the possible benefits of public policies and programs as macro-interventions on employment rates of individuals with disabilities in other countries, including the United States.

POLITICAL ENGAGEMENT

People with disabilities (like other marginalized groups) were historically excluded from voting, however, civic participation is a predictor of QOL (Kelly, 2013). Disabled people in the United States are deeply impacted by public policy and legislation (Andrews et al., 2019). The Voting Rights Act (1965) was the first federal legislation that guaranteed individuals who needed assistance with voting for reasons of disability be permitted to get assistance from a person of their choice (Matsubayashi & Ueda, 2014). The most recent legislation, the Help America Vote Act (2002) was enacted to make polling places accessible to disabled persons, in a way to make participation in voting more similar to nondisabled people in terms of privacy and independence (Matsubayashi & Ueda, 2014). Matsubayashi and Ueda (2014) identified mandated accessibility of voting places and other measures designed to make voting easier (i.e., vote by mail, early voting) as macro-interventions and have analyzed voting data to determine the impact of these changes on voting participation among disabled people. Findings of their analysis of population data in the United States from 1980 to 2008 revealed a consistent gap in voting participation between disabled and nondisabled people. Voting trends noted increased voting participation by both groups starting after the 1996 election, with no change in the gap during the time period examined despite the new legislation introduced. Further analysis revealed that individuals with cognitive and mobility impairments were the least likely to vote, and that the likelihood of voting by mail was higher than voting in person for individuals across disability groups. Researchers concluded that vote by mail is effective in increasing participation for persons with disabilities, and that greater attention to voting accessibility is needed (Matsubayashi & Ueda, 2014).

Rehabilitation counselors and professionals are much more accustomed to considering micro-interventions as they work to positively influence the well-being of their clients. However, consistent with the person-in-environment philosophical tenet of rehabilitation proposed by Lewin, practitioners must also consider how the context may support or threaten well-being. Bhattarai and colleagues (2020) argue that the path to addressing health and well-being disparities experienced by disabled people is identifying population-level interventions that will result in improved life circumstances as a social justice mandate. This view is consistent with those experienced within the disability community, where activists promote a civil rights view on disability, suggesting the disadvantage due to disability is caused by the fact that the world was not created with disabled people in mind. The appropriate interventions to address disadvantages, therefore, are to society, not the person (Burke & Barnes, 2017).

IMPLICATIONS FOR COUNSELING PRACTICE

In this chapter, we have emphasized the importance of internal and external contributors to well-being and quality of life as well as how rehabilitation counseling professionals can intervene at both the micro- and the macro-level to enhance these far-reaching outcomes. As noted, rehabilitation counselors tend the emphasize micro over macro in efforts to increase well-being and quality of life. This tendency is justified in situations and circumstances when individual change is most needed. However, there is a potential for harm that comes from emphasizing micro-level well-being interventions when a macro-level approach is warranted.

For example, a rehabilitation counselor focusing exclusively on coaching an individual living in a poor neighborhood to focus on social networking, without acknowledging that their network may not produce job leads to the same degree of those with more privileged networks is likely causing harm. The same potential for harm applies when rehabilitation counselors emphasize macro-level well-being interventions when a micro-level approach is warranted. For instance, a professional who places all their focus on making a local gym accessible while ignoring things their clients can do to maintain their health outside the gym is missing opportunities to enhance well-being. We proceed with discussion of how person-centered principles can be used to effectively understand sources of strain on individual well-being and conceptualization of possible interventions at both the micro and macro levels.

Customized Well-Being Interventions

In reality, many unmet needs or desired change leave room for some combination of micro- and macro-level interventions. For most people, there is almost always something that can be improved at the individual level to increase well-being. For clients with marginalized identities, there is also likely to be systemic factors limiting opportunities and negatively impacting well-being. The first step in pursuing a customized approach to well-being interventions is to acknowledge that not all micro- or macro-level barriers to change or success are within the control of the counselor. In fact, few are. This may be particularly important for macro-level barriers that can often feel overwhelming. Key to this effort is recognizing that the commitment to acknowledging macrom-level barriers does not require fixing them. In the example of the rehabilitation counselor selecting the single approach of networking when the client's social networks are not well-suited for job leads, just a recognition of difference in privilege at the macro-level and incorporating multiple approaches to address the employment need can lead to more healthy and helpful interactions.

THE DETERMINATION OF MICRO, MACRO, OR BOTH

Any well-being or quality of life intervention suggests the need for change or achievement in functioning, social connections, social roles, autonomy, health, leisure, or any number of other life domains. The question we address here is where the emphasis should be placed in facilitating the desired outcome. Rehabilitation counselors may benefit from taking any goal for improving well-being and considering the following questions:

1. How much are the currently unmet needs of the client the result of inequities in resources or privilege?

2. What is the client's perspective on the sources of well-being strain?

3. Can skills, habits, or personal changes address the unmet needs?

4. How has legislation or policy (or the lack thereof) impeded the clients ability to make the desired change or achievement up to this point?

5. How does the client's community impede the client's ability to make the desired change or achievement up to this point?

6. How might commonly held societal beliefs have impeded the client's ability to make the desired change or achievement up to this point?

7. How might my own experiences and perspective prevent me from recognizing the macro-level influences that could be impeding my client in creating successful change or achievement?

There is nothing difficult or complex about these questions, and yet, the personal experience of these authors suggests that without a consciousness effort to incorporate both micro and macro-level considerations, rehabilitation counselors will continue to be unbalanced in their approach. This tendency is, of course, not limited to rehabilitation counselors. The well-established concept of actor-observer bias has shown that we all have a tendency to ascribe the actions of others to internal factors while allowing our own actions to be explained by external factors. The application of this tendency to rehabilitation counseling is to assume that the solution to improved well-being lies within the person, and if we can identify the area of needed growth and support them we will find success. This view ignores the role of external barriers to well-being, and the risk of reinforcing social messages that anything can be overcome with hard work or the right supports.

To support the application of these ideas, we consider the case of Michelle, a 57-year-old women with Multiple Sclerosis who is seeking rehabilitation counseling services for support during a stressful transition. Her doctor referred her because she endorsed a high number of depressive symptoms at her last appointment. When you first meet Michelle, she denies feeling depressed, just stressed because of her recent MS-related exacerbations, an unsuccessful job search after being laid off last year, and the risk of eviction from her apartment because of her unemployment. Michelle explains that not only is she feeling unwell because of her symptoms, but her disability is becoming more noticeable in her speech and gait and is now harder to "hide." She feels this is getting in the way of being hired because employers do not understand MS, and she doesn't feel confident to explain it to them. She strongly suspects that she is not hired for jobs that she is clearly qualified for because she sounds and looks "different." She is also not able to take care of herself as well as she could before, particularly with her diet and exercise because she can't afford to. Since she lost her job, she is buying less expensive foods and stopped her gym membership. She received an eviction notice this month and is worried about losing her apartment, and where she will go if she needs to move out.

Michelle's difficulties in finding a job have been particularly troubling given the low unemployment rate in her area and the many business advertising the need for workers. As a rehabilitation counselor—and a human being prone to actor-observer bias—your first inclination may be to cut Michelle's complaints about an unfair labor market short with a pep-talk designed to encourage her to focus on her job search strategies or simply to write her off as unmotivated when the pep talk does not help. After all, much of this stress would be abated (and her well-being improved), if she could find a stable job again. However, with macro-level considerations fresh in your mind, you determine to give the questions above some reflection.

First, you consider how much Michelle's unmet needs are the result of inequities in resources or privilege? In this reflection, you appreciate anew the difficulty Michelle must be having to remain positive about her job prospects when her unemployment has resulted in an eviction notice for the apartment she has been living in for several years. Next you consider how legislation or policy (or the lack thereof) might be impeding Michelle's ability to find work. You appreciate in this thinking that the fact that there is anti-discrimination legislation for people with disabilities highlights the widespread discriminatory beliefs and practices that Michelle is likely facing. In a more nuanced reflection, you appreciate that some companies may even view Michelle as more high risk because of false beliefs that they would not be able to fire her because of her disability if she does not prove to be a good fit for the company. Her age may also be a factor in hiring decisions, with employers preferring someone younger who can be paid less. You also recognize that Michelle may benefit from financial resources to take some of the pressure off of her until she is able to find stable work. Reminded of her description of her diet, you connect her with a food assistance program to increase her access to healthier food.

Next, you consider Michelle's perspective on the source of strain on her well-being. She prioritizes her job search as causing some of her other stress, but also notes that disability-related exacerbations are impacting her. It may be that she needs some additional medical intervention, physical or occupational therapy, or adaptive technology to help her maintain her health and function and ability to continue with her daily activities independently. You move ahead with connecting her with an independent living center to find resources for adaptive equipment and to learn more about accessible housing options. You also encourage her to ask her doctor for a referral to an Occupational Therapist, to help her with balance and independence in her daily activities. Michelle is also describing, but not naming, disability-stigma when she talks about her disability becoming more obvious and the negative impact it has on her. It is possible that providing a place for her to process some of her feelings about her MS, and the visibility of her disability and how that impact her self-concept would be helpful. You also consider whether skills, habits, or personal changes can address the identified strains on well-being. Michelle identifies that she could use some help practicing how she might address her disability with possible employers, or even friends and family members in a way that makes her feel comfortable and empowered. Michelle also recognizes that she used to practice mindfulness and journal. She feels that while these approaches will not address her imminent financial problems, they might help her maintain a more positive outlook and continue to persist through her difficult circumstances.

As part of this process, you reflect deeply on how your own experiences and perspective may be preventing you from recognizing the macro-level influences that could be impeding Michelle in her job pursuits. Primed by the previous questions, you realize that you have never been in a situation where an eviction seemed eminent, and you had nowhere else to go. Or perhaps you appreciate all the more the privilege you experienced in getting the lead for your current job from a well-connected family friend. These considerations ground you in balancing the micro-level issues with the contextual or macro-level issues that are also relevant in addressing Michelle's well-being. When you meet with Michelle next, you lean into her description of the difficulties she is experiencing by sitting with her in the likelihood of macro-level inequities and resistance. This acknowledgement has a positive impact on Michelle, she notes that she appreciates feeling heard and listened to.

Within a short time, she is ready to consider the alternatives for both macro- and micro-level interventions. With an increasingly person-centered and macro-level perspective, you support Michelle in her job pursuits by using the employer openness survey to identify companies that appreciate disability as a valued form of diversity in the workplace (Gilbride et al., 2003, 2006). Although many employers did not reply, and others provided a more neutral one, a few in the community provided a quick and positive response. Sharing this information with Michelle increased her sense of hope that she would be given fair consideration at those companies. Recognizing that anti-discrimination legislation may make employers hesitant to say it if they experience discomfort or doubts about someone with disabilities in their workplace, you also work with Michelle to practice impression management techniques that have been shown to improve employer perceptions of disability (e.g., Lyons et al., 2018). Michelle's disability is quickly identified in how her MS affects her movement and speech. However, in practicing disclosure you learned that Michelle tends to avoid talking about her disability because she feels embarrassed by her speech difficulties now compared to how she was before her diagnosis. You find that supporting her to process these feelings increases her confidence, and that addressing her disability directly seems to be producing a more positive response in her initial interviews after beginning to use this strategy. Finally, based on your earlier reflections and the lack of employers who responded as being open to hiring employees with disabilities, you determine it is time to engage in your local chamber of commerce again and offer to provide them with updated data showing the benefits that are associated with companies who target the hiring of disabled employees (e.g., Accenture, 2018; Fraser et al., 2011; Hindle et al., 2010; Kesselmayer et al., 2022; Lindsay et al., 2018; Ochrach et al., 2022; Thomas et al., 2021).

Michelle's example shows the interplay of micro-level and macro-level impacts on well-being and how they might interact within an individual. It is through considering multiple domains of life, and how disability, health, functioning, cultural, social, and economic circumstances are supporting or hindering well-being that we understand the most appropriate interventions. In Michelle's case, appreciation of disability stigma, the impact of unemployment and economic hardship, disruptions to health and function, and disability-related discrimination leads us to a multi-faceted approach to supporting increased well-being.

CONCLUSION

Interventions to increase well-being can take many forms, and may be most useful to clients at the micro-level, or by addressing macro-level issues that disproportionately impact the disability community. Outcome studies have demonstrated positive impacts of interventions designed to improve well-being by addressing disability-related barriers, increasing personal strengths to address challenges, and reducing economic and social marginalization. Counselors seeking to positively impact clients' well-being should consider individual perspectives, and pursue approaches based on the sources of strain and the importance of the life domain to the person's conception of QOL. Broadening our focus to include macro-level interventions is a growth area for Rehabilitation Counseling, with much potential for improving social and economic conditions that threaten well-being in the disability community.

CLASS ACTIVITIES

In small groups, consider the following:

1. What are some questions you might ask clients to better understand their well-being?

2. How might you learn more about barriers to well-being as you consider appropriate interventions?

3. What is the difference between counseling interventions designed to treat symptoms and those intended to increase quality of life? How are they similar?

REFERENCES

The full references appear in the digital product on Springer Publishing Connect™: https://connect.springerpub.com/content/book/978-0-8261-5111-7/part/partV/chapter/ch22

Bhattarai, J. J., Bentley, J., Morean, W., Wegener, S. T., & Pollack Porter, K. M. (2020). Promoting equity at the population level: Putting the foundational principles into practice through disability advocacy. *Rehabilitation psychology*, *65*(2), 87–100. https://doi.org/10.1037/rep0000321

Braveman, P. A., Kumanyika, S., Fielding, J., LaVeist, T., Borrell, L. N., Manderscheid, R., & Troutman, A. (2011). Health disparities and health equity: the issue is justice. *American journal of public health*, *101*(S1), S149-S155.

Chou, C. C., Chan, F., Phillips, B., & Chan, J. Y. C. (2013). Introduction to positive psychology in rehabilitation. *Rehabilitation Research, Policy, and Education*, *27*(3), 126–130.

Deiner, E. (2009). *The science of well-being: The collected works of Ed Diener* (Vol. 37, pp. 11–58). Springer Science and Business Media.

Rashid, T. (2015). Positive psychotherapy: A strength-based approach. *The Journal of Positive Psychology*, *10*(1), 25–40.

Seligman, M. E. P. (2011). Flourish: A visionary new understanding of happiness and well-being. Free Press.

Vladisavljević, M., & Mentus, V. (2019). The structure of subjective well-being and its relation to objective well-being indicators: evidence from EU-SILC for Serbia. Psychological reports, 122(1), 36–60.

CHAPTER 23

USERS OF ASSISTIVE TECHNOLOGY: THE HUMAN COMPONENT

HUNG JEN KUO, ANNEMARIE CONNOR, AND MICHAEL YEOMANS

LEARNING OBJECTIVES

After reading this chapter, you will be able to:

- Define assistive technology
- Differentiate assistive technology devices from assistive technology services
- Identify models of assistive technology
- Identify ethical concerns surrounding the provision of assistive technology services
- Discuss the importance of universal design and how it is different from assistive technology

PRE-READING QUESTIONS

1. What is assistive technology?
2. What are some examples of assistive technology?
3. What are some possible challenges when implementing assistive technology?
4. What is the role of the rehabilitation counselor in assistive technology service?

WHAT IS ASSISTIVE TECHNOLOGY?

Assistive technology comes in many different shapes and sizes. The devices and services that encompass assistive technology can also vary in their technological complexity; from the simple magnifying glass to the more advanced hearing aid, assistive technologies represent an essential aspect of the rehabilitation counselor's toolbox. It is crucial for rehabilitation counselors to be familiar with the operational definitions of assistive technology and relevant legislation, statistics about their use and availability, and the impact that assistive technology has on the lives of individuals who use them.

Assistive technology is defined as "any item, piece of equipment, or product system, whether acquired commercially off the shelf, modified, or customized, that is used to increase, maintain, or improve functional capabilities of individuals with disabilities" (Technology-Related Assistance for Individuals with Disabilities Act, 29 U.S.C. 2022 § 3, 1988). Whereas the definition is widely used, the meaning may not always be clear. For instance, something that may not traditionally be regarded as assistive technology (e.g., a calculator in the classroom) can be considered as such if it allows an individual to accomplish a task that is otherwise impossible. For some students, the calculator may provide an easier, faster way of solving a math problem; however, for students with certain physical and/or intellectual disabilities, the calculator may be essential to their ability to solve the same problem (Center on Technology and Disability [CTD], 2018). In addition, people tend to perceive "technology" as something high-tech. However, an assistive technology device can be as low-tech as a cardboard template or a pencil holder. The concept is less about the item itself and more about how it is used. In the previous example, a calculator can be considered an assistive technology or otherwise, depending on a combination of the task to be achieved and the person who is using it.

History and Legislative Influence

The Technology-Related Assistance to Individuals with Disabilities Act of 1988 was passed by Congress with the intent to increase access to, availability of, and funding for assistive technologies through state efforts and national initiatives (Disability Rights Ohio [DRO], 2013). This was the first of many pieces of legislation to acknowledge and address the need for assistive technology in the United States. By July 1990, the Americans with Disabilities Act (ADA) was signed into law, providing civil rights protections against discrimination for individuals with disabilities. From an employment perspective (Title I), the ADA protects individuals with disabilities from discrimination based on the disability alone if they are qualified to perform the essential functions of the job, with or without reasonable accommodations. These accommodations may include the use of assistive technology and technology access unless the changes create what is considered to be an undue hardship for the employer (DRO, 2013). Title IV of the ADA addresses assistive technology specifically, as it requires that telephone companies provide the necessary services to allow people who are deaf or hearing impaired to use telecommunications devices (CTD, 2018).

While originally signed into law in 1973, the Rehabilitation Act has undergone several amendments that extend its protections to include aspects of assistive technology and their service delivery. The 1992 amendments place a greater emphasis on achieving employment goals and specify the ways in which state vocational rehabilitation programs need to describe and report which assistive technology devices and services will be provided as part of an assessment for determining individual eligibility and vocational rehabilitation needs (Rehabilitation Act Amendments, 1992). The 1998 amendments include regulations for federal agency procurement of electronic and information technology that allow individuals with disabilities to produce and have access to information and data in a manner comparable to that of individuals without disabilities (Rehabilitation Act Amendments, 1998). In other words, Section 508 of the Rehabilitation Act requires that all websites, video and audio tapes, electronic books, televised programs, and so on developed and used by any federal government agency must be accessible to people with disabilities (CTD, 2018).

To meet the growing demand for assistive technologies and services, Congress has expanded upon its work since 1988. Using the Technology-Related Assistance for Individuals with Disabilities Act of 1988 as a framework, the Assistive Technology Act of 1998, or the "Tech Act," provides federal funds to assist states in developing consumer-responsive systems of access to AT, services, and information. Specifically, three types of programs are supported by the Tech Act: (a) the establishment of assistive technology demonstration centers, information centers, equipment loan facilities, referral services, and other consumer-oriented programs; (b) protection and advocacy services to help people with disabilities and their families as they attempt to access the services for which they are eligible; and (c) federal/state programs to provide low-interest loans and other alternative financing options to help people with disabilities purchase needed assistive technology (CTD, 2018).

The most recent legislation pertaining to assistive technology is known as the Individuals with Disabilities Education Act (IDEA). IDEA works to ensure that eligible children and youth with disabilities have free appropriate public education, including special education and related services (IDEA, 2004). Originally referred to as the *Education for All Handicapped Children Act of 1975*, the act did not include language about or definitions of assistive technology devices and services. This was remedied with the 1990 Amendments to IDEA, specifically with the addition of Section 300.5, which includes the most widely accepted definition of assistive technology: "Assistive technology device means any item, piece of equipment, or product system, whether acquired commercially off the shelf, modified, or customized, that is used to increase, maintain, or improve the functional capabilities of a child with a disability. The term does not include a medical device that is surgically implanted or the replacement of such device" (Section 1401; IDEA, 2004).

Importantly, there is no federally "approved list" of assistive technology devices and services covered by IDEA. The determination of assistive technology for a student with a disability must be made on an individual basis. However, it is worth noting that the language in IDEA extends the the definition of assistive technology beyond devices to related services. Specifically, the act mandates that "students with disabilities must be provided supplementary services and aids that permit them to benefit from their education" (Section 300.42; IDEA, 2004).

Needs and Usage Rates

According to the Centers for Disease Control and Prevention (CDC, 2023), 89 million or 27% of adults in the United States have some type of disability. Research has found that many individuals with disabilities use assistive devices in their daily lives (Berardi et al., 2021; Russell et al., 1997). A study conducted by Russell et al. (1997) found that the use of assistive devices increased dramatically from 1980 to 1994. They found that among those surveyed, 7.4 million persons reported using assistive technology to compensate for mobility impairments, more than any other general type of impairment (Russell et al., 1997). More recent studies conducted in Canada report similar high usage statistics, with 95% of the 3,775,920 Canadians with a disability using some form of assistive technology (Berardi et al., 2021). The WHO and United Nations Children's Fund 2022 Global Report on Assistive Technology estimates that 2.5 billion people need one or more assistive products, such as wheelchairs, hearing aids, or apps that support communication and cognition (WHO & United Nations Children's Fund, 2022).

WHO and United Nations Children's Fund (2022) estimate the prevalence of the need for assistive products in the global population is 31.3%. They found that two-thirds of the global population of people aged 60 years and older need at least one assistive product, with the need being lower in younger age groups (WHO & United Nations Children's Fund, 2022). Prior reports have estimated that the unmet need for assistive technology remains high. In 2018, WHO reported that there were 200 million people with low vision who did not have access to assistive products for low vision. The need for wheelchairs and hearing aids was similarly unmet, with only 5% to 15% of the population in need receiving the necessary equipment (WHO, 2018).

The most frequently reported barrier to assistive product access is affordability, followed by a lack of support and lack of availability (WHO & United Nations Children's Fund, 2022). The variety of assistive technology devices can include low-, middle-, and high-tech devices and, as such, the costs for these devices can vary. In an educational setting, the most common forms of assistive technology are relatively inexpensive, ranging from $10 calculators and reading glasses to more expensive frequency modulation (FM) listening systems that can cost over $500 (Hearn et al., 2016). Mobility aids like walkers and wheelchairs can range in price depending on the level of complexity. A standard walker can cost as little as $30 and as much as $100, with other premium models that offer more features costing as much as $600 (Sellars, 2022). Wheelchairs vary similarly in price. The average cost of a standard manual wheelchair is around $500; however, powered wheelchairs can cost anywhere between $1,500 and $30,000, with an average cost of $7,132 (www.costhelper.com, 2022; Rentschler et al., 2004). The cost of assistive technology is also correlated with disability severity. For example, depending on the needs of individual visually impaired persons, the average cost can vary from approximately $1,000 to as much as $20,000 (Uslan, 1992). Recent research on the affordability of hearing aids in the United States reports an average bundled cost of $2,500 (Jilla et al., 2020). It is worth noting that the U.S. Food and Drug Administration (FDA) recently announced a rule on August 16, 2022, that a prescription is no longer required for purchasing a hearing aid. This is in response to the underutilization of hearing aids due to the high cost. It is estimated that this new rule will significantly reduce costs to the individual (Jewett, 2022).

IMPACT

Assistive technology has caught attention in recent years among rehabilitation practitioners due to its promising effect in improving the quality of life for persons with disabilities (Kuo & Kosciulek, 2021). These positive influences can be seen in many aspects of a person's life, including education, employment, and leisure and community activities.

Education

Assistive technology can be found in classrooms of all levels, helping students with disabilities achieve their educational goals. For younger children in elementary and middle school, assistive technology devices are primarily used to help with the development of particular skills. Research has demonstrated that assistive technology devices can be effective tools to aid in the development of literacy and mathematics skills in children with disabilities (Bouck et al., 2020; Stauter et al., 2019). Such tools include access methods (e.g., adapted computer mouse), computers (e.g., laptops, desktops, tablets), augmentative and alternative communication, and software applications. Recent research has even demonstrated that specialized robotics can be used to enhance the social skills of children with autism spectrum disorder (ASD; Syriopoulou-Delli & Gkiolnta, 2022).

In higher education, assistive technology often fosters the inclusion of students with disabilities and aids in their engagement with their academic work. Research has found that students with disabilities rate their own academic performance and satisfaction higher after making use of assistive technologies. Specifically, students found that academic tasks such as reading, writing, note-taking, test-taking, and studying were all improved with the use of assistive devices (Malcolm & Roll, 2017).

At the college level, assistive technology is particularly valuable in facilitating access to information, fostering an environment that can broaden access, and improving collaboration and networking (Lyner-Cleophas, 2019). In addition to helping students with disabilities achieve their academic goals, the use of assistive technologies can promote positive psychological and social changes. Students who use assistive technology devices are more autonomous, motivated, and confident, thereby increasing their social interactions and promoting engagement in clubs or groups (McNicholl et al., 2021).

Employment

Assistive technology can also be found in workplaces around the globe, allowing individuals with disabilities to perform tasks that may otherwise be difficult or impossible. Examples of commonly used workplace assistive technologies include handheld computers; wearable technology (e.g. smart watches); portable electronic devices (e.g., iPods, cell phones); mobility devices (e.g. wheelchairs, canes, or walkers); prosthetics and orthotics, environmental controls; and seeing, listening, and communication devices. In particular, handheld computers and portable electronic devices have demonstrated effectiveness in increasing the work performance of individuals with intellectual disabilities (Collins & Collet-Klingenberg, 2018; Morash-Macneil et al., 2018). Specifically, Morash-Macneil et al. (2018) found that use of assistive devices produced meaningful gains in the work-related domains of productivity, navigation, time management, and task completion. Assistive technology devices are particularly valuable for facilitating independence among individuals who have intellectual or cognitive disabilities (Collins & Collet-Klingenberg, 2018; Sauer et al., 2010). Assistive cuing systems available on portable electronic devices can provide timely instruction on when and how to complete tasks, reducing the need for external prompting by a job coach, which in turn fosters autonomy and improves the social experiences of workers (Collins & Collet-Klingenberg, 2018). A recent study conducted by Duncan et al. (2020) found that rehabilitation technology, among other vocational rehabilitation services, is one that increases the odds of employment for persons with an amputation. Those with physical disabilities working with the aid of assistive technologies report numerous benefits, including increased productivity, self-esteem, better attendance, and more paid work hours (Stumbo et al., 2009).

Leisure and Community Involvement

Assistive technology can also help individuals with disabilities participate in numerous leisure activities and be more active members in their communities. Experienced users of assistive devices often describe benefits of increased levels of internal satisfaction, independence, and social participation in society (Lenker et al., 2013). Assistive devices for daily use, such as an adapted mouse for a computer, can be invaluable supports for individuals with limited hand dexterity for their leisure communication and engagement with others (Stasolla & De Pace, 2014). Findings of recent research suggested that everyday assistive products are highly relevant for engagement and performance in sports. Geppert et al. (2022) evaluated the 50 priority assistive products on WHO's Assistive Products List and found that all, to some extent, facilitated the participation of sport at all levels, from occasionally watching to competitive play.

CATEGORIES OF ASSISTIVE TECHNOLOGY

Assistive technology devices are generally categorized by their intended purpose (aids for mobility, vision, hearing, speech, language, etc.) or by the degree of technical complexity. Three commonly recognized categories include low-, mid-, and high-tech devices.

Low-Tech

Low-tech assistive technologies are relatively simple devices, often with few mechanical parts that do not require a power source. Adapted handles for tools or grips for pens and pencils are prime examples of low-tech assistive devices. Other examples include magnifying glasses or eyeglasses for the visually impaired, canes and walkers to assist with mobility, and sensory input items such as fidgets and squishy balls. Generally, these devices do not require much training to use effectively and may be less expensive and more accessible compared to their mid- or high-tech counterparts (Chazen, 2019; Piltingsrud, 2018). However, low-tech assistive devices may not be sufficient without other supports.

Mid-Tech

Devices that are considered to be mid-tech are more mechanically complex than those defined as low-tech and may require an internal or external power source. Manual wheelchairs are often regarded as the most common mid-tech assistive devices. Other examples include calculators, electronic organizers, audiobooks, adapted computer mice and keyboards, and many more. Mid-tech assistive devices are relatively low cost and are generally accessible. However, some training or technical knowledge may be necessary to make effective use of these devices (Chazen, 2019; Piltingsrud, 2018). Furthermore, the user may not be able to complete a given task if the device fails.

High-Tech

High-tech assistive technologies are comparatively complex, are often composed of sophisticated electronics, and may even be computerized. While the manual wheelchair is the premier example of a mid-tech assistive device, the powered wheelchair represents the shift to high-tech. Other examples include digital hearing aids, speech recognition and text-to-speech software, and eye gaze–controlled computers. High-tech assistive devices can facilitate educational or vocational goals that may otherwise be challenging for individuals with disabilities. While these devices may have more quality-of-life features, their cost is also higher than their counterparts. In addition to extensive training and technical knowledge, access to follow-along technical support is often necessary when utilizing high-tech assistive devices (Chazen, 2019; Piltingsrud, 2018). Furthermore, users may abandon the devices due to difficulties in configuring and modifying the settings (Petrie et al., 2018).

AN ETHICAL ORIENTATION TO ASSISTIVE TECHNOLOGY SERVICES

Assistive technology consultation is an essential function of the rehabilitation counselor (Kuo & Kosciulek, 2021; Scherer et al., 2005). Therefore, rehabilitation counselors have an ethical obligation to develop entry-level competence in using the counseling process to support clients in the selection, application, and maintenance of assistive devices that support participation in employment, independent living, and social participation. However, the obligation to support does not imply that counselors can be, or should be, continually up-to-date on all the latest technologies. Rather, counselors must possess competence in the assessment of clients' technology needs and preferences and either the ability to competently provide direct assistive technology services or possess the necessary knowledge and skills to effectively refer clients to skilled assistive technology providers (Connor et al., 2018). This chapter describes a broad range of assistive technology service provision models and details Connor et al.'s biopsychosocial model of assistive technology service delivery, which guides counselors in determining whether a medical model of device selection and support is necessary, thereby assisting counselors in knowing when device trials can be explored by the counselor and when referral and consultation with licensed healthcare providers is necessary for safe and effective service. The need for assistive technology team collaboration is emphasized throughout.

Estrada-Hernandez and Bahr (2021) delineate six aspects of assistive technology service provision that may pose ethical dilemmas related to the protection of consumers' privacy, autonomy, and decision-making. These six aspects can be divided into client factors (autonomy, access, consumer's cultural views) and external factors (qualification of the provider, stigma and obstructiveness of the device, and privacy). To protect consumer *autonomy*, the counselor must consider how the consumer can communicate choice in the process to a level considered "enough-informed" (p. 289) given the consumer's cognitive and communicative abilities in conjunction with consultation with their trusted network of personal and professional supports. To facilitate *access* to assistive technology, counselors must consider geography and cost, which have been identified by multiple authors as the main barriers to assistive technology (Dorsten et al., 2009; Peterson & Murray, 2006; Zwijsen et al., 2011). For example, rural residents have decreased access to university-hospital assistive technology research and clinical services, and many devices are cost-prohibitive without insurance funding. Moreover, counselors should consider not only the initial cost of adopting a device but also its ongoing maintenance or need for upgrading. Medicare, for example, will never replace a wheeled mobility device sooner than 5 years from the date that use began, even as needs change. For instance, the client may be using a manual wheelchair but is seeking employment in a kitchen where Occupational Health and Safety (OSHA) rules dictate that workers handling food cannot concurrently self-propel a wheelchair. In such an instance, powered mobility may be a solution, but may not be accessible to the client unless they can pay out of pocket for the new chair, which can cost anywhere from $1,500 to $15,000! In addition to respecting consumers' ability to pay, cultural considerations are important to device acceptance and retention. To respect consumers' *cultural views*, counselors must be willing to accept that their appraisal of the best device may not be an acceptable choice to the consumer due to differing cultural attitudes. For example, the culture of the family may dictate that carrying the family member with mobility needs to a second-floor bedroom is preferable to installing a motorized chair-lift on the stairs if the family values physical closeness and their effort as an ethic of care over convenience.

Regarding external factors, the *qualification of the provider* is paramount. As discussed earlier, an ethical approach to service provision requires that the counselor knows when, how, and with whom to consult and/or refer out for competent and effective service. Estrada-Hernandez and Bahr (2021) define qualified assistive technology providers as professionals with a rehabilitation degree and the Assistive Technology Provider (ATP) credential bestowed by the Rehabilitation Engineering Society of North America (RESNA). While the RESNA ATP designation is not a requirement for entry-level practice in assistive technology, knowledge of best practices related to the population of interest is both necessary and essential for rehabilitation counselors. The ATP designation is assurance of an advanced level of expertise. A second external factor (Estrada-Hernandez & Bahr., 2021) is the potential *stigma and/or obstructiveness* that the tool may impose in addition to any functional gain. For example, Dos Santos et al. (2022) interviewed students with low vision regarding the perceived stigma of the white cane versus smart glasses and found that smart glasses were more acceptable to the population due to their modern aesthetics and association with nondisabled users, whereas the white cane, despite its simplistic utility, was less acceptable due to its clear association with visual impairment. It should be noted that consumer perceptions of aesthetics are not superficial, as using a device that clearly identifies the user as a person with a disability can result in real or perceived danger related to vulnerability. For example, users of long canes to aid low vision may worry that the cane marks them as potential targets of crime, such as muggings. In response to this fear, Branham et al. (2017) described a need for assistive technology that helps people with low vision identify threats in the environment, such as an individual with a weapon, or to help locate a police officer. Finally, *privacy* must be considered when recommending any device. For example, Estrada-Hernandez et al. (2021) caution that devices, such as fall monitors, tracking devices, video cameras, and even digital organizers, can all be used to violate a consumer's privacy. Specifically, a prudent counselor will weigh the benefits of safety or convenience against the cost to the consumer in privacy.

In sum, ethical delivery of assistive technology services requires that the rehabilitation counselor preserve and facilitate the privacy, autonomy, and decision-making capacities of the consumer. To facilitate this stewardship, counselors must understand their role and scope of practice as it relates to assistive technology, along with those of related professionals, such as occupational therapists and special educators, who are often involved in the provision of assistive technology and adaptive equipment (Connor et al., 2018). Beyond understanding the role and scope of the team players, counselors should appreciate that team collaboration around assistive technology service provision results in better outcomes for consumers (Gierach, 2009; Peterson & Murray, 2006; Terpenny et al., 2006).

ASSISTIVE TECHNOLOGY MODELS

Advanced and novice practitioners alike will find utility in the following models of assistive technology service delivery. Among the models presented here, some are contextually specific (SETT), person-centered (HATT), psychosocially focused (MPT), or integrated across medical and psychosocial approaches (BMAT). Each should be selected intentionally by the rehabilitation professional in relation to the needs and context of the AT consumer.

Student, Environment, Task, and Tool Model

As clearly delineated in the IDEA, assistive technology service provision is critical to the learning of students with disabilities in school. The effect of assistive technology provision in the school system is evident in a report generated by the National Council on Disability in 1993, in which it claimed that almost three-quarters of school-age children with disabilities could remain in regular classes if appropriate technology could be offered. In addition, when appropriate assistive technology was provided, a 45% reduction in school-related service needs was observed. Traditionally, students were provided with assistive devices based on their abilities in relation to the learning objectives of the curriculum. Therefore, a student with memory deficits may be provided with a notebook as a task reminder, and a student with a cognitive disorder may be aided with a calculator to solve mathematical problems. Whereas the ability-objective focus of assistive technology implementation is useful in certain cases, it suffers some drawbacks. As Zabala (1995) described, the siloed focus of individual ability and task objective may lack consideration of context. Therefore, an AT solution that is useful for a given task may only be applicable in a given environment and lack scalability. At best, the AT provision and implementation may solve only a given problem in a given situation; at worst, the AT solution may not be feasible for real-life use. In addition, Zabala also emphasized the cumbersome nature of learning to use an assistive technology device that is context specific. "How much time and effort would anyone put toward using a tool that did not fit the task or the environment in a useful, meaningful way," Zabala asked and answered, "Not much" (Zabala, 2020, p. 20).

In response, Zabala (1995) introduced the SETT model to guide the provision of assistive technology devices and services to students with disabilities in the school system. Specifically, the four letters of the model stand for *Student, Environment, Tasks, and Tools*. The *Student*, which is the only singular term in the acronym, focuses on the individual. The premise is that each individual is unique, even when compared to others who may have the same disability diagnosis. Zabala emphasized that when a student is asked to identify the desired outcomes from the assistive technology service, theymay respond in general terms, such as "walk" or "talk." The specificity of these objectives must then be further explored by considering *The Tasks*. The *Environments*, as labeled in a plural form, emphasize the multitude of locations and situations in which the student will utilize the assistive technology solutions. Whereas the targeted environment may still be within the school, the differences among the classroom, playground, cafeteria, hallway, and transportation stops could be significant and require considerable attention. A typical example is an electronic device that needs to stay plugged in and therefore may be suitable and useful in the classroom setting but not so much in others. *The Tasks* focus on the skills to be built with help from the assistive technology solutions. It should be noted that assistive technology is not to be used to replace the student to perform the task. Therefore, a critical question to ask is whether the assistive technology helps the student learn the skills. One helpful way to determine *The Task* is to break down a given objective into steps. Once the steps that hinder a student's learning are identified, one can further investigate what specific elements or barriers are causing the hindrance and build the assistive technology solution accordingly. *The Tools*, labeled in a plural form, emphasize generating workable options. It is not uncommon that the student is prescribed a specific solution with a take-it-or-leave-it mentality. For any given desired outcome, there should be "no-tech," "low-tech," and "high-tech" options available, among which the student can exercise choice. Ultimately, it is the student who will be using the assistive technology, and if they do not perceive it as valuable, they may abandon it. Combining these four aspects facilitates the rehabilitation professional in organizing their approach to clinical reasoning and more effectively

TABLE 23.1 **Questions guiding the SETT model**

Student	• What does the student need to do? • What are the student's special needs? • What are the student's current abilities?
Environment	• What materials and equipment are currently available in the environment? • What is the physical arrangement? • Are there special concerns? • What is the instructional arrangement? • Are there likely to be changes? • What supports are available to the student? • What resources are available to the people supporting the student?
Tasks	• What activities take place in the environment? • What activities support the student's curriculum? • What are the critical elements of the activities? • How might the activities be modified to accommodate the student's special needs? • How might technology support the student's active participation in those activities?
Tools	• What no-tech, low-tech, and high-tech options should be considered when developing a system for a student with these needs and abilities doing these tasks in these environments? • What strategies might be used to invite increased student performance? • How might these tools be tried out with the student in the customary environments in which they will be used?

making assistive technology decisions. A series of questions, provided by Zabala, may be asked to gain insight into each aspect (see Table 23.1).

Although not explicitly listed in the model, Zabala (2020) stressed the need to have a team consider not only the assistive technology devices but also the assistive technology services. Zabala's question list should be considered instrumental to the service delivery team for activities such as selection, acquisition, and facilitation of the effective use of assistive technology devices in school-based settings. Importantly, the four constructs of the SETT model require continuous monitoring and updating in order to meet ever-changing individual abilities and learning outcomes, as well as addressing the need for device updating and maintenance as necessary.

Human Activity Assistive Technology Model

Similar to the SETT model, the HAAT was originally created to describe a process for prescribing assistive technology solutions that can optimally serve individuals with disabilities (Cook & Hussey, 1995). The model was based on Bailey's (1989) Human Performance model (HP), which incorporates three elements, including Human, Activity, and Context. In the original HP model, the focus is on how the individuals perform certain tasks in a given context, and assistive technology was not explicitly delineated. Cook and Hussey (1995) then modified the model and generated the first version of the HAAT, which incorporates four elements, including the Human, the Activity, the Assistive Technology, and the Context. As can be seen in Figure 23.1, the Context element from the original HP model was replaced by the Assistive Technology element and a rectangle (i.e., context) was added to enclose the entire circle. This is to illustrate that assistive technology uniquely interacts with human and task both directly and interdependently (Giesbrecht, 2013). In addition, context is not just an element but an overarching existence that influences every aspect of the model. As Giesbrecht (2013) described,

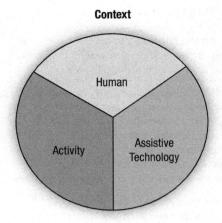

FIGURE 23.1 HAAT model

context should be conceptualized beyond location and physical conditions and include aspects such as social, cultural, and institutional factors. In the most recent version of the book *Assistive Technologies: Principles & Practice* (5th ed.), Cook et al. (2020) again revised the presentation of the model while retaining the same four elements. Specifically, the original two-dimensional graph was replaced by a three-dimensional ball sitting on a rectangular box. The change is mainly to emphasize the interlocking nature and the dynamic relationships of each element (see Figure 23.1).

It is important to note that although the HAAT model is mainly used to guide assistive technology service delivery, Cook et al. (2020) emphasized that the focus should be on the person and the activity. The philosophy is to start the service by identifying that "someone" will be doing "something" "somewhere" with the help of assistive technology. The emphasis of the order is to promote a focus on the person, rather than the technology, at the center of the service. Therefore, instead of the person trying to adapt to the technology, the technology must accommodate the person's needs in that specific context. For example, a technology-proficient person living in a northern state (e.g., Michigan, Wisconsin) can choose a higher-tech device that is cold tolerant; on the other hand, a novice technology user who lives in a southern state (e.g., Florida) may choose to use a device that is heat resistant and simple to operate. Ultimately, the assistive technology solution is to complement the person for the task in the specific environment.

While an emphasis on the person-first approach is ideal, it should be noted that challenges exist. For example, options of technology that are readily available may be limited to meet a wide spectrum of individual needs. In addition, practitioners' knowledge and experience in assistive technology may also be limited. Often assistive technology solutions are prescribed based on familiarity rather than feasibility and necessity. In other cases, clients may need to go through a significant amount of training, and fitting before an assistive technology solution can be helpful in day-to-day use. This process, while necessary, may hinder users' willingness to try the prescribed solution.

Matching Person and Technology

Although assistive technology can be an effective intervention for individuals with disabilities to pursue their life goals, it has its own challenges. Among these challenges, one that is particularly alarming is the high abandonment rate (Petrie et al., 2018; Phillips & Zhao, 1993; Sugawara et al., 2018). Specifically, Phillips and Zhao (1993) reported that 29.3% of users abandoned their assistive technology devices prematurely. When looking into factors that caused the high abandonment rate, Phillip and Zhao found four major reasons, including (a) change in user needs, (b) easy device procurement, (c) poor device performance, and (d) a lack of consideration for users' opinions. Interestingly, of the four reasons, only one, poor device performance, has to do with the device itself and one has to do with the process of procuring the device. Perhaps not as intuitive, the easier the process is for procuring the device, the more likely the users would abandon their device. As Phillip and Zhao (1993) explained, just because the device is readily available, it does not mean it is the best fit for the users. In fact, the "standard procedure" of prescribing a certain assistive technology device, such as a wheeled walker or long-handled reacher, to a disability population, as commonly seen in the hospital, may overlook the nuances of individual differences and ultimately lead to device abandonment. Importantly, the other two reasons for high assistive technology abandonment have to do with the nature of the individuals' needs, both physically and psychologically. A lack of forward thinking may overlook the changing nature of individuals' disabilities. Hence, when the physical or cognitive capacity of the individual changes, the AT device may no longer be applicable. Lastly, users' opinions should be included in the assistive technology decision-making process. In fact, Phillip and Zhao (1993) argued that assistive technology service provision and solution implementation should be a team effort with various experts included, and most importantly, the user should be part of the team. Without a careful assessment of what users really want, abandonment is likely.

In response to the need for carefully assessing individual differences and needs, the Matching Person and Technology (MPT) model was created (Scherer, 2004). Scherer et al. (2007) stated that the provision of an assistive technology service used to be guided by a traditional medical view of disabilities, with the focus placed on addressing functional limitations to the exclusion of psychological needs or social context. Shifting from a medical model, Scherer et al. (2007) claimed that MPT adopts a social model of disability and a consumer-driven philosophy. As Scherer (2004) described, the MPT model emphasizes three components: (a) the characteristics of the person, (b) the milieu, and (c) the features of the technology. Each component may uniquely contribute to users' willingness to engage and the effectiveness of using technology, either positively or negatively. Therefore, a technology may seem suitable for a person, but it may still be discarded when the environment does not support the use. To guide assistive technology service providers and increase the consumers' engagement, MPT operationalized the entire process into seven steps: (a) identify goals; (b) identify supports used in the past; (c) match with the specific technology; (d) the consumer and professional discuss factors that may indicate problems with optimal use of the technology; (e) after problem areas have been noted, the professional and consumer work to identify specific intervention strategies; (f) the professional and consumer work to devise and document an action plan to address the problems; and (g) a follow-up assessment is conducted to determine any adjustments or accommodations needed. Each step comes with associated assessments to help service providers better conceptualize the situation.

The Matching Person and Technology model was created by Dr. Marcia Sherer as a result of a funded project from the National Science Foundation. Throughout the years, the model has grown and been validated. The breadth of its impacts and knowledge made the MPT its own study in the field. A plethora of information about how to effectively implement MPT can be found from the official website of MPT: https://sites.google.com/view/matchingpersontechnology/.

Biopsychosocial Model of Assistive Technology Team Collaboration

In addition to the assistive technology process models outlined in this chapter, Connor et al. (2018) describe a biopsychosocial model of AT team collaboration (BMAT; 2018). In response to rehabilitation counselors' perceived lack of preservice preparation to provide assistive technologyservices and drawing from clinical experience in vocational rehabilitation and special education settings, the authors provide a training model intended to improve rehabilitation counselors' readiness to address clients' assistive technologyneeds by understanding the roles and scopes of practice of the various disciplines involved in assistive technology service provision. The model is unique in that it encompasses both medical and psychosocial aspects of AT and includes a temporal component that guides the rehabilitation counselor to first address medical aspects through referral and consultation with the appropriate professional (occupational therapist [OT], physical therapist [PT], physiatrist, etc.) as necessary, while concurrently and continually assessing the psychosocial aspects of the client's need for technology through the use of traditional counseling assessments, such as interviewing and behavioral or situational assessment, along with specific assistive technologyassessments, such as the MPT (Scherer, 2004). Some of the challenges to effective assistive technologycollaboration suggested by Connor et al. (2018) include differing use of assistive technologyterminology by rehabilitation professionals and high rates of device abandonment.

NEED FOR COMMON TERMINOLOGY ACROSS REHABILITATION PROFESSIONS

Connor et al. (2018) caution that the term *assistive technology*, while defined along a continuum from low tech to high tech, is commonly used to connote high-tech, powered, and often chip-based devices, such as electronic communication devices or screen readers. As part of the rehabilitation team, counselors should consider that other rehabilitation professionals who align more with a medical model of service (e.g., OTs and PTs, physiatrists, nurse practitioners) will commonly use the term *adaptive equipment* or *durable medical equipment* (DME) to refer to low-tech assistive technologyitems, such as passive seating and positioning devices, long-handled reachers, walkers, or simple task aids, such as sorting templates that help a consumer complete a job task more independently. In essence, the lack of shared terminology across professions is a barrier to interdisciplinary teaming, while the extant literature has long identified teaming as a factor contributing to improved client outcomes with assistive technology(Gierach, 2009; Peterson & Murray, 2006; Terpenny et al., 2006). Therefore, it is recommended that rehabilitation counselors be clear with their language by differentiating between assistive technologyand adaptive equipment in order to promote more effective interdisciplinary team collaboration.

NEED TO ADDRESS HIGH RATES OF DEVICE ABANDONMENT

As Kuo (2013) emphasized, assistive technologyabandonment can be detrimental to consumers not only because of the added cost to individuals and agencies but also the loss of confidence in assistive technologythat may ensue when devices are used only briefly. As Scherer et al. (2007) noted, the lack of consideration of a user's psychological need often leads to assistive technologyabandonment. There are a variety of different reasons for individuals with disabilities to abandon their assistive technologydevices. As Sugawara et al. (2018) explained, reasons can range from personal (e.g., the user's health condition changed, for better or worse), to intervention-related (e.g., the device causes discomfort), to product-related (the device no longer functions as designed), to environmental (e.g., device use was not perceived favorably in work, home, or community settings). The complexity of these factors makes providing effective assistive technologyservices under a strictly medical model difficult, highlights the need for consideration of the psychosocial aspects of assistive technology(Scherer et al., 2008), and further reinforces the need for team collaboration and an integrated biopsychosocial approach to reduce abandonment and improve acceptability of assistive technology(Connor et al., 2018).

DEFINING ASSISTIVE TECHNOLOGY TEAM COLLABORATION

BMAT differs from other models in that it mainly focuses on the process of how rehabilitation professionals should communicate and collaborate in assistive technologyservice delivery. To fully grasp the model, the concepts of multidisciplinary, interdisciplinary, and transdisciplinary collaboration have to be understood. While all three approaches involve some level of communication and cooperation, the core belief is different (Collin, 2009). Multidisciplinary collaboration involves each professional addressing their unique professional role, scope of practice, and assigned tasks in parallel or sequentially with other disciplines. The main idea is that each profession stays within their disciplinary boundary. For example, a physician may assess an individual's physical condition and overall health after an injury and identify weakness as a presenting issue but will refer the patient to a PT to implement a muscular strengthening program. Interdisciplinary collaboration pertains to members of different professions working toward a shared goal (Mallon & Burnton, 2005). The main difference between multidisciplinary and interdisciplinary collaboration is that there is active communication and recognition among the professions in the latter case. Therefore, in interdisciplinary collaboration, practitioners are aware of each discipline's intervention plan with a given client and actively update plans based on what other team members are addressing. However, it is worth noting that each discipline is still only working within their traditional scope of practice. Transdisciplinary

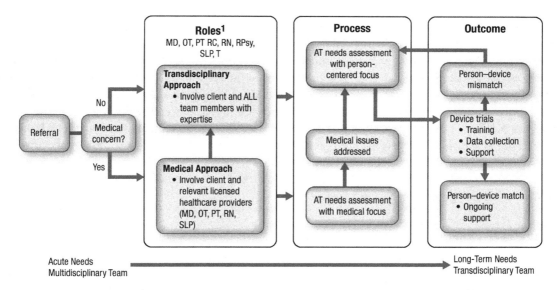

FIGURE 23.2. The biopsychosocial model of assistive technology team collaboration depicts an iterative, collaborative process addressing medical and psychosocial needs of clients within a temporal framework.

MD, medical doctor; OT, occupational therapy; PT, physical therapy; RC, rehabilitation counselor; RN, registered nurse; RPsy, rehabilitation psychology; SLP, speech language pathology; T, teacher

Source: Connor, A., Kuo, H.-J., & Leahy, M. J. Assistive Technology in Pre-Service Rehabilitation Counselor Education: A New Approach to Team Collaboration. *Rehabilitation Research, Policy, and Education, 32*(1), 20–37. https://doi.org/10.1891/2168-6653.32.1.2032.

collaboration, being the highest level of collaboration, emphasizes that members of different disciplines work with a "shared conceptual framework, drawing together discipline-specific theories, concepts, and approaches to address a common problem" (Rosenfield, 1992, p. 1351). The advantage of transdisciplinary collaboration lies in better integration of each discipline's expertise, which creates a more seamless experience for the client. Valuing the benefit of transdisciplinary collaboration while recognizing that transdisciplinary teaming requires familiarity among and regular communication between professionals, Connor et al. (2018) suggested that assistive technologyservice can be most effectively addressed through multidisciplinary collaboration in the more acute or medically complex stages of rehabilitation and gradually move into a more comprehensive, transdisciplinary approach after acute medical needs are addressed (see Figure 23.2).

BIOPSYCHOSOCIAL MODEL OF ASSISTIVE TECHNOLOGY PROCESS EXAMPLE

As illustrated in Figure 23.2, when a medical concern, such as a musculoskeletal, neurological, or integumentary issue, presents, the medical team (e.g., doctor, rehabilitation nurse, OT/PT) will address the acute medical needs of the patient. Once the immediate medical needs are satisfied, practitioners from various disciplines will then work as a transdisciplinary team that incorporates knowledge of the medical need while further addressing nonacute physical needs and psychosocial concerns. As previously noted, it is particularly important to recognize that a successful assistive technology implementation requires that the team address more than just the physical and functional demands, lest abandonment occur (Scherer et al., 2007). An assistive technology device, for example, that leads to stigma or discrimination will likely be discarded.

According to BMAT, ideally, once the comprehensive needs are identified, the collaborative and transdisciplinary team will communicate through processes such as case conferencing, include the consumer as a member of that team, and provide the individual with appropriate AT options. To further reduce abandonment, opportunities should be made for the consumer to trial the recommended devices. The intention of the AT trials is to ensure a better person and device match. If a match can be identified, service providers can prescribe the AT solution to the person and provide ongoing support, such as troubleshooting, software updates, and hardware maintenance; if no match can be found, service providers can revert back to the previous step and arrange additional assessment for a better understanding of what the person's needs are. As Connor et al. (2018) mentioned, assistive technologyservice should not be a one-and-done process. Consumers' needs may change, and technology will evolve. Therefore, ongoing monitoring and service updating are required for a successful, long-term assistive technologyoutcome.

Universal Design

The term *universal design* (UD) was coined by an architect named Roland Mace, who is also a wheelchair user. When Roland was pursuing his degree in architecture at the North Carolina State University School of Design, his experience of inaccessible facilities on campus inspired him to conceptualize UD and to advocate for accessible building design on campus. UD was defined as "the design of products and environments to be usable by all people to the greatest extent possible without the need for adaptation or specialized design" (Center for Universal Design, 1997, para. 1). To understand the essence of UD and its difference from assistive technology, one can look into the term *handicap* developed WHO. Specifically, in their International Code of Impairment, Disease, and Handicap (ICDIDH), WHO defines the term *handicap* as the interference experienced by a person with disability in a restrictive environment (Vash & Crewe, 2004). Therefore, the term *handicap* is used to describe the environment, the building, the transportation, or the system for their lack of accessibility, instead of the person. A person with a disability, in order to navigate through the restrictive environment, has to rely on certain tools (assistive technology). However, if the environment was designed and built with diversity, equity, and inclusiveness in mind at the outset, the accessibility concern would be minimal, and assistive technology, along with the stigma inherent in its presentation, becomes irrelevant. Therefore, in a learning environment, instead of using visual-based learning materials and expecting individuals with visual impairment to use a screen reader to navigate through, materials that integrate video, audio, and tactile learning should be used to accommodate different learning styles.

UD offers the most comprehensive and universal approach to increasing accessibility and participation. However, it may be difficult, or even impractical, to implement universal design within every aspect of the environment. UD should be prioritized, as much as is practically possible, over individual solutions such as assistive technology. Work, home, and social environments evolve rapidly in our current technological landscape. This rapid evolution may limit our opportunities to look back and redesign how we build and structure our living. As an example, commercial technology such as the smartphone will keep growing, and if research and design teams do not include UD as they innovate, gaps in accessibility for individuals with disabilities will only widen. Assuming that assistive technology will be able to continually generate work-arounds is not only inefficient but also ethically problematic. While the sociopolitical implications of UD are broad reaching, a full discussion of the need for and applications of UD is beyond the scope of this chapter. However, readers should recognize that assistive technology can offer only temporary, individual-level solutions, whereas UD is the ultimate egalitarian approach to maximizing participation in work, home, community, and school environments.

CONCLUSION

This chapter provides an introduction to assistive technology terminology, historical and legislative evolution, ethical considerations, and models that guide the effective implementation of assistive technology services. It should be noted that throughout this chapter an emphasis has been placed on the necessity of considering the personal and contextual aspects of technology use as a means of empowerment and increased autonomy for persons with disabilities. Further, all technology, not just assistive technology, is designed to help individuals accomplish tasks. Therefore, rehabilitation professionals should emphasize mainstream devices over potentially stigmatizing and/or narrowly applicable specialized technology. Along the continuum from low to moderate and high technology, parsimony is key; thus, the simplest potential solution should be explored before additional complexity and costs are incurred. Moreover, the practice of assistive technology should never be reduced to the devices themselves; assistive technology is a *service* that requires skilled evaluation of the client's strengths and needs; training on device use; and follow-along supports that include new uses of the device across environments, device maintenance and updates, and anticipation of client needs over time. Most of all, rehabilitation professionals must place the client at the center of the assistive technology team and work collaboratively across professions to maximize the client's long-term use, enjoyment, and success with assistive technology.

DISCUSSION QUESTIONS

1. What can rehabilitation practitioners do to advocate for the use of assistive technology?

2. What can rehabilitation practitioners do to ensure that the assistive technology service provision is ethically sound?

3. What are some of the challenges for a successful assistive technologyimplementation?

4. What are the differences between an assistive technologyapproach from universal design?

5. What is the role of a rehabilitation counselor in the spectrum of assistive technologyservice provision?

CLASS ACTIVITIES

Case Study

Mike is a 20-year-old college student in the accounting program. His teacher describes him as an enthusiastic and spontaneous student who is always on top of things. He has a very introverted personality, but he has a few close friends from his cohort. Due to his hearing loss, Mike has requested some accommodations through the resource center on campus. The accommodations range from live captioning for online classes and requesting that professors use a microphone in large in-person classes to providing a sign language interpreter. These accommodations have been working effectively and smoothly for Mike in both online and in-person classes. As he is approaching graduation from the program, he starts to work with a public vocational rehabilitation counselor to identify and pursue his career goal to be a corporate accountant. One thing that worries him a lot is the frequency with which he will need to communicate with his clients. While he has found ways to communicate effectively at school, he worries that the level of support will not be the same once he graduates. Mike's counselor plans to investigate assistive technology options while working on identifying job opportunities for him.

In small groups, please discuss the following questions:

1. What are some of the key factors that will influence the assistive technologyservices provided to Mike?

2. What model(s) would you use to help conceptualize Mike's assistive technology implementations?

3. What are some assistive technologydevice options for Mike?

4. How will you help Mike to go through this transition from school to work?

KEY REFERENCES

Only key references appear in the print edition. The full references appear in the digital product on Springer Publishing   Connect™:   https://connect.springerpub.com/content/book/978-0-8261-5111-7/part/partV/chapter/ch23

Connor, A., Kuo, H.-J., & Leahy, M. J. (2018). Assistive technology in pre-service rehabilitation counselor education: A new approach to team collaboration. *Rehabilitation Research, Policy, and Education, 32*(1), 20–37.

Cook, A. M., & Hussey, S. M. (1995). *Assistive technologies: Principles and practice*. Mosby.

Estrada-Hernandez, N., & Bahr, P. (2021). Ethics and assistive technology: Potential issues for AT service providers. *Assistive Technology, 33*(5), 288–294. https://doi.org/10.1080/10400435.2019.1634657

Kuo, H. J., & Kosciulek, J. (2021). Rehabilitation counsellor perceived importance and competence in assistive technology. *Disability and Rehabilitation. Assistive Technology*, 1–7. https://doi.org/10.1080/17483107.2021.2001062

Phillips, B., & Zhao, H. (1993). Predictors of assistive technology abandonment. *Assistive Technology, 5*(1), 36–45.

Scherer, M., Jutai, J., Fuhrer, M., Demers, L., & Deruyter, F. (2007). A framework for modelling the selection of assistive technology devices (ATDs). *Disability & Rehabilitation: Assistive Technology, 2*(1), 1–8.

Zabala, J. (1995). *The SETT framework: Critical areas to consider when making informed assistive technology decisions.* https://eric.ed.gov/?id=ED381962

CHAPTER 24

RELIGION AND DISABILITY

BRYAN O. GERE, NAHAL SALIMI, ROY K. CHEN, AND UZOAMAKA OKORI

LEARNING OBJECTIVES

After reading this chapter, you will be able to:

- Describe the history and definitions of spirituality and religiosity in the United States
- Describe how disability is understood and how persons with disabilities have been perceived and treated in the major world religions throughout history
- Identify and discuss research findings related to the influence of spiritual beliefs on adjustment and adaptation to a disability and the importance of religion and religiosity in the lives of people with disabilities
- Identify and discuss some approaches that rehabilitation counselors can use to incorporate and discuss religion/spirituality as part of therapy

PRE-READING QUESTIONS

1. What do spirituality and religion mean to you?
2. In what ways are religion and spirituality connected to clients presenting problems in counseling?
3. How would you explore religion and spirituality in counseling treatment, and what is one question you could ask a client in order to initiate a discussion that explores the client's religious beliefs or spirituality?
4. How would you integrate religion and spirituality themes into counseling?

Disability is part of the human experience. The term is often used interchangeably with the word *handicap*; however, these two terms have different meanings. Under the Americans with Disability Act Amendment (2008), *disability* is defined as a physical or mental impairment that substantially limits a major life activity or major bodily function. *Handicapism,* on the other hand, is a disadvantage resulting from an impairment or a disability for a given individual, one that prevents the fulfillment of a role that is considered normal (depending on age, sex, social, and culture factors) for that individual. Smart (2016) stated that disability can be defined from a medical, functional, or social perspective. From a medical perspective, disability is defined as a physical or mental impairment that makes it difficult for a person to perform certain activities and interact with their environment (Smart, 2016). This definition views disability as a problem that exists within a person's body, one which can only be addressed through medical treatment. Over the last six decades, the medical definition of disability has been criticized as being too restrictive and paternalistic (Haegele & Hodge, 2016; Koller & Stoddart, 2021).

The functional or interactional perspective defines disability as a limitation in the ability of an individual to function or perform functional activities due to physical or mental impairment (Haegele & Hodge, 2016). According to Smart (2009), the physical environment in which an individual lives amplifies functional limitations and therefore can be modified to facilitate their capabilities or functioning. This perspective has influenced the introduction of architectural or environmental modifications (ramps, handrails, lifts, and bathroom and other home modifications), Universal Design for Learning (UDL; Smart, 2016), and other forms of assistive technology that enhance the functioning of people with disabilities (PWDs).

The social perspective of disability defines it as resulting from negative attitudes and from exclusionary sociocultural practices that impact the ability of individuals with disabilities to live independently, achieve community integration, and meet their economic and social needs (Smart, 2016). Specifically, sociocultural beliefs about the environment in which a person with disability resides, including religious perspectives on disability, have significant implications for how individuals with disabilities are perceived and treated within their society. These perspectives shape ableist attitudes as well as cultural and social acceptance of PWDs. They also impact the fundamental legal rights of PWDs (Pardeck et al., 2012; Smart, 2011) and prevent these individuals from accessing opportunities and participating in community (Mukushi et al., 2019).

MAJOR RELIGIONS IN THE UNITED STATES AND THEIR PERSPECTIVES ON DISABILITY

Religion and the United States

The *Merriam-Webster Dictionary* (2022) defines religion as a personal set or institutionalized system of religious attitudes, beliefs, and practices. However, most scholars believe religion is related to culture (Guthrie, 1996). Guthrie (1996) posited that there is no convincing general theory of religion because the different interpretations given to religion resemble each other due to the human-like features in things and events. The assumption underlying this notion is that religion is seminal and pervasive because it defies boundaries and shares the nonhuman universe that is significantly like humans. Guthrie (1996) suggested that students of religion view it from the scope of anthropomorphism, which informs their thoughts and actions more than they recognize and which engenders a view of religion as a family. On the other hand, Geertz (1993) viewed the cultural concept of religion as "denoting a historically transmitted pattern of meanings embodied in symbols, a system of inherited conceptions expressed in symbolic forms through which men communicate, perpetuate, and develop their knowledge about and attitudes toward life" (p. 89). The explication of these concepts widens, broadens, and expands the definition of religion toward a better understanding.

Founders of the United States, coming from different religious backgrounds, thought the best way to protect religious liberty was by separating the government from the state. They drafted the First Amendment, which was adopted in 1791. The amendment prohibits the federal government from making any law interfering with a person's religious beliefs or practices (Onion et al., 2018). The common understanding of the First Amendment is that various religious groups should be allowed to maintain and develop their faith and beliefs within U.S. society (Scroupe, 2019). Although the country is religiously diverse, its national identity and patriotism lean toward Christianity. For instance, the rhetoric of "God Bless America" and the statement "In God we Trust" found on the currency denote a blend of religion and patriotism, a mix also observed during major holidays such as the Fourth of July and Thanksgiving ceremonies (Scroupe, 2019).

U.S. religious diversity can be viewed as a product of immigration, for instance, in the wave of Jewish immigration in the 19th century and onwards due to persecution, which introduced Judaism. Members of other nationalities or cultures also had reasons to migrate to the United States, bringing their religions with them (Scroupe, 2019). Therefore, religion has become a powerful tool for inducing patterns of general interest in cultural geographers (Shortridge, 1976).

The United States, being a land of religious freedom, attracted even newer religions among people who were previously atheists. For instance, the United States is the home of the New Atheism movement, which was sparked by atheist writers Richard Dawkins and Sam Harris (Scroupe, 2019). This sect is present on large internet platforms such as Reddit, where it has about 2 million followers and which acts as a meeting place for atheists in the United States and globally (Scroupe, 2019).

Although many Americans are Christians, there are people of many religions and faiths in the country. According to Byaruhanga (2022), there are five main religions in the United States, accounting for about 75% of the population of 329.5 million. About 230 million people practice Christianity, 4.17 million identify as Buddhists, 3.45 million are of the Islamic faith, 7.5 million observe Judaism, and 2.5 million practice Hinduism (Byaruhanga, 2022). Other religions in the United States include the Amish, Universalist, Jehovah's Witness, Latter-day Saint (Mormon), Church of Scientology, and others classified as nonaffiliated (Pew Research Center, 2012).

Major Religions in the United States

The advent of religion in the United States started with Catholicism in the late 16th century, introduced to Florida and New Mexico by Franciscan friars. In the mid-18th century, Catholicism was practiced in California. The missionaries converted the then Native Americans, who incorporated their cultural practices into their newly adopted religion, making it distinct from the European version (Byaruhanga, 2022). Then Protestantism came to the United States through Protestants who settled on the East Coast. Members of other branches of Protestantism, like Presbyterianism, Puritans, and Baptist sects, later arrived and settled in New England (Byaruhanga, 2022). Religious and ethnic persecution experienced by Jewish people caused their migration to the United States. The Spanish monarchy expelled the first group from Spain in 1492, which later ended up in what is now South Carolina. The second group was removed from Brazil in 1654 and arrived in present-day New York. In 1881, following the massacres of Jews in the Russian Empire, more than 2 million migrated from Eastern Europe to the United States (Byaruhanga, 2022).

Buddhist religion came in the 1840s when Chinese laborers settled in the western part of the United States. By 1893, the World Parliament of Religions had arrived in Chicago to demonstrate the "Eastern" religions to the American audience. Buddhist Churches of America was established in 1899, and Buddhist teachers began spreading to Canada and Europe to establish centers (Byaruhanga, 2022). Most enslaved people brought into the United States as early as 1776 were African Muslims. Although one of the American founding fathers, Thomas Jefferson, accepted their faith, they abandoned their religion and converted to Christianity. Due to the Industrial Revolution, the influx of Muslims from Eastern Europe, the Middle East, and Asia in the late 19th and early 20th centuries began to develop small community organizations around the United States. Many African Americans began to turn to Islam because they saw it as a lost part of their heritage (Byaruhanga, 2022).

Hinduism was one of the "Eastern" religions introduced in the 1893 World Parliament of Religions. Later, in the 1900s, Hindu missionaries and Indian immigrants settled on the West Coast as they began to arrive in the United States. Because the newcomers were men who worked in agriculture, lumber, and on the railroad, there was no opportunity for them to start families; the Hindu religion did not significantly impact American society until the beginning of the 21st century (Byaruhanga, 2022).

DISABILITY AND WORLD RELIGION

Religion helps PWDs quickly adjust to disabilities. They draw strength from the exhortation of the word accompanied by rituals performed during meetings. Having observed religion's neglect and reductive treatment in disability studies, Imhoff (2017) called on scholars to pay attention to the intricacies of religious beliefs, practices, texts, and communities. He pointed out that PWDs are often religious, reporting in current figures that 80% to 85% of PWDs say that faith is fundamental in their lives, a proportion equal to that for nondisabled people (Ault Jones, 2010; Disabilities & Faith, 2016; as cited by Imhoff, 2017). Religion is central to how people interpret and cope with chronic pain. Edward et al. (2016) explained what PWDs refer to as a "positive framing of pain" as helping them find the strength to manage and cope with their pain. They also noted that religious beliefs provided answers to difficult existential questions and influenced the cognitive appraisal of circumstances, reducing their impact on distress and anxiety and increasing one's sense of control over them. Imhoff (2017) speculated that religion forms an integral part of meaning-making for PWDs as it relates to all the models of disability.

Imhoff (2017) posited that for devotees of the social model of disability, religious ideas, texts, communities, and practices must be considered part of the social discourse that constructed the disabled body. For those using the medical model, religious beliefs, texts, communities, and practices really affect mental and bodily status. And for those open to new models, religious studies offer a space in which they can begin to think about the meaning and experience of chronic pain as a disability (Imhoff, 2017). In summary, religious studies always have new insight concerning disability studies. Anderson (2008) observed that the religious community is one of the largest networks of inclusion in the United States.

ADJUSTMENT/ADAPTATIONS TO DISABILITY

The World Health Organization (WHO) approximates about 15% of the world's population (WHO, 2011) as living with disabilities, so it is necessary to document the spiritual beliefs and views surrounding their disabilities. Salkas and Gill (2016) noted that Christians tend to develop positive interpretations of negatively themed biblical texts, which keep them going even in the face of adversity. On the other hand, atheists with disabilities are less likely to see religion as an essential facet of their lives (Hendershot, 2006; as cited by Salkas & Gill, 2016). Research on disability and spirituality by Chen et al. (2011) found that spiritual beliefs can influence one's disability. Because religious beliefs mediate life experiences, attitudes, and cognitions about them, they create religious perceptions of the self and the world that can influence one's sense of self, thereby causing the link between spirituality to seem like a broader concept, making religion and disability less obvious (George et al., 2000; as cited by Salkas & Gill, 2016). Findings on adjustment and adaptability to a disability, as revealed by Salkas and Gill (2016), indicated that PWDs persevered through negative issues associated with their disabilities by using what is termed *secular* proactive measures. Secular proactive measures include taking medications and avoiding anything that would trigger symptoms, meditation, or prayer while seeking a connection with others. The authors confirmed the same findings of Chen et al. (2011), who reported that how people deal with a disability has much to do with their level of spirituality. Using meditation and avoiding triggers of symptoms appeared to be intrapersonal ways of coping with disabilities. While Christians reported the importance of feeling connected to their spiritual congregations and to God, atheists reported that the feeling of being connected to the human race was important to them (Salkas & Gill, 2016).

CONTEXTUAL FACTORS AND TRENDS AND THEIR INFLUENCE ON RELIGIOUS PERSPECTIVES OF DISABILITY

The term *context* has various meanings; however, for the purposes of this chapter, it means the interconnected conditions in which a phenomenon exists or occurs. People's culture, the environment in which they live, economic conditions, the level of technological development, and religious practices are all contextual factors that can influence individuals' perspectives on disability (Bunning et al., 2017; Imhoff, 2017; Mukushi et al., 2019). A trend is the direction of change in the conditions of a phenomenon, which results in something new or different. Societal trends reflect and are influenced by sociocultural changes. Thus, an individual's personal religiosity may also be related to the prevailing sociocultural trends (Almond et al., 2011). Similarly, there are several aspects of religious beliefs that involve myths and superstitions, and as society advances in technological development, there is increased understanding of formerly unexplained and less understood phenomena, resulting in shifts in religious beliefs. Consequently, the extent to which an individual's religious perspective is shaped by contextual factors and trends appears to be mediated by the extent to which the person is exposed to these factors.

Religious perspectives and teachings on disability vary across different settings, with underlying rationales and justifications. In some cultural contexts, PWDs are perceived and treated poorly, whereas in others, they are considered and treated as special human beings (Cohen et al., 2016; Miles, 2002; Mukushi et al., 2019). Religious organizations would go to great lengths to legally codify and enforce these beliefs (Adamczyk, 2017; Beit-Hallahmi, 2014). Scholars have noted that religion is inherently cultural in nature (Cohen, 2015; Cohen et al., 2016). Culture and religion share reciprocal influences (Beyers, 2017). For instance, the prevalent culture within a context will have a strong influence on shaping the focus, intent, and requirements of any given religion, including religious education and experiences. Associatively, the religious beliefs of a community could serve as a medium for the development of social structure, cultural identity, social norms, and values (Gala & Gershevitch, 2011). Studies have posited that African traditional religious views of individuals are influenced by folklore, animism, nature, and beliefs in ancestral spirits (Bayat 2015; Eskay et al., 2012; Nyangweso, 2018; Ojok & Musenze, 2019; Umeasiegbu et al., 2016). Bayat (2015) suggested that these perceptions are similar to those traditional African religion adherents hold of illness, affliction, and other health-related conditions. Interestingly, there is a parallel religious view of disability in Africa characterized by outside influences (e.g., Christianity, Islam) that attribute disability to "fate," the will of God, a gift, or a punishment from God (Bunning et al., 2017). Many non-Western religious perspectives on disability, such as those found in the Middle East, Asia, and the Pacific, are similar to those of traditional religions (Mohamed Madi et al., 2019; Miles, 2002). In some contexts, the religious perspectives of disability are drawn from a mixture of beliefs, which sometimes results in conflicting responses (Stone-Macdonald & Butera, 2012).

The geographic location in which an individual lives impacts their alignment with a particular religion or culture and shapes their religious perspectives on disability (Brown & Eff, 2010). Studies have indicated that those who live in rural areas display greater religiosity than their urban counterparts (Thomas et al., 2015). The major religions of the world can be found in different regions. However, many religions are associated with the region from which they emerged or where they have the largest number of adherents. For instance, Buddhism is prevalent in East and Southeast Asia; Islam is the dominant religion in Central Asia, West Asia, North Africa, the Sahel, and the Middle East; and Christianity is prevalent in North and South America, as well as sub-Saharan Africa (Pew Research Center, 2012). Individuals who live in these regions may display greater religiosity than counterparts in other areas of the globe. This could be the case for individuals who live in countries that officially favor certain religions over others. For instance, a report by the Pew Research Center (2017) indicated that more than 80 countries worldwide have state-sanctioned religions. Many of these countries are in the Middle East and require adherents to hold views that are strict, orthodox, or traditionalist. Depending on the type or nature of the disability, individuals who live in a rural setting or in an area where there are strong religious views may express more stigma and discrimination toward PWDs. Conversely, individuals within these societies are more likely to express religious views that are more tolerant or accepting of PWDs (Bunning et al., 2019).

The prevailing sociopolitical spheres also impact religious perspectives on disability. In America, for instance, faith-driven progressives insist that society and governments uphold the fundamental notion that all people are equal in God's eyes and deserve basic dignity, freedom, political rights, and economic opportunities (Smith, 2020). The religious perspectives of populists on disability are rooted in "identity" and compartmentalize individuals into "good," "bad," or "dangerous" categories, and according to which PWDs are getting an unfair advantage for contributing nothing to society (Smith, 2020). Additionally, religious leaders' positions on social issues, including disability, may significantly shape adherents' religious perspectives on disability (Al-Aoufi et al., 2012). For instance, Al-Aoufi et al. described the actions and attitudes of past Muslim leaders such as Omar Ibn Al-Khattab and Walid ibn Abd al-Malik in the second Islamic state in Damascus, which significantly shaped Muslims' religious attitudes toward PWDs. These leaders also built the first hospital that accommodated people with intellectual disabilities and assigned them individual caregivers (Al-Aoufi et al., 2012).

However, even with all these contextual influences, scholars (Al-Aoufi et al., 2012; Bayat, 2015; Bunning et al., 2017; Etieyibo & Omiegbe, 2016; Nyangweso, 2018) have argued that people's religious perspectives on disability reflect their own understanding of their religion and not necessarily the exact meaning inherent in their religion or its interpretation. It is also likely that an individual's religious perspective on disability simply reflects their cultural values. For example, Al-Aoufi et al. (2012) noted that some Muslims with children with disabilities (CWDs) often use religion to address issues of social embarrassment and stigma within their immediate communities.

RELIGION AND FAMILY PERSPECTIVES ON DISABILITY

The terms *religion* and *spirituality* are used most of the time interchangeably, but they have different meanings. Johnstone et al. (2007) described religion as an external experience of formal expression with associated systems of worship, traditions, practices, doctrines, beliefs, moral codes, and accompanying dogmas that represent specific ideologies shared by the faith-based group. Conversely, spirituality is an internal experience of personal cultivation motivated by one's interest in meaning, purpose, and significance (Johnstone et al., 2007). Put simply, spirituality is more of a personal practice and has little to do with one's religious inclination, while religion, such as Islam, Christianity, and Buddhism, relates to a group's beliefs and practices. Religion and spirituality are, then, two separate entities; a person can be religious without being spiritual and vice versa. It is a common belief that PWDs find solace in religion, since the nerve of every religion is to practice what is preached and participate in activities associated with the religious community (Bunga et al., 2022).

In exploring worldwide religions and their attitude toward disability, Miles (2002) noted that Judaism has a negative view of PWDs. He explained that Jewish priests would examine sacrificial animals to ensure they were without blemish. Furthermore, individuals with visual impairment could not serve in priestly office. By contrast, Islam honored men with visual impairments by giving them the task of memorizing sacred texts on public and private occasions (Miles, 2002). Christianity recorded several healings, which denotes compassion and acceptance. Miles (2002) noted that the Buddhist community provided asylums for PWDs in Sri Lanka. Hinduism's texts contain many references to disabilities. Some are exhortations, while others recommend excluding PWDs, suggesting they be fixed in the undesirable position of receiving charity (Miles, 2002). Bunga et al. (2022) highlighted the importance of religion and religiosity in the lives of PWDs. The authors reported that PWDs use positive religious coping strategies rather than negative ones (Shogren & Rye, 2005). PWDs in the United States were more likely than the general public to pray several times a day (Hodge & Reynolds, 2019). Imhoff (2017) stated that religion helped people interpret pain more positively, as noted by Bunga et al. (2022).

The religious community generally plays a vital role in the inclusion process of people with disabilities. Bunga et al. (2022) posited that religiosity positively affected parents of PWDs. Parents' ability to accept the challenges they faced, trust in God, and discover spiritual meaning in their troubles were fundamental resources in helping them overcome adversity (Hatun et al., 2016). In Indonesia, parents of CWDs were able to cope with their hardships. Religion was a protective factor in their lives because it provided hope and much-needed care for both parents and their children (Kiling et al., 2019).

Family Perspective on Having a Child With a Disability

Reichman et al. (2008) defined disability as broadly including most types of physical, developmental, and emotional disorders or, more narrowly, specific conditions and their degrees of severity. Under the Americans with Disabilities Act, one has a disability when a physical or mental impairment substantially limits a major life activity. While defining disability as a physical or psychological condition that limits a person's movements, senses, and activities, the etiology of the disease should also be considered. According to the 2019 American Community Survey, over 3 million children (4.3% of the under-18 population) in the United States had a disability in the survey year (Young & Crankshaw, 2021). The authors suggested that the advances in neonatal care technology have increased the survival rates of infants with deficient birth weight infants and infants with severe congenital disabilities and have created more room for children with long-term health problems or cognitive deficits.

Childbirth and early development are one of the most critical stages in every human being's life, and they may be accompanied by risks. Although the causes of developmental damage may vary, caring for a disabled child is difficult. A CWD represents a heavy psychological, physical, social, and economic burden for a family. It is crucial to support the whole family and not only the CWD. A CWD could adversely affect the family's psychological well-being and become an economic burden. Regardless of its cause, and in addition to its damage to the child, disability destabilizes the entire family—parents, siblings, and in some cases, the extended family members. The disability's impact on the family will depend on its type and severity, as well as the family's physical, emotional, and financial conditions.

Ferguson (2002) examined family reactions to childhood disability by exploring two basic questions: "What is the nature of parental reaction to having a child with a disability?" and "What is the source of this reaction?" He categorized the nature and the source of parents' reactions as attitudinal or behavioral. The attitudinal categories are the psychodynamic and psychosocial approaches. On the other hand, the behavioral categories are the functionalist and interactionist approaches (Ferguson, 2002). The psychodynamic approach is characterized by a neurotic parent who expresses displeasure with the doctors and other professionals over their lack of adequate support, or a passive parent who feels guilty and refuses to acknowledge the reality that something is wrong with the child (Ferguson, 2002). The passive parent would rather reject whatever terminology or labels are assigned to the child. The functionalist approach is characterized by a dysfunctional parent who will institutionalize their child identified as being mentally challenged or having other types of disabilities. The dysfunctional parent feels more relaxed, harmonious, and integrated into marital life. According to Ferguson (2002), "the psychosocial approach emphasized the interplay of parental emotions with the environmental circumstances in which the family found itself. Guilt, anger, and denial were replaced by stress, loneliness, and chronic sorrow" (p.127). The interactionist approach is characterized by a powerless parent who is burdened with the socially imposed outcomes of impoverishment, disempowerment, stigma, and fatigue (Ferguson, 2002).

The Impact on Families of Having a Child With a Disability

Caring for a child with special needs requires expertise, especially at a young age. According to a United Nations International Children's Emergency Fund (UNICEF) report, sub-Saharan Africa is home to a large number of CWDs, who lack access to basic healthcare services. Adugna et al. (2020) pointed out the limited healthcare and rehabilitation services in rural areas. Regular preventative vaccination and essential treatment for basic illnesses such as fevers are not always available to those living in rural areas. Mothers in rural parts of developing countries, who have few or no resources for attending to their needs, tend to travel to urban areas to receive basic healthcare. Reichman et al. (2008) cite the positive and negative impacts of having CWDs on parents. On the positive side, the family's perspective is broadened as its members become aware of their inner strengths, become closer, and strengthen their connections to community groups or religious institutions. On the negative side, time and financial costs, physical and emotional demands, and logistical complexities have far-reaching effects on the family. Having a CWD makes it difficult for parents to deal with decisions about work, having more children, and relying on public support; the latter may be associated with guilt, blame, or lowered self-esteem. The out-of-pocket costs of medical care and other services could be enormous, having repercussions on the quality of the parents' relationship, their living arrangements, any future relationships, and their family structure. Having a disabled child affects parents' allocation of time and financial resources to their healthy children, their parental practices, and their obligations to the child's grandparents and other extended family members (Reichman et al., 2008). Studies indicate that having a CWD increases the likelihood that parents will divorce or live apart, that mothers will not work outside the home, and that the family will rely on public assistance. Having a CWD could also reduce the father's work hours. Reichman et al. (2008) referred to another study that found that parents of CWDs have lower rates of social participation than parents without CWDs and are less likely to have large families. CWDs affect the well-being of grandparents and peer activities. Furthermore, cognitive development scores seem to be lower for the siblings of CWDs, low socioeconomic status and maternal depression are frequent, and negative financial impacts and caregiving burdens are explicit. Psychologically, the parents and siblings of a CWD are stressed out mentally, resulting in poor mental health outcomes (Reichman et al., 2008).

Demographic Factors in Having a Child With a Disability

Family responses to having a CWD depend on the family's unique characteristics, socioeconomic situations, and cultural backgrounds. In a study investigating the challenges faced by families of CWDs in Ethiopia (Disasa, 2022), a mother recounted how she cared for and raised a child with a mental problem who later failed to walk and was sick most of the time. She was fully engaged in transporting the child to different health centers and different holy water (Disasa, 2022). Another mother recounted how she could not leave the child's side, as the child would cry ceaselessly; the mother lacked sleep most nights as she tried to stop him from crying. The child would tear his clothes and roll in mud; the mother would wash and mend the torn clothes. This mother had no time for herself because her entire life was tied to the child. Another family had difficulty expressing the financial burden that taking care of their CWD had placed on them. They wished the child's medical treatment could inform them as to whether or not the child would be cured. They also tried traditional healing, where they would send him for weeks and months without a remedy. They had to resort to borrowing money, but their child's situation worsened as the child began to run around naked most of the time.

In exploring the caregiving experiences of Muslim mothers of CWDs, Othman et al. (2022) emphasized that Muslim cultures enact family values that are deeply rooted in patriarchal practices. In other words, mothers are responsible for meeting dependents' physical and psychological needs, including providing care for family members with disabilities. The authors explained that although the Quran does not explicitly mention disabilities, it does imply that the disadvantaged should not be blamed for their condition; rather, the disadvantaged and their caregivers should be treated with kindness and respect. Some mothers of CWDs consider their caregiving role as a responsibility assigned to them by God under a pretext that God knows they would do a perfect job. Some Muslim mothers of CWDs try to hide the condition of their CWDs, especially of children with mental health issues, because they do not want to become the topic of neighborhood discussion. Some mothers expressed that they could no longer participate in pleasurable outings with friends or family due to the demands of caregiving. However, most of the maternal experiences Othman et al. (2022) investigated were positive, because the U.S. mothers could get good support and referrals from families and friends. It is likely that because this particular Muslim community is in the United States, these mothers received more help than their counterparts in other parts of the world.

PROGRESS TOWARD DEFINING AND CLASSIFYING DISABILITY

Disability categories have proven to be essential to theory and practice among professions that deliver disability services (Smart, 2016). For instance, agencies, national organizations, and laws that support the rights of PWDs (e.g., the 1990 Americans with Disabilities Act) tend to have their own definitions of disability (Smart, 2016). Disability literature has shown that understandings, definitions, and responses to disabilities vary, one key reason being that the concept of "disability" is constructed in multiple ways (Liachowitz, 2010; Marks & Jones, 2021; Smart, 2016). While numerous factors have been said to substantially shape individuals' understanding of what is considered disabled or not, religious and spiritual beliefs and practices have been shown to have a historical role in perceptions of health and ill-health. This has led to a growing need for research focusing on religion and spirituality and their ties to health and human sciences.

Spirituality, Religion, and Disability: A Growing Movement in Research

For years, the relationship of religion and spirituality with health and disability was omitted from the growing research literature. One key reason for this was found to be the negative experiences of many PWDs and their family members with religious attitudes and practices surrounding the naming and origin of disability (i.e., the moral and religious model of disability; Gaventa, 2018). As attitudes toward disability and toward individuals with disabilities began to change, the fear, anxiety, shame, and uncertainties surrounding disability and living with a disability began gradually to change as well (Salimi & Crimando, 2020; Smart, 2016; Thurneck, 2007; Yuker, 1988). Moreover, the rise and expansion of advocacy movements and community support created small societies that value and welcome positive spiritual beliefs, norms, and practices (Gaventa, 2018; Proescher et al., 2022; Smart, 2016). These communities have focused primarily on matters such as disability rights, PWDs' quality of life and personal goals, and the importance of the environment in PWDs' lives (Gaventa, 2018).

Spirituality and Religion: Definitions

There is a myriad of literature and scholarly works that tend to define religion and spirituality. This is primarily because these concepts have been historically used in different fields and disciplines such as philosophy, psychology, medicine, and sociology. Common among all definitions is that both concepts are characterized by trying to find the "truth" and attempting to find ultimate answers to life and the nature of the universe (Fallot, 2008; Vail & Routledge, 2020). However, they may take different paths in this capacity. Similar to the concept of disability, spirituality can also be seen as a social construct, a concept that every human may experience differently, and as such, multiple factors may shape its definition and perspective (Fallot, 2008; Gaventa, 2018). Some prefer to see or define spirituality through a more functional lens. For instance, Dr. George Fitchett and his colleague in the book titled *Spiritual Care in Practice: Case Studies in Healthcare Chaplaincy,* (2015) described the functional aspect of spirituality by analyzing medical case studies. Through the analysis of each case and by applying spirituality assessments through interviews, they tried to illustrate that spirituality was a way for patients to find meaning and purpose in their lives.

Although spirituality is a universal concept that is unique to each individual and requires a multi-disciplinary approach to be studied or explained (Gaventa, 2018), defining religion seems to be more objective. Significant advances have been made in different disciplines or sciences such as philosophy in order to understand spirituality and religion. For most scholars, the definition of religion is close to that of the *Oxford Dictionary*: a particular and systematic set of beliefs in the existence of a su-perhuman power (a god or gods) and the desire to worship this power (Gunn, 2003; Horton, 1960). Although some literature treats spirituality and religion as interchangeable concepts that exist on a continuum, rather than as a separate type of beliefs or practices (Koenig, 2015), others argue that religion must be discerned from spirituality (Hill et al., 2000; Worthington & Sandage, 2001). These definitions commonly seem to conclude that religion can control what humans cannot (Hill et al., 2000; Pargament, 2001; Worthington & Sandage, 2001).

SPIRITUALITY, RELIGION, AND INDIVIDUAL PERSPECTIVES

Compared to the literature surrounding other identity markers, the literature on disability and religion or spirituality is a bit broader. Religion plays a critical role in determining how disability is understood among a particular population that practices specific religious values or beliefs. Religion and spirituality may also influence individuals' general attitudes toward disability and PWDs. Thus, religion may affect the process of seeking disability treatment (Johnstone & Oliver, 2007; Salimi & Crimando, 2020; Yuker, 1988). Although books and research from a Christian standpoint have dominated the discussion related to the intersection of religion and disability, literature on other religions has begun to grow in the 21st century. In past decades, there has been a debate about the decline of religiousness in the modern world. One key reason is the assumption that in industrial times being religious means that an individual must comply with the principles and standards of one's religious tradition and rituals (Gaventa, 2018). However, for many people, religion or other ways of relating to the sacred help them cope with stressors (Gaventa, 2018; Pargament, 2001). A significant and growing body of research examines the relationship between spirituality and religion and disability as well as their links between spirituality and religion and positive health outcomes or recovery-enhancing effects (AbdAleati et al., 2016; Koenig, 2015; Koenig, et al., 2012). In this scope, the primary goal was to address subjects such as: Do different religions define disability differently? Are spirituality or religion a source of strength to those with disabilities? If so, does the type of disability matter? As it relates to coping or responding to disabilities, are there any differences between those who hold spirituality or religious beliefs compared to others? (AbdAleati et al., 2016; Koenig, 2015; Koenig, et al., 2012).

Numerous studies have been conducted to address these questions. For instance, in terms of world religions and disability perspectives, numerous findings illustrate different standpoints regarding dis-ability among world religions. For example, Islam is a religion practiced by approximately 1.8 billion people worldwide (Rehman et al., 2021). Muslims adhere to their holy book, the Qur'ān, also spelled

Quran and Koran (Firestone, 2019). Muslims believe that their holy book was revealed by the angel Jibrīl (Gabriel in English) to the Prophet Muhammad in the Arabian towns of Mecca and Medina beginning in 610 and ending around 632 to 635 CE, with Muhammad's death. The Qur'ān is believed to be the word of God—an authentic collection of divine pronouncements revealed to the Prophet Muhammad and from him to all humankind (Valkenberg, 2020). Islam teaches that disability is a natural part of humankind. Both well-being and sickness originate from God. From a Muslim point of view, health is one of the benevolences God required Muslims to maintain by forbidding them to consume certain foods or alcoholic beverages and forbidding them to waste food (Towards Understanding the Quran, 5:90; 7:31; 7:152–157; 20:81)

The word *marad* (illness), which is the opposite of *sihha* (health), is used in the Qur'ān frequently. Only *marad* signifies an illness (possibly both physical and mental) that may hinder a person from participating in *jihad* (fighting against injustice). Another word is *saqim* (sick), which is used in the Qur'ān only a few times. The reason for imposing sickness upon humans is God's willingness to test one's belief or truthfulness (Schumm & Stoltzfus, 2016). The Prophet Ayyub (Job), for instance, is the personification of persistence and patience in the Qur'ān. Ayyub suffered long-lasting pain and illness but because of his perseverance and faithfulness, God eventually healed his disability and rewarded him by restoring his health and wealth (McAuliffe, 2001; Schumm & Stoltzfus, 2016). The Qur'ān asks Muslims to be patient, emphatic, and caring toward those with illness and encourages them to make *dua* (pray) for those with illness. Although Islam does not ask Muslims to replace healthcare with prayer for major issues, it encourages prayer to calm the body and mind (Schumm & Stoltzfus, 2016).

SPIRITUALITY, RELIGION, AND OTHER CONSIDERATIONS IN THE BODY OF DISABILITY LITERATURE

Due to the multidimensional nature of spirituality and religion, their relationship with health is not consistently positive and exceptions always exist (Koenig et al., 2012). However, spirituality and religion have received attention as potential recovery-enhancing resources or coping strategies among individuals with disabilities and their families or caregivers (Baetz & Bowen 2008; Braun et al., 2022; Puchalski et al., 2014). Braun et al. (2022) conducted a study among patients with fibromyalgia syndrome (FMS) to examine the relationships between several demographic variables, including spirituality, religion, and disabilities. Participants were Catholics, Protestants, and Muslims, with the majority of them reporting belief in a higher existence. Examinations of the influence of religiosity on coping and health outcomes have revealed some connections between the variables. Those who reported higher use of "religious coping" received higher scores in the religious and spiritual dimensions. Exploration of the influence of psychological, physical, spiritual, and demographic variables on FMS-related disability indicates lower importance of any dimension of religiosity for disability. Braun et al. also shared that some patients reacted aversively when they were asked about their opinions on religiosity. Researchers received comments such as "why should God exist when I suffer from pain all day long?" Later, researchers concluded that such comments in their cohort indicate that religion was a positive source of strength for the participants, but doubts and the feeling of being abandoned by God were also reported and may influence the application of successful coping strategies. Lastly, the authors argued that those conclusions were consistent with some related previous research.

Hodge and Reynolds (2019) examined the relationship between eight dimensions of spirituality and religion and people with four different types of disability: hearing, vision, physical mobility, and emotional or mental disabilities. Their findings reveal that those participants with hearing, physical, and emotional disabilities were more likely to report religious or spiritual practices such as daily prayer. The results also show that people of all disability groups were more likely to report having a turning point when they became less committed to religion or spirituality. Starnino (2014) conducted qualitative research to examine the role of spirituality in the lives of those with severe mental disabilities. In this study, spirituality was often reported as a source of strength and a central factor in facilitating adjustment and wellness. In a similar study, Counted et al. (2022) examined the relationship between hope and religious coping in promoting well-being during periods when strict stay-at-home orders were in place in Colombia and South Africa. Their findings indicate that higher levels of religious coping were associated with higher levels of well-being. In a qualitative study that examined the role of religion and spirituality in the lives of individuals with developmental disabilities, their families, and caregivers, Liu et al. (2014) found three main themes: the importance of expressions of faith, the importance of faith and spirituality as a personal affirmation, and the impact of faith and spirituality on the participants' self-identity as individuals with a disability. The findings reflect the importance of faith and spiritual expressions in their lives. Participants also shared their acceptance and identity as individuals with disabilities in the context of faith.

Dein et al. (2020) conducted a research study related to mental health and religion during the COVID-19 pandemic. In their work, they also discuss some religious doctrinal responses to the COVID-19 pandemic that were counterproductive and led to the spreading of infection. For instance, they argued that some religious groups may believe that the pandemic is not simply an unusual disease but apocalyptic. Dein et al. also provide several examples of responses to COVID-19 in different religions such as Christianity and Orthodox Judaism. One example is the leader of a church and his followers in South Korea. The leader promised a new heaven and a new earth, and he banned wearing face masks, stating that doing so was disrespectful to God. The governor of Seoul later ordered prosecutors to charge the religious group's founder with causing harm and violating the Infectious Disease and Control Act (Dein et al., 2020).

Two other religious groups have not taken COVID-19 prevention measures. The first is Haredi Jews in Israel. The pandemic for them is a punishment for inadequate religious adherence (Halbfinger, 2020). The second is Muslims in Malaysia. Despite the public outcry, the worshippers (8,700 people) met in tents and held the Tablighi Jamaat movement, the largest Islamic missionary movement in the world, which emphasizes returning to the way the Prophet Muhammad used to live, praying and eating together in mosques. *"None of us have a fear of Corona,"* one participant said (Beech, 2020). Research also suggests that caution is needed when working with individuals with psychosis. Individuals diagnosed with psychotic spectrum disorders frequently experience delusions or hallucinations with religious content. Furthermore, some researchers have found that individuals whose delusions or hallucinations are overtly religious are less likely to respond to treatment outcomes. Attempting suicide or murder in response to command hallucinations has also been reported by clinicians. In this regard, a close examination of the person's religious delusions and the cultural context is shown to be essential when working with those with psychosis (Fallot, 2008).

REHABILITATION COUNSELORS AND APPROACHES TO DISCUSSING RELIGION/SPIRITUALITY AS PART OF THERAPY

Religion and spirituality are personal and important aspects of an individual's cultural identity that facilitate closeness to the transcendent and increase the capacity of individuals to derive meaning from life's circumstances and to cope with difficult challenges (Beyers, 2017). In rehabilitation counseling, clients' religious beliefs and spirituality are critical sources of meaning, strength, and healing as they cope with their immediate vocational and mental health problems and across their life span (Vieten & Scammell, 2015). Although a little controversial, more and more counselors are considering the exploration or discussion of religion and spirituality in counseling (Diallo, 2013; Diallo et al., 2021;

Nosek, 1995). Some scholars have even argued that neglecting clients' religious and spiritual beliefs is unethical, given that they are an integral part of a client's culture and that such explorations are essential for the delivery of culturally competent treatment services for many client groups (Elliot, 2012).

There is a growing awareness of the importance of and consideration for clients' religious and spiritual practices in rehabilitation counseling settings, although these are often not the primary focus of treatment (Stewart-Sicking et al., 2017). Spiritual and religious issues may be relevant to the underlying issues that prompt clients to seek services, or they may be a source of strength to help clients adjust to the daily challenges of living with a disability and achieve treatment goals (Smart, 2011). However, only counselors who have clinical competence or experience should be encouraged to engage in such discussions. Previous studies have found that respondents were willing to deal with religion or spirituality if the counselor was knowledgeable about the specific religion or spirituality of the client (Diallo, 2013).

Clients' religion and spirituality can be discussed at various points in therapy. For example, counselors can discuss issues related to clients' religion or spirituality during intake, in regular counseling sessions, or through the use of formal assessments (Nichols & Hunt, 2011). In exploring clients' background, contexts, worldview, and all the factors that contribute to clients' presenting problems during intake, rehabilitation counselors can obtain useful information about clients' religious or spiritual beliefs and where they are situated in each client's life (Colling & Davis, 2005). When counselors provide a welcoming environment, the exploration becomes easier, even when the counselor and the client do not espouse the same beliefs. Providing a welcoming environment when exploring religious and spiritual beliefs also communicates to the client that the counselor is interested in the client's whole experience. In other instances, counselors may find during the provision of vocational rehabilitation or mental health counseling service that there is a direct connection between the client's problems and their religious beliefs or commitments. In such instances, counselors may need to intentionally focus on understanding clients' spiritual backgrounds and identities (Diallo, 2013; Stewart-Sicking et al., 2017). Once the counselor has determined the importance of religion and spirituality in the client's life, the counselor can implement some spirituality assessments.

Scholars have proposed the use of formal paper-and-pencil assessments or the use of spiritual genograms to analyze the spiritual heritage of clients and their influence on clients' psychosocial functioning (Elliot, 2012; Nichols & Hunt, 2011; Şahin, 2017). Nichols and Hunt (2011) noted that the use of assessments at the inception of services can help to reinforce spiritual legitimacy, whereas at later stages, it could help to assess issues related to spirituality as well as how clients utilize spirituality as a support or resource. Some examples of spirituality assessments are the Spiritual Assessment Inventory (SAI) designed by Hall and Edwards (1996), which assesses the individual's awareness of God and the quality of relationship with God, and the Spiritual Experience Index, developed by Genia (1997), which consists of the spiritual support and the spiritual openness subscales. Spiritual ecograms (Hodge, 2005) have also been used as tools that highlight the spiritual and religious strengths within clients' families. Such tools depict how multigenerational dynamics inform current spiritual functioning, and they are commonly used in psychology and healthcare settings.

CONCLUSION

The conception of disability across social and cultural contexts has significant implications for how PWDs are accepted and treated within their societies. Spirituality and religion, like disability, are human experiences and constructs that have their own core elements and dimensions that need to be studied. Research showed that many individuals with disabilities utilize these social constructs as a source of confronting and dealing with disability and its possible limitations. For instance, evidence shows that spirituality has shown to be a strong coping method for parents of those with intellectual and developmental disabilities. The focus of this chapter has been to review the major religions in the United States and their perspectives on disability. Specifically, we examined the history and definitions of spirituality and religiosity in the United States, how disability is understood, and how PWDs are perceived and treated in the major religions. In addition, we identified and discussed the research findings related to the influence of spirituality on adjustment to a disability and the importance of religion and religiosity in the lives of PWDs. We also identified and discussed some approaches rehabilitation counselors can use to incorporate and discuss religion/spirituality as part of therapy. These include exploring clients' backgrounds, contexts, worldviews, and all the factors that contribute to clients' presenting problems during intake; counselors providing a welcoming environment; intentionally focusing on understanding clients' spiritual backgrounds and identities; and using spiritual genograms to analyze the spiritual heritage of clients and their influence on clients' psychosocial functioning.

CASE STUDY

Agilo and his family were referred to a pediatrician, who delivered their baby girl Arere 1 month ago. The couple are Nigerian immigrants from the Niger Delta region who moved to the United States less than 5 years ago and practice a traditional African religion. Arere was born 3 months earlier than the expected delivery date. Due to the preterm birth, the baby developed an intellectual disability, cerebral palsy, and asthma. The mother, Binibiriere, experienced some complications during the pregnancy due to some traditional medicine that she was taking for anxiety. Binibiriere developed anxiety as a result of the family's sudden immigration to the Unitd States. The family was living in a part of the Niger Delta where there was communal conflict due to oil exploitation. Following the birth of the baby, the doctor informed the parents, Agilo and Binibiriere, that the child would need significant long-term healthcare and support. The doctor also informed the parents that the condition resulted from the preterm birth, which was caused by the mental health challenges of the mother during pregnancy. However, the parents are convinced that the condition results from their failure to perform the cleansing sacrifices expected of persons traveling outside of their ancestral homes to other lands or countries.

A therapist, Dr. Ali, a second-generation American of Middle Eastern descent, is meeting with Mr. Agilo and his family for the first time. Dr. Ali is a devout Muslim who works with families with personal and interpersonal problems as well as mental health issues. He is also a trained multicultural counselor who works with clients from diverse cultural backgrounds. During the first initial interview, Dr. Ali realized the strong role of religion and spirituality in this family, and he is aware that religion is used by many individuals with disabilities and their family members to help them adjust to their disabilities. He also acknowledges that by ignoring or avoiding spiritual beliefs within the family, he would only be endangering the therapeutic relationship and possible interventions. Therefore, one of his tasks as a counselor is to identify the degree of spiritual and religious development and affiliation present in Mr. Agilo and his family and their potential effects on their counseling relationship, as well as their effects on the process toward meeting goals and objectives. He may also consider working with this family to discuss some coping strategies that might help them adjust to their daughter's impairments and give new meaning to their lives. To achieve this goal, Dr. Ali may consider discussing the possibility of Mr. Agilo's family collaborating with community organizations that can help the family connect with their religious and spiritual roots.

DISCUSSION QUESTIONS

1. What areas of spirituality and religion are of particular interest to you, or what areas are you familiar with? In what ways will these areas of interest or knowledge be useful to you in your role as a rehabilitation counselor, now or in the future?

2. Having read this chapter, what are some additional areas of spirituality or religion that you would like to know more about? What can you do to gain knowledge about these areas?

3. How can rehabilitation counselors use knowledge from religion and spirituality to work with diverse clients with disabilities to address the rehabilitation counseling needs?

CLASS ACTIVITIES

Family Religious/Spirituality Activity

Directions:

1. Divide the class into groups of two or three individuals, such that students are able to work with others in the group.

2. Each student should have their own writing materials to answer the following questions:

   a. What are/were the ritual/spiritual/religious practices of your ancestors?

   b. What are your current or present spiritual/religious beliefs or practices?

   c. How does your spirituality/religious beliefs shape your view of health and disability and the factors that contribute to health problems or disability?

   d. In what ways do you think that spirituality/religious beliefs influence your perceptions of treatment for disability conditions?

3. Ask the students to switch their papers in which they have written their answers or responses to the questions.

4. Ask the student to identify a few things they all have in common and one thing that is unique to each of them.

5. Ask the students this question: What did you discover about yourself as a result of this exercise?

KEY REFERENCES

Only key references appear in the print edition. The full references appear in the digital product on Springer Publishing Connect™: https://connect.springerpub.com/content/book/978-0-8261-5111-7/part/partV/chapter/ch24

AbdAleati, N. S., Mohd Zaharim, N., & Mydin, Y. O. (2016). Religiousness and mental health: Systematic review study. *Journal of Religion and Health*, 55(6), 1929–1937. https://doi.org/10.1007/s10943-014-9896-1

Al-Aoufi, H., Al-Zyoud, N., & Shahminan, N. (2012). Islam and the cultural conceptualization of disability. *International Journal of Adolescence and Youth*, 17(4), 205–219. https://doi.org/10.1080/02673843.2011.649565

Almond, G. A., Appleby, R. S., & Sivan, E. (2011). *Strong religion: The rise of fundamentalisms around the world*. University of Chicago Press.

Baetz, M., & Bowen, R. (2008). Chronic pain and fatigue: Associations with religion and spirituality. *Pain Research and Management, 13*(5), 383–388. https://doi.org/10.1155/2008/263751

Braun, A., Evdokimov, D., Frank, J., Pauli, P., Wabel, T., Üçeyler, N., & Sommer, C. (2022). Relevance of religiosity for coping strategies and disability in patients with Fibromyalgia Syndrome. *Journal of Religion and Health, 61*(1), 524–539. https://doi.org/10.1007/s10943-020-01177-3

Cohen, A. B. (2015). Religion's profound influences on psychology: Morality, intergroup relations, self-construal, and enculturation. *Current Directions in Psychological Science, 24*(1), 77–82. https://doi.org/10.1177/0963721414553265

Counted, V., Pargament, K. I., Bechara, A. O., Joynt, S., & Cowden, R. G. (2022). Hope and well-being in vulnerable contexts during the COVID-19 pandemic: Does religious coping matter? *The Journal of Positive Psychology, 17*(1), 70–81. https://doi.org/10.1080/17439760.2020.1832247

Etieyibo, E., & Omiegbe, O. (2016). Religion, culture, and discrimination against persons with disabilities in Nigeria: Opinion papers. *African Journal of Disability, 5*(1), 1–6. https://doi.org/10.4102%2Fajod.v5i1.192

Ferguson, P. M. (2002). A place in the family: A historical interpretation of research on parental reactions to having a child with a disability. *The Journal of Special Education, 36*(3), 124–131. https://doi.org/10.1177/00224669020360030201

Gaventa, W. C. (2018). *Disability and spirituality: Recovering wholeness*. Baylor University Press.

Gunn, T. J. (2003). The complexity of religion and the definition of religion in international law. *Harvard Human Rights Journal, 16*, 189–195

Haegele, J. A., & Hodge, S. (2016). Disability discourse: Overview and critiques of the medical and social models. *Quest, 68*(2), 193–206. https://doi.org/10.1080/00336297.2016.1143849

Hall, T. W., & Edwards, K. J. (1996). The initial development and factor analysis of the Spiritual Assessment Inventory. *Journal of Psychology and Theology, 24*(3), 233–246. https://doi.org/10.1177/009164719602400305

Hill, P. C., Pargament, K. I., Hood, R. W., McCullough, J. M. E., Swyers, J. P., Larson, D. B., & Zinnbauer, B. J. (2000). Conceptualizing religion and spirituality: Points of commonality, points of departure. *Journal for the Theory of Social Behaviour, 30*(1), 51–77. https://doi.org/10.1111/1468-5914.00119

Liachowitz, C. H. (2010). *Disability as a social construct: Legislative roots*. University of Pennsylvania Press.

Othman, E. H., Ong, L. Z., Omar, I. A., Bekhet, A. K., & Najeeb, J. (2022). Experiences of Muslim mothers of children with disabilities: A qualitative study. *Journal of Disability and Religion, 26*(1), 1–25. https://doi.org/10.1080/23312521.2021.1911734

Pargament, K. I. (2001). *The psychology of religion and coping: Theory, research, practice*. Guilford Press.

Puchalski, C. M., Blatt, B., Kogan, M., & Butler, A. (2014). Spirituality and health: The development of a field. *Academic Medicine, 89*(1), 10–16. https://doi.org/10.1097/acm.0000000000000083

Towards Understanding the Quran: Surah Al-A'raf 7:152–157. https://www.islamicstudies.info/tafheem.php?sura=7&verse=152&to=157

CHAPTER 25

SOCIAL JUSTICE, OPPRESSION, AND DISABILITY COUNSELING

IRMO MARINI, KERRA LAJOY DANIEL, UZOAMAKA OKORI, AND TORI LIVINGSTON

LEARNING OBJECTIVES

After reading this chapter, you should be able to:

- Identify the many areas in life where persons with disabilities who are/are not persons of color are oppressed and discriminated
- Examine the many contributing factors facilitating oppression of persons with disabilities and other minorities
- Examine how other countries treat persons with disabilities
- Review the differences between the opportunities of those with privilege versus those who are oppressed
- Identify key factors that make up social justice counselors and the rules that they serve for and with their clients

PRE-READING QUESTIONS

1. What are the statistical differences in terms of living environment, treatment, and quality of life for individuals deemed privileged versus those with disabilities and/or are a minority?
2. How do persons with disabilities fare in terms of governmental support and societal attitudes in other countries, particularly industrialized versus Third World countries?
3. What are some of the barriers faced by persons with disabilities who may or may not also be persons of minority in the United States?
4. Define the nuanced differences in job duties of individuals who are social justice counselors.

Inequality is perhaps America's most egregious, embarrassing, and least desirable trait as an industrialized nation. Although some would argue the United States ideally upholds egalitarian values and traditions, its history chronicles a plethora of contradictions dating back to the country's formation (David, 2014; Fox & Marini, 2012; Hughes & Avoke, 2010; Liu, 2011; Ramsey & Marini, 2016; Smiley & West, 2012; Stiglitz, 2013). If Gandhi, Churchill, Hubert Humphrey, Pope John Paul II, Dostoyevsky, and others' observations that a society is judged by how it treats its most vulnerable members (paraphrased) is accurate, then the United States has surely failed. Indeed, with the greed and corruption of corporate America embedded and arguably controlling the political system, with financial contributions supporting their causes, there is no voice to advocate for its poor and most-in-need citizens (Huffington, 2003, 2010; Marini & Stebnicki, 2012; Ramsey & Marini, 2016; Smiley & West, 2012; Stiglitz, 2013; Warren, 2014).

The root causes of social injustice are in part centralized around wealth inequities, politicians, and legislation favoring the wealthy; discrimination; and a Darwinian mentality (Greenwald, 2011; Marini, 2012b; Warren, 2014). Whereas Darwin and his followers in the late 19th century espoused natural selection in that the strong will survive and the weak shall perish regarding eugenics, Marini (2012b) states the 21st-century mantra has morphed into a more surreptitious "survival of the financially fittest" social psyche (p. 490). The eugenics movement in its extreme during Hitler's Nazi regime murdered an estimated 300,000 German citizens with disability deemed "undesirables" and "useless eaters." Survival of the financially fittest in today's era, however, is much less conspicuous in the overall harm it afflicts on its most vulnerable citizens. When the life expectancy for Americans living in one ZIP Code differs by 20+ years compared to those living several miles away in another code due partially to wealth disparities, it behooves us as a society to solve such social and moral problems (Bloch, 2013).

In this chapter, we explore the ramifications of social injustice in America and other parts of the world, focusing on those with disabilities. The ripple effect of poverty, oppression, and disability and its subsequent deleterious impact for equitable treatment and opportunity are discussed. Beginning with prevalence statistics regarding poverty in general and disability specifically, the chapter segues into an exploration of the domino and vicious cycle effects of inequitable education, employment, healthcare, and health. The resulting psychosocial impact on minorities and those with disabilities is a reciprocal occurrence between these populations interfacing with an arguably apathetic societal and political populace. Finally, a dialogue regarding the social justice counselor and strategies for counseling and advocating for this most ignored and disenfranchised population in America is discussed.

SOCIAL INJUSTICE AND POVERTY IN OTHER PARTS OF THE WORLD

In most parts of the world, social injustice is a common phenomenon, primarily experienced by the poor and people with disabilities. While Naami and Mikey-Iddrisu (2013) likened poverty to people with disabilities because their problems tend to be multifaceted, Trani et al. (2016) noted that disability is associated with deprivation in several other dimensions besides poverty. In their research to compare the national prevalence and wealth-related inequality among persons with disability across many countries from all income groups, Hosseinpoor et al. (2013) noted that disability is defined as having difficulties in completing everyday tasks, also known as *activities of daily living* (ADLs). They stressed that disability spans such dimensions as education and a medical condition that compromises one's physical, mental, and social functioning abilities. In pointing out that persons with disabilities experience worse socioeconomic outcomes than persons without disabilities, Hosseinpoor et al. (2013) suggest that disability correlates with disadvantage that has multidimensional causes and often statistically leads to poverty and oppression.

Carew et al. (2019) cite abundant literature suggesting that persons with disabilities are the most disenfranchised and vulnerable group, often being marginalized and denied their human rights. Carew et al. (2019) note that there is evidence that people with disabilities in developing countries have poorer access to education, employment, and transportation and are at risk of social exclusion within their communities, especially in the Global South (Carew et al., 2019). Although it is expected that persons with disabilities in developed and wealthy nations should receive better and more equitable care across the board regarding healthcare, transportation, employment, and other areas, that is not always the case, since even in wealthy nations like the United States, the majority of persons with disabilities live under the poverty line and are largely unemployed, at approximately 70%.

Beliefs and Religious and Cultural Practices in Some African Countries

Etieyibo and Omiegbe (2016) pointed out some beliefs about disabilities being attributed to witchcraft, sex, the supernatural, charms, amulets, and spells, otherwise known as juju, in West Africa. People with disabilities are seen as hopeless and helpless, and disability is often viewed as a curse (Etieyibo & Omiegbe, 2016; as cited by Desta, 1995). Some local myths see people with disabilities as social outcasts serving punishment for the offenses of their forefathers. Other cultural practices recounted by Etieyibo and Omiegbe (2016) include trafficking and killing persons with mental illness, people with oculocutaneous albinism and angular kyphosis, raping of women with mental illness, and the use of children with disabilities for alms-begging.

Despite the outcry by people with disabilities and their families regarding the denial of human rights, the interventions attempted thus far have proven to be unsuccessful in minimizing the stigma and discrimination toward disability (Scior & Weiner & Scior, 2015). For example, Arimoro (2019) noted that in Nigeria, people with disabilities were largely unemployed because employers assumed they would be an economic burden to their company. Unfortunately, these same sentiments are found among many employers in the industrialized world as well, speculating that hiring even qualified persons with disabilities still may lead to a decrease in work productivity, frequent absenteeism, and increases in workers compensation costs. The sentiments have largely been demonstrated empirically as being untrue.

The worldwide stereotypes, prejudice, and stigma contribute to the discrimination and exclusion experienced by people with disabilities and their families. Rohwerder (2018) postulated that the drivers of disability stigma in developing countries include lack of understanding, lack of awareness about the causes of disabilities, and misconceptions about the nature of the disabilities rooted in the cultural and religious beliefs of the people. He found that this stigma is particularly compounded and difficult regarding women. Christian fatalism is the belief that disability is a punishing act of God for past misdeeds of the individual or their ancestors and affirmed by Stone-McDonald and Butera (2014). Specifically for women and girls with a disability in India, Marchildon (2018) found many were regularly beaten at home, 25% of those with intellectual disabilities were raped, and approximately 6% had been forcibly sterilized.

In other African countries such as Cameroon, Ethiopia, Senegal, Uganda, and Zambia, societal attitudes regarding those with disabilities view it as an ancestral curse deserving of individuals with disabilities (Division for Social Policy and Development [DSPD], 2016). As previously noted by Rohwerder (2018), cultural and religious beliefs of those societies view disability as demonic witchcraft, with such beliefs even held by parents and particularly mothers of these children.

The different beliefs and understandings about the causes of disabilities have led to several consequences of the maltreatment of individuals with disabilities. Inguanzo (2017) found that infants born with an impairment in countries like Kenya, Guinea, Niger, Sierra Leone, Togo, and Nepal are sometimes believed to be the result of the family being punished or that the infant is a nonhuman spirit; however, there is no empirical evidence or data that supports these beliefs. Statistics show, however, that in such households, others will often abandon the family, leaving the mother the sole responsibility of caring for the child (Ditchman et al., 2016). The low numbers of children with disabilities in official statistics are often attributed to the stigma surrounding the disability, which makes children with disabilities go unreported (Bond Disability and Development Group [DDG], 2017). Njelesani et al. (2018) reported that the negative beliefs associated with children with disabilities make them vulnerable. They face a greater risk of violence in Guinea, Niger, Sierra Leone, and Togo. Children with disabilities are mocked and bullied due to their disabilities into adulthood because of a belief that they are not humans (Aley, 2016). The DSPD (2016) reported that countries such as "Ethiopia and Sierra Leone recommend violent 'cures' for psychosocial disabilities such as epilepsy and other mental illnesses: the forcible ingestion of contaminated water and being thrown into a pit with one or more starved hyenas with the belief that the hyenas would scare away the evil spirit that inhabit the person" (p. 7). The surveys conducted in Cameroon, Ethiopia, Senegal, Uganda, and Zambia indicated that "38% of respondent caregivers of children with disabilities reported hiding them away away or forbidding them to take part in social activities owing to stigma and shame, to protect them from perceptions and stigmas" (Mostert, 2016, p. 7).

In Nepal, Inguanzo (2017) reported the belief that the disability of a child was due to God's will, preventing families from accessing healthcare or appropriate education for their children because they were ashamed of their children or did not see the benefit of sending them to school. Sometimes, the stigma ostracizes the entire family because of the belief that the disability is associated with punishment for previous immorality (Parnes et al., 2013).

However, some of these cultural beliefs about disabilities in Africa are positive, as many families take care of their children with disabilities (Mosart, 2016). The Chagas in East Africa see children with physical disabilities as pacifiers of evil spirits. The Benins in West Africa select people with physical disabilities as law enforcement personnel; the Turkana of Kenya perceive them as gifts from God to be well taken care of to avoid the wrath of God (Stone-Macdonald & Butera, 2014).

The belief that these treatments are meted out to individuals with disabilities in these cultures is rooted in the fact that these populations should be free from poverty (Trani et al., 2015). They suggest that civil society organizations should take the lead to promote awareness of the social and emotional well-being of persons with disabilities for inclusion in society to enjoy the benefits of others in the community. Because these false beliefs about disabilities and their nature are challenging to overcome, they change and evolve when interventions to address disability stigma are implemented. Rohwerder (2018) suggested that these interventionstend to be effective when implemented at the intrapersonal and familial levels, including self-help, advocacy, and support groups. Bond DDG (2017) reported the nongovernmental organizations' success in reducing and eliminating stigma by providing information and support through self-help groups, peer support, and parental training groups. Also, empowering people with disabilities is vital for overcoming internalized stigma (DSPD, 2016). One final point to consider with many of the developing countries is that the negative attitudes and in some cases maltreatment of infants and children with disabilities are largely found among those families who were poorly educated and are much less prevalent among the educated population.

POVERTY AND DISABILITY IN AMERICA

Poverty in America has remained relatively unchanged during the past 5 years. In the Current Population Survey (2015), the U.S. Census Bureau indicates that more than 46 million, or 14.8%, Americans continue to live in poverty. It is interesting to note that poverty rates did edge up between 2013 and 2014 for individuals with disabilities, those with bachelor's degrees or higher, and married couples, indicating that even those with a postsecondary education or perhaps two incomes were at risk. As with previous years, approximately one in five children lived in poverty according to federal guidelines. The 2014 U.S. federal poverty rate for single younger persons under 65 was $11,670. For single parents, the rate was $15,730 with one child, with 30.6% were female single parents and 15.7%

were single male parentd. For two-parent households with two children, the poverty rate was $23,850 per year. As in previous years, minorities had significantly higher poverty rates. African Americans led the way at 27.4%, Hispanic/Latinxs at 26.6%, Asian Americans at 12.1%, and Caucasians at 9.9% (U.S. Department of Health and Human Services, 2014).

For persons with disabilities in 2014, the poverty rate differed depending on one's age. For children younger than 5 years, 34% of their primary caregivers surveyed lived in poverty (Annual Disability Statistics Compendium, 2014). This rate dropped to 32.6% between ages 5 and 17 years and lowered further to 28.2% for those between 18 and 64 years of age. For the same adult age group of persons without disabilities, the comparative rate was only 13%; therefore, the rate for those with disabilities living in poverty was more than double that for those without disabilities with the same demographics. A similar near-doubling trend was also observed between those with and without disabilities at the other age groups as well. The prevalence with which persons with disabilities require some type of assistance gradually increases with age; roughly less than 10% at age less than 15 years and more than 50% at age 80 years or older (Brault, 2012).

When combining disability and minority status, persons with disabilities who are a minority are by far the largest population living in poverty, and especially so for disabled female minority parents (Brault, 2012; Hughes & Avoke, 2010). Greater than one in four children with disabilities live below the poverty level, with the greatest prevalence being single female minority families (Parish et al., 2010). Smiley and West (2012) cite the vicious cycle of poverty begetting poverty and the difficulty that impoverished individuals have climbing out of the cycle of poverty. Fremstad (2009) argues that although the poverty and disability literature overlap significantly, they are rarely jointly discussed or connected. He cites that not only are persons of minority with disabilities more likely to be unemployed or surviving off government benefits, but they are also more likely to incur medical costs not otherwise covered by Medicare or Medicaid. The connection between disability, minority status, poverty, and oppression is further detailed subsequently.

THE SOCIAL AND ECONOMIC COST OF OPPRESSION AND DISENFRANCHISEMENT

The cost of inequitable treatment of persons with disabilities and/or minorities is deleterious not only to these populations but society as well, both socially and economically. During any election cycle, Medicare, Medicaid, and Social Security are always topics of discussion, generally with politicians acknowledging the increased costs, but few are willing to take any steps to actively address solutions. Brault (2012) noted that approximately 59% of working-age adults with severe disabilities receive some form of public assistance in terms of Social Security, subsidized housing, food stamps, and cash assistance. Approximately 20% receive Supplemental Security Income (SSI), which is the Social Security Administration's income assistance for persons with disabilities who qualify as being poor. Ouellette et al. (2004) further note that simply citing poverty rates does not fully capture the material hardship that individuals endure. The nuances of living in poverty include housing instability, food insufficiency, living in unsafe neighborhoods, the ongoing stress of potential utility and telephone disconnection, and inadequate or no healthcare.

Nam et al. (2012) note the racial and ethnic disparities in America regarding food insufficiency. They and others cite that approximately 17.2 million families in the United States suffer long-term effects of not having enough food and the uncertainty of being able to feed one's family on a daily basis. This, in turn, has a negative effect on children's physical and cognitive development and ability to fight chronic diseases, impairs academic achievement, contributes to higher dropout rates, and hurts one's potential for competitive employment in adulthood (Jyoti et al., 2005; Whitaker et al., 2006). The overrepresentation of minorities with disabilities generationally living in a cycle of continued poverty is alarmingly high and contributes to the large life expectancy discrepancy noted earlier between the haves and have-nots in America (Stiglitz, 2013).

The social cost to persons and/or minorities with disabilities is that they become "stuck" in a continuing ill-conceived poverty cycle, which does not allow SSI recipients to be competitively employed and keep their medical coverage (Marini & Reid, 2001; Marini & Stebnicki, 1999). In addition, the social cost to one's self-concept and self-esteem is diminished by not being a contributing member to society (Marini, 2012a). The American work ethic has long since been idealized as a primary pathway from rags to riches and simplistically thought by many to be easily determined by one's drive, perseverance, and motivation to succeed. Although there are social programs that facilitate these efforts (Ticket to Work), there are also government policies (Medicare work restrictions) that fiscally inhibit the efforts of those with disabilities from entering the workforce (Marini & Reid, 2001; Marini & Stebnicki, 1999).

In addition to the self-esteem costs to unemployed individuals who otherwise would like to work is the ever-continuing shaming and negative societal attitudes toward those who are perceived as living off the system (Rose & Baumgartner, 2013). Rose and Baumgartner (2013) studied what we today term *public shaming* regarding media coverage of almost 50 years regarding poverty in the United States. Specifically, the authors cite numerous media outlets (newspapers, magazines, books, etc.) as well as politicians who frame topics that sway public opinion. They note that the framing of the poor in the 1960s was projected as the poor being victims of living in an unfair economic system with poor health options, attending underfunded dysfunctional schools, and being subject to racial discrimination. The result of such attitudes and media framing culminated in the War on Poverty, and the government's response to eradicate poverty was immediate and effective, reducing the poverty level from 22% to 12% within 15 years as social program assistance increased from 3% to 8%.

In the early 1970s, however, the discourse on poverty began to change, largely when Ronald Reagan was campaigning for president. Politicians and the media began framing persons living in poverty as lazy, cheaters, and welfare queens having children who were also living off the system (Hancock, 2004; Rose & Baumgartner, 2013). Much like disability, concepts related to the poor are socially constructed and subsequently can shape public policy. Hancock (2004) believed this new discourse largely impacted President Clinton's 1990s Welfare Reform, which saw funding cuts and 5-year maximums for persons on welfare. This sentiment continues to exist today, especially among so many in the Republican Party, as Mitt Romney demonstrated in a 2012 Florida speech to wealthy donors, citing about 47% of Americans who live off the system. During the same 2012 campaign, House Speaker Newt Gingrich's famous sound bite that President Obama would be "the best food stamp President in American history" also demonstrated the disdain toward the poor and those in government who are perceived as enablers of free taxpayer giveaways to the poor. Although many see the issue of poverty as a rather simplistic dichotomous personal choice of being lazy or alternatively motivated to work, we next turn to how this topic is much more complex when considering the impact of social injustice and oppression in America.

Education

Researchers of social economics who focus on the economic complexities of social policies and their impact begin to unravel the stark differences between the haves and have-nots, and the impact of oppression and inequalities, from an early age (Hughes & Avoke, 2010; Liu, 2011; Stiglitz, 2013). These and other authors argue there is a ripple effect for families living in poverty. Poor families typically live in low-income neighborhoods with low property tax revenues to adequately finance local public schools. Hughes and Avoke (2010) note that poorly funded schools may be dilapidated, have poor heating, are underfunded and understaffed, have lower teacher expectations, and statistically experience higher dropout rates. These schools are predominantly in low-income minority neighborhoods, and Balfanz and Legters (2004) cite a 50% dropout rate among African American students and a 40% dropout rate among Hispanics from such neighborhoods.

Conversely, in many developing countries, children with disabilities do not have such opportunities of being educated. Out of the estimated 1 billion of the world's population living with disabilities, an estimated 80% of them live in developing countries. People with disabilities are not likely to be employed, go to school, or participate in life. According to Marchildon (2018), about 264 million children in developing countries are out of school due to barriers such as conflict and violence, gender inequality, and poverty. Although it is estimated that 90% of children living with a disability in developing countries are not in school, there is little data to support the claim.

For students with disabilities, the statistics are equally grim. A U.S. Department of Education (2009) report found that minority students with severe disabilities were more likely to be placed in special education and segregated from the general education population. The curriculum in special education ideally is supposed to focus on developing self-determination and essential job skills needed for employment; however, the special education curriculum often falls far short of curricular expectations (Wehman & Kregel, 1997). Without the opportunity for a quality education or to learn entry-level job skills for the competitive labor market, students with disabilities from underfunded low-income neighborhoods essentially have no skills to become employed. Newman et al. (2009) found that after high school, youth diagnosed with a developmental disability had only a 31% mostly part-time employment rate, 14% lived independently or semi-independently, 26% had a checking account, and 7% attended some postsecondary education. Newman et al. concluded that disability and poverty combine for poorer educational opportunities, lower graduation rates, higher dropout rates exceeding 50%, and ultimately poor employment options and rates among youth with disabilities, particularly those of minority status.

Overall, there are statistically poorer economic and employment outcomes for children with disabilities living in low-income neighborhoods who attend underfunded schools when compared to nondisabled children in better-funded schools. The dropout, graduation, and ultimately employment rates are drastically different for low-income children with disabilities, and their opportunity to climb out of poverty is marginal at best. Attempting to learn while one is hungry or cold due to insufficient school heating becomes difficult, as is the ability to concentrate on one's studies when living in low-income, unsafe neighborhoods.

Employment

The ripple effect of a poor or inadequate education for the variety of reasons noted previously ultimately impacts one's ability to gain competitive employment. Braddock and Parish (2001) cite an 80% unemployment rate among adults with disabilities raised in poverty conditions in the United States. Being a minority female with a disability ranks highest among those most unemployed. Brault (2012) indicates that employment opportunities for persons with disabilities who have not been afforded a quality education and an opportunity to obtain a postsecondary education are relegated to largely entry-level minimum wage occupations performing primarily physical labor. This is not the case for those with mobility impairments, but rather those with cognitive or developmental disabilities if they are capable of performing competitive employment. For those with mobility but no cognitive impairments, there continues to be an approximate 70% unemployment rate overall for this group as well.

One of the major disincentives Marini and Reid (2001) have previously argued, however, is that in the majority of states where the minimum wage remains at $7.25 per hour or just more than $15,000 per year (without deducting income tax), combined with the likelihood of losing one's medical benefits, it is simply not worth the risk for those collecting disability benefits for a minimum wage job. For those single individuals collecting SSI benefits, their maximum earnings are $733 per month. As such, for most individuals collecting SSI amounting to $8,800 per year with medical benefits and given the choice to earn a few thousand dollars more working 40 hours per week with minimal, if any, medical benefits, it is simply not worth taking the risk. Of all beneficiaries historically on the Social Security roles, less than 1% ever leave to return to the workforce (Marini, 2012a). This same Catch-22 exists for persons with physical impairments who require home care assistance to complete ADLs. All states have maximum daily limits regarding the number of hours per week of home care assistance; one must be homebound, and services are not provided for those who want to or can work and/or drive. Although the archaic Medicare homebound rules allow for an individual to attend adult day care, they are not allowed to work to qualify for ADL-related home care services. The incentive should be to support employment efforts by providing such assistance rather than penalizing those with disabilities who want to work but need home care assistance to do so.

Healthcare and Health Costs

Individuals without health insurance decreased from 2013 to 2014 largely due to the Affordable Care Act and the mandate for insurance companies to provide coverage for those with preexisting conditions. There was an approximate 23% decrease of uninsured Americans from 41.8 million people in 2013 down to 33 million in 2014 (Current Population Survey, 2015). In her book, *Money-Driven Medicine*, Mahar (2006) cites healthcare practices and costs that demonstrate approximately 7 of 10 personal bankruptcies filed by Americans are due to extraordinary medical bills that most hospitals are elusive at attempting to explain. Several days of hospitalization for relatively minor surgery can easily exceed more than $100,000, and for the majority of Americans poor or otherwise without adequate insurance, these costs can never be paid. An estimated 15% of private hospitals have also been known to practice "patient dumping" whereby high-cost patients who have been stabilized but do not have insurance are literally dumped off at the door of another hospital or elsewhere (Rice & Jones, 1991). The authors note that the uninsured are made up largely of minorities who generally do not seek medical services until it is an emergency.

As noted earlier, the overall significance of social injustice toward poor minorities with disabilities can result in more than a 20-year difference in life expectancy between this population and those with greater wealth. Although living a long and healthy life is partially an individual's responsibility, statistics cannot ignore the higher mortality rates among poor minorities who have a disability living in lower-income housing, obtaining poorer healthcare, having an insufficient income to eat healthy, and living in unsafe or hazardous environments and neighborhoods. A two-tier system of inequitable treatment in healthcare, housing, employment, and education between the haves and have-nots ultimately ends with higher and younger mortality rates for the have-nots (Brault, 2012; Liu, 2011; Mahar, 2006; Smiley & West, 2012; Stiglitz, 2013).

Environmental Inequities

Persons with disabilities and other minorities have been subtly subjected to social injustices via environmental and social barriers as well. Again, these inequities are related to low socioeconomic status where statistically a majority of minorities and those with disabilities reside. These populations are more likely to live in unsafe neighborhoods without a nearby grocery store or park for recreation and exercise (Liu, 2011). The stark diversity in urban planning between wealthy and poor neighborhoods creates an unhealthy environment for those living in poverty. Individuals living in low-income neighborhoods without a vehicle must travel many miles to a local grocery store and have difficulty purchasing healthy foods. As such, these neighborhoods typically have convenience stores stocked with high-calorie, high-sugar, inexpensive foods that are more affordable and available. Obesity and the multitude of secondary health-related complications (e.g., diabetes, hypertension, cardiovascular disease) from being obese are much more prevalent among those living in poverty and in impoverished neighborhoods (Ramsey & Marini, 2016; Romero & Marini, 2012).

Those living in low-income housing also face other environmental hazards. Johnston et al. (2016) cite the decades-old common practice of environmental injustice, whereby environmentally hazardous industries take up residence in low-income, mostly minority areas. The authors cite a disproportionately higher number of waste disposal facilities across the country, including oil and gas wastewater disposal wells. The recent publicity of contaminated water wells and the deleterious health impact on the cognitive and physical development of children and adults is appalling. Similarly, although the poisonous health impact (e.g., seizures, mental retardation, nervous system abnormalities) of lead paint has been known for more than 75 years, corporate lead paint proponents successfully lobbied to keep using it, particularly in low-income housing developments, up until the late 1970s (Ludden, 2016).

Pathak (2021) explored the disparities between Native American/Alaskan Native women in terms of employment as compared to White mothers. They cite childhood poverty rates for Native American and Alaskan Native households to be upwards of 40% and overall poverty at 23%, which has been a consistent pattern for the past 30 years. Unfortunately, this population also has the lowest participation in the labor force due to decreased wages and underrepresentation (Pathak, 2021). In a similar vein, more than 55% of Native households are managed by a single breadwinner, usually the woman, in comparison to 37% of White mothers. Educational achievement is also much lower with only 24% of Native Americans/Alaskan Natives having completed a degree-granting program at the associate's level or higher when compared to 42% of White students. Furthermore, 21% of Native Americans/ Alaskan Natives under the age of 18 lived in a house with a family member who completed a bachelor's degree compared to 52% of White households. Housing conditions for many American Indians on nongaming reservations are also dismal, with a reported 58 out every 1,000 Native American households lacking plumbing in comparison to 3 out of 1,000 White households. There is no adequate healthcare coverage on the reservations, leaving families often having to travel great distances to a public hospital. Native Americans have a much higher than average risk for advanced cancer, cardiovascular disease, substance abuse, and suicide. Like other minorities, they too have been exposed to hazardous waste sites from commercial and military toxic waste facilities being built around the communities where they reside.

For persons with disabilities, environmental barriers continue despite the now 33-year-old Americans with Disabilities Act (ADA) of 1990. Recent studies of Americans with disabilities show they continue to express their daily frustration with pockets of noncompliance across the country in the areas of transportation, public accommodations, employment protections, and healthcare access (Graf et al., 2009; Marini et al., 2009). From medical facilities having inaccessible exam tables for wheelchair users to hospitals and/or medical clinics not offering translators for persons who are deaf, these entities continue to be in violation of the law. ADA filings under the Equal Employment Opportunity Commission (just Title I) since 1997 to 2015 have ranged and gradually climbed from approximately 15,000 to almost 27,000 complaints annually regarding alleged employment discrimination alone (U.S. Equal Employment Opportunity Commission, n.d.). Public accommodations complaints have exceeded these numbers. For most entities that have not made the appropriate ADA changes by now, many of them have taken an apathetic "so sue me" type attitude, which conversely affects one's ability to earn social currency or capital. Social capital is essential to positive social experiences and is earned through social engagement as well as networking. However, social capital has only been studied in relation to "in-person" experiences. There is growing attention among researchers studying social networking platforms that social capital may also be earned without in-person contact. The next section will explore the experiences of individuals with disabilities and social media.

NAVIGATING SOCIAL MEDIA THROUGH A LENS OF DISABILITY

For people with disabilities, social networks have meant a considerable improvement in their quality of life by facilitating their access to education, enhancing their leisure time, and enhancing their interactions with others (Bonilla del Río et al., 2022). Nonetheless, gaining the full involvement of this group in a society that is becoming increasingly technology-focused remains difficult, since digital inclusion is influenced by various factors and the diversity of experiences. Moreover, the opportunities provided by social networks for people with disabilities to define their profiles and choose how they wish to present themselves in the digital realm also enable the overcoming of the appropriation of disability, which has resulted in a social image that does not always correspond to the reality portrayed by influencers on social networks (Bonilla del Río et al., 2022).

Influencers with disabilities, and disabled women in particular, are typically excluded from narratives of beauty because they are perceived as dependent, fragile, and asexual. However, there have been stands on this within this community creating a movement called the *body positive movement*. The body positivity movement has often been seen as synonymous with fat acceptance (Hill, 2022). However, as Darwin and Miller (2021) indicate, this is not always the case, and because the body positivity movement is broad and complex, there are numerous tensions within it. While this greater diversity is much needed, it is vital to recognize that popular body positivity discourses continue to place an emphasis on physical attractiveness and privilege whiteness. Self-representations that are seen as "too difficult" are frequently met with animosity, either from other social media users or the moderation procedures of the social media platform, which flag such content as undesirable (Hill, 2022). The body is discursively separated and compartmentalized into dualistic categories, such as adolescent and adult, healthy and sick, fat, and thin, attractive, and unattractive, abled and impaired, and male and female. Each of these categories is governed by societal standards (Hall, 2018).

In Western countries, typical bodies are characterized as young, able, muscular, and/or low in body fat (Hall, 2018). As innumerable television shows, newspapers, and magazine exposés would have us think, deviations from these norms are typically viewed as "freaky" or hazardous. Hinz et al. (2021) found that a popular fitness practice known as yoga is not considered representative or inclusive of women with disabilities from a content analysis of 800 yoga practitioners. Researchers collected and analyzed Instagram posts using several variations of hashtags, including the word *yoga* (i.e., #yogabody, #yogapractice, #yogawoman). Of the 800 analyzed posts, 100% of the posts appeared to be that of an able-bodied person, 80% classified as athletic/thin build, less than 15% showed visible body fat, 90% were perceived to be under 40, and more than a quarter were perceived as White. The exclusion of individuals with disabilities and their visibility in yoga practices is reinforced by the absence of visual representation on social media (Hinz et al., 2021). Moreover, the disabled body is relegated as nonsexual, and deviations from this social norm are frequently rejected. Given this context, it is not surprising that positive and empowering discourses regarding disability and sexuality are either invisible or nonexistent (Hall, 2018). Hill (2020) argues that it is crucial for women with disabilities to stress the need for physical acceptance and enable others who defy normative values, such as disabled persons, to come forward and achieve visibility.

Visibility is essential to postfeminism and is synonymous with the term *empowerment*. According to Banet-Weiser (2018), the politics of visibility, in which the demands of marginalized groups to be seen lead to the acquisition of various civil rights, has shifted toward "economies of visibility" in which "visibility becomes the end rather than a means to an end." Within economies of visibility, "empowerment" is frequently attained through attention to the visible body, and marginalized bodies are placed in postfeminism's regulatory "luminous spotlight," which is "literally designed for social media" (Banet-Weiser, 2018, p. 27). In her study of disabled girlhood on YouTube, Todd (2016) argues that social networking sites invite "disabled people to 'perform' their disabled identities that are not possible elsewhere." However, "disabled people are called to narrate their bodies, experiences, and feelings in ways that render disability understandable, palatable, and sexy" (Todd, 2016, p. 45).

Therefore, disabled individuals are encouraged to come forward on the basis of "neoliberal inclusionism" (Banet-Weiser, 2018, p. 26). Neoliberal inclusionism makes disabled people visible by adopting various diversity-based practices on the condition that they can appropriate "historically specific expectations of normalcy" based on ideals of able-bodiedness, rationality, and heteronormativity (Banet-Weiser, 2018, p. 26). The term *heteronormativity* is the assumption that heterosexuality is the standard for defining normal sexual behavior and that male–female differences and gender roles are the natural and immutable essentials in normal human relations (Robinson, 2016). People with disabilities are expected to "blend in" by "passing as non-disabled, or at least not too disabled." As a result, self-representations of disability are expected to adhere to the logic of social media self-branding within economies of visibility in which "inclusion" is defined as "expanding an existing set of norms" (Banet-Weiser, 2018, p. 26).

In sum, social media is an opportunity for users of any ability status, race, religion, age, gender, or sexual orientation to explore and engage with other people. Regrettably, people with disabilities are not wholly represented in the social media arena unless able-bodied people render them appropriate or worthy (Banet-Weiser, 2018). Notably, the same can be said of person-to-person engagement which does not reach the threshold of full inclusion due to the ableist ideals and the assumed monolithic experiences of those with disabilities (David, 2014; Goethals et al., 2015).

THE PSYCHOSOCIAL COST OF OPPRESSION

David (2014), in his edited book *Internalized Oppression: The Psychology of Marginalized Groups*, notes the impact of oppression on persons of minority status and those with disabilities. David et al. note how after years of discrimination and microaggressions, many marginalized individuals succumb to feeling, and ultimately believing, that they are devalued or second-class citizens. Wright (1988) similarly addressed this concept of succumbing. Ramsey and Marini (2016) also address the psychosocial impact of being devalued and dehumanized by negative societal attitudes. Dohrenwend (2000) found a correlation between perceived discrimination and higher levels of depression and anxiety among minority groups. David (2014) similarly found that individuals who internalized oppression also experienced stress, depression, and anxiety.

Aside from feelings of low self-worth, persons with disabilities who perceive they are discriminated against also report to be less likely to socialize with friends and family, less likely to go to the movies or a restaurant, and more likely to perceive their lives will become worse rather than better (National Organization on Disability, 2004, 2010). Many persons with disabilities living under the poverty level worry about their health and well-being, finances, limited community support, and unsafe or unhealthy living conditions (Cooper et al., 2009). Besides such daily worries for those minorities with few resources, persons with disabilities continue to experience daily hassles and frustrations dealing with inaccessible businesses, fragmented medical services, and the perceived negative attitudes of others (Graf et al., 2009; Li & Moore, 1998; Marini et al., 2009).

In further exploring the mental and physical health implications for individuals who are, or perceive to be, oppressed and/or discriminated against, a number of interesting studies show the significance of the person–environment interaction and its implications. Aguinaldo (2008), for example, studied the concept of gay oppression as a determinant of gay men's health, citing the premise that "homophobia is killing us." In his literature review, Aguinaldo notes the mental and physical health problems of gay men living in a society that oppresses, discriminates, and is blatantly prejudiced toward them. The resulting fear, physical and verbal abuse, felt hatred, and anger gay males often endure by others carry a heavy psychological toll, sometimes resulting in depression, anxiety, a lack of self-worth, shame, self-destructive behaviors such as suicide, inferiority, and self-defeating behaviors (Dempsey, 1994).

Generalized stress and stress-related illnesses have also been linked to others who are oppressed and feel discriminated against (Turner & Avison, 2003). Turner and Avison found that African Americans reported higher occurrences of discriminatory experiences, including violence, death, and daily discrimination, resulting in chronic stressors when compared with White study participants. Perlow et al. (2004) noted how discrimination negatively impacts one's sense of control, and feelings of hopelessness can ultimately lead to a variety of mental health disorders.

If societal discrimination and oppression simply stopped there, the negative physical and mental health impact of oppressed individuals would be alarming in and of itself. Unfortunately, the peripheral implication of perceived prejudice toward an individual or group has further negative ramifications that can exacerbate health problems (Kessler et al., 2003; Krieger, 1999). Numerous studies show the resulting ripple effect of discrimination, including unemployment or underemployment, lower socioeconomic status, poorer healthcare, lower educational attainment, and poverty (Eaton & Muntaner, 1999; Kessler et al., 2003; Krieger, 1999; Ramsey & Marini, 2016; Williams et al., 1997).

Hughes and Avoke (2010) describe the elephant in the room in relation to poverty, disability, and unemployment or underemployment of persons with disabilities. They note that individuals who live under these circumstances are chronically exposed to inadequate housing opportunities, educational opportunities, transportation, poor finances, and concerns about their health or well-being. Current public policies have failed to remedy many of these ongoing problems despite decades-old fair housing legislation, the Individuals with Disabilities Education Act, and the ADA. Much like the 1964 Civil Rights Act has taken decades to gradually remedy the impact of oppression and discrimination, the full equal rights of minorities and those with disabilities have yet to be reconciled and continue to be violated to this day. Marini (2012b) poses the question as to whether the glass is half-full or half-empty concerning the human rights of persons with disabilities.

In measuring the pulse of American politics regarding disability equal rights, the ADA, in all probability, will remain in effect for the foreseeable future to be the last major effort to better the lives of persons with disabilities. In the 2016 presidential race, for example, neither party campaigned on any further improvements to nor strengthening of the civil rights of persons with disabilities. Even with such promises, the gaps in the law and the lack of legal oversight to enforce the law leave much of it relatively ignored across parts of the country and left up to individual citizens with disabilities to police their own law and file suits.

INTERNALIZED OPPRESSION

Although major legislation has granted people with disabilities and other minorities more access, rights, privileges, and protections on varying levels, the lingering effects of oppression are commonly known as *internalized oppression*. David (2014), contends that internalized oppression stems from the intermingling of negative attitudes and beliefs that are synonymous with cultural or social norms centered in inferiority. Power structures and the perpetuation of oppression are fueled by an individual's disparagement of self and those in their respective social groups (David, 2014). Social groups are categorized by but not limited to race, gender, sexual orientation, and ability. Several researchers agree that internalized oppression is a consequence of oppression passed down through generations and engenders a more substantial psychological disruption than conspicuous acts of oppression such as discrimination and hate speech (Paradies, 2016; Szymanski & Henrichs-Beck, 2014). Gordijn and

Boven (2009) postulate that internalizing negative stereotypes subverts one's self-concept. Generally, people with disabilities are immediately evaluated for what they are unable to accomplish, a peculiarity that follows them in most social settings (Goethals et al., 2015). These stereotypes are underpinned through microaggressions, microinvalidations, and microinsults, which result in notable resistance in highlighting the joys, strength, and/or power of living with a disability (Chen & Lin, 2016; David, 2014; Garland-Thomson, 2017). Although strides have been made to change attitudes and encourage inclusivity, the experience of a person with a disability is still convoluted by ableist ideals, opinions, and attitudes in addition to merely existing in a restrictive society (Slater & Liddiard, 2018).

The Impact of Ableism on Overall Health and Well-Being

People with disabilities are expected to humbly accept their places or conform to ableist ideals, which are rooted in the "normalcy" of the human body to exist without defect. Unfortunately, navigating the world as a person with a disability has the potential to create detriments on overall well-being and health. Health and well-being are defined in broad terms that encompass psychological, social, and physical aspects that intersect and overlap, forming complex interactions in people with disabilities (Johannsdottir et al., 2021). However, the paucity of health and well-being studies as it relates to people with disabilities is unintentionally setting the stage for other fields to set the precedent for this area of research, which may likely be rooted in the medical model of disability (Brown & Leigh, 2018; Livingston & Boyd, 2010). Campbell (2009) contends that ableism is more concerning than unpretentious ignorance or negative attitudes; it is an impractical idea of perfection and an unrealistic view of how human bodies should look and perform. One researcher examined 311 adults with disabilities and found a negative relationship between ableist microaggression and positive mental health outcomes. In short, the higher the number of ableist microaggressions experienced by a person with a disability, the lower the positive mental health outcomes (Kattari, 2020).

People without disabilities who perpetuate ableist ideals oftentimes engage in the nondisabled gaze and intercorporeality comparisons (Loja et al., 2013; Shogo, 2015). Researchers assert that the nondisabled gaze is a stare or gaze from people without disabilities that repudiates the normalcy of people with disabilities. Loja et al. (2013) conducted a study where participants interpreted the gazes from nondisabled people as sorrowful, curious, a person in need of help, or a disabled hero. Other encounters with the nondisabled gaze brought on feelings of vexation, humiliation, and feeling like an object of commiseration in respondents (Loja et al., 2013). Intercorporeality aligns with the ideas of ableism and impacts the way people with disabilities view their bodies in relation to others without disabilities (Shogo, 2015). Intercorporeality and the nondisabled gaze may cause people with disabilities to struggle when building social capital, a hinderance that also undermines the ability to build economic, cultural, and emotional capital (Bourdieu, 2008; Shogo, 2015). Relatedly, a large-scale study by Mithen et al. (2015) evaluated the relationship between social capital and self-rated health status in a sample of 15,028 adults with and without disabilities. Of the 15,028 participants, 3,734 of them reported a disability. Notably, social capital is referred to as assets obtained through social settings that can be used for personal interest (Mithen et al., 2015). Researchers found that people with disabilities ranked lower in social capital and reported poorer health than individuals without disabilities. The largest difference in social capital between the two groups were found in emotional and financial capital (Mithen et al., 2018).

Factors Contributing to Internalized Oppression

David (2014) contends that internalized oppression is exacerbated by those intentional and unintentional microaggressions that can act as a catalyst for self-blame. Furthermore, internalizing ableist ideals on a daily or consistent basis can lead to devastating mental health issues (i.e., anxiety, depression, isolation, and negative body image). Blame and responsibility for one's disabling condition and the negative or positive responses from others have received little attention in the literature. However, researchers suggest that the stigma attached to the reason behind a condition or marginalized social identity is perceived by others as controllable or uncontrollable, thereby justifying self-blame, rejection, and isolation from the dominant group (Ramierez-Valles et al., 2013; Schwarzer & Weiner, 1991). For example, African American women with disabilities are viewed as untrustworthy and undeserving of sexual affection according to a study by Syndor-Campbell (2017). The findings are indicative of how racist and ableist ideals create a less-than-stellar representation of a person who is ill intentioned or has decreased moral character based on their marginalized identities. LaChappelle et al. (2014) maintain that the invisibility and degradation in terms of race and ability act as a catalyst for diminishing positive self-appraisals, thereby increasing the likelihood of internalizing oppression and devaluation of oneself. Giordano (2018) highlights shame as a precursor to anxiety in addition to depressive symptoms. Johannsdottir et al. (2021) also cite shame as a social determinant that renders disability as unacceptable or inferior to the general population. Slobodin (2019) cites shame as a by-product of alienation and defeat, which may be the body and mind's natural defense mechanisms.

While negotiating one's existence as valid or invalid based on ability status, some people with disabilities enlist coping mechanisms. In particular, Ahmed (2017) suggests that when bodies do not correspond with traditional norms and beauty standards, they are interrogated and devalued if they cannot exhibit power to overcome the disability. More importantly, Johannsdottir et al. (2021) assert that people with disabilities feel as though they must blend in, fit in, or ascribe to an identity that is not their own in order to be accepted. Ahmed (2017) refers to the process of taking on identity that is not your own as "passing," which is used as a survival skill or safety tactic to avoid negative interactions with those outside of your social group. Mitra and Doctor (2016) find similar survival and coping tactics in males who identify as gay and who utilize passing as heterosexual to avoid negative experiences with others.

In sum, people with disabilities are expected to exist in an ableist-, racist-, sexist-, heterosexist-driven world and accept constant evaluation of their abilities, gender, race, and sexual orientation in order to be seen as acceptable, powerful, valuable, or autonomous (Johannsdottir et al., 2021). Negative stereotypes associated with people in marginalized groups are heightened by microaggressions (David, 2014), intracorporeally (Massmann, 2022), nondisabled gaze (Loja et al., 2013), and sustained generationally by familial, cultural, and societal norms (David, 2014).

SOCIAL JUSTICE

The American Counseling Association (ACA) has led the way only recently in considering social justice to be a valid counseling specialization. Specifically, in its 2014 revised code of ethics, the ACA cites "when appropriate, counselors advocate at the individual, group, institutional, and societal levels to examine potential barriers and obstacles that inhibit access and/or growth and development of clients" (ACA, 2014, p. 5). The ACA has also approved the new Division for Counselors for Social Justice within the ACA. On its 2010 home page defining what social justice counseling entails, the Division for Counselors for Social Justice cites:

> Social justice counseling represents a multifaceted approach to counseling in which practitioners strive to simultaneously promote human development and the common good through addressing challenges related to both individual and distributive justice. Social justice counseling includes empowerment of the individual as well as active confrontation of injustice and inequality in society as they impact clientele as well as those in their systemic contexts. In doing so, social justice counselors' direct attention to the promotion of four critical

principles that guide their work: equity, access, participation, and harmony. This work is done with a focus on the cultural, contextual, and individual needs of those served. (Counselors for Social Justice, American Counseling Association, n.d., para. 5)

Greenleaf and Williams (2009) discuss the view that the counseling profession has been largely driven or entrenched by the medical model paradigm, one that focuses exclusively on the individual and treating his or her impairments. This represents a pathological orientation to diagnosis and treatment described earlier and is perhaps no better evident than our reliance on the *Diagnostic and Statistical Manual of Mental Disorders* (5th ed., *DSM-5,* American Psychiatric Association, 2013). However, to truly consider a holistic approach toward working with people with disabilities, we must consider the 81-year-old writings of Lewin (1936) concerning the person–environment interaction discussed in Chapter 5. Specifically, our behavior is a function of our individual traits and characteristics in response to our interactions with our environment ($B = f[P \times E]$). Numerous empirical studies have shown that regardless of how strong a character someone has, with a perceived discriminatory social environment, the individual's physical and mental health may be negatively affected (Dohrenwend, 2000; Gee, 2002; Li & Moore, 1998; Ramsey & Marini, 2016; Rumbaut, 1994; Williams & Williams-Morris, 2000).

The Social Justice Counselor

The paradigm shift in how we work with clients must extend beyond simply working with them and their families to ultimately exploring what, if any, societal and environmental barriers may likely block their goals (Neville & Mobley, 2001). It has been suggested that social advocacy is the "fifth force" within the counseling profession, essentially an extension of and complement to the multicultural movement (Ratts et al., 2004, p. 28). The ecological approach to counseling acknowledges the impact that an unfriendly environment can have on the well-being of clients (Wilson, 2003). Ivey and Ivey (1998) describe the developmental counseling and therapy model, noting how external stressors can impact intrapsychic changes in clients. The authors cite the progression and reciprocal effect of these interactions, including (a) environmental or biological insult, which may lead to (b) stress and physical/emotional pain, which may lead to (c) sadness/depression, which may lead to (d) defense against the pain and possibly mental disorders.

In providing a holistic approach to helping clients with disabilities, counselors must be willing to not only acknowledge that social injustice exists but also willing to go the extra mile to do something about it. As the Division for Counselors of Social Justice web page indicates, "Social justice counseling includes empowerment of the individual as well as active confrontation of injustice and inequality in society as they impact clientele as well as those in their systemic contexts." In defining exactly what "active confrontation of injustice and inequality in society" means, counselors must be aware of what their job's contractual limitations are, if any, regarding congressional letter writing, advocacy, peaceful protests, and other legal remedies to confront injustice and inequality. The ACA has been quite effective over the years in rallying its 43,000+ constituents by providing them with legislative alerts, synopses of relevant legislative bills being introduced for passage, who their congressional leaders are, and sample letters for counselors to use as a template. The ACA Advocacy Competencies (Lewis et al., 2003) concerning social justice advocacy in counseling recognize the ecological model; oppression and discrimination are socially constructed and have a damaging physical and mental health impact on individuals who are functioning within a toxic reciprocal person–environment atmosphere (Bronfenbrenner, 1977; Wilson, 2003).

Several recent school counselor education publications have addressed active steps in preparing counselors for social justice (Bemak & Chung, 2008; Steele, 2008). Bemak and Chung (2008), for example, describe ACA advocacy competencies in relation to promoting systems advocacy, student empowerment, identifying specific advocacy strategies to communicate to colleagues, and stressing the need to further disseminate information to other constituents. These competencies emphasize strength in numbers and group action in promoting equality in educational funding, adequate resources, and a safe learning environment. To passively sit back and counsel students in a dysfunctional or antiquated learning environment is inadequate. The authors cite potential counselor concerns as to why they may not want to become involved in remedying social injustice problems. Some obstacles include general apathy, being labeled a troublemaker, fear of retribution, a sense of powerlessness, and anxiety that can lead to guilt for not advocating. Bemak and Chung offer recommendations to assist counselors; for example, aligning social justice advocacy with organizational mission and goals, using data-driven strategies, having the courage to speak out, taking calculated risks, recruiting colleagues and others in the cause, developing political partners, becoming politically knowledgeable, and keeping faith (Bemak & Chung, 2008, pp. 379–380).

In considering social justice regarding persons with disabilities, counselors and case managers can influence a number of possible inequities in healthcare, education, housing, and employment. Persons with disabilities and especially those of minority status are statistically the most disenfranchised population in the United States (National Organization on Disability, 2004). Counselors have to acknowledge environmental inequities as well as the implications that oppression and discrimination can have on clients who can succumb to and give up trying (Dempsey, 1994; Dohrenwend, 2000; Gee, 2002). Thesen (2005) discusses how he and other physicians often knowingly or unknowingly treat patients in a dehumanizing and oppressive manner. He indicates that this type of behavior is counterproductive to patient health and can leave them feeling powerless and without any control. Thesen calls for medical professionals to instead empower their patients by including them in the decision-making process, educating them, and acknowledging their concerns. Bham and Forchuk (2008) illustrated empirically Thesen's (2005) premise in their interview of 336 current and former psychiatric and/or physically disabled clients. Specifically, the authors found that patients with comorbid conditions of a psychiatric and physical disability perceived themselves to be more discriminated against and oppressed by healthcare professionals. This, in turn, positively correlated with psychiatric problem severity, self-rated general health, and poorer life satisfaction and well-being. Counselors should be prepared to step in and advocate for clients when they witness the negative attitudes of healthcare professionals.

In other life domains concerning clients with disabilities, counselors and case managers should be prepared to tackle social injustice issues that impede client progress in the social and vocational realm. Despite the 20-year-old ADA, environmental barriers still exist that have been shown to result in some persons with disabilities feeling frustrated, angry, socially anxious, and depressed at times (Charmaz, 1995; Di Tomasso & Spinner, 1997; Graf et al., 2009; Hopps et al., 2001; Li & Moore, 1998; Marini et al., 2009). Counselors can assist clients in constructing letters to business owners demanding removal of access barriers, filing complaints with the Office of Civil Rights, referring clients to Client Assistance Programs (CAPs), and finding an ADA lawyer if necessary (Blackwell et al., 2001; Blankenship, 2005; Marini et al., 2009). There appears to be little doubt from numerous empirical studies showing negative or perceived hostile environmental conditions can, and do, have a negative impact on client well-being. For counselors to concern themselves just with assisting clients to deal with living in an able-bodied world, it is a job that is left unfinished or incomplete.

ADVOCACY

Social justice and advocacy are sometimes used interchangeably and are often considered synonymous concepts. The primary difference, however, is that social justice is a broader concept recognizing unequal power, unearned privilege, and oppression (Alston et al., 2006). Advocacy is more behavioral and action oriented and is an activity that often involves actions to correct some social injustice. As such, several authors discuss social justice advocacy in relation to some perceived social inequity. O'Day and Goldstein (2005) interviewed 16 disability advocacy and research leaders regarding the top contemporary advocacy issues concerning persons with disabilities. Disability advocacy organizations, such as the Consortium of Citizens with Disabilities (CCD), Not Dead Yet (NDY), Americans with Disabilities for Attendant Programs Today (ADAPT), American Association of People with Disabilities (AAPD), and others, are involved with grassroots advocacy, ongoing events, rallies, and information dissemination regarding important legislative issues toward enhancing full inclusion of persons with disabilities. O'Day and Goldstein found the top five contemporary issues were affordable and accessible healthcare, employment, access to assistive technology, long-term care, and civil rights enforcement concerning Titles II and III (public services and public accommodations) of the ADA. Similar concerns have been reported elsewhere (Graf et al., 2009; Marini et al., 2009).

Advocacy can take several forms in terms of action. The simplest form of advocacy involves letter writing to local and state constituents in attempts to bring attention to some social inequity, such as accessible housing. Arguably, more extreme forms can involve peaceful protests, such as occupying lawmakers' offices and sometimes subsequent citations for trespassing. The group ADAPT has been relentless and fairly successful over the past several decades in promoting disability rights, with its successful start in the early 1980s fighting for accessible public transportation in major cities, including city buses, subways, and Greyhound bus lines. The group would organize; primarily the wheelchair users would block buses, chain themselves, and otherwise occupy legislators' offices to be heard. In time, the majority of their efforts were successful in bringing major change across America, where persons with physical disabilities were unable to use public transportation. During the past decade or so, ADAPT has focused its fight on community-based care, whereby persons who require assistance with activities of daily living do not have to live in a nursing home. Their motto is "free our people," arguing that more than two-thirds of federal and state monies are successfully lobbied into nursing homes instead of the money following the person who chooses to live at home. For counselors and case managers who work for the state or federal government, the central question becomes whether this type of advocacy to support such causes has any job repercussions. If conducted on our own time, there generally is no adverse impact; however, counselors are encouraged to be familiar with their agency's workplace policies. Too often when we advocate, we do so for our own interests and to protect our jobs or territory and disguise it as client beneficence.

Ericksen (1997) indicates that advocacy is conceptually a cross between public policy, public relations, and conflict resolution. Lee (1998) defines advocacy as becoming the voice of the clients and taking action to make environmental changes that may impede barriers to a client's career, academic, personal, or social goals. Semivan and White (2006) noted that the skills needed for effective advocacy include passion, fact-finding, knowledge, data-based research, and goal-oriented concrete objectives. They must also know the limits of their professional roles and be able to separate highly charged emotions from their actions. Stewart et al. (2009) cited practical advocacy strategies to include (a) identifying the target population and the nature/facts of the injustice; (b) developing a rationale as to how advocacy will affect the advocate and target population chosen; (c) developing clearly and concisely how advocating will fit the therapist's role and fits within the scope of practice or ethics for the counselor; (d) conducting research on the background and nature of the social injustice thoroughly, including speaking to individuals who have been affected by it; (e) developing a list of references and resources for dissemination; (f) outlining the broader and then individual measurable goals of the advocacy project and reviewing them regularly for refining if necessary; and (g) after selecting goals, determining what the first steps are and whose responsibility it is to carry out each activity (Stewart et al., 2009).

So how can rehabilitation educators, researchers, and counselors either directly or indirectly become better advocates for persons with disabilities? For educators, teaching students about relevant advocacy community services, such as CAPs, legal aid, guardianship, and services provided by Centers for Independent Living (CILs), becomes important in knowing about nonmedical services that can help in social injustice situations (Blankenship, 2005; Marini et al., 2009). In addition, educators can teach students about legislation pertaining to persons with disabilities, provide legislative alerts, and show students how to write to legislators on behalf of persons with disabilities. Two organizations that are extremely effective in providing information and education on these topics are the National Rehabilitation Association and the ACA. Educators can also have letter-writing campaigns for important legislation as part of a class grade and/or attend or develop local information sessions about impending legislation. Overall, teaching students how to advocate effectively can then be passed on to teaching clients with disabilities once students graduate.

For rehabilitation education researchers, studying the impact of teaching and empowering persons with disabilities about how to advocate for themselves can minimize years of dependency on others who have traditionally made decisions for them (Brinckerhoff, 1994). Brinckerhoff noted how teaching adolescents affected by learning disability self-advocacy skills regarding effectively managing their college experience can be self-empowering and enhance self-esteem (Van Reusen & Bos, 1990). Research topics could include a control and experimental group design; provide the experimental group with tangible training skills to become more proficient at some self-advocacy task; and then measure the psychosocial impact of empowerment, locus of control, and self-efficacy. Anecdotally, it would seem self-evident that individuals who are taught skills to become more proficient in mastering or controlling parts of their environment would enhance client self-esteem and self-confidence.

Counselors working directly with persons with disabilities in a variety of settings and in a variety of ways can work with clients directly regarding advocacy and self-empowerment issues. Although many counselors have been empowering clients for years regarding job clubs, job search strategies, interview skills training, and so on, others may tend to "do for" rather than "do with" clients, which can be counterproductive. Brodwin et al. (2007), for example, discuss the importance of including clients in selecting assistive technology or adaptive equipment, because without client input, many clients will not use or will discard the device. As noted with educators, counselors can refer clients to appropriate advocacy agencies, assist in writing letters of complaint or letters to congressional leaders, and teach assertiveness and advocacy skills in presenting their case.

CONCLUSION

In many ways, rehabilitation and other counselors have become somewhat desensitized to the unchanging 70% plus unemployment and underemployment rate among persons with disabilities (Houtenville, 2000, National Organization on Disability [NOD], 2004), alarmingly high dropout rates for students (NOD, 2004), higher poverty rates (Hughes & Avoke, 2010; McNeil, 2001), poorer and inadequate healthcare (Berk et al., 1995), social oppression and discrimination (Ratts et al., 2004), and ongoing physical access barriers for persons with disabilities (Graf et al., 2009; Marini et al., 2009). The social justice counselor is a relatively new breed of counselor who actively advocates for change in the community and among policy makers when part of the client's issues has an environmental basis. Counselors in training should not only learn about how to assist clients with disabilities with coping skills to live in an able-bodied world but also empower and actively assist clients to combat social injustice and oppression in their lives.

CLASS ACTIVITIES

1. Have the class engage in a discussion to write out on the blackboard all the reasons they can think of as to why persons with disabilities who are/are not a minority may not fare well in American society.

2. Have students write down without a signature, so their responses are anonymous, whether they think a large part of individuals living in poverty is their fault or society's unjust discriminatory practices.

3. List on the blackboard all of the common myths and misconceptions about persons with disabilities and those of other minorities, including Native Americans, African Americans, Asian Americans, Middle Eastern Americans, and Mexican Americans.

KEY REFERENCES

Only key references appear in the print edition. The full references appear in the digital product on Springer Publishing Connect™: https://connect.springerpub.com/content/book/978-0-8261-5111-7/part/partV/chapter/ch25

Alston, R. J., Harley, D. A., & Middleton, R. (2006). The role of rehabilitation in achieving social justice for minorities with disabilities. *Journal of Vocational Rehabilitation, 24*, 129–136.

Annual Disability Statistics Compendium. (2014). *Poverty in the US.* https://disabilitycompendium.org/sites/default/files/user-uploads/Archives/PreviousDisabilityCompendiumReleases/2014%20Compendium%20Release.pdf

Bham, A., & Forchuk, C. (2008). Interlocking oppressions: The effect of a comorbid physical disability on perceived stigma and discrimination among mental health consumers in Canada. *Health & Social Care in the Community, 17*(1), 63–70.

Braddock, D., & Parish, S. (2001). An institutional history of disability. In G. Albrecht, K. Seelman, & M. Bury (Eds.), *Handbook of disability studies* (pp. 11–68). Sage.

Carew, M. T., Colbourn, T., Cole, E., Ngafuan, R., Groce, N., & Kett, M. (2019). Inter- and intra-household perceived relative inequality among disabled and non-disabled people in Liberia. *PLOS One, 14*(7). https://doi.org/10.1371/journal.pone.0217873

Cooper, E., Korman, H., O'Hara, A., & Zovistoski, A. (2009). *Priced out in 2008: The housing crisis for people with disabilities.* Technical Assistance Collaborative. http://www.tacinc.org

Counselors for Social Justice, & American Counseling Association. (n.d.). *What is social justice in counseling.* https://counseling-csj.org

David, E. J. R. (2014). *Internalized oppression: The psychology of marginalized groups.* Springer Publishing Company.

Fox, D. D., & Marini, I. (2012). History of treatment toward persons with disabilities in America. In I. Marini & M. Stebnicki (Eds.), *The psychological and social impact of illness and disability* (pp. 3–12). Springer Publishing Company.

Greenleaf, A. T., & Williams, J. M. (2009). Supporting social justice advocacy: A paradigm shift towards an ecological perspective. *Journal for Social Action in Counseling and Psychology, 2*(1), 1–12.

Greenwald, G. (2011). *With liberty and justice for some: How the law is used to destroy equality and protect the powerful.* Metropolitan Books.

Johannsdottir, A., Egilson, S., & Haradsdottir, F. (2021) Implications of internalized ableism for the health and well-being of disabled young people. *Sociology of Health and Illness, 44*, 360–376.

Li, L., & Moore, D. (1998). Acceptance of disability and its correlates. *Journal of Social Psychology, 138*(1), 13–25.

Liu, W. M. (2011). *Social class and classism in the helping professions: Research, theory, and practice.* Sage.

Naami, A., & Mikey-Iddrisu, A. (2013) Empowering persons with disabilities to reduce poverty: A case study of action on disability and development, Ghana. *Journal of General Practice 1*(2), 113–120. https://doi.org/10.4172/2329-9126.1000113

Ramsey, W., & Marini, I. (2016). Social justice and counseling the oppressed. In I. Marini & M. Stebnicki (Eds.), *The psychological and social impact of illness and disability* (pp. 585–591). Springer Publishing Company.

Stiglitz, J. E. (2013). *The price of any quality: How today's divided society endangers our future.* W. W. Norton.

Turner, R. J., & Avison, W. R. (2003). Status variations in stress exposure: Implications for the interpretation of research on race, socioeconomic status, and gender. *Journal of Health and Social Behavior, 44*(4), 488–505.

Williams, D. R., & Williams-Morris, R. (2000). Racism and mental health: The African American experience. *Ethnicity & Health, 5*(3–4), 243–268.

Williams, D. R., Yan Yu, Jackson, J. S., & Anderson, N. B. (1997). Racial differences in physical and mental health: Socio-economic status, stress and discrimination. *Journal of Health Psychology, 2*(3), 335–351.

CHAPTER 26

THE IMPACT OF SOCIAL MEDIA INFLUENCE ON MENTAL HEALTH

RIGEL MACARENA PIÑÓN AND KERRA LAJOY DANIEL

LEARNING OBJECTIVES

After reading this chapter you will be able to:

- Understand the important role social networking sites play in current society
- Identify different uses for different platforms and their effects on mental health
- Become familiar with maladaptive behaviors manifested in users and create awareness of detrimental effects
- Discuss and consult with both individuals and other professionals the different interventions that can be utilized with different age groups and other populations in efforts to promote moderation

PRE-READING QUESTIONS

1. Why might it be important for rehabilitation and other counseling professionals to understand social media, its benefits, and overall implications?
2. What might be some of the considerations for rehabilitation and other counseling professionals when working with digital natives, Generation Z, and Millennials?
3. How might counselors integrate moderating techniques for social medial use?
4. How might counselors tactfully help create self-awareness in the world of work and culturally concerning the impact social media may have on its users?
5. How can counselors understand the rising challenges that rehabilitation professionals will face as technologies continue to evolve and merge into our everyday life?

Social media has become a ubiquitous part of modern life with billions of people around the world using platforms like Facebook, Instagram, Twitter, and TikTok to connect with friends, family, and virtual communities. These digital spaces have become a normative part of current global culture, following the release of the smartphone, notably enabling a monumental increase in online participation before, during, and after the COVID-19 pandemic. Further, social media has become one of the most significant drivers of economic change, transforming the way people and businesses interact with each other. The rise of social media platforms has also created a new era of opportunities for entrepreneurs by transforming traditional industries, creating new careers and the affordability of remote work (Campbell, 2019). Another industry that has been transformed by social media is the media and entertainment industries, considering platforms make it easier for individuals and businesses to create and massively distribute content, including music, movies, and television shows. This new era has also provided new opportunities for content creators to disrupt traditional economic distribution models with the intent to maximize content profit. Further, as social media continues to evolve, it is likely that its impact on the economy will only become more pronounced. Nevertheless, as the digital world continues to expand to areas and countries that once did not have access to technology, there has been a rise in overall mental health concerns. Even though social platforms have had a positive significant impact on human relationships by changing the way people communicate and interact with one another, including the creation of virtual communities, it has also contributed to a decline in face-to-face communication, a decline in empathy and emotional intelligence, and a new "life on the screen" (Turkle, 2011). According to a recent digital data report, there are 7.96 billion people living on Earth, 5.03 billion are internet users and 4.70 billion use social media (Kemp, 2022). This means that now most of the world's population is virtually connected, with the latest global total being equivalent to 59% of the world's total population. To date, the average person spends a collective 2 hours and 55 minutes on social media platforms daily (Kemp, 2022). Further, as per the World Health Organization (WHO), the approximated average global time a person will dedicate to social media in their lifetime is the equivalent of 6 years and 8 months (WHO, 2019). For comparison, the Bureau of Labor Statistics (2021) reported people spend more time on social media than they do in everyday activities. According to the Bureau of Labor Statistics (2021), over the course of a person's lifetime (73.4 years), daily activities such as sleeping take up a total of 25 years and 5 months, followed by watching TV (8 years and 4 months), then is social media (6 years and 8 months), next is eating and drinking (3 years and 7 months), followed by shopping activities (2 years and 2 months), then socializing (1 year and 11 months) and finally housework (1 year and 8 months; U.S. Bureau of Labor Statistics, 2021). Consequently, the key question is no longer whether our audiences are using these technologies, but rather what they are using them for and with what purpose.

Social networking sites have metamorphosed into a key tool for amplification of marketing, organizing around social and political movements, and overall influencing the masses. Such advances in digital communications have revolutionized present economical climates and served as powerful tools for social activism for underrepresented groups, including disability advocacy, racial equality, reproductive rights, and humanitarian organizations, among other issues, through both formal and informal communication. Such efforts are intended to bring historically ignored narratives into public consciousness to shed a light on overlooked injustices (Sommerfeldt & Yang, 2017).

TIME SPENT ON SOCIAL MEDIA

As of 2022, in the United States, YouTube, Facebook, Instagram, and TikTok are the top most used social networking platforms, with each user averaging a total of 6 years and 8 months throughout a lifetime. In 2019, Facebook had a total of 3.48 billion individual users, with 53.6% of its users being between the ages of 18 and 34 (Auxier et al., 2019; Auxier & Anderson, 2021). The second most used social media network is YouTube, comprising 86% of total internet users who spend their days watching entertainment and information content through a variety of clips in the form of movies, news shows, and personal videos (Auxier, 2019). Instagram has over 1.47 billion monthly active users, with an average of 95 million photos and 400 million stories uploaded daily (Miles, 2013). Instagram is an online platform that allows an instantaneous way for people around the world to share life moments with friends through a digital lens. According to Miles (2013), this often includes a compilation of filter-manipulated pictures and videos organized with tags and location information. It is through browsing that users can access trending content and follow other users to add on their personal profile feed to keep people continuously interrelated. Lastly, TikTok, founded in 2016, has over 80 million users with 3.3 billion downloads and 62% of its users being between the ages of 10 and 29 (Auxier, 2019).

Mass social media usage and the amount of time people engage on social platforms demonstrated a steady growth in 2012, where people spent approximately 90 minutes per day on social networking sites (Auxier, 2019). In 2019, the number rose to 144 minutes per day and 2020 statistics showed an average of 153 minutes spent per day (Auxier, 2019). Consistent with previous research, a 2019 study conducted by the Pew Research Center composed of 2,002 U.S. adults found the social media landscape to be dominated primarily by Facebook, absorbing 58 minutes of a person's day, YouTube users averaging 53 minutes per day, Instagram consuming a median of 35 minutes, TikTok 32 minutes, Snapchat 26 minutes a day, and lastly Twitter with 15 minutes of engagement per day (Iqbal, 2020). To date, social media platforms are the most frequently used venues for augmenting online visibility despite geographic location, ultimately reducing the distance among people in creating a global community (Kietzmann et al., 2011).

SOCIAL CONSTRUCTS MEDIATED BY SOCIAL MEDIA

Facebook, Instagram, and TikTok are the fastest-growing social networking sites worldwide with 91% of updates primarily composed of photos (Wagner, 2015), making it the key platforms for online monetizing and social currencies. Social currency is a societal value placed in a virtual world based on reputation, taken in the form of likes and comments (Ging & Garvey, 2018). Because of its interactive features and worldwide acceptance, users can disseminate information, likability, and mass influence. Following 2020, approximately two-thirds of Americans using social media shed a light on the disproportionality of opportunities available to marginalized groups such as systemic oppression, thereby giving the opportunity for their voices to be heard (Coyne et al., 2020). However, the success of social media is contingent upon the capacity to connect while influencing a virtual community of like-minded people to act in solidarity. Presently, social media users have overtly exercised their collective influential power to create social constructs on a global scale. As discovered by Sundar and Limperos (2013), this has afforded the digital convenience to communicate and thus shape, customize, and redirect online virtual communities for better or worse.

Interestingly, numerous studies suggest an association between increased time spent on social media and an increase in mental health disorders, including anxiety and depression (Banjanin et al., 2015; Barry et al., 2017; Pantic et al., 2012; Woods & Scott, 2016), body image concerns, lower self-esteem (Koff et al., 2001), eating disorders (Holland & Tiggemann, 2017), substance abuse (Wilson, 2000), sexual dysfunction (Fredrickson & Roberts, 1997), and suicidal ideation (Brown, et al., 2020). In addition, other newly recognized disorders currently known as *internet communication disorder* (Wegmann et al., 2017) and *social networking site addiction* (Choi et al., 2015) are now recognized by researchers exploring this phenomenon. Further, the association between time spent on social networking sites and mental health has also been biasedly promulgated by high-profile news articles with headlines such as "Have Smartphones Destroyed a Generation?" as well as "Social Media Linked to Rise in Mental Health Disorders" (Charles, 2019; Twenge, 2017; Twenge et al., 2018). However, other studies challenge any connection between social media use and associations with mental health concerns. For instance, recent meta-analysis findings suggest that the relationship between social media and mental health is mixed and debatable (Best et al., 2014; Huang, 2017). Recently, Charles

(2019) suggests that the effect of screen time (social networking sites) on mental health was as large in effect size as the impact that eating potatoes has on mental health.

Taken together, the relationship between social media use and mental health is complex, as studies tend to find a mixed pattern of relationships (Coyne et al., 2020). One explanation can be that social media use does not impact self-esteem for the majority of the (digital) population considering specific within-person effects. Contrastingly, Orben and Przybylski (2019) state that quantifiable minorities do experience some form of positive and negative effect, suggesting a true relationship between social media use and mental health disorders (i.e., lower self-esteem, body image concerns, depression, anxiety), which can be explained by person-specific individual susceptibilities.

THEORETICAL FRAMEWORKS

Another potential explanation for our innate need to engage in these maladaptive behaviors is elucidated by the theoretical framework of intrasexual competition, a phenomenon model derived from Darwin's theory that suggests sexual selection is grounded in an evolutionary context, providing a better understanding as to why people participate in social comparisons through social networking sites (Darwin, 1888). The theory hypothesizes that women, more so than men, participate in appearance-related comparisons as a baseline to assess their own attractiveness in contrast to their gender counterparts in efforts to entice and keep partners with superior physical attributes (Suls & Wheeler, 2013). Notably, this impulsivity to engage in social comparison is mediated through social networking sites, as it is deeply rooted in our evolutionary history as a powerful biological mechanism that implies human beings possess an innate tendency to compare their own aptitudes and abilities with the attributes of others (Festinger, 1954; Garcia et al., 2013; Tiggemann & Slater, 2004).

Taken into context, social comparison theory (Festinger, 1954) argues that women evaluate their own appearance by comparing themselves with the sociocultural thin ideals of beauty presented in the media. Strahan et al., (2006) and Want (2009) posit the problem lies in the upward social comparison specifically made when women compare their physical features with another female who is perceived to have higher-quality attributes than their own. Such comparisons occur in a manner such that women purposely contrast their bodies with a slimmer ideal, creating a discrepancy between their own self-image (Bessenoff, 2006) and leading to negative assessments of their own appearance (Hendrickse et al., 2017). Moreover, other motivators for upward social comparisons include gaining accurate self-perception (Kruglanski & Mayseless, 1990), self-enhancement (Wood, 1989), and self-improvement (Wood, 1989) as a form of coping mechanism for mood regulation (Wood et al., 1985). The growing problem for most female users engaging in upward social comparison is that they internalize images that are often photoshopped and distorted from a realistic body ideal.

Contrastingly, other studies suggest downward social comparison motivators are contingent upon a variety of variables that encompass specific personality traits as well as circumstantial components (Wheeler, 1966; Wills, 1981). As a result, researchers posit that subsequent emotions experienced after engaging in social comparisons are associated with pity, fear, worry, sympathy, or contempt (assimilative emotions); *schadenfreude* (pleasure derived by someone from another person's misfortune; Smith, 2000); or pride (contrastive emotions; Tesser, 1991). However, there is also an upside for some users engaging in viewing upward social comparisons, which includes feeling inspired (Brickman & Bulman, 1977) and optimism or a sense of admiration (Lockwood & Kunda, 1997). Yet this can also lead to assimilative emotions such as depression, shame, envy, and resentment (Crosby, 1976). This social comparison culture paradox is best termed in Brown's (2021) latest book, *Atlas of the Heart: Mapping Meaningful Connection and the Language of Human Experience* as "trying to simultaneously fit in and stand out" to "be like everyone else, but better." This often creates internal conflict with oneself in many dimensions and a lack of clarity in terms of self-awareness (p. 20).

EFFECTS OF SOCIAL MEDIA ON MENTAL HEALTH

Time spent on platforms has been shown to have parallel negative psychological reactions that have generated emerging new terminology, including iDisorders (Rosen et al., 2012), fear of missing out (FOMO; Przybylski et al., 2013), Metaverse (Mystakidis, 2022), social currency (Ging & Garvey, 2018), Facebook depression (Kross et al., 2013; Selfhout et al., 2009), Facebook fatigue (Rainie et al., 2013), and Vaguebooking (Child & Starcher, 2016), to name a few. With the emergence of the smartphone and the internet, a recent study postulates that the need to overengage is attributed to new social constructs known as the highlight reel, social currency, and FOMO, which serve as mediators between psychopathological symptoms and negative consequences of social networking sites (Oberst et al., 2017). This new influential term widely known as people sharing their best moments in life is often ascribed as the highlight reel—individuals want their followers to believe that they are living this amazing life and that their life is perfect (Hannah et al., 2017). Another phenomenon is the desire to obtain *social currency* such as social media likes, comments, shares, and so on, frequently used as a form of currency to determine self-value both in real life and on social networking sites. Another contributing factor accentuating overengagement is recognized as FOMOO, generally referred to as the pervasive apprehension that friends are doing fun activities without you (Przybylski et al., 2013).

New and Old Terminology

iDisorders: The negative relationship between technology usage and mental health (Rosen et al., 2012).

Fear of missing out (FOMO): The pervasive apprehension that friends are doing fun activities without you (Przybylski et al., 2013).

Highlight reel: When people share their best moments in life, imposing the fake ideal that life is perfect (Hannah et al., 2019).

Body dissatisfaction: The negative subjective evaluation of the weight and shape of one's own body (Hendrickse et al., 2017).

Body surveillance: The habitual monitoring of the one's body's appearance (Frederickson & Roberts, 1997).

Social currency: Value placed in the virtual world based on reputation, taken as a unit of trade in the commercial blog industry, contingent on the number of "likes," "follows," "retweets," "favorites," "friends," and comments (Ging & Garvey, 2018).

Social comparison theory: The idea that individuals determine their own social and personal worth based on how they stack up against others (Festinger, 1954).

Facebook depression: The affective result of spending too much time on social platforms that results in the subsequent decline of overall subjective well-being (Kross et al., 2013; Selfhout et al., 2009).

Facebook fatigue: Voluntarily taking a break from the social networking site due to excessive gossip, negativity, conflict, and drama (Rainie et al., 2013).

Metaverse: Presently known as the convergence of technologies that enable multisensory interactions with virtual environments, digital objects, and people such as virtual reality (VR) and augmented reality (AR). It is an interconnected web of social and networked immersive environments in persistent multiuser platforms (Mystakidis, 2022).

Vaguebooking: A unique form of strategic posting that creates ambiguity on Facebook (Child & Starcher, 2016).

This recurring attraction to appearance-focused content is pursed with the intent to receive social currency, a new form of external validation described earlier. For example, users may unconsciously satisfy reassurance and self-worth needs through compulsive mindless scrolling and/or incessant notification checking for social currency. This enhances time spent on social platforms, increasing their chances of being cyberbullied or developing detrimental mental health disorders.

Interestingly, researchers in this area have also found parallel behaviors between substance use disorders and behavioral addictions, as well as substance use disorder (SUD) and other emerging diagnoses, including social networking site addiction (Choi et al., 2015) and internet communication disorder (ICD; Brand et al., 2014; Brand et al., 2016; Kuss & Griffiths, 2011; Wegmann et al., 2017). Social networking site addiction has become an increasing concern due to smartphone technological advances that facilitate compulsive checking behaviors and excessive engagement without any form of moderation, enabling a user to remain online for hours at a time (Choi et al., 2015; Montag et al., 2015). Separately, ICD is referred to as the utilization of social networking sites as a coping mechanism to deter loneliness and social anxiety by satisfying primal physiological needs such as social support and sense of belonging (Rademacher et al., 2014). More importantly, Griffiths (2005) and Spada (2014) suggest that users with behavioral addictions are at higher risk of developing ICD, considering both disorders' criteria overlap in symptomology in terms of loss of control, relapse, withdrawal, tolerance, preoccupation, and neglect of interests in addition to decline in daily functioning. According to the Substance Abuse and Mental Health Services Administration (SAMHAS, 2020), following 2020, more than 40 million Americans are currently living with a substance use disorder, a figure that doubled from 2019, with an estimate of 20 million people (SAMHSA, 2020). The same study also found that about half of adults ages 18 and older in 2020 with a co-occurring SUD and any mental illness (AMI) in the past year received either substance use treatment at a specialized facility or some form of mental health service (50.5%), with only 5.7% receiving both (SAMHSA, 2020).

Mental health has increasingly become needed following the COVID-19 pandemic; however, not enough services or attention is being directed toward these rising co-occurring concerns, including social media. Moreover, several study findings suggest a variety of motivators and expectations were being met through social networking sites interactivity, such as fulfilling social needs, regulation of negative emotions, and receiving external validation from peers. This is due to neurotransmitter activation in the brain that occurs when we are supported and rewarded. An example would be when seeing someone smile (Rademacher et al., 2014), confiding in a friend (Fareri et al., 2012), feeling socially accepted (Izuma et al., 2008), or self-disclosing something meaningful (Tamir et al., 2015).

Psychological appearance–gratifying needs compel spending more time on platforms to escape personal problems and congeal with social norms. Research indicates that given the cumbersome virtual presence and reliance of young adults, specifically young women, it is imperative that attention be placed on the adverse ways that social media influences perceptions of body image and impacts mental health. Ging and Garvey (2018) found that when social currency is not obtained through likes, shares, and comments, further body surveillance takes place in the form of body dissatisfaction and body shaming, resulting in potential eating disorders and other mental health concerns that are often more prevalent in females. Moreover, the negative effects of media exposure have generally been attributed to the process of social comparison (Levine & Murnen, 2009; Want, 2009). Social comparison theory (Festinger, 1954) argues that women evaluate their own appearance by comparing themselves with the sociocultural thin ideals of beauty presented in the media. Prior to the internet, individuals used to only be able to compare themselves with others in their local community, schools, and at work, but now we can compare ourselves with others across the globe. This potentially increases the amount of body image and appearance concerns.

Social media use also varies in relation to demographics such as race, age, gender, marital status, and level of education. While 78% of all women in the United States use social networking sites, men fall short, with only 65% of social networking site engagement, considering preceding studies found women allocate aggregated time to administering social media accounts in the form of updates, manipulation of photos, and editing of video filters in contrast to their male counterparts (Stefanone et al., 2011). This emergence of these psychological disorders is now referred by researchers as "iDisorders," defined as negative relationships between technology usage and psychological health (Rosen et al., 2012). Notably, due to the immediate accessibility, millions of users around the world interact daily on social networks for a variety of reasons. Several study researchers have found that the overexploitation of platforms has been shown to detrimentally affect subjective well-being and perceived life satisfaction (Kross et al., 2013; Verduyn et al., 2015) as a result of the vast opportunities it provides for unflattering social comparisons. In addition, another consequence of overengagement is experiencing Facebook fatigue, which is taking a voluntary break from the social networking sites due to excessive gossip, negativity, conflict, and drama (Rainie et al., 2013).

WOMEN AND BODY IMAGE

Researchers of social networking sites are finding that some women, particularly adolescent girls, can be very susceptible to body image issues that can negatively influence their mental health cognitions, behaviors, and emotions (Koff et al., 2001). As a result, women of all ages and particularly those under 25 may be at higher risk of developing depression, anxiety, substance abuse problems, eating disorders, suicidal ideation, sexual dysfunction, and internet addiction (Choi et al., 2015; De Wit et al., 2011; Fredrickson & Roberts, 1997; Holland & Tiggemann, 2017; Roy et al., 2020; Wegmann et al., 2017; Wilson, 2000). Cross-sectional (Botta, 1999) and longitudinal studies (Harrison & Hefner 2006; Kross et al., 2013; Levine & Harrison, 2009) continue to find that media exposure increases body dissatisfaction, thin body ideals, body objectification, and overall decline in subjective well-being (Kross et al., 2013) among preadolescent girls and young women (Stice et al., 1994). According to researchers, this is partially attributed to the dominant westernized ideal feminine body image constructed for the purpose of objectifying women from a viewer's perspective (Fredrickson & Roberts, 1997) and to be sexually gazed upon (Spitzack, 1990). Taken together, this sociocultural context teaches women about self-objectification (Fredrickson & Roberts, 1997; McKinley & Hyde, 1996), an internalized view of their own body manifested in habitual monitoring of one's appearance known as *body surveillance* (Moradi & Huang, 2008). Existing research supports that body surveillance leads to body shaming when cultural body ideals are not met (Tiggemann & Slater, 2001), increasing the risk of generating body image issues among women. The gender difference is more pronounced among women (36%) than men (24%), where platforms such as Instagram provide an opportunity for users to touch up and manipulate their best self-presentation online with the hopes of gaining praise/social currency as a form of gratification (Rainie et al., 2012). Therefore, promoting emphasis on the present perspective can heighten understanding of how distorted body image ideals enhance social comparisons and internalization of the idealized thin female, resulting in body dissatisfaction (Cash, 2011; Thompson et al., 1999; Tylka & Calogero, 2011).

Eating Disorders

Fitzsimmons-Craft and Bardone-Cone (2012) posit that when social currency is not obtained, further body surveillance leads to body objectification and body dissatisfaction, thereby increasing the possibility of potential eating disorders and other mental health concerns often more prevalent in females. Williamson et al. (1995) suggest that in order to reduce one's perceived body dissatisfaction and associated negative self-assessments, young women tend to engage in risky health behaviors (anorexia and bulimia) to fit the perfect thin body ideal by purging or restricting their food intake. Additionally, diverse evolutionary researchers surmise that going through cosmetic surgery (Arnocky & Piché, 2014) and restricting food consumption are considered appearance-enhancing strategies for maladaptive behaviors being adopted by many women currently in our society and abroad (Abed, 1998). In this regard, expectations vary in relation to users' age, gender, and level of interactivity on social networking sites, taking into consideration that receiving feedback congruent to participants' expectations is significantly associated with increased emotions of euphoria and connectedness (Grinberg et al., 2017). This sense of connectivity in the form of "likes" leads many users perceive it as positive societal support, which contributes to self-perceived satisfaction (Wohn et al., 2016). Moreover, the negative effects of media exposure have generally been attributed to the process of social comparison in reference to how users experience positive or negative affect as a result of the social comparison outcomes (Levine & Murnen, 2009; Want, 2009).

Collectively, the interactive features of social media platforms, such as the strong peer presence and myriad number of content exchanges in the forms of visual images, raise concerns of social comparisons and regulated psychological processes. Moreover, the predisposing individual vulnerability characteristics can enhance overengagement and negatively impact mental health, self-esteem, and overall quality of life.

TREATMENT APPROACHES

Literature exploring social media and mental health disorders or addiction is scarce, therefore limiting the availability of interventions and techniques for behavioral addiction for professionals such as counselors, psychologists, psychiatrists, other clinicians, and researchers (Andreassen, 2015). However, this section offers already known traditional approaches to treat overlapping prior approaches to depression, eating disorders, and substance addictions in the interim (Andreassen et al., 2013).

Intervention for Behavioral Change

Motivational interviewing (MI) has traditionally been used as a method to assist people with addiction disorders in changing their behavior (Lundhal et al., 2010). MI is a human-centered method that relies on strategies curated and guided by the counselor to encourage inherent changes in behavior. However, the relationship between counselor and client is collaborative in nature and requires each party to take an active role in the sessions and can be applied to varying populations, regardless of age, gender, disability, stage of addiction, and addiction type (Miller, 2010). The idea or overall goal of MI is to move a person from the precontemplation stage of change to the action stage (Miller, 2010).

A literature review conducted by Weiss et al. (2013) examined 119 studies focused on MI as an intervention tool over the course of 25 years. The results indicated MI as a worthwhile treatment over a comprehensive range of abusive tendencies such as substance abuse, eating disorders, and addictive behaviors. Of the 119 studies reviewed, 75% reported some improvement on different levels. Of that 75%, some participants experienced moderate or more noticeable change (25%) and others revealed a small or more subtle change in behavior (50%).

People with eating disorders are noted for being indecisive toward treatment with little to no intrinsic motivation to change. In essence, it is highly valued and suggested to highlight the advantages of MI in this population (Cassin et al., 2008). These researchers studied 242 women with binge eating disorder (BED) and two methods of intervention. The researchers compared women with BED who received a self-help book and one adapted motivational interviewing (AMI) session to women with BED who only received the self-help book as treatment. Follow-up phone interviews were conducted every 4 weeks over the course of 4 months post-intervention. AMI was found to be effectual for this population whereby individuals in the AMI group illustrated higher levels of self-efficacy in relation to change more so than in the group who only received the self-help book. Cassin et al. (2008) found additional effects of AMI included notable positive changes in self- esteem and decreased depressive episodes among women in this group.

Cognitive Reframing Interventions

CBT is the reframing of abnormal or dysfunctional thinking (Beck, 1979; Hofmann et al., 2012). CBT is versatile in that it is used for a broad scope of mental health disorders. It is one of the more scrutinized methods of psychotherapy and called upon by researchers, practitioners, and students to assist or understand people suffering from disorders affecting eating, emotions, mood, and body image. Due to CBT's adaptability, there is a plethora of evidence-based studies solidifying the validity of the method of psychotherapy with varying clients, with more favorable mental health results compared to other therapies (Farrell et al., 2006).

Researchers have found that eating disorders such as bulimia or anorexia nervosa are generally preceded by body image disturbance and/or body dissatisfaction (American Psychological Association, 2013; Butters & Cash, 1987; Nye & Cash, 2006). Although there are definitive methods outlined to treat body image dissatisfaction or disturbance, some researchers advocate for CBT as an effective method of treatment that decreases undesirable thoughts or affect relating to body image, reduces nonadaptive perspectives in terms of body image, and promotes self-esteem (McLean et al., 2011; Perpiñá et al., 1999).

If practitioners are attempting to sequester body image disturbance or dissatisfaction as a predominant condition or precursor to eating disorders, they should consider the modified CBT model. The modified CBT model includes a VR component which provides the opportunity for participants to modify or adjust the dimensions and proportions of various body parts (i.e., buttocks, arms, thighs, stomachs) of 3D computer-animated humans (Perpiñá et al., 2003). Participants are allowed to manipulate the 3D figures into idealized body types. Multiple studies support the efficacy of modified CBT with VR in several populations of women. The results suggest that attitudes relating to body image improved when confronted with reality-based scenarios in the VR world. Furthermore, researchers found notable differences in eating habits posttreatment, improved interest in treatment, and increased CBT change processes (Clus et al., 2018; Ferrer-Garcia & Gutierrez-Maldonado, 2012; Marco et al., 2013).

Interventions for Improving Overall Well-Being

Self-compassion intervention (SCI) is an empirically sound intervention tasked with creating a positive effect on resilience and well-being for people with mental health disorders such as stress, anxiety, and depression (MacBeth & Gumley, 2012). SCI challenges an individual to practice handling oneself with care, concern, and compassion amid personal failure, deficits, or stressful life situations. SCI is based on three elements: self-kindness as compared with self judgement, humanity as compared with isolation, and mindfulness as compared to overidentification (Moffit et al, 2013; Neff, 2003). Similarly, Albertson et al. (2015) examined 263 women with body image disturbance or dissatisfaction and found that increased self-compassion mediates the influence of body image–related discrepancies (i.e., body mass index, society beauty standards, and self-imposed shame). They also found that participants who scored higher in self-comparison and lower in self-worth ranked lower in self-compassion (Albertson et al., 2014). Accordingly, implementing SCI with young women and girls experiencing body image disturbance or dissatisfaction may prove helpful in sustaining body-positive perceptions during the previously mentioned discrepancies facilitated through the limitless lens of social media site access (Homan & Tylka, 2015).

In a similar vein, researchers in one study examining the use of self-compassion intervention in a randomized group of women found that those who received SCI showed a 43% increase in self-compassion while concurrently reducing stress, emotional avoidance, and depressive symptoms. Additionally, results were proven to be sustainable with postintervention follow-up calls at 6 months and 1 year that suggest results were long-lasting (Neff & Germer, 2013). Several additional studies support SCI as a proven method for treating eating disorders and reducing symptoms such as internal shame, binging, and inhibitory eating practices (Ferrerira et al., 2013; Webb & Forman, 2013).

Since the invention of the internet, social networking sites and cellular phones, billions of individuals globally have become daily users in an era of 24/7 access to limitless and instantaneous information. The advancement of technology and the ability to connect online has accelerated our understanding of ideals and concepts that were once only available through libraries or printed literature as well as our experiences in our community. On the other hand, this technological treasure trove does not always positively influence those who use its amenities such as social media sites. In particular, women are more vulnerable to the negative impact on mental health from social media due to their usage, which is greater in comparison to men (Asano, 2017). As researchers continue to decipher the origins of mental health issues and social media usage, practitioners and clinicians will be better positioned to assist individuals presenting with similar symptoms.

CONCLUSION

Social media has become an integral part of modern life, with billions of people around the world using platforms like Facebook, Instagram, Twitter, and TikTok to connect with friends, family, and communities. While these platforms have brought numerous benefits, including increased connectivity and access to information, they have also had a profound impact on the current culture, the economy, and overall mental health. Numerous studies have shown that excessive use of social media can lead to anxiety, depression, screen addiction, sleep disturbances, cyberbullying, eating disorders, and lower self-esteem, which are often more pronounced among digital natives and younger audiences. Therefore, it is important for individuals and society to critically assess the impact that social media and technology are having on our lives and culture and to make informed decisions regarding age-appropriate parameters, content consumption, and overall usage. It is important to understand that social media is a powerful tool and that setting healthy boundaries and parameters (age limits) and creating a no-tolerance policy is critical for the enhancement of this growing digital culture for younger individuals and adolescent girls. The conversation starts at home and with each other regarding the uses as well as consequences of not knowing how to use these platforms and technologies. As rehabilitation professionals, the best we can do is create awareness and apply techniques for moderation across all forms of technologies to ensure the emotional and overall psychological well-being of our clients with and without disabilities.

CLASS ACTIVITIES

1. Choose a social media platform and write a two- to three-page reflection on your reason for using it. Observe your algorithm and discern the content on your page and the people/accounts you follow and evaluate if there are any triggers. Write about the

kind of content you follow, how it makes you feel, whether it is good or bad, and why you are drawn to that platform.

2. Interview two different parents, one who regulates screen time and another whp does not, then write about how they handle parameters around screen time and why. What insight did you gain from this exercise?

3. Do some research on the top five most used social media platforms, what they are used for, what age group uses them most, and the current digital population of each platform.

4. Write a two- to three-page paper on how social media has impacted your life.

5. Interview an older individual in your life who doesn't use social media regularly and find out their experience with social media platforms. What is their insight? Does that limit or help their life in any way?

6. What are some parameters or guidelines you believe social media must implement? Is it for everyone? Should there be an age limit? If so, what age is appropriate? Do you believe a specific platform should or should not exist? What have you learned from using your own platforms?

KEY REFERENCES

Only key references appear in the print edition. The full references appear in the digital product on Springer Publishing Connect™: https://connect.springerpub.com/content/book/978-0-8261-5111-7/part/partV/chapter/ch26

Auxier, B., & Anderson, M. (2021). Social media use in 2021. *Pew Research Center, 1*, 1–4.

Auxier, B., Rainie, L., Anderson, M., Perrin, A., Kumar, M., & Turner, E. (2019, November 15). *Americans and privacy: Concerned, confused, and feeling lack of control over their personal information.* Pew Research Center: Internet, Science & Tech (blog). November 15, 2019. https://policycommons.net/artifacts/616499/americans-and-privacy/1597151/

Brown, Z., & Tiggemann, M. (2016). Attractive celebrity and peer images on Instagram: Effect on women's mood and body image. *Body Image, 19*, 37–43. https://doi.org/10.1016/j.bodyim.2016.08.007

Darwin, C. (1888). *The descent of man, and selection in relation to sex* (Vol. 1). Murray. https://doi.org/10.5962/bhl.title.110063

Festinger, L. (1954). A theory of social comparison processes. *Human Relations, 7*(2), 117–140. https://doi.org/10.1177/001872675400700202

Fredrickson, B. L., Roberts, T. A., Noll, S. M., Quinn, D. M., & Twenge, J. M. (1998). That swimsuit becomes you: Sex differences in self-objectification, restrained eating, and math performance. *Journal of Personality and Social Psychology, 75*(1), 269–284. https://psycnet.apa.org/doi/10.1037/0022-3514.75.1.269

Tiggemann, M., & Slater, A. (2004). Thin ideals in music television: A source of social comparison and body dissatisfaction. *International Journal of Eating Disorders, 35*(1), 48–58. https://doi.org/10.1002/eat.10214

Twenge, J. M., Joiner, T. E., Rogers, M. L., & Martin, G. N. (2018). Increases in depressive symptoms, suicide-related outcomes, and suicide rates among US adolescents after 2010 and links to increased new media screen time. *Clinical Psychological Science, 6*(1), 3–17. https://doi.org/10.1177/2167702617723376

CHAPTER 27

REFLECTIONS AND CONSIDERATIONS

IRMO MARINI, ALLISON FLEMING, AND MALACHY BISHOP

PART A: IRMO MARINI

In some ways, not much has changed specifically concerning people with disabilities since our 2018 seventh edition, but overall, for everyone, the world has changed in many ways that directly and indirectly influence those of us with disabilities. From my perspective anyway, since Drs. Fleming and Bishop have their own opinions to follow, I try to view the world looking at it from the space station, then bring it back to a more United States local level. It is difficult to look at us (the United States) in isolation without considering the continued interconnectivity of all of us globally and how the world is changing. Having reread my 2018 reflections piece, none of those issues have changed for the better in a noticeable way, but have perhaps amplified for the worse.

Some of the major events since 2018 with the COVID-19 pandemic affecting the global economy and millions of lives lost from it, the impact continues its death toll, and the economy moves closer to a global recession. The death of George Floyd in May 2020 also ignited worldwide marches in protest of police brutality and demonstrating the power of mobilizing millions with social media. We also were witnesses to the defiance of a peaceful transfer of power and the resulting exacerbation of a fractured American societal divide over race/ethnicity and increasing partisan toxicity. The war in Ukraine and threats of nuclear war from Russia have also captured global attention. Finally, the alarming increase of climate change refugees migrating to safer countries with more resources is another threat. Although most of these world events do not directly impact persons with disabilities, a couple of them will in the not-so-distant future.

Of specific interest is the rapidly increasing number of climate change refugees across the globe from the natural disasters, massive drought, and drying up of lakes and rivers that will never be fruitful again. Ida (2021) reports that there are currently more than 21.5 million climate refugees, expected to rise to over 1.2 billion people by 2050. Here in the United States, several million Guatemalans, Hondurans, and Salvadorans make the journey into the country annually, some to escape gangs and violence, many others from hurricanes and drought that have ravaged their landscape to where nothing grows for the poor rural people who live off the land. Sea-level rise due to melting ice caps is also expected to get worse by 2050 for poor developing countries living on islands as well as coastal residents of various continents who either live off the fishing industry for survival or choose to live on the ocean.

The Ecosystem Threat Register released a report in 2018 (cited in Ida, 2021) stating that in 2019, the top five countries that experienced displacements from natural disasters included India, with over 5 million displaced; the Philippines, China, and Bangladesh, each with over 4 million displaced; and the United States, with 916,000 displaced citizens (not including immigrants). Kehinde (2021) reports that desertification in African countries like Nigeria and Ethiopia has led to increasing numbers of climate refugees due to the lack of water and food from at least 3 years of drought. In 2010, it was estimated that approximately 10% of global migrants hailed from Africa. Millions of other displaced Africans are unable to leave the country, particularly for the aged, the disabled, and the poor. Tens of thousands of children have died from malnutrition, with professionals and charities coming in to help but still extremely lacking in personnel and medical aid in assisting the growing masses coming to tent camps.

There are currently over 7.9 billion people across the planet and an expected growth of over 9 billion by the year 2050 (Roser et al., 2019). The highest rate of growth reached 2.2% in 1963, and the growth rate has been dropping ever since, but we continue to have children. Without global scientists trying to solve the growing world food and water shortages due to unsustainable growth in numbers vying for the remaining resources across the globe, this slow-moving crisis will eventually affect everyone, not just developing countries. This brings us back to some of my same concerns in this section with our 2018 edition.

Specifically, millions of Americans with disabilities who are unable to work and live off of Social Security benefits continue to live under the poverty line. Although America is fortunate to be one of the wealthiest countries and as such has excellent purchasing power, as demonstrated in first purchasing millions of COVID vaccines for the United States, many of the developing countries were, and continue to be, less fortunate with large swaths of populations still without any vaccine access. With that said, however, ongoing lack of resources will eventually arrive at our door. When that happens years or decades from now, the poor, as has repeatedly historically shown, will be the first to experience the ramifications. Social inequities continue to impact the poor in every country, particularly minorities with a disability. I have coined this as "survival of the financially fittest" in past editions based on Darwin's theory and espoused by eugenics proponents.

Millions of disenfranchised poor and minority Americans with and without a disability have experienced social inequities for hundreds of years. In HBO's four-part documentary series *The Weight of the Nation* (Hoffman et al., 2012), Centers for Disease Control and Prevention physicians and related obesity and city planning scientists cite specific causes of social inequity based on ZIP Codes and higher mortality rates. The poor and disabled in some areas living within 10 miles of those living in a wealthier ZIP Code have a much higher mortality rate—up to 25-year differences. This is attributed to ill-conceived community planning, grocery store deserts, fast food restaurants flooding poorer communities, fewer hospitals, and fewer playgrounds and parks for exercise, among other things. These ongoing social inequities continue to negatively impact the mental and physical health of low-income Americans largely composed of those with disabilities and/or of minority status.

Kamdar et al. (2021) accessed the National Health and Nutrition Examination Survey database from 2007 to 2016 of 2,630 U.S. veterans regarding their health and living status. They found veteran suicides were proportionally almost double that of the general population, attributed to mental illness, homelessness, food insecurity, depression, and chronic pain. Stramondo (2021) similarly argues that when a society restricts the rights and privileges of people with disabilities leaving them with few options for living a satisfying life and negatively affecting their quality of life, some individuals will contemplate suicide. Kellett et al. (2021) found that when surveying 1,566 individuals with physical, cognitive, and emotional disabilities who were moved from an institutional setting to community-based living and then surveying them at 6, 12, and 24months post placement showed that the vast majority of participants echoed a much-improved quality of life and life satisfaction. For those persons with disabilities who did not report improved life satisfaction, they related it was due to no improvement in health coverage, low income, no accessible transportation, and poor access to assistive technology.

Case and Deaton (2020) as well as Tilstra et al. (2021) show that those who live under oppressed and poor living conditions have a higher likelihood of dying from substance and drug abuse overdose as well as suicide as a result of low-income resulting in poor quality of life and life satisfaction. The authors coin this national epidemic of opioid overdoses and alcohol-related liver disease as individuals living "lives of despair" that lead to "deaths of despair." Despite such dismal statistics, Stramondo (2021) and similar researchers (Terlazzo, 2016; Tsai et al, (2021) indicate that many persons with disabilities living under dismal living conditions still tend to adapt to their surroundings as best they can, a concept known as *adaptive preferences* regarding quality of life.

Finally, in relation to the COVID-19 pandemic is the approach and hospital policies followed by emergency room (ER) physicians and related first responders in terms of triage at thousands of emergency rooms in the United States inundated with patients in the ER. Physicians needed to make quick life-and-death decisions as to who would, and would not, most benefit from lifesaving medical care during the pandemic. Prior to the pandemic, however, was the 2005 Office of the Surgeon General report encouraging physicians to acquire additional competencies to better treat persons with chronic disabling conditions. Past and present research findings surveying physicians have consistently found preconceived bias that many physicians have regarding the perceived quality of life of persons with severe disabilities. Gerhart et al. (1994), for example, surveyed 153 ER physicians, nurses, and residents regarding the level of care they would provide to individuals with high-level spinal cord injuries (SCIs). The authors reported that 41% of the first responders believed resuscitating individuals with SCI was too aggressive, 28% opined the individual's quality of life should be considered first, 22% indicated they would not want to use resuscitative measures, and 23% indicated such patients should only receive pain relief and no lifesaving measures. More recently, Iezzoni et al. (2021) found that 82% of practicing U.S. physicians perceived people with severe disabilities have a poor quality of life, but 40% of them felt that they could still provide quality medical care to such patients. Although there will never be a factual accounting of how many individuals with chronic disabilities may have been denied ventilators during the pandemic, wartime triage has generally been left up to ER physicians to determine who does, and does not, receive lifesaving measures.

Overall, people with disabilities have generally been perceived and resulting often treated like second-class citizens in the United States and elsewhere. They have also been perceived as helpless, incapable, and noncontributing members of society. As resources continue to diminish worldwide that will ultimately really impact the United States, our history dictates that the wealthiest of individuals will continue to thrive, while the disenfranchised among us will continue to succumb to a higher mortality rate. There has to be a quantum shift in societal attitudes to oppressed individuals with and without disabilities in America if there is any hope of improving the quality of life and lowering mortality rates for this vulnerable population.

PART B: ALLISON FLEMING

I would like to begin with recognition of my positionality as a nondisabled, White, cisgender woman, which limits my understanding of the experience of disability, ableism, and its impact. I offer this reflection with that caveat. I have chosen to use both person-first and identity-first language in this reflection out of respect for both academic tradition and preferences expressed by some in the disability community. As it pertains to this updated text, I extend my most sincere gratitude to Dr. Irmo Marini for his leadership on this project and to the authors for their wonderful contributions. This updated text includes works from some of the very best writers and thinkers in our field, and the volume provides comprehensive coverage of the psychological and social aspects of chronic illness and disability. In his reflection, Dr. Marini raised some hard truths and realities of our current context—particularly related to economic inequality and the striking correlation between poverty and disability in the United States. I agree with him that we are at the point where we can no longer ignore the outcomes of deepening structural inequality within our borders and around the globe. It is an inconvenient truth that many people coming to the United States to seek refugee status are in harm's way as a direct result of our foreign policy and involvement in the politics and governance of other nations in our sphere. Developing countries are experiencing the harshest results of climate change, caused largely by the pollution and environmental exploitation of developed countries like ours who have profited off of natural resources for some time. As Dr. Marini noted, in the United States we are only beginning to see the consequences.

As someone trained as a rehabilitation counselor, I continue to believe the work we do with individuals is critical and important. However, as Desmond Tutu famously offered, "There comes a point where we need to stop just pulling people out of the river. We need to go upstream and find out why they are falling in" (Shannon, n.d., para. 8). Dr. Marini has pointed out the evidence that disabled people are falling in and cited some of the reasons. What we must also confront is that many of our social programs and policies are built upon the assumption that they will fall in, as though this is inevitable and somehow due to a personal failing. These outcomes are not inevitable, and framing them this way is incredibly dismissive and damaging. In the United States, the public dollars spent on medical and cash benefits for disabled people far outweigh resources put in to education and vocational training that would set people on a path to opportunity (Houtenville & Brucker, 2014). This choice to fund the most minimal of financial support over making an investment in people and their potential is striking. It calls back to the beginning of social welfare policies in the United States where disabled people were counted among the "deserving poor" and those who needed assistance and care to survive. The decision that disabled people must be cared for sends the message that disability translates into being incapable and dependent and disenfranchises individuals from having autonomy, control, and full community access. The result has been what Dr. Marini described: social inequity driving reduced mental and physical health and quality of life for many people, disproportionally impacting individuals with disabilities and other minoritized persons. The question for me is: How do we shift away from these ideas that are so engrained in our country's history and social policy that they seem intractable?

Bhattarai et al. (2020) call on rehabilitation counselors and related professionals to prioritize promoting equity for disabled people in our work. This way of thinking is entirely consistent with founding philosophical views on rehabilitation counseling and statements that have been around for some time. An example is found from Tamara Dembo (1982) in an address she provided to an audience unfamiliar with rehabilitation psychology where she outlined her views on inequity experienced by people with disabilities. She clarified that most of the problems disabled people have are not caused by their disability, but by the devaluation of disability and exclusion from community life. She argued that we as individuals are representatives of our culture, and when the culture does not value disabled people, we will not either. This is just as true for rehabilitation counselors and other professionals as the general public. As clarified in his chapter on ableism, Dr. Dana Dunn points out that these values can be internalized by professionals and also disabled people. In the next paragraphs, I aim to center the ideas of several scholars (many of whom identify as disabled) and their suggestions on how to shift how we view our role in promoting equity for disabled people.

The disability community is our first place to look to join advocacy efforts and center their priorities as we work to promote equity and disability justice. As noted by Dunn et al. (2016), there are concrete ways to do this in our education, counseling, and research efforts. For starters, we can commit to integrating identity-first language, promoting disability culture and identity, and increasing meaningful stakeholder engagement in research design and implementation to ensure the results are usable and helpful to those most impacted. These ideas, of course, have been present in the discourse for many years—taking many forms and varied terminology along the way. Several authors in this volume discuss aspects of disability culture and identity-affirming approaches (Chapter 4, Mueller et al.), ableism (Chapter 5, Dunn), and the impact of language including microaggressions (Chapter 11,

Aydemir-Döke) that provide guidance for counselors and disability professionals looking to become better and more effective allies. Another important aspect is increasing representation of disabled counselors and professionals, scholars, and faculty. Data on disability identity is not easily found, but evidence suggests that people with disabilities are starkly underrepresented in psychology trainees (Lund, 2022) and likely rehabilitation counseling and leadership. Finally, Hartley and Saia (2022) call on us to amplify the voices of the disability community through our professional organizations as a way to ensure that our actions and priorities are in service of disabled people. Historically, alignment between the disability community and rehabilitation counseling organizations was much closer, but professionalization movements seem to have distanced the professional associations from grassroots disability advocacy. A critical part of this will be self-examination and combatting of ableist practices, committing to providing real access in our spaces, and valuing disabled voices within our membership (Hartley & Saia, 2022).

Second, despite the fact that the majority of our training is centered on effective practices to work with individuals, we have been called to prioritize systemic advocacy into our role to support the disability community (Bhattari et al., 2020). Many years ago, Dr. Nancy Crewe introduced the idea that the underlying goal of all rehabilitation interventions is to improve quality of life (Crewe, 1980). There are many types of rehabilitation interventions, and her suggestion of quality of life as a shared principle is helpful to find commonality across a diverse discipline. Her principle also helps us see that how we approach interventions is steeped in assumptions of what is needed to improve quality of life. Consider the differences between the medical model and the social and diversity models that provide greater recognition of the social impact of disability, where environmental barriers are highlighted and disability is valued as a natural part of the human experience (Hartley & Saia, 2022). Under the medical model, we would approach the person. In the latter models, we would look to the environmental barriers and social context as places to intervene. Bhattarai et al. (2020) encourage us to look beyond the individual and to the context as the avenue for equity and leverage macro interventions to address many of the situations that Dr. Marini raised in his reflection. Macro interventions are varied, but common features include community organizing and partnerships, social action, or legislative action and policy change to increase the well-being of individuals in communities (Ferguson et al., 2018). Considering the significant marginalization of disabled people in the United States and globally and the threats associated with ongoing poverty, social isolation, and poor health, macro interventions appear to be a promising avenue for improving quality of life. The macro view on interventions is also consistent with the need to consider intersectionality, as disability status alone is not sufficient to understand marginalization. Disabled people of color, LGBTQIA+ disabled people, and those otherwise marginalized will experience different kinds of oppression and have different avenues for improving quality of life (Withers et al., 2019).

As counselors, we pursue this kind of work because we like helping and may see our primary role as being there to "pull people out of the river." I believe we have unique and important skills to be able to do this well. However, pulling people out is much less effective than preventing them from falling in to begin with. It is clear that without a significant shift, counselors will never be able to counteract the deepening inequality and marginalization experienced by people with disabilities and others. We need to listen to the disability community to understand why people are falling in and work toward meaningful policy change to address the causes.

PART C: MALACHY BISHOP

When Irmo asked me to assist with this edition I was extremely honored, but also anxious. Working on this text is a great responsibility. For decades, this book has been an important touchstone for the profession. The literature of a profession is a statement of current knowledge and identity, as well as its professional memory. For 45 years and through eight editions this text has marked, for good or bad, our progress. It has reflected the issues on which we have chosen to focus in terms of the psychological and social impacts of chronic illness and disability and the changing perspectives through which rehabilitation professionals and individuals with chronic illnesses and disabilities have experienced and defined and responded to these impacts. The editions in this series show a profession in constant transition but constantly committed to seeing and understanding the realities of the psychological and social impacts of disability, struggling with new questions and problems (and sometimes with old and intransigent problems in new ways), and challenging readers to respond with action.

This series has also been played a large part in my own development as a rehabilitation counselor. I mark personal and professional milestones in terms of its various editions. This series introduced me to some of the most important writers and thinkers in rehabilitation. I write this reflection 45 years after the first edition was published in 1977. The third edition of Marinelli and Dell Orto's *The Psychological and Social Impact of Disability* marked my entry into the profession and has been on my bookshelf for over 30 years, since it was the required text in my first master's-level course in rehabilitation counseling. (Thank you, Hanoch, and thank Providence for letting my path find yours.) Through this series I was introduced to, inspired by, and challenged by the ideas of Zola, Schontz, Hahn, Dembo, Leviton, Wright, Stubbins, Anthony, Dell Orto, Livneh, Kerr, Vash, Nosek, and Siu, among others.

This series has always challenged me. The carefully selected papers in the earlier versions (many of which are still as original, important, and meaningful as when they were first published) and the newly developed chapters in the later editions have explored the limits and limitations of rehabilitation and challenged readers with the "much work [that] remains to be done" that Marinelli and Dell Orto described in their preface to the first edition (1977, p. xiii). Under the editorship of Irmo and Mark Stebnicki, the commitment to challenging perspectives and portrayals and to present the current research on topics of importance to rehabilitation professionals and people with disabilities continued. The current edition has evolved in a period of significant social and professional change, as Irmo has delineated. The impacts of these changes on the lives of people with disabilities feel new and often daunting. Others are familiar, daunting, and frustrating. The effects of significant change and unchanging challenges in the lives of people with disabilities and chronic illnesses are reflected in the chapters in this edition and, as always, in some new ways, they challenge us as rehabilitation professionals and as humans. In this period of transition, however, there are important themes that are also present in the chapters of this text that, as I have reflected on them over the many months of working with the authors, give me optimism.

The first is a changing perspective on the meaning and definition of disability. This change is implicit in several chapters and explicit in the chapter by Mueller et al., who describe "a new understanding of people with disabilities themselves as agentic and involved in co-creating, defining, and growing disability as an identity and cultural category." The second is the ways rehabilitation has evolved, and is continuing to evolve, by challenging existing assumptions and expectations, exploring questions from new, more diverse perspectives, and advocating for change in historically inequitable and unjust environments and relationships. This evolution, if rehabilitation is to be relevant, must increasingly be driven by the priorities of those whose lives it affects. The fact that progress remains to be made in this sense is clear in the chapters of this text. However, a review of prior editions provides, at times, a compelling juxtaposition. Finally, I am excited by the new minds, new research, and new perspectives represented among the authors. It has been a privilege and honor to work with them. They have created a text that, consistent with prior editions, both informs and challenges us to respond with action. Irmo and Allison, I know you both feel as strongly as I do about this series. Your wisdom, passion, hard work, and brilliance made this edition what it is, and it is a worthy addition. Thank you for allowing me to participate.

KEY REFERENCES

Only key references appear in the print edition. The full references appear in the digital product on Springer Publishing Connect™: https://connect.springerpub.com/content/book/978-0-8261-5111-7/part/partV/chapter/ch27

Bhattarai, J. J., Bentley, J., Morean, W., Wegener, S. T., & Pollack Porter, K. M. (2020). Promoting equity at the population level: Putting the foundational principles into practice through disability advocacy. *Rehabilitation Psychology, 65*(2), 87–100. https://doi.org/10.1037/rep0000321

Case, A., & Deaton, A. (2020). *Deaths of despair and the future of capitalism.* Princeton University Press.

Dunn, D. S., Ehde, D. M., & Wegener, S. T. (2016). The foundational principles as psychological lodestars: Theoretical inspiration and empirical direction in rehabilitation psychology. *Rehabilitation Psychology, 61*(1), 1–6. https://doi.org/10.1037/rep0000082

Houtenville, A. J., & Brucker, D. L. (2014). Participation in safety-net programs and the utilization of employment services among working-age persons with disabilities. *Journal of Disability Policy Studies, 25*(2), 91–105. https://doi.org/10.1177/1044207312474308

Ida, T. (2021). *Climate refugees: The world's forgotten victims.* www.weforum.org.

Kamdar, N. P., Horning, M. L., Geraci, J. C., Uzdavines, A. W., Helmer, D. A., & Hundt, N. E. (2021). Risk for depression and suicidal ideation among food insecure US veterans: Data from the National Health and Nutrition Examination Study. *Social Psychiatry and Psychiatric Epidemiology, 56,* 2175–2184. https://doi.org/10.1007/s00127-021-02071-3

Kehinde, M. (2021). *Climate refugees on the rise in Africa!* Leafgreen Africa. https://leafgreenafrica.org/climate-refugees-on-the-rise/

Kellett, K., Ligus, K., & Robison, J. (2021). "So glad to be home": Money follows the person: Participants' experiences after transitioning out of an institution. *Journal of Disability Policy Studies, 33*(2), 22–132. https://doi.org/10.1177/10442073211043519

Stramondo, J. A. (2021). Bioethics, adaptive preferences, and judging the quality of a life with disability. *Social Theory and Practice, 47*(1), 199–220. https://doi.org/10.5840/soctheorpract202121117

Terlazzo, R. (2016). Conceptualizing adaptive preferences respectively: An substantial account. *Canadian Journal of Philosophy, 45* (2), 179–196. https://doi.org/10.1111/jopp.12062

Withers, A. J., Ben-Moshe, L., Brown, L. X. Z., Erickson, L., Gorman, R., da S., Lewis, T. A., McLeod, L., & Mingus, M. (2019). Radical disability politics. In *Routledge Handbook of Radical Politics* (pp. 178–193). Taylor & Francis. https://doi.org/10.4324/9781315619880-15

V

PERSONAL PERSPECTIVES

Available to the authors are the many dynamic stories of those who use different coping strategies to live and to grow despite a serious disability or illness. These personal perspectives are living illustrations of how to be productive while experiencing significant life challenges. We wish to include some personal perspectives here that can broaden the reader's understanding of living with and beyond an illness or disability and also show that different perspectives of coping and living only enrich an understanding of the dimensions of the total human experience. These personal perspectives enlarge on Irving Kenneth Zola's conviction, clearly stated in the foreword of the third edition of *The Psychological and Social Impact of Disability* (Marinelli & Dell Orto, 1991): "Disability was not merely a personal problem to be solved by individual effort . . . as much a social problem created and reinforced by social attitudes and prejudices whose solution would require governmental resources, protections, and interventions" (p. xv).

These personal statements also further emphasize and extend the implications of the disability-related issues identified throughout the book. The personal journeys of Robert Neumann and Tosca Appel that you will read illustrate both the material discussed in the chapter in Part II on psychological adaptation to chronic illness and disability and the chapters in Part III on family issues in illness and disability. These family issues are further highlighted by the narrative experiences of Judy Teplow, Karen's mother, and both Chris and his mother. Paul Egan's poignant account brings to life many of the concepts identified in the chapters in Part II. With the description of David's experience, all of these personal statements provide the reader with an opportunity to understand the varied models of disability, discussed clearly in the chapter by Mueller, Andrews, and Minotti in Part I.

REFERENCES

Marinelli, R. P., & Dell Orto, A. E. (1991). *The psychological and social impact of disability* (3rd ed.). Springer Publishing Company.

MY EXPERIENCE AS A DEAF WOMAN

CASSANDRA CANTU

Music, dancing, and gathering at our house with loud close family and friends is what I grew up with. It did not occur to me until I was a teen that the reality of my hearing disability had begun to show its true colors. To describe my experience as a Deaf woman involves judgement, challenges, neglect, and the feeling of being taken advantage of; however, these negatives have shaped me into the person I am today.

My mother recognized right away that I was deaf, but there were no answers back then. To this day I just became gradually deaf, whereas today babies take their hearing test. Immediately, I was put into a speech school and deaf program. However, I was one of five groups that were selected to move from the deaf program to mainstream, which included an extra teacher, and we were required to wear hearing aids with cable wire and box wrapping around our body and to use verbal and learning signs at the age of 5. I was told that I would not be able to graduate from college because my reading level was at a sixth-grade level. Today, I've accomplished associate, bachelor's, and master's degrees, and I am currently taking rehabilitation counseling classes for another master's degree and hopefully my PhD, God willing. I would never imagine myself coming this far, but others always have.

As a person who is deaf, the challenges will always surround us. I'm talking about our community's lack of resources, the neglect most of us go through, costs considered over accommodating our disability, our voices not being heard, or even the ongoing lack of education that "mute" is incorrect and offensive and the perspective that most persons who are deaf don't want to achieve due to a closed-minded society.

I sometimes describe my deafness as a lost dog. I look both ways to see who's talking and yet voices are still muffled. Here is an example of what every day as a student is like:

I need that person to face me because I rely heavy on lip reading. No, show me what you're talking about because I need to see what you mean. Wait, where? What did I miss? Okay, what could that be the connection to? I am wanting to ask for clarification but okay, never mind, the interpreter misread what I said and the classroom is staring at me. I'll just review this when I get home. Alright, let me open the book. Whoa, where did all this information come from? Wait a minute, what does that mean? Let me get the dictionary. Oh, wow, let me write it down. Its 2:12 a.m. already? I can't quit, I need to finish this chapter. I don't get it. I'll start fresh tomorrow. New day starting and yet there's no time to finish my homework. Okay, my homework is done let me review it but I don't have time. Back in class and Uh-oh, I don't like that reaction. They're looking at me like I'm stupid. Okay they're asking me what I mean—but I couldn't explain better. I know! I need to work on my grammar. I've been told this for many,many years! This is getting annoying. If only they knew the difference when using ASL. They don't understand that I am trying to pay attention to the interpreter and when he/she is stating something, I try to see what they're showing over the PowerPoint/internet/video, and I have already missed that information or what interpreter was signing and he or she is not using the terms from books like in ASL. And in advising and counseling signing like ASL, one sign can have different meanings. I need to have the PowerPoint ready before class so I can know what they're talking about in class. English grammar is very hard and they have no idea how many times I had to type and delete all of this all over again and I am still being told to fix my grammar 5 or 10 times. I am losing hope. I see many red "X's" on my writing. They do not know that I had to create my own index card to study vocabulary or rewrite the vocabulary after telling me that I don't try hard enough. I end up having to bug my family or friend what this chapter talks about and asking if they can just break it down with simple summary. Yes, all this is taking me three times as long to study for just one class. I need to speak up for myself. Here we go. Okay I think that went well! What! No, that's not what I'm talking about. I guess the interpreter must have said something else again. I'll take the grade. I'm tired already.

I have become the face of people who are deaf for events. The pressure to become the leader when everyone else is afraid to take charge. The pressure to set up events because no one wants to be responsible. Everyone wants their voice to be heard but won't step up, and that's where I've been put, in the front and center. My journey has been a bumpy road full of obstacles and setbacks, but these lessons have taught me to give back by working for educating others about the Deaf and hard of hearing.

DISCUSSION QUESTIONS

1. Have students describe how they would feel if they were placed into a class where the professor taught in an entirely different language that they didn't know or understand.

2. Ask students to describe which activities they would miss the most and why if they suddenly became deaf.

3. Have the students discuss how they might feel and think and what they might consider doing if they learned their newborn child was deaf.

FIRES ARE NOT DRILLS

DONELLE HENDERLONG

I was 6 years old when society first looked me in the face. It was fire drill day in first grade, and I had been rehearsing the steps in my head all morning for the afternoon excitement: *When the alarm sounds, listen to the teacher, get in line quietly, head outside and wait.* As we anticipated the impending ruckus, my classmates and I were sitting in our music class awaiting the alarm when my teacher came over to me and said softly,

"Donelle, since this is only pretend, we don't have to make a fuss to get you outside. You just stay here and we will be back in a little bit."

Upon hearing this, my mind slowly erased the protocols that my fellow students and I had been rehearsing in the previous days: "When the alarm sounds, listen to the teacher, get in line quietly, head outside and wait." Instead I was now given my own set of rules; a hybrid of the complete opposite of the rules that my classmates were being told would protect them in the event of an emergency, along with the same original underlying thread:

Listen to the teacher, she is supposed to keep you safe.

I didn't get in line. I didn't head outside. At 6 years old, I sat in a room by myself quietly and waited.

The casual observer in this situation may side with the teacher's good intentions here. It's within reason to think, "There was no actual fire, it was only more convenient. There will be a million other fire drills over the course of her school career, she will have the opportunity to learn at some point. Had there been a real fire, they would have gotten her out."

It is equally reasonable to conjecture that while I was waiting for my class to return from their practice, at 6 years old in a room alone, an actual fire could have broken out and I would have had no knowledge of keeping myself safe and a teacher who was away keeping others safe.

All social justice movements operate on a "start and stop" mechanism. The majority group gets a desire to slightly let the minority group infiltrate the mainstream world by controlled osmosis. That is, to allow a slow dripping of diversity into society so that a change is noticeable enough that the majority can be praised for realizing that a segment of the population was thirsty, but don't turn the faucet on so much that the majority can't control what happens. When they are ready, the majority will turn the faucet on, but not enough to allow the minority to quench their thirst on their own.

Such was the case in 1996, the year of the first fire drill. I was one of the only kids with a disability in my community enrolled entirely in mainstream school, which also happened to be the newest (and really only, at least to my needs) accessible school in our community. The school was built with ramps across the school, perfect for my pink wheelchair to go up and down. An orange school bus with a wheelchair ramp picked me up every day. The community had done their due diligence and all was settled. I should have been satisfied. In reality, social change does not settle. Did they have protocol in place for me at the time should there have been an actual fire? Perhaps, but perhaps not. And while I am sure they would have found a proper exit for me, protocol is not meant to be taught during the emergency for which it is protocol. Did I have the right to say something? Absolutely, but I was 6 and 6-year-olds know to listen to authority, a parallel to the adult marginalized population, particularly those who have disabilities.

Thankfully, my parents spoke up, learning about it after I told them when I got off the bus, saying, "Mommy. If there is a fire at school during music class, I need to stay inside and burn in the building because I don't know how to leave."

I was included in every school fire drill from then on, but that didn't exclude me from having to learn how to navigate the continuous fires that would come up in my adult life.

Take, for instance, the fire for ambition, namely the concept of gainful employment. Coming out of my master's degree program in 2015, I had been taught as part of the curriculum how to negotiate and, even more progressively, how to negotiate to ensure equal pay as a woman. What I was not taught about was the economic stigma that having a disability would place on me, including how to tactfully ask for less money than was offered to me in order to meet my personal care needs.

You read that right: In order to survive as a person with a disability, I cannot earn a competitive wage.

I currently utilize the Indiana MEDWorks system, a division of the Indiana Family and Social Services Administration that allows state citizens with disabilities the opportunity to work and receive traditional Medicaid insurance and benefits by paying a monthly premium. If I were to be paying out of pocket for the necessary daily aide care that I need in order to survive (assistance with showering, toileting, dressing, physical body transfers, and food prep), it would be close to $31,000 annually. Being as there was once a time where it was unheard of for people with disabilities to work, our state should be proud of this advancement; however, the current system still controls exactly how much I advance. Actually, in order to advance in my career, I've had to take steps back. At my highest-paid position, a mid-level higher education administrator position at a university I had been with for 4 years, I was only $804 away from making the salary cutoff to receive the Medicaid benefits I needed: a cash amount of $42,804. I was forced to turn down raises despite good performance reviews, making the decision to not be forced to live on $11,804 a year after my aide care was paid.

After turning down several pay increases, I ultimately made the decision to take a substantial pay cut at a university closer to home in order to cut down my commute and save some gas money. I started once again at an entry-level position so I would be able to have the opportunity to be compensated fairly for an increase in skill level. The somewhat unfortunate irony of this is that this university does not currently offer merit pay raises.

Most recently, there has been a merging of sorts between these two fires in my mind, a true wildfire that all of us are aware of, though we never seem to extinguish as it leaves horrendous destruction in its path. I first became aware of it at 9 years old as it raged through Columbine High School. I gasped in tears in my college dorm room as I packed to go home for Christmas, lamenting that 27 people would never again do the same. I lit a candle in a church in Michigan with my mother on the morning after the Pulse nightclub shootings, a mixed sigh of sorrow for the lost lives and gratitude that I had been lucky enough to not recognize a name on the news. I recalled the fear of not feeling safe in high school during an emergency lockdown while I watched as students in Parkland, Florida, exited the building, stripped of an innocence that so many of us have been able to keep. After Uvalde, I began to panic.

I currently work at a small private university in an office that oversees implementation of various types of accommodations to remove barriers for students with disabilities. Many of these students have physical limitations like myself, but we also serve several students who are neurodiverse, who experience stimming by means of vocalizing or other outward sounds or movements while in stressful situations. It became clear to me that the typically advised protocol of "run, hide, fight" during an active shooter situation may provide a chance of safety for the average able-bodied individual, but it left both me and my students exposed and alone with an ableism gap spanning the confines of life and death.

I have spent the better part of several workdays poring over articles from the Federal Emergency Management Agency (FEMA) to local newspapers, looking for accessible alternatives to "run, hide, fight." I am terrified. I am terrified that out of all of the articles I have looked at published post–Americans with Disabilities Act and post-shootings, the most inclusive guidance I have been able to find involves barricading myself with heavy surrounding objects that I am not able to lift or using my medical equipment as a weapon. My power wheelchair is indeed heavy and has run over a few feet, but it will stop operating the second its operator is shot in the chest. The seatbelt will disengage as soon as an assailant presses the button to lift my 120-pound body out of the chair, removing so easily the thing that is supposed to act as my only tool in this situation. Moreover, this is not just a matter of personal safety anymore. I am now in the role that my teacher was in so many years ago. It is my job to keep my students safe. I have found no guidance on best practices for safety for neurodiverse persons, but I have found that police and many other first responders have also not received training on how to best communicate with those who are neurodiverse or cognitively impaired, choosing to escalate their voices, rather than deescalating the anxiety of the distressed individual so that they are able to listen to instructions and trust safety personnel. Do our law enforcement and first responders know basic American Sign Language to communicate safety protocols in an emergency, or will the Deaf community just be expected to be intuitive? These are now the fears that plague me daily, as I am not the educator who will tell her students to "just stay here."

Maybe after reading this, a fire has ignited within you. Is it a fire of anger? A fire of urgency for social justice? Either way, these are good fires, and good fires must be stoked. Good fires are stoked with leaves of continuous education in arenas that reach beyond that of one's surroundings, of asking questions, and having a persistence of dissatisfaction for the current social system. These fires are all too quickly extinguished by complacency, exhaustion, and discouragement; they must continue to be lit as soon as the foot which has tried to stamp them out has lifted. I only wish I had more time to tell you of the good fires I experience, those of warmth, of passion, of platonic and romantic love, of desire. They do exist but cannot be fully appreciated until the harmful fires are acknowledged and controlled, knowing that neither type of fire, even if dormant for a time, will never cease to exist.

How are you currently responding to the fires in you or around you as you read this? How will you respond to them the second you close this text? It is okay if you need time to assess where you are needed; after all, no one expects you to rush into a burning building.

However, the system *is* on fire.

We, the People with Disabilities, are burning with good fire in the midst of harmful fires everywhere.

As citizens, we sit and wait for the teachers, who now take the form of government officials and agencies, to tell us what to do while the alarm goes off because they are supposed to keep us safe. Sometimes, the inaction by those who call for action ignites the fire.

It's not a drill, nor has it ever been. If you hear the alarm, how are you helping to control the burning?

DISCUSSION QUESTIONS

1. Thinking back to your own experience in school, how was disability addressed in emergency preparedness?

2. Consider one of your current classroom buildings. Devise an accommodation plan for a fire or extreme weather that would allow people with physical disabilities, sensory disabilities, and intellectual disabilities to escape safely.

3. How can emergency responders be supported to communicate effectively and be prepared to rescue people with various kinds of disabilities?

4. How does our Federal Emergency Management Agency account for disability-related needs in their guidance for response to extreme weather, evacuations, and other emergencies?

MY STORY OF BECOMING BLIND

MACARENA PENA

After 24 years of being blind, it is difficult to pinpoint the beginning of my rehabilitation process. It's a question as paradoxical as asking what came first, the egg or the chicken. Clearly, quite challenging to determine! As I wrote this story, many forgotten memories came back to life and allowed me to reminisce in my story and how my journey began. The truth is, I lost my sight at the age of 35, in a matter of 2 weeks, due to retinal detachment in both eyes, which was ultimately a complication of diabetes. I was living in Monterrey, Mexico, at the time, a married mother of two, who was now completely blind. I haven't spoken much to anyone about this really considering that during the first 3 to 4 years of living with my visual impairment, I made no effort to seek any form of rehabilitation such as mobility training, assistive technology, or any form of rehabilitative counseling. I did not have access to such resources, nor was it encouraged or recommended by any of my medical specialists treating my eyes. These initial years had me in limbo. In all honesty, deep down, a big part of me was waiting for a miracle; I still had hope that I would recover my sight and therefore avoided accepting my reality by keeping my mind and heart busy. At the time, I was taking care of my 1-year-old son and newly adopted 5-year-old daughter with a husband who worked all day. We were living in Monterrey, Mexico, with zero relatives in the area, without any eye doctors who could competently treat my condition.

As a U.S. citizen living relatively close to the border, we had the ability to travel to Houston, Texas, for regular treatment by the best eye specialist we could find. A manifestation of my deeply rooted belief is that one day I would recover my sight and everything would go back to normal. Backtracking a bit, I have been diabetic since birth, although diagnosed at age 13. I was a huge baby who weighed almost 14 pounds during an 8-month pregnancy, being the youngest of eight. Genetically, my mother was diagnosed with diabetes at 36 and passed away at 66 after surviving several strokes and spending almost 15 years in a wheelchair. Despite living through this, I still did not learn my lesson. I remember growing up and repeatedly being told not to pay much attention to my diet because it wasn't a severe medical condition. It wasn't until later adulthood that I learned to manage diabetes, which included adjusting my body to 400 to 500 glucose levels, and to this day I continue to learn new things about myself and how my body works. Fast-forward to 1999. It was when I turned 30 that I realized there was a problem with my vision when I began having issues reading my son's birthday cards. Slowly but surely, everything progressively became blurry in a matter of 2 weeks, until I was totally blind. That was the end to a new beginning. Shortly after, the first of 11 surgeries took place in Houston, Texas, only to be told "There is nothing more we can do at this point, sorry ma'am."

I will forever be grateful to my sister Patricia who during this time became my designated driver, nurse, companion, and cheerleader throughout my journey. Her love for me allowed her to drive from Saltillo, Coahuila, to pick me up in Monterrey and drive another 8 hours to Houston, Texas, making it a 13-hour drive, just so I could see an eye specialist. She was never tired, sad, mad, or negative. She was one of my strengths during this time of uncertainty. Never missed an eye surgery and appointments. Even after my devastating final diagnosis where all I could do was cry, she was there in this moment with me. I genuinely felt miserable, afraid, mad, distraught, and very angry. I remember, Patricia just sat there quietly, not doing anything, without a word, just stood still in time with me. She waited until I finally composed myself and asked her "Are you going to say anything?" which resulted in the least expected answer. "You are not just a pair of eyes; we tried it, but it did not work our next step is training," she said. It's been 24 years, and to this day I still use this quote as a form of encouragement with the people who are currently navigating their newly acquired disability. Today, I am grateful for her wise words and unwavering strength. Now I understand that despite my loss, I came to the realization that I am more than just a pair of eyes.

It was now 2001; 3 years had gone by since I became completely blind, and nothing had changed despite our efforts. We finally made the decision to move to the United States, specifically McAllen, Texas, to be closer to family and have better access to healthcare. The kids and I moved first and spent the first 6 months alone while my husband found employment and adjusted to new life. Max was almost 4 and Rigel almost 8. Interestingly, although we were closer to our family, everyone worked, and my recovery still felt quite lonely and unknown. Despite all these changes, Rigel started school right away and Max stayed home with me. During this time, I can truly say transportation was the greatest challenge even though I have a cane, I did not have mobility training or assistive technology, nor did I have the slightest idea they existed! Several times I fell after missing a step or hitting a curb and little by little started creating my new way of life. This is exactly why I did not hesitate when I finally learned about mobility training or the benefits of using a cane. Interestingly, for me it was never a "disgrace" to be seen with a white cane, maybe because I thought it to be a wonderful tool that provides independence, confidence, and personal freedom. This allowed me to perform most activities of daily living, and slowly but surely, I came to master it. With two small children to take care of, I never once abandoned my duties as a mother and incrementally made time to apply newly learned skills of my own, including having to relearn how to cook, clean, do laundry, assist in homework, coordinate transportation, and everything else that comes with motherhood.

Once someone asked if my blindness affected my kids. My first answer was NO. But after reflecting, I can admit that it did. I am aware that it allowed my kids to be compassionate, kind, and understanding of other people's needs. Despite me being in a new home, new country, new friends, and closer to family, I knew quite nothing about the world of the blind and how much I had yet to learn about myself and my journey. Back then, I truly believed that I was so independent! Just because I could bake a cake and memorize information right off the top of my head. Little did I know how much I would break many beliefs and be forced to relearn my lifestyle. I guess a milestone in my rehabilitation process occurred when I realized there were others like me. Going through the same emotions and uncertainty provided a form of normalcy, belonging, and identity. I wanted to meet other blind people and explore the many ways of life. I had so many questions and couldn't ask them fast enough. I wanted to know their approach to things and exactly "how did blind people go about grocery shopping?" also "how do blind people use a computer?" and "was it possible for people like us to work?" This was my first taste, and that was enough; I began feeling restless and hungry to do more with my life.

I then contacted the local rehab agency, and my real recovery began. Initially, I had a visit from a vocational rehabilitation counselor who assessed my needs, wants, and vocational goals, which was essential to recovering my newly found identity. Throughout all this my husband was uneasy and concerned, which made this transition challenging. Don't get me wrong. I have the most amazing husband and partner considering we have been together for almost 28 years. When I spoke with him for the first time about attending the Criss Cole Rehabilitation Center for the blind in Austin, Texas, for 3 months, he hated the idea. That night he told the kids, 8 and 12 at the time, that mommy wanted to go away and leave them. You can just imagine that the kids cried all night and slept on top of me, making it clear that it was something our family could not do at the time. Despite the resistance, long talks, and many tears, I was able to attend Criss Cole Center and proudly graduated from their program in May 2007. To this day I still keep in touch with my cohort, and the sad reality is that as of today I am the only one who is actively working. It does baffle me to think that we all attended the same trainings and classes, had the same instructors, and had similar experiences yet had different outcomes. What was the difference between me and them? From my personal experience I believe the difference was embracing challenges as opportunities with a positive attitude and accepting that any decision requires a certain level of risks, and with the right support system, anything is truly possible.

Subsequently, in 2008, I was hired by the Department of Assistance and Rehabilitation Services (DARS) the Division for Blind Services (DBS) department as an independent living program caseworker. While training for this new position I faced many unfamiliar challenges considering my job duties included doing home visits with individuals age 55 and older who had acquired a new disability and desperately needed independent living training. In this work, I found my purpose. It was challenging to say the least because for one, I knew about performing activities of daily living, but helping others accept their condition was an entirely different ball game. From a vulnerability perspective, this was a level of acceptance I am still working on. Since then, I have come to terms with my condition. First, I do not consider myself disabled. I am just blind. Second, in my heart, I still believe that this is temporary. One day, I do not know when or how, but I will see again. Most importantly, I do not like to be blind, yet every day I make the conscious choice of being a very happy blind person.

There is something I always say to my customers/clients: "It is not important what I say, the most important is what you do with what I say." In the rehab process, there are ups and downs. I tell them sometimes I will carry you, other moments I will push you, and always know that I will be close to you. That is the kind of support that has made the difference in my life.

My support system and environment are what made me who I am today. My children wanted a "normal" mom. As children, they did not understand that mommy was blind; therefore, they expected the same as any other child who had sighted moms. Yet I never backed down and I did everything in my power to be the best mom I could be for them despite my limitations. My husband was my rock; even when we both feared the future, he always supported me. I am also blessed with a group of friends who trusted me and gave me the benefit of the doubt to care for their children, organize parties and trips, and be the life of the party. Fortunately, my siblings have always treated me as their sister and not as a blind person, and God who has always given me the strength to keep learning and growing. For that I am humbly grateful. This became my second chance.

So, when people tell me how wonderful and independent, I am, I just laugh. It is not me; it is where God placed me. I am surrounded by love, support, and a lot of high expectations.

Gabriel

We had been married for only 4 years when my wife started losing her sight. At first it appeared as if it was a temporary situation and after seeing the best doctors in Houston, she would see 20/20 again. Nevertheless, we were constantly told that every time she had laser treatment, she was losing more sight. We never truly addressed how serious our situation was and the implications of it but made it our goal to face every challenge with God's grace. Now after almost 25 years, we know that diabetes is the number one cause of blindness in Hispanics. When the treatments did not improve the eyesight, I became more and more scared for my family. Although Macarena always tried to stay positive and active, I could see her limitations and was scared for my small children. We did not have family and no close friends to help. We lived a day at a time. My job was to make the house "safe" for the kids and for my wife; meanwhile, she was the mother of my children. I can now see that it is the motherly instinct that allowed her to "see" things as a mom. I learned to trust her and to feel confident when I was at work. Also, thank God for phones because we were always in communication with each other and more so when it mattered most. After many procedures, 11 surgeries, and many prayers later, we learned to live with "limited" vision. The kids learned that Mom could not see very well and guided her in many things. At the early age of 2, our son Max learned to say "step" to warn Macarena that a curb or step was in sight. My daughter learned to use the microwave, change diapers, and serve food very early in life because that is what families do. We stick together, and we all learned to work as a team. It was hard to let her go to Criss Cole; however, it became an essential part of her rehabilitation journey and for that I am grateful. After 27 years married, I can honestly say that I wouldn't change anything about the life we have built. Yes, we lived some rough moments together and made some permanent adjustments, but our life is beautiful just as it is. We have learned to inspire, educate, and live many moments as a family, and despite any challenge what unites us is our resilience and love for one another.

DISCUSSION QUESTIONS

1. What values are apparent within the family dynamic that helped adjust to the acquired disability? What are your present values? How do your values play a role in your own family?

2. What are the key elements that are crucial for a positive rehabilitation process? Which elements can hinder or enhance this process? Examples include family, friends, or a spouse.

3. What insight did you gain from this relationship and the decisions made following the disability?

4. As a rehabilitation counselor, what other two resources, trainings, or services would you have recommended if this were your client? What resources are available now that didn't exist 15 years ago?

5. What are your thoughts on parents with a disability raising a child? What if both parents had a disability? Should this limit them from forming a family? What additional barriers could they face?

6. If you were the person who lost their sight would you have moved to a different country and start anew, considering the availability of new resources? How would you have done things differently?

7. What did Macarena mean when she realized she is "not just a pair of eyes"? What are other components in a person's identity?

MULTIPLE SCLEROSIS: NOT JUST SURVIVING BUT THRIVING

JESSICA HENRY

In December 2011, I moved to Pittsburgh, Pennsylvania, to begin an internship at the Office of Vocational Rehabilitation (OVR). At that time, I was 26 years old and nearly finished with my 2-year master's program at Alabama State University. Grateful for the opportunity to change careers and still serve people with disabilities, I accepted an offer to intern in a new vibrant city located close to my family and home state. However, my excitement did not account for what was slowly happening with my health.

The transition from Alabama to Pennsylvania was exciting yet stressful. In the weeks before moving into my new apartment in Pittsburgh, I drove 12 hours nonstop, from Montgomery to Cleveland in my small Volkswagen Jetta. I was exhausted from the drive, so I attributed the numbness in my hands and feet to the long journey. Moving into my new place located just a few miles from One PNC Plaza was exciting because I moved in on New Year's Eve, just in time to count down the new year and watch the fireworks. I credited the blurry vision I was experiencing to the higher altitude of roughly 1,300 miles above sea level, which was well above the elevation in Alabama and Cleveland. Of course, being the strong Black woman that I am, I kept going despite how sick I truly felt. Since New Year's Day fell on a Sunday, I had one extra day to *get it together* before I started orientation on January 3. That day as I ran a few errands, I attributed the fatigue and vertigo to my apprehension about starting a new career.

Neurological impacts of multiple sclerosis (MS) were present during the first month of my new job. While I wanted to make a good impression, my hearing was fleeting, and I could not make logical sense of what was happening around me. As an intern, I struggled to apply the things I had learned to support consumers during my training program because I was sick most of the time. One evening, after work, I called 911 because I was too weak to drive myself, and being in a new city, I had not yet identified a reliable social network. After spending hours at the hospital with a diminished ability to walk, doctors discharged me but not before adding a false and potentially harmful diagnosis of "alcohol poisoning" to my medical records. This particular diagnosis is especially risky to a state employee and highlighted bias. Despite my health, the show had to go on, meaning each morning, I would arrive at work on time, making my best effort to assist consumers to achieve their employment goals from intake and eligibility to assessment, follow-up, and case closure while I simultaneously wrestled with thoughts about if I was truly capable and competent.

In February 2012, I recall a night that, when told with the proper lighting and horror sound effects, reminds me of a psychological thriller. I recall the night vividly as my symptoms worsened and gained new intensity. I went to bed as normal and woke up feeling like I had just taken a ride on the famous Cleveland amazement park ride, The Rotor. Due to extreme vertigo, I felt like the floor became the ceiling and the ceiling became the floor. This time I called my parents, worried that my life was coming to an end, and they drove 2½ hours to take me back to the hospital. This time they were present as my care advocates (note: this was a critical missing piece to my first emergency room visit).

With their support, doctors initiated a series of tests, including magentic resonance imaging (MRI), a computed tomography (CAT) scan, spinal tap, and blood tests, to determine the cause of my illness. The results of all the tests came back consistent with MS. MS is a neurological condition in which nerve damage disrupts the pathways that send and receive messages between the brain and body. Symptoms can ultimately be exacerbated when stress and anxiety are high due to information overload. With all that was happening in my life, there was now an explanation for what I was experiencing. When the doctor delivered the diagnosis, I remember releasing a sigh of relief that there was finally proof that I was not faking an illness.

My neurologist took two important steps once we had a formal diagnosis. First, he removed the incorrect alcohol poisoning diagnosis from my medical record. He also conveyed concern that the chart could be detrimental to my career. Second, he prescribed a medication that was known to slow the progression of the disease. At my job, I evolved from just a provider of vocational rehabilitation supports to a recipient of services. This assistance allowed me to get back to work, finish my internship hours, graduate from my master's program, and go on to start a PhD program in August 2012. To the readers of this story, please note that my journey to living with MS was not as straightforward as it seems. There were many days when I felt defeated and like an imposter. Even with the medication I was still experiencing neurological complications such as numbness, gait issues, changes to cognitive functioning, and memory loss.

During this time of my life, I had to navigate the eight stages of adjustment to disability: (a) shock, (b) realization, (c) denial, (d) depression, (e) anger, (f) hostility, (g) acknowledgment, and (h) adjustment (Dutta & Kundu, 2007). There were times when I would lose my vision and hearing, but naturally put aside my health problems to complete whatever task set before me. I was unaware that I ultimately lacked the skills to rest and recover for fear that I might be looked down upon as weak or incapable. I later discovered that this ideology derived from what is known as the Superwoman schema/trope introduced by Michelle Wallace in 1978 and focalized to health disparities and stress among African American women by Woods-Giscombé in 2010. Eventually I learned that external triggers, such as stress, intensified and made disease symptoms more frequent.

Early in my story you may recall moments in my life that were overlooked by the untrained eye, so I became the trained eye by focusing my dissertation and research agenda on understanding wellness and disease management. To conclude my PhD requirements, I conducted a phenomenological research investigation and wrote a dissertation on the experiences of stress on symptom management among Black women with MS. My work fills a gap in research on specific impacts and health outcomes for a historically marginalized group. Ultimately, I took advantage of what happened to me from healthcare treatment to healthcare management and made it work for me. Currently, as a college professor, my goal and commitment are to train future helping professionals on best practices when serving individuals with disabilities. I encourage the readers of this textbook to consider how healthcare bias and failure to consider all aspects of the consumer's background can negatively influence how we individualize and tailor services to their needs. Although people with MS or disabilities are not a monolith, my story may help better put in context the concepts of supporting people who are adjusting to disability to not just survive with a disability but also thrive by creating a new normal.

DISCUSSION QUESTIONS

1. The author describes seeking medical care after experiencing significant symptoms for about a month. How does this align with the typical process of being diagnosed with multiple sclerosis?

2. Consider the role of healthcare bias in this author's story. How was she harmed by her first visit to the emergency room?

3. How does this author manage her symptoms? What do we know about the role of stress in exacerbation of symptoms for individuals with multiple sclerosis?

CHRIS AND HIS MOTHER: HOPE AND HOME

CHRIS MOY

The following personal perspective presents the often irrational life experience that can test and strengthen the human mind, body, and spirit. A son and his mother share their journey, as well as the hopes and dreams that had to be let go and those aspired to.

Chris's Perspective

Before my injury in July 1991, my family had endured its share of trials and tribulations. I guess you could say we were a typical middle-class family. At least we considered ourselves middle class. Actually, we were on the low-income end of middle class, but we were happy. We never felt deprived of anything; even though we didn't have a lot of money for clothes or extras, we never went without.

Reprinted from Power and Dell Orto (2004).

My two older brothers and I shared many wonderful times with our parents. Everyone was always very close: church every Sunday, dinners together, and always discussions on how things were going. My parents, to my knowledge, never missed a sporting event or school function. Everyone was treated fairly, given the same opportunities, and encouraged to grow and learn by experiencing new things. We were always given the freedom to choose our activities, but we were expected not to quit halfway through. If we started something, we were always expected to give it a fair chance before deciding not to continue with it. I guess that's where I developed much of my determination.

My father and mother shared the responsibilities of keeping the household going. When my father lost his job, he took over all the household chores and my mother continued to work full time. Dad was always the athletic type, and he instilled in us the belief that hard work, determination, and self-confidence would not only help us athletically but later in our lives as we began to go out into the world. Our friends were always welcome in our house. I'll never forget how my Dad would fix lunch every day for me and my best friend during our senior year. There aren't too many guys who would want to go home every day for lunch, but I always felt very comfortable with it.

Mom has always been the matriarch of the family. Being an optimist, she was able to see the good in everything. Although she's a petite woman, she had a quiet, gentle strength about her. I never tried to "pull one over on her," as she always had a way of finding things out. When one of us boys would do something we shouldn't have, Mom always found out. This still amazes me.

My oldest brother was always quiet and kind of shy. Acting as a role model for me and my other brother, he worked hard in school and pursued extracurricular activities. At the time of my injury, he was out of school and living on his own. As the middle child, my other brother was more aggressive and outgoing. Striving for independence, he couldn't wait to be out on his own. As the youngest of the three boys, I was always on the go. I was very popular in school and gifted athletically. I had just graduated from high school and had secured a baseball scholarship at a nearby university. It had always been my dream to play professional ball. It seemed I had been preparing my whole life to play in the "big show." Little did I know that I was really preparing for the challenge of my life.

After graduating from high school, I was carefree and looked forward to a great future. I was planning on attending Walsh University, where I had been awarded the baseball scholarship, where I would major in business. I could not wait to start college, become independent, and meet new people. New challenges and new opportunities occupied my thoughts.

The summer after my graduation was a time I remember vividly. Playing 80-odd games in 6 weeks and enjoying my new freedom with friends, I thought I had it all. I figured as long as I had baseball, friends, and family, I had everything I would ever need. What I did not figure on was losing baseball, being separated from friends, and becoming almost completely dependent on my family.

On July 29, 1991, a friend and I went to the mall to do some school shopping. Afterward we decided to hang out at the local strip and see what was going on. We ran into two of our friends, Valerie and Bobby Joe. The four of us talked and cruised around enjoying the cool summer night. Around 10:30 p.m., we decided to stop off at Taco Bell to go to the restroom and get some drinks. When we entered the Taco Bell, I noticed nothing unusual so we proceeded to order. It was supposed to be a fun night out on the town, and it probably would have ended that way had the conclusion of the night not found me lying in a coma, fighting for my life.

As we were leaving the restaurant, I still hadn't noticed anything unusual. As I proceeded out the door a couple of steps behind my friends, I was struck in the face by a fist. Swinging around to see who had struck me, I was disoriented. As soon as I swung around, I felt a glass bottle shatter over my right temporal lobe. I immediately fell to the ground where I was kicked and beaten for what felt like an eternity, but was actually only a few minutes. Afterward, I slowly tried to regain consciousness. I was rushed to the hospital where I fell into a coma for a month.

Emerging from my coma was the greatest challenge of my life, a challenge I will never forget. It called for every resource I had if I were to breathe and walk again. It was like I was alone in a dense, thick fog groping for a familiar hand yet unable to find anything concrete and strangely aware of a vast emptiness and solitude. This is a faint reflection of my coma. As I lay there, I experienced repeated flashes of light . . . my brain inevitably reacted. I wondered where the light came from! Had I really seen it or was it only a figment of my imagination? I convinced myself that the flash of light was real and thus my only hope of finding my way back home. From a great distance, I heard the distinct voices of my mother, father, and brothers and Amy, the girl next door. Each time I heard their encouragement, I drew one step closer to the light. Although I felt like falling into despair, a word of love from God, my family, and my friends urged me forward. Without such love I would not have advanced even one step. Along with these words of love, I also heard the muffed voices of doctors and the high-pitched whispers of nurses as they wondered what they could do to help me. Eventually, they concluded that I would not make it. I was determined to prove them wrong.

Every day, I fought the coma with all of my might. Every day, I drew a little closer to the light. Finally, the day came when I opened my eyes and saw the heartbroken tears of the people I loved and longed to be with. Meanwhile, I could not move a single muscle in my body. I could not even talk. However, this did not bring my spirits down; somewhere deep within I knew that I had just answered the greatest challenge of all, the challenge of coming back from virtual death.

After awakening from my coma, I slowly began to realize what had happened. I went from a fully functional young adult to practically a vegetable in a blink of an eye. I was left totally immobile, not able to talk, and my world had seemed to crumble to dust. My family and friends were there to support me; if not for them, I think I would have died.

During the ensuing weeks, the doctors and nurses gave me little hope for recovery, but through persistent pleading, my mother convinced the doctors to give me time before decisions were made to institutionalize me. My family and I vowed to meet this brain injury head on and give it our best. I slowly regained mobility and could see gradual improvements. The doctors also saw my progress and decided to send me to a rehabilitation hospital to continue therapy.

It was at the rehabilitation hospital that my attitude and commitment to recovery preceded all other thoughts. My family, friends, therapist, nurses, and doctors were my team, and they were counting on me to bring them to victory. You see, it was the ninth inning, the game was tied, the bases were loaded, and I was at the plate facing a full count. It was the kind of situation I thrived on. It was do-or-die time. I could dig in, face the challenge, and try, or I could drop my bat, strike out, and die.

The choice was mine. What did I do? Well, I stepped up to the box, dug my feet in, and my mind focused on the pitcher, or in this case, the injury. I saw the ball coming; it was like a balloon. I stepped toward the ball, made a smooth swing, and then I heard a crack. The ball ricocheted off my bat like a bullet from a gun. I just stood there and watched it soar high and long; I knew in an instant it was gone. As I touched each base, a part of my recovery passed, and before I knew it, I was home, starting school, and enjoying life again.

Although my recovery is not yet complete, I play a game every day in my head, and with every hit, catch, and stolen base, a part of my recovery passes. My next home run could be the one that brings me full circle. The pursuit of this dream is encompassed by the determination and hope that one day I will make it back to my ball field. All I can do is try and pray that everything will turn out right, and if it does not, I will still go on because I know I gave it my best.

The road to recovery has been long and wearisome, but I have already put many miles behind me and I know I will emerge completely triumphant. This experience has taught me many valuable lessons. Above all, it has convinced me that the human will can overcome obstacles that many consider insurmountable. I have walked through the valley of the shadow of death and have come out, not unscathed but undaunted. I am among the few people who can say that they have experienced near-death and were able to live and talk about it. I consider myself lucky and remain grateful to all who have helped me recover from this disaster. My experience has indisputably helped make me the person I am today.

Although many things helped my family overcome this catastrophe, the most helpful was first and foremost our faith in God and belief that He would make everything all right. Second, it was the over-whelming support we received from family and friends. How could we not make it with such kindness and compassion? The third thing was becoming knowledgeable about brain injury. This seemed to make us feel more in control of the situation, instead of relying on doctors and nurses for details of what was happening. Throughout the injury, we kept a positive outlook on life, knowing that we would pull through. The family as a whole had a kind of inner strength, which told each member that things would work out in the end. Finally, we came to accept the situation and the consequences it has brought. The past cannot be changed, but the present and future can.

Intervention was never offered to my family. I often wonder why, but I guess no one ever thought to ask what the family needed. Interventions that would have been helpful to my family include:

- A team of doctors who would offer in-depth knowledge on the subject of head injury or offer literature or reading material in a layperson's terms

- Counseling for the family because just being able to talk to someone about what was happening would have helped; information on support groups and meeting other families who have experienced such trauma would have been extremely soothing

- Someone offering assistance with a list of attorneys, if needed, or other medical facilities better equipped and able to help a patient progress

- Someone who would have been able to structure a program that would have fit my family's needs, for example, phone numbers of groups or organizations that offer help, and, if out of town, assistance with lodging, meals, churches, and so forth

After reading and realizing the lack of professional help my family had, I have to wonder what really helped us get through this experience. It seemed that everything that was needed by the family, the family provided. I thank God for giving us the strength, courage, and wisdom to endure each day and for watching over us as we struggle through my head injury.

His Mother's Perspective

I remember lying in bed the night we got the phone call. I was wondering why Chris was late. It was 10:30 p.m. He had gone school shopping at the mall with a friend. It wasn't like him not to call if he was going to stop somewhere else.

Just the weekend before, he had finished up a grueling summer baseball schedule, playing 80-odd games in 6 weeks. He had worked so hard on getting a scholarship, and we were very proud of him. I remember his last tournament game. When they lost, he quickly tossed his uniform, like only a ballplayer could, to get ready for the drive to Walsh University where he would be attending in the fall. It was orientation weekend, but he had come back to play his final game. His dad had said, "Well, Chris, that was your last game." A strange feeling passed through me, and I quickly added, "Until you get to college." As we later drove to the hospital that night, that conversation kept floating through my thoughts.

We really didn't know how bad things were until we arrived at the hospital. When they told us he was having seizures and would need immediate brain surgery, we were devastated. Some friends of ours had gone through a similar experience just the year before, so we were all too aware of the seriousness of the situation. As friends and family gathered at the hospital to keep a constant vigil, the pain and devastation set in. So many questions kept going through our minds. Would he live? If he did, how would he be? Why was this happening to us? The nurses were very helpful and brought much-needed comfort during the long weeks while he was in a coma. My husband and I could not bear to leave the hospital. The doctors did not seem to be educated enough to deal with the situation, so we finally had to make the agonizing decision to have him moved. All along we prayed to God to give us the strength, courage, and wisdom to make the right decisions.

My husband was offered a job, and the decision was made for him to go to work as I stayed with Chris. My husband quickly took over all the responsibilities of working and running the household, plus handling all the stacks of paperwork. I, on the other hand, was learning, right along with Chris, about therapy. Together we struggled to help him get better. For him, it was a matter of working relentlessly to make his body do what he wanted it to do. For me, it was the anguish of watching and being there for my child, but not really being able to make it all better. It was a feeling of helplessness. I was determined to learn everything I could about head injury. Somehow being more knowledgeable on the subject made me feel more in control. I always tried to keep a cheerful, encouraging face on for Chris even though my heart was breaking. My other two sons were great. The middle son remained at home with his father and did everything he could to help out. My oldest son visited Chris daily and opened his bachelor apartment, which he was sharing with two other guys, to me.

Although the outlook was bleak, we never gave up hope that Chris would return to normal. But as we've learned, nothing is ever normal. Our lives are constantly changing. As Chris begins to have more and more control over his body, he seems more content. When Chris started school again after his injury, I never imagined he would do this well or go this far. Having him transferred so far from home has been hard on the whole family, but he seems so happy that it's hard not to be happy for him. From the beginning, he was always accepted for who he was, not for what his body had trapped him into. The son we had was taken from us, but the son we were given back is even better in so many ways. Chris is a constant inspiration to all who come in contact with him. There is not a doubt in my mind that he will succeed in life.

As I reflect back, the pain and hurt will never go away, but I developed a tolerance for it. Life for all of us in this world is a challenge. You draw strength to meet those challenges through those around you. Things are so unpredictable, but would we really want to know how things will turn out? All we can hope for is to be surrounded by love and the courage to face what life has to offer. A Garth Brooks song better explains this point: "Yes my life is better left to chance. I could have missed the pain, but I'd had to miss the dance" (Arata, 1990).

DISCUSSION QUESTIONS

1. If you were engaged and your fiancé/fiancée had a traumatic brain injury, what would you do? What would your family suggest?

2. How would you respond if you or a family member were brain injured as a result of violence?

3. Discuss the athletic frame of reference that Chris had and how it was an asset in his treatment, recovery, and rehabilitation.

4. Why was Chris's family able to rally in a time of crisis?

5. If your loved one were not expected to survive, what would you do if faced with the decision concerning the use of life supports?

6. After reading this personal perspective, would you consider rehabilitation at any cost?

7. What did Chris mean when he stated, "I know I gave it my best."

8. How can people learn to adapt to change as Chris and his family did?

KAREN—MY DAUGHTER FOREVER

LINDA STACEY

Medical History: Karen

I am the mother of Karen. Although it is she who must bear the trauma, the pain, and the limitations, it is I who suffer with her and sometimes, truthfully, because of her.

After writing Karen's brief medical history (see table), I thought I would try to compute the hours spent in and traveling to and from hospitals. I found it impossible—the hours are uncountable. Worse, I think, is the life-or-death surgery with comparatively little follow-up or routine orthopedic surgery, which requires trips to Boston (20 miles one way) three times a week for physical therapy. It has been almost a year since the last surgery, and we are still making the trip twice a month. The exercises are never-ending, the casts must be continually replaced, and trying to motivate acceptance of these responsibilities by Karen was, until recently, next to impossible.

AGE	MEDICAL PROBLEM
4 weeks (4½ pounds)	Open-heart surgery
10½ months	Cerebral palsy diagnosed
2½ years	Brace on leg to allow for walking
6 years	Heel cord surgery
7 years	Open-heart surgery
10 years	Muscle transplant—arm

She is mine forever, I sometimes think. I will never forget the doctor's response when I asked when all this would stop. His answer was to the point: "When her husband takes over." To him, she is not a person but an arm or a leg, depending on where the problems lay at the time.

I think back to her day of birth—thrilled with another girl. Karen was preemie weight but full term. Because she nursed well, she was allowed to come home with me. Symptoms began to appear within a few weeks, but nothing that seemed too unusual. A doctor who cared enough saw her once or twice a week to check and called me often when I didn't call him. Because he cared enough to keep a close watch, he was able to diagnose a congenital heart defect before it was too late—he saved her life. I had never dreamed of a problem of such magnitude.

The diagnosis was a septal defect in the heart. In other words, a hole in the heart that allowed oxygenated blood to mix with deoxygenated blood. Emergency surgery was needed to repair the defect. The doctors would not give us any odds on Karen's survival of the surgery, but she had no chance at all if surgery was not performed. Karen was at the time one of the smallest (although not the youngest) infants to survive this surgery. We thought our problems were over until we discovered (when she was 10½ months old) that Karen had cerebral palsy. It was years before I could say those last two words: cerebral palsy. I always said that she had damage to the motor area of the brain. Somehow that didn't seem so bad.

The cause will always remain unknown. It could be congenital, it could be due to a lack of oxygen before the corrective heart surgery, or it could have happened during the surgery at a time when

---

Reprinted from Power and Dell Orto (2004).

techniques were not perfected for working on such a small child (she was hooked up to an adult-sized heart–lung machine, for example). The cause is unimportant. It is the effects that we must deal with.

At first, the attention a family gets in these circumstances is unbelievable. You're special, everyone wants to help, and there is a certain amount of glory or martyrdom involved. "How do you manage?" they ask. They could never do it. Well, the answer to that is you do it because you have to. There is no one else to do it for you. You only wonder how you managed after the latest crisis has passed. Then it's on to the next crisis—always another one to look forward to. It's almost as if this child will be mine forever—in the sense that I will always be responsible for her. Although this may sound selfish, I can't imagine any parents wanting to keep their children with them for the rest of their lives. Cop out? Maybe it is, but I can't help it.

How do we feel about Karen? It was a long time before I could say that sometimes I hate her for all the problems she presents. A parent cannot easily voice this emotion regarding a child, especially a handicapped child—it's almost inhuman. Karen's sisters could say "hate" much easier—children's feelings are much closer to the surface than those of adults.

On the other hand, these same sisters who sometimes hate her will rise to her defense when they see that she is treated badly. She is not, however, an easy child to get along with. Although Karen functions well in school with a great deal of supportive help (resource room, counseling, etc.), she is socially immature and has no real friendships to rely on. It is we at home who care for her who must bear the brunt of her frustrations—acting out and generally behaving abominably.

Of course, we love Karen, but it is often difficult to show openly. A child of Karen's temperament can drain your emotions. The more affection and attention you give, the more she wants. I often feel as though I am bled dry. She is all-consuming.

Sometimes, I feel pity. What will she be able to do? Because she appears almost normal, people expect normalcy from her. For that matter, so do we, for I am always afraid of selling her short. We demand that she perform tasks that are within her capabilities—even more. If I tie her shoes for her now, who will do it when I'm not here? She needs to know how to tie shoes with one hand. She must learn in spite of herself.

Often I feel compassion. How do you console a child who has no "real" friends? What playmates she does have are not above tormenting her in insidious ways. What do you say when she tells you that the kids at school call her "mental"? How does it feel knowing that if someone comes to call for you, it is only because no one else can come out to play? Telling her not to pay attention is almost ludicrous. These things hurt us both, but it is very difficult to build self-image in a child who is "different" and intelligent enough to know it.

I always feel guilty—not because I've somehow done this to her, but because she is so much better off than other victims of cerebral palsy. Cerebral palsy can be devastating to the point of total immobility and retardation. Karen is neither. Why then should I complain? I guess I can only say that this is our problem, and it is we who must deal with it.

At night, I cry when I see her sleeping. She sleeps relaxed, the spasticity is gone, and the cerebral palsy seems to have disappeared for 12 hours or so. But in the morning, Karen still limps, her hand is still misshapen, and she still has trouble with school work and social adjustment. I cry now.

What will Karen be when she grows up? My head knows that there's a place for her somewhere—my heart wonders if she'll find it.

Update: 30 years later, Karen is married and is working.

DISCUSSION QUESTIONS

1. What role do siblings play in the developmental process of a sibling who is disabled?
2. What role does birth order play in the area of sibling rivalry for an adolescent with a disability?

3. How can the family be a liability in the school-to-work transition for an adolescent with a disability?

4. How has the AIDS issue created additional concerns for families of adolescents with special needs?

5. How would you and your family feel if you had a child like Linda's child and who was making great strides in managing the particular disability but then was diagnosed with another debilitating disease?

6. What advice, help, or insight would you give a family member who may not stop focusing on what he or she has lost because of the caring demands associated with the severe disability of a child?

LIVING IN SPITE OF MULTIPLE SCLEROSIS

TOSCA APPEL

Multiple sclerosis (MS) was something I knew nothing about or even considered being part of my life. Even if I did, it was more an illness for those who were young adults. However, I was one of those rare cases of MS that occur before the age of 20 years—I was 11 years, 9 months old when my first symptom occurred.

My first attack of MS took the form of a lack of motor coordination of my right hand. I was unable to hold utensils, and my hand was turned inward. My parents, in their concern, rushed me to the emergency room of the hospital. The intern who saw me at the emergency room told my parents without any exam that I had a brain tumor. Needless to say, this shocked my parents because, other than this attack limited to my right hand, I was otherwise normal and healthy. I was admitted to the hospital, where I stayed for 12 days. Ten days after the initial attack, the symptoms abated. Two days later, I was discharged from the hospital and was totally back to normal. The doctors had put the blame of the attack on a bad case of nerves. Before the attack, I was enrolled in Grove Lenton School of Boston. This was a very high-pressured school. From my A average in grammar school, my grades had dropped to roughly a B average. I was worried, and I spent many sleepless nights crying myself back to sleep. I could not handle the pressure of going to a private school. Consequently, I transferred to a public junior high school. Without the pressure, my grades went up to an A average. I was happier and everything was fine.

My second attack occurred when I was 16 years old and in the 11th grade. My mother and I were planning my Sweet 16 birthday party. My mother rented a room in a nightclub. I was all excited, planning who I was going to invite, what it was going to be, and what the room was going to be like. One day before the party, my history teacher asked me a question. I stood up to answer, and my speech

Reprinted from Power et al. (1988).

came out all garbled. I was unable to string the words into a sentence. I was even unable to utter words. All that came out were sounds. I clutched my throat to help the words come out easier. At times they did, but at times it came out a garbled mess. I remembered the teacher's look. He looked at me in utter surprise and a little bit helplessly. In total utter shock, my attempts at speech sounded so ludicrous to me—so totally as if it did not belong to my head and so totally foreign that I started laughing hysterically. I couldn't be serious about the sounds I was making. Again, my parents rushed me to the hospital where again another intern did his initial workup on me. However, the sounds that came out of me were so funny that I again started laughing almost hysterically because I was well aware of what I wanted to say and I was also well aware that it was not coming out of my mouth right. The intern, in his wisdom, thought that this behavior was an attention-getter. He thought I was faking the whole thing.

After the first attack, my mother had decided that this time she would not let me be admitted to the hospital. I was then not admitted, but I was instead seen on an outpatient basis. The inability to speak lasted roughly 2 weeks. I had the party and had a good time. But pictures were taken during this time, and I hated them. Why? My smile came out cockeyed. I smiled with the left half of my mouth, without moving the right side. To me it was quite ugly. After my speech returned, the doctors said that the right side of my mouth and tongue were numb and paralyzed, thus making it very hard for me to talk. Overall, I do not remember the attack. Two weeks after this attack, I again went into complete remission.

In 1967, at the age of 19 years, I applied to and was accepted at Northeastern University. However, during the fall term, I started having trouble seeing. My father drove me to the train station so that I would be able to take the trolley to school. But after I got on the trolley, I took it beyond my stop and went to the Massachusetts Eye and Ear Infirmary to have my eyes checked out. I did not tell my family about my concerns because I did not want to worry anybody. A doctor put me through a whole eye workup, and he said that he could not promise how much sight I would get back in my eye but that he would do all he could. Considering that I was an English major and I loved to read, this freaked me out. I asked him if glasses would help, and he said no, that he might be able to get all my sight back or none of it, but that he could not promise me anything. I had to call my mother after I left him. I first went into the restroom and cried. I controlled myself long enough to call my mother. I got off the phone with my mother as quickly as possible and left for school on the train.

During the ride, I was attempting to figure out if it would have been better to have been born blind and never have seen anything than to lose sight after having it and know what you are missing. As a result of this thinking process, I came to the conclusion that it would have been better for me to have been born blind, because I now knew the beauties of a sunset, of reading, of a flower, of all the things that people who have sight take totally for granted. I do not know how I would rationalize it now.

When I got to school I went into the cafeteria, sat with my friends, and began crying. Once I stopped crying, I got it all out of my system, and my friends and I decided that crying would not solve anything and the best thing I could do was to go home, take some medication, and see if my sight returned. When I returned home, I did not initially tell my parents what the doctor had said about the possibility that my sight might not return. I decided that my parents always got very nervous when something happened to me and that there was no need to worry them about me.

So, I did not say anything until my mother mentioned that she had spoken to my neurologist. At this time, unbeknownst to me, I was diagnosed as having MS. My neurologist had told my mother of the diagnosis and told her to tell me. My mother had refused. The doctor then told her that I would never forgive her if she did not tell me. She said that was something that she would have to deal with and did not want to tell me. Consequently, following my mother's wishes, the doctor naturally did not tell me.

The loss of sight in my left eye lasted 3 weeks, and then I went back to college and continued the daily routine of living. Still my mother had not told me about the MS. She bore it alone and did not tell anyone for 6 months after she knew. The only person she spoke to about my MS was my older sister, who is 6 years older than I am. When my mother would become depressed, she would call my sister and cry about the injustice of this happening to me rather than to herself.

My mother's rationale for not telling me was basically twofold. First, she felt that she should not burden me with the knowledge of my chronic degenerative disease because the knowledge of MS could deter me from doing what I wished to do. Second, when my mother saw me running out of the house to go on a date or to a party, she would get scared and sad, thinking about the day that I would not be able to go out and enjoy myself. My mother felt that the knowledge would hang like a cloud over my head, so she made it her responsibility that I was not to know.

However, this conspiracy of silence put my doctors in a difficult position when I went to see them. I would beg the doctor to tell me what was wrong, but he could not because of a promise made to my mother. Because I remembered when a doctor had told me I might have had a brain tumor, which was incorrect, I asked my neurologist if I was going to die of a brain tumor—to which he said, "You can only die of a brain tumor if you have a brain." This may have been a joke to him; it was not for me! The worry about the brain tumor was a preoccupation of mine. My fingers would tingle or I would feel something go wrong with my balance, and I would be worried that it might be caused by a brain tumor. I was really worried about dying. I found no comfort in the silly remark that I would need a brain to have a brain tumor. At the time, I told the doctor that I was not kidding and that I was very worried. To that, he replied that they did not know what was wrong with me, but when they discovered a pill for it they would rush it to me. I left his office feeling very depressed, very alone, and not understood.

Finally, when my mother told me I had MS, I was sad and confused, but also very much relieved. Now there was a basis for my physical concerns. Because I had long periods of remission over the next 10 years, there were the low points of exacerbation but the long periods of life, living, and the pursuit of happiness. It was great to be a young adult who was living life and running ahead of the long-reaching shadow of MS.

At age 28 years, I reached a major crisis point in my life. I was faced with the reality of ongoing deterioration. My sight reached the point where I was not able to read the newspaper. In addition, I lost what functional use I had in my left hand. Although these losses may not seem to be catastrophic issues to the nondisabled, they were catastrophic to me. The reason was that they reaffirmed the reality that I had little control of my body and of what was happening to it.

The feeling intensified when I had to resign myself to the fact that I needed to use a wheelchair. To me, this was an admission of defeat and that my disease was getting the best of me. Although I made the cognitive decision to continue to struggle, it was very difficult when the little physical control I had was slowly eroding away. As a result, I made the choice to live rather than to deteriorate or die. Although this is easy to verbalize, it is often not easy to implement. I can choose to actualize myself, but I am limited by physical and emotional resources to follow through completely in that process.

My unique situation is that I was dependent on my family, with whom I lived. I was also dependent on my mother to provide me with the assistance I needed, such as cooking and partial dressing. Even though I wanted to live independently, I had to accept that I had a wonderful home life, caring parents, and a loyal sister and brother.

The next major transition occurred when my father and mother died, both within the same year. While initially having to deal with the impact of the loss of people I care about, I also had to face the question of what would happen to me. Fortunately, when my parents became ill, I made the choice to get an apartment and to develop the independent-living support systems I would need. Another possibility for me was to extend the relationship with my boyfriend, to whom I was once engaged and whom I had been dating for 15 years. However, this possibility was questionable, for there were reasons we did not get married and they are still real concerns.

This is my response to the disease that has plagued me for 24 years and has altered the course of my life. I will not let it beat me. What motivates me is the memory of my parents and the knowledge of my heritage. My mother and father spent years in a concentration camp, and many of my other family members perished there. I feel the obligation to make the best of my situation and draw on the strength of those persons who suffered far more than I am suffering. As I see it, the key to my ability to survive is the memory, support, and encouragement of others. They have made the difference, accepting me as I am and helping me to resolve my feelings about not being what I was or could have been.

DISCUSSION QUESTIONS

1. What is your reaction to how Tosca was told about her MS?

2. What are the family issues with Tosca that helping professionals should be aware of?

3. After reading her personal perspective, if you were in Tosca's situation, would you consider marriage or having a child?

4. How do societal roles and expectations create stress for women with disabilities?

5. Do you think that the mental health needs of women with disabilities are different from those of men with disabilities? If so, please explain in what way(s)?

6. How would you feel if your parents decided, when you were 17 and had a crippling disability, to place you in another caring environment so that better care could be given to your sibling who also had a devastating illness?

SURVIVING AMYOTROPHIC LATERAL SCLEROSIS: A DAUGHTER'S PERSPECTIVE

JUDY TEPLOW

Betty Miller: Beloved Wife, Mother, and Grandmother, September 4, 1986, Age 70 Years

In the early spring, when the ground is soft, I will lay a marker on my mother's grave, a permanent marker to commemorate the life of a very special lady. The inscription will be short, impersonal, and incomplete—and somehow not befitting a woman who courageously struggled against a devastatingly cruel terminal illness.

I cannot inscribe her story in stone, but I can set it on paper as a lasting tribute. I hope it will be a comfort to those who are afflicted with a serious or terminal illness and a help to the families and health professionals who are involved in their care and treatment.

Reprinted from Power and Dell Orto (2004).

It was going to be an unbearable, oppressive day, but my mother had no intention of sitting in her small, air-conditioned apartment. She set out early with her walking buddies on their 5-mile jaunt and, as usual, took the lead. She was amused that her companions, who towered over her 5-foot frame, could not keep up with her brisk pace.

Everything seemed to be going well for her and my dad. Retirement for them was not a sedentary life, but rather one that was full and gratifying. In a few weeks, they would return to their apartment in Boston for 5 months of relief from Florida's intolerable heat.

But for now, Betty was enjoying her walk and thinking about how rich her life was. As she turned the bend, her thoughts were cut off abruptly by a stiffening in her left leg—perhaps a cramp—but she did not have the pain associated with a cramp. Her gait slowed down considerably, and in a minute she found herself lying on her side. She was stunned by this unexpected interruption. She did not stumble over a rock or a crack in the roadside. What should she attribute this weakness to?

It took 5 months for the doctors to make an accurate diagnosis. An electromyogram was performed at the Brigham and Women's Hospital, and it was this test that ultimately determined that my mother had amyotrophic lateral sclerosis (ALS), Lou Gehrig's disease, a progressive, degenerative disease that is terminal. It is probably the most dreaded neurological disease and is one with no known cause or cure.

Within 1 year of the first visible symptom, Betty would be a virtual paraplegic, confined to a wheelchair, unable to talk or to feed herself. Breathing and swallowing would become progressively more difficult. At no time would the disease affect her mental faculties, and she would always be aware of the creeping paralysis.

My initial reaction to the diagnosis was one of disbelief, devastation, and helplessness. How could such an active and health-conscious person be stricken with such a catastrophic illness? I felt a sadness for my parents, and I had real concerns about my dad's health also. It was conceivable to me that this tragedy could destroy him as well, and I prepared myself for the worst.

The family and doctors were in total agreement as to how much to tell my mother. She had always been petrified of doctors and hospitals and was by nature very nervous and anxious. We knew that she could not cope with such outrageous news.

She was told that she had a chronic neuromuscular disease and that she would need intensive therapy. We did not offer her hope of a cure, nor did we inform her that she was terminally ill. She asked very few questions, wanted to know as little as possible about her disease, and became adept at tuning out whatever she was not ready to hear.

Like my mother, my aunt, my father, and my brother went to great lengths to avoid the truth. Denial became a protective measure they were to use effectively throughout the course of the illness. As much as I tried to beat through this barrier, I was met with resistance. It was this resistance that was to become a great source of frustration and anger for me. My aunt held out the longest, talking about the research, cures, and the possibility of people living several years. My brother, who never coped with adversity too well, did not become an integral part of the team, and his visits to the nursing home were often sporadic and brief.

I had to know all the medical aspects of the disease, so I asked a lot of questions and read many books on ALS and on death and dying. Someone had to take charge, to plan, and to carry the family through this crisis.

From the Brigham and Women's Hospital, my mother was transferred to the Braintree Rehabilitation Hospital. It was there that she was put on a daily regimen of physical, speech, and occupational therapies. She was extremely tense and frightened, but the staff was very professional and experienced and knew how to respond to her emotional and physical needs. This was really not a time for rehabilitation as much as a time for enormous adjustment. It also allowed the family to make plans for home healthcare. I wished that my mother could stay at Braintree indefinitely, for I feared that the support systems at home would not be adequate.

My fears were well founded. She was not home 2 months when all systems began to break down. My mother required constant attention, and the Visiting Nurse Association and private-home health professionals were not able to keep up with her demands. Oftentimes, my father was left without help, and he had to assume the role as a primary caregiver. Tensions mounted and tempers began to flare, and what was once a very happy marriage now appeared to be very strained. My dad's health was deteriorating as well as my mother's, and they looked to me for a quick solution.

I knew that my mother required round-the-clock care in a skilled nursing facility, but I did not want to be responsible for initiating the search. I could not find it in my heart to do this to her, especially when she threatened to commit suicide before she would enter a nursing home. My grandmother had taken her own life because she could not cope with a painful illness, so I was worried about my mother's intentions. I began to get pressure from her sister also, in defiance of any plan to move my mom from her home. We were in a crisis, and we needed help quickly.

I was fortunate to find a psychologist who would help me accept and confront problems that were difficult and painful. He helped me see issues more clearly when everything seemed overwhelming and confusing. It was through him that I began to understand the complexities surrounding chronic and terminal illnesses. His continued support and genuine concern were to sustain me through some very difficult times, the first of which was my mother's move to a nursing home.

The transition from the apartment to the nursing home was traumatic for the family. Ostensibly, the home was attractive and meticulous, with spacious rooms and beautiful furnishings. In sharp contrast to this orderliness was a picture of deterioration—of very old people in their 80s and 90s ravaged by debilitating diseases, marked with permanent deformities, hooked up to life-supporting machines, impaired by mental illness—an aura of sadness and loneliness and a sense that many of these people were deserted by their families.

I wished that I could put blinders on my mother's eyes—to shut out a world that was so unreal but yet only too real and disheartening. My mother was only 69 years old and looked 10 years younger. How could we do this to her! I knew that there was no alternative, but I was stricken with guilt, a guilt that was to stay with me for a long time. It took a good 3 months before I could walk into the nursing home without feeling sick—without feeling very, very shaken.

I don't think my mother ever adjusted to nursing-home life. I think she resigned herself to her fate. I know she often felt very sad, lonely, and misunderstood, but I do not think she felt abandoned. She knew that the family was there for her, and it was this prevailing sense of security that kept her from slipping into a deep depression.

A schedule was worked out, wherein one or two family members would visit daily. This was arranged, mostly out of love, partly out of guilt, and out of an acute awareness that strangers would not minister to her needs the way family would. We also knew that if we were going to survive this ordeal, we would have to share the responsibilities, for each of us had a history of medical problems. Often, the burden of responsibility rested on my shoulders, and at times I felt overwhelmed. But I also felt that if my mother could cope with the effects of a very disabling disease, I could deal with any problems that arose.

I do not know how she endured all the suffering, and I do not understand what held her together. She certainly did not triumph over her disease—she did not write a book, or paint by mouth, or engage in anything that was extraordinary. She just tried to get through the day. There were many tears and many moments of anguish, but even in her despair, she insisted on getting up, getting dressed, and—above all—having her hair done weekly. Thank God there was a hairdresser on the premises, and thank God she still cared about her appearance. Throughout her illness, she never lost her sense of humor or her ability to smile and laugh. But the laughing was done for the staff, and most of the crying was done with the family.

We tried to maintain a sense of equilibrium, but it was difficult to keep control when all systems were failing. The disease was progressing at an alarming rate, and we knew she would need the strong support of the family and the specialized services of many healthcare professionals. Some services were effective, but most fell short. Many professionals were not familiar with or could not cope with the demands of ALS. They were uneasy in treating a terminally ill patient or clearly had an attitude problem toward the sick and the elderly. I must acknowledge, though, that most people did try to help, and I cannot fault them for their human limitations in dealing with a very difficult case.

I also believe that my mother's inability to speak had a lot to do with the quality of care she received. This was a great source of frustration for her and for the health professionals who worked with her. The family members were the only ones who had the patience to make use of the communication boards. We acted as liaison between my mother and the staff, so our involvement in her care was crucial.

We also acted as her advocates and protectors. There were aspects of nursing-home care that were unsettling, but because we had a very good working relationship with the staff, most of our grievances were worked out. I can only think of one incident that was offensive and repulsive, and it was due to a personality conflict between my mother and an aide. An aide had lost control and, out of anger and impatience, threw a sheet over my mother's head. This was a gross violation of my mother's right to be treated as a living human being until the day she died.

The only other situation that disturbed me occurred outside the home. A week before my mother died, her doctor was called to check on her deteriorating condition. To our dismay, we learned that the doctor was on vacation and had left instructions for the covering physician. Her doctor had promised to leave explicit directions regarding heroic measures. This was not an insignificant oversight. I had chosen this doctor because he had been highly recommended by another physician and was on staff at a hospital directly opposite the nursing home. Because of his close proximity, I thought that he would be accessible to my mother and the family, but unfortunately we found him to be very impersonal and distant.

Without the encouragement and concern of a handful of people, the experience would have been unbearable. There were three exceptionally caring people who made a great impact on my mother.

Janet, a nurse's aide, became my mother's guardian angel, and she was to watch over her and attend to all her needs while she was in the nursing home. There was such a strong attachment between them that on the day my mom died Janet was unable to work.

Margaret, the assistant director of nursing at the nursing home, had lost her mother to ALS, and she was familiar with the disease and its effects on the family. She was always available to us, and it was not unusual for her to interrupt a busy schedule to explain what comfort measures should be used. She was also instrumental in educating the staff about the nature of the disease. She was my inspiration and a great source of strength.

Bobby was a close friend of the family. He had experienced the loss of a loved one, so he was no stranger to personal tragedy. He attended many workshops with Elizabeth Kübler-Ross and was involved in hospice, and he knew how to relate to the terminally ill. Bobby showered my mother with gifts and flowers and made her feel very special. He was the only one who could talk to her about death and life after death and ultimately helped her accept her mortality. He was a good friend to me also, and I was able to talk with him about my greatest fear—the use of life-support systems.

The issue of support systems was always a source of great pain and anguish for me. My anxiety was heightened by my mother's refusal to discuss these matters and the inability of family members to agree on a specific course of action. I personally believed that the use of heroic measures in my mother's case would be cruel and inhumane—a prolongation of inexorable suffering pain—and an interference with the natural order of things.

But I had to know where my mother stood on these issues for, ultimately, it was her life and her decision. Three months before her death, she began to make her wishes known. She slowly spelled out the word die every day. She made it quite clear to me that she could no longer tolerate living. She finally came to terms with her death, knew it was imminent, and had an urgency to express her grief and fears about dying. Once she accepted her death, she became more tranquil.

I did not want my mother to die in the arms of strangers, nor did I want her to experience death alone. I was fortunate to be with her at the final moment of death. My aunt and I sat by her side and held her hands, and except for a brief interruption by staff, this was a family affair. We exchanged a few words of support and comfort, but we were mostly caught up in remembering and recollecting. I wondered if my mother saw her life flashing before her and if she were passing through the dark tunnel toward Omega, but I could not be sure.

DISCUSSION QUESTIONS

1. What aspects of Judy's mother's transition from the apartment to the nursing home were most traumatic for the family?

2. How does the slow deterioration of an elderly parent emotionally affect the immediate members of his or her family?

3. What is the meaning of the statement: "My mother's inability to speak had a lot to do with the quality of care she received"? What is the relationship between those two factors?

4. Are there additional roles, other than advocate and protector, that an adult child of a chronically ill parent must play during the illness?

5. Of the three "exceptionally caring people who made a great impact on my mother," who would you choose if you could only select one to care for your own mother who may be chronically ill and needs caregiving efforts?

6. If you were in a similar situation with an elderly, chronically ill parent, what would be your reaction to the statement, "She made it quite clear to me that she could no longer tolerate living"?

MY LIFE WITH A DISABILITY: CONTINUED OPPORTUNITIES

PAUL EGAN

For me life began very comfortably more than 57 years ago in a then-affluent suburb of Greater Boston. I was the third son of a prominent up-and-coming general contractor. I also had an older sister. A month before I was born, tragedy befell the family when the firstborn son, then aged 6 years, died of diphtheria. So, when I arrived healthy and sound, I was a most welcome addition to a grieving mother and father. Just before I turned 2, another brother was born.

In September 1944, I entered the U.S. Navy, and after completing boot camp, I was initially assigned to motor-torpedo boats in the Philippines. I was then assigned to a yard minesweeper with a team of 22 officers and men. Our assignment consisted of sweeping (dragging) the shipping channels and ports of the Philippine Islands. During this time, my job performance was classified as outstanding, and I received many promotions. However, my life suddenly came apart. While I was moving a keg of concentrated ammonia across the deck, it blew up in my face. The ammonia burned my eyes, the linings of my nose and throat, and also the skin around my facial area. I was rendered unconscious,

---

From Power et al. (1988). Reprinted with permission.

and on regaining consciousness 3 days later, the doctor told me that my eyes were badly burned and that I would have to be patient and pray for a miracle to take place.

One year, seven hospitals, and several operations later, vision returned to my right eye to the degree of 20/70 with corneal scarring. Other complications emerged as my head and my right hand had a constant tremor. This ailment was incorrectly diagnosed as a nervous anxiety reaction. So I became a psychiatric bouncing ball. In May 1947, I was discharged with a 70% Veterans Affairs (VA) compensation.

I immediately went to work for a friend, pumping gas in a gas station. But I had greater ambitions, and I enrolled at Boston Business Institute in a business administration curriculum for 2 years. Shortly after I returned to school, my mother developed cancer and passed away on December 15, 1947. This was a profound loss to all of us, as my mother was always on hand with her guidance and sense of fortitude. She was always there to listen, to encourage me to make the most of myself, and to go back to school. In fact, in the initial stages of my readjustment to civilian life and to my own disability, it was Mom's positive attitude, including her expectations for me, that inspired me to move forward. Her philosophy of making one's residual assets work for the fulfillment of goals is one that I have adopted in my own life.

In June 1948, I married Marietta, a girl I had known before I entered the service. Around this time, my father went on a trip to Newfoundland, his place of birth, and came back a few months later, married. He had married his brother's housekeeper, a plain-appearing woman who was 25 years younger than he was. They immediately isolated themselves from all family and friends for years to come.

In June 1949, I graduated from business school and started experimenting with the real world. Although I was very fortunate in not being unemployed for more than a month during the next 24 years, my choice of expanding my horizons was limited greatly by an uninformed business environment. Time after time when applying for positions for which I was qualified, ignorance, fear, stigmatization, and prejudice were barriers I found most difficult to overcome.

During the next 20 years, my wife gave birth to five daughters, we moved to a larger house, and I was employed in various jobs. Shortly after the birth of our first daughter, I began a series of operations on my left eye. These operations climaxed with an unsuccessful corneal transplant, which resulted in the surgical removal of my left eyeball. Soon after the birth of our second daughter, I had a laminotomy. I understood this operation as involving the transaction of the thin layers of connective tissues around the optic nerve. The pain and suffering endured were the most excruciating of my life. But I was able to get through all of this because of the support of my wife. We didn't think about the past or about my other disabilities. We focused on the present, and together we often discussed our mutual concerns. This was a tremendous help to get through my own sufferings. But in 1968, my tremors got worse, and I went into a VA hospital for a brain operation. After doing an encephalogram, the doctor thought that the risks were too high. Instead of the operation, a new experimental drug was tried, but that increased the body involvement and was quickly discontinued.

Moreover, a trauma occurred in our family on a night in January 1970 when the temperature was 25 degrees below zero and our oil-burning furnace exploded, destroying our home and all of our possessions. All of our neighbors came to our support, and they held a fundraising party for us that resulted in not only a substantial amount of money but also in donations of services in our efforts to rebuild. Another factor in our rebuilding effort was that after an absence of more than 20 years, my father reappeared and lent us the remaining necessary funds to rebuild. After we had made a few repayments he said, "You've shown good faith," tore up the note, and then chose to go back into hibernation with his wife. I tried on numerous occasions to visit with him on his 90-acre farm, but he was always "out" or had to go some place in a hurry.

After getting settled into our new home in June 1970, our life returned to a semblance of normalcy until late in 1973 when I lost my job. My employment was not the only loss, however, for I also lost my sense of dignity and self-respect, and I drifted aimlessly in a sea of self-pity and depression for nearly 4 years. Though my family was very supportive of me during this time, I knew this was my own struggle and they themselves had to survive. My daughters were married and had their own families, but seemed to be there when I needed someone to share my feelings.

In June 1977, I was classified as blind. That November I entered the VA Blind Rehabilitation Center at West Haven, Connecticut, and from that time on life took on a new perspective. After 14 weeks of intensive training and guidance, I was again doing things for and by myself. The educational-testing evaluations done at the center indicated a potential for higher education. So in September 1978, I returned to school with the goal of becoming a social worker. In May 1982, I received my BS from Suffolk University, and then in 1984, I earned an MS from Boston University. In April of that year, I began a new career as a field representative and outreach-employment specialist with the Blind Veterans Association. Yet as I look back now on all of these years of family life, of living with my disabilities, and then finally becoming blind, I often think of my own family, with their patience and understanding. They made the difference so often during my many rehabilitation efforts. Even when I became depressed, they urged me to continue, for somehow they appreciated what I could still do. Probably I would never have gone back to school without their encouragement. Even my father, who died in 1978 and who really never got over the shock of seeing his first financial empire disintegrate, was there one time when we really needed some assistance. To all of my family, I say thank you.

DISCUSSION QUESTIONS

1. After reading the personal perspective by Paul Egan, at what time during the progressive deterioration of his eyesight do you think that family intervention would have been most effective?

2. After reading the chapters in Part IV related to intervention approaches and resources, what do you consider the role of spirituality and could it be applicable to Paul Egan's family?

3. If disability or a severe illness occurred in your own family, and considering Brodwin et al.'s chapter "Users of Assistive Technology: The Human Component," how would you access the resources that could provide assistive technology?

4. Discuss the issues related to the following statement: "I really can't have any effective contact with a family that is living with a disability situation unless I have a degree in family counseling or family therapy."

EXPERIENCING SEXUALITY AS AN ADOLESCENT WITH RHEUMATOID ARTHRITIS

ROBERT J. NEUMANN

It was a walk I'd taken many times before, down to the train station of our town in suburban Chicago to watch the sleek yellow Milwaukee Road streamliners pass through. Usually it was nothing for the healthy 12-year-old kid that I was. Just seven or eight shady, tree-lined blocks—but today it felt like miles. With every step, my right knee was aching more, feeling more stiff.

My friend Terry was walking along with me. I gritted my teeth against the rising pain and struggled to maintain a steady gait. I didn't want Terry to know. I sensed that this was no ordinary ache, and I feared he would not understand. I was right on both counts.

Finally, I could stand it no longer. "You know, Terry, my right knee's feeling awfully stiff and sore," I said.

Without missing a beat, my horror-film-aficionado friend shot back, "Must be rigor mortis!"

Happily, rigor mortis it wasn't, just rheumatoid arthritis. Yet it would be 5 painful months before I and my family had even the small comfort of that diagnosis. But, in a way, Terry was right: It was the demise of the lifestyle I had known for my entire previous 12 years.

By my 12th birthday, I was just beginning to feel that things were going really well. I enjoyed getting out of the house by taking long rides on my bicycle; the guys were actually beginning to seek me out to play baseball with them; I was positively ecstatic when my parents allowed me to take my first long-distance train trip all alone to visit an aunt in Pittsburgh.

The arthritis changed all that. Literally within days my right knee became so stiff, swollen, and sore that it was all I could do to hobble from bedroom to bathroom to kitchen. I began seeing a bewildering succession of doctors who could not even arrive at a diagnosis, much less an effective treatment. They hypothesized tuberculosis or cancer of the bone. Their treatments were progressively more drastic: aspiration of the knee, a leg brace, exploratory surgery. None accomplished much more than aggravating the condition physically and sending me emotionally even deeper into fear and depression. This was the late 1950s, and apparently in those days even the medical profession was less aware that rheumatoid arthritis can and does affect people of all ages, young and old.

Early in 1960, I went to the Mayo Clinic, where my arthritis was diagnosed at last and where more appropriate treatment was prescribed. Nonetheless, even this was not able to halt the progression of the disease to my other joints. First, it was my other knee, then my ankles, then my fingers, then my elbows, then my neck, then my hips, then. . . . With a sort of gallows humor, I'd say I had joined the Joint-of-the-Month Club. But behind this facade, I was terrified at how my body was progressively deteriorating before my eyes. Actually, I would avoid seeing it—or letting others see me—as much as possible. I would refuse all invitations to go to the beach or park for fear I would have to wear shorts that would expose my spindly, scarred legs. I would wear hot, long-sleeved shirts on even the most blistering summer days to avoid anyone seeing my puny arms.

One day, almost by chance, I could avoid it no longer. I caught a good look at myself in a full-length mirror and was appalled at what I saw. I had remembered myself as having an able body. The person I saw looking back at me had a face swollen from high doses of cortisone, hands with unnaturally bent fingers, and legs that could barely support his weight.

I felt devastated. But as I look back on it now, I believe that experience of seeing myself as I really was, was the first step in becoming comfortable with the person I am. Of course, what I did not realize then was that I was a victim not just of a disease but of that even more insidious social phenomenon that Beatrice Wright (1983) has identified as the idolization of the normal physique. As a society, we celebrate the body beautiful, the body whole. As Dion et al.'s (1972) research has demonstrated, we believe that what is beautiful in conventional terms is good, and we equate physical attractiveness with greater intelligence, financial success, and romantic opportunities. Media images of all types reinforce the notion that being young, active, and attractive is the ticket to the good life. Lose that attractiveness, lose that physical perfection, the images imply, and gone as well are the chances for success in love and life. This is definitely not the type of foundation on which an adolescent's fragile self-concept is likely to develop a solid, confident base.

From Power et al. (1988). Reprinted with permission.

But painful as it was, looking at myself in the mirror and seeing myself as I really was, was the prerequisite for self-acceptance. It was acknowledging the physical facts, if not liking them. It was not until years later when I was in graduate school that I attended a seminar given by a marvelous person named Jesse Potter and came to understand that our culture's body-beautiful emphasis is only one way—one narrow, constricting way—of viewing reality. She helped me redefine my experience and understand that a person's attractiveness, a person's value, depends on who one is, not on how one appears. Simple as it sounds, for me that was a revelation and a liberation to realize that in the words of the *Velveteen Rabbit* (Williams, 1975), "once you are real, you can't be ugly—except to those who don't understand."

If my rheumatoid arthritis was a trauma for me, its effects also extended to stress other members of the family. My mother was a quiet source of support and preferred to keep her feelings about the disease to herself. Often she would cry alone in her room; she told me this only years later. But nowhere were the effects of the disease more evident than on my father. A traveling salesman with stubborn ways and a volatile temperament, my father would frequently return from business trips edgy, angry, and generally out of sorts. This in turn caused me to dread these homecomings because as an adolescent I had no way of predicting what mood he might be in or what might set him off. It was only after I had moved from home and was employed as a hospital-based psychologist that he felt free enough to tell me how he could do nothing but think of me at home while he was spending those long hours driving the expressways and lonely country roads, worried by how sick I was and frustrated by his own powerlessness to do anything about it—if only he had been able to express those feelings openly and directly 20 years earlier.

One subject my father was able to express himself directly on was the topic of education and my future. He put it in his customary unvarnished manner: "Bob, you don't have much of a body. But you got a good mind. If you're going to succeed, you've got to use it." And as I was growing up, there never was any question I would succeed. It was simply assumed I would do well in school, go on to college, and get well-paid employment. Clearly, I internalized these expectations for academic success even more than my father intended. But there is no doubt his high expectations functioned as a self-fulfilling prophecy. In large measure, I owe the PhD after my name, the jobs I have had, and many of the wonderful people I have met to my father's simple belief that I could and would. And today, when I work with clients, it is a particular frustration to see how many parents needlessly limit their disabled children's life possibilities through well-intentioned but misguided protectionism or realism that lowers expectations for success by focusing on all the problems rather than on the potentials.

During my high school days, my social life was virtually nonexistent. Because I received physical therapy at home in the afternoon and because my stamina was poor in any event, I only attended school until about 1 p.m. This eliminated any possibility of interacting with peers in extracurricular activities. To complicate the situation further, because my life revolved around classes and studying, I routinely received unusually good grades and routinely broke the class curve, much to the animosity of those peers I did interact with. But perhaps most significant, the school I attended was a Catholic, all-boys high school. This removed me from any contact whatsoever with the female part of the population at a time when my interest was anything but dormant. I literally had only one date, with the daughter of family friends, during my entire 4 years of high school. This situation bothered me enough that I eventually discussed it with my biology teacher. A layman, he suggested that things would be better when I got to college, a response that was only partially more reassuring and accurate than that of the priests who counseled cold showers when issues like these arose.

These less-than-satisfying experiences have led me to be a strong advocate of mainstreaming. From one perspective, I was fortunate to have experienced a limited form of mainstreaming in an era before the advent of Public Law 94–142. At least the interactions I had with male peers gave me a basic idea of how able-bodied adolescent males view the world. Unfortunately, neither the school authorities nor my parents understood how important it was to ensure that deficits in social skills would not develop through lack of informal, out-of-classroom socialization with male peers and the total lack of contact with any female ones. Meanwhile, I unsuspectingly continued to study and dream of the day I would start college and the active love life I had fantasized about for so long.

Finally, the big day arrived. Armed with a body of knowledge about women derived solely from TV, James Bond movies, and the *Playboy* magazines my younger brother smuggled in, I arrived at a small Midwestern college never dreaming I was, in reality, as green as the lovely pines that graced the campus.

It took only a short while before I noticed that my actual accomplishments with women were falling far short not only of my expectations but also of the experiences of my friends and acquaintances. Within a few months, most of the people I knew, both men and women, had developed ongoing intimate relationships. Everywhere the couples were obvious: sitting together in classes, dining together in the cafeteria, partying together at dances, studying together, walking together, and sleeping together. I, on the other hand, became frustratingly adept at performing all these activities alone.

Actually, I was quite good at developing nonsexual friendships with women, especially those who had other boyfriends. I could relate well to them because there was no need for me to do the mating dance, no need for me to call on sociosexual skills I had never learned. These friendships were a mixed blessing. They provided emotional support and the beginning of much-needed learning about the opposite sex. But inevitably there were many poignant moments when my friend would go off to her lover, and I would go off alone. As unpracticed as I was in picking up social cues, I continually confused friendship and romantic messages when meeting apparently available new women. A poem I wrote at that time unintentionally reflected the confusion:

> LOST
> I like you
> when we joked and laughed 'bout people that we knew. I wanted
> you
> when you softly said
> that you must have love too. I love you
> then you took his hand, and oh, I knew, I knew.

It was a depressing pattern. A woman would express an incipient interest; I would misread the cues and respond inappropriately, then feel crushed when the relationship died. Rejection and depression became themes that were only too familiar. I became convinced I was unlovable.

Finally, my roommate Michael decided to do something about the situation. A self-styled ladies' man with the body and bravado of a Greek god, Michael appointed himself my teacher. My first assignment was to read a book he provided me with called *Scoremanship* (Gray, 1969). Once I had finished the book, Michael proclaimed me ready for field experience. It was late on Friday afternoon, and Michael and I were having an early supper in the cafeteria.

"Bob," he nudged me. "Isn't that that Jane over there you've been wanting to go out with?"

"Yeah," I responded dubiously, looking at a woman several tables from us. "Well, remember the book. Just go up and ask her to go to a movie tonight." "Tonight?" I nearly choked. "But it's too late. She's probably got ten dozen things to do."

"Self-defeating talk is unknown to the Scoreman," Michael smiled serenely. "Just go and do it!"

Michael would not let me back out, so I figured I had no alternative but to go forward and experience my next rejection. Slowly I walked over to her table. "Oh, hi, Jane!" I said, as if I'd just noticed her. "You know, uh, seeing you here reminds me. I was thinking of going to a movie tonight. Would you like to come?" Listening to myself, I was sure she'd never buy this one. "Why I'd love to!" she enthused. "Pick me up at my dorm in a half-hour!"

I could hardly believe it. I rushed back to our table. "My God! She actually said yes. She actually said yes! What do I do now?"

Michael gazed at me with a smile of patient superiority. "You take her to the movie. Then you bring her back to our room. I'll fix everything up. Don't you worry about a thing."

The date itself was fine. The movie was enjoyable, and the conversation relaxed and friendly. She even agreed to come back to the room for a drink.

I put the key in the door. As I opened it, I discovered just how much fixing Michael had done. Out billowed clouds of incense. Inside the room, candles everywhere cast their flickering light on *Playboy* magazines that had been artfully strewn about and opened to the most suggestive pages. Clothes and books were piled high on all the furniture except my bed. (So she would have to sit right beside me, Michael later explained.) But the crowning touch came when I noticed that on the night table beside my bed, Michael had arranged a little altar, complete with candles, a small *Playboy* calendar, and an opened package of condoms. I could have died.

Needless to say, seeing all this, Jane instantly developed a headache that required her immediate return to her dorm. After she had set out for her dorm, and though Michael had been trying to be a friend, I was embarrassed and set out to find him and relate my feelings.

Obviously, my role models were not always the most appropriate. And being the only disabled person on that small campus meant I did not have the benefit of interacting with and learning from other disabled peers. Nonetheless, I was learning, observing which things I did worked and which did not. Over time, even I could see that I was gradually improving my relationships.

My senior year eventually arrived, and I celebrated my 21st birthday—still without ever having experienced a physical relationship. Chronologically, I had come of age, but emotionally I still felt insecure, lacking the physical experience that symbolized manhood. I assumed my disability was largely to blame, since by then I knew I could develop nonsexual friendships with ease. Increasingly I came to view my virginity as a barrier in need of being surmounted. But this was not just a matter of desire, a stirring of hormones. To me it was also a matter of self-worth and self-esteem. For as long as I was valued by others only for my companionship and intelligence, I still was not being related to as a whole person, a person with sexual dimensions and emotional, intellectual, and spiritual ones—and I feared for whether I ever would be a whole person.

As it happened, that doubt was soon to be laid to rest in a manner I could never have foreseen. It was a Saturday night, and my friend Justin and I had just finished viewing an on-campus theatrical production by the Garrick Players when we encountered Sarah in the foyer. Justin had been friends with her for some time, but I knew her only peripherally from having shared a class or two and an occasional meal in the cafeteria. Generally, Sarah traveled in a different circle from mine. But tonight she was alone, so after some discussion we three agreed it would be fun to drive to town to get a drink.

We stopped at the Nite-N-Gale, a popular campus hangout, and had a couple of glasses of wine. But mostly we just talked. The conversation was good: comfortable and convivial, a pleasant mix of the light-hearted and the more serious. After a while, we headed back to Sarah's room on campus and continued in the same vein. Midnight arrived, and Justin declared himself tired and left for his room, leaving Sarah and me alone.

The conversation turned more serious. She asked me what it was like to live with arthritis. I told her about the Joint-of-the-Month Club and looking in the mirror. She in turn shared some of the hurts she felt in growing up in poverty with parents in ill health. Finally, I noticed it was approaching 2 a.m. "Well, I guess it's time to go," I said.

"You don't sound too wild about it, Bob."

I was surprised she had picked up on a reluctance I thought I was not showing. "Yeah, you're right," I sighed. "It's just that when I get back to the room I'll find Michael there with his girlfriend. It's damn depressing. Hell, I met her before he did! I liked her too!"

For a long second, Sarah just stared at me. Then a smile, warm and tender like I had never before seen, began to cross her face. "Bob, you know you don't have to," she said.

I will never forget Sarah, perhaps more than most people will never forget their first. What we shared was physical, but also far more. With her, I did not have to worry about how to handle the issue of my disability because to my astonishment, she did not view my disability as an issue: The mere fact that our relationship was physical confirmed as nothing else could that this, too, was possible. The effect on my self-esteem was tremendous. As a disabled colleague once remarked, "When most of your problems have been on a physical level, it's on the physical level that you're most strongly reassured." That statement has always stayed with me, even though I would amend the thought somewhat. Self-esteem is most enhanced when one's positive expectations converge with the reality of one's experience. Lack one or the other, and the individual suffers. At any rate, I still recall how brilliantly the sun was shining the next day as Sarah and I walked across the campus.

DISCUSSION QUESTIONS

1. What was your reaction to the statement by Neumann: "Self-esteem is most enhanced when one's positive expectations converge with the reality of one's experiences"?

2. Who should be responsible for sex education programs for adolescents coping with disabilities?

3. What role has society played in the formulation of attitudes toward the sexuality of persons with disabilities?

4. Would there be a significant difference in the critical issues with a young woman who has had an experience similar to that of Neumann as related in his personal perspective?

5. How is an adolescent's search for self-identity complicated by a serious, chronic disability?

6. What is the role of the health professional in working with parents concerned about the sexuality of their children?

MY LIFE WITH MUSCULAR DYSTROPHY: LESSONS AND OPPORTUNITIES

ROBERT P. WINSKE

I am 41 and the middle son of three boys born with a rare form of muscular dystrophy known as *nemaline rod myopathy*. To date, there is still little information known about the disease, as was the case at the time when we were born in the early to mid-1960s, though it is clear that it is a progressive condition and is passed from mother to son. At the time of each of our births, what made the case more baffling to the doctors was how this occurred. As I stated, muscular dystrophy is a congenital

Reprinted from Power and Dell Orto (2004).

impairment that is passed through the X chromosomes of the mother. To my mother's knowledge, however, she herself didn't have the disability.

When my older brother was born, the doctors requested that my parents check the family tree and see whether there was anyone on either side of the family who may have had muscular dystrophy. As requested, my parents, with the assistance of their parents, did check each side, and their efforts proved unsuccessful. To their knowledge, no one on either side of the family had ever been diagnosed and treated for any form of the impairment. Though my mother did have a physical disability, to her knowledge it was polio, not muscular dystrophy. She became sick as a young child in the late 1940s, which was at the height of the polio epidemic that extended into the early 1950s. Growing up, my mother always talked about getting sick when she was a young girl when her muscles got weak, especially in her lower extremities, and was told by her parents that it was polio. She had no reason to doubt this information because her mother was a registered nurse. She was also treated in hospital wards where several children her age were being treated for the same condition, and some were worse than she was. My mother was still able to walk, which was not so for most of the children.

As there were no signs of the disease found on either side of the family, the doctors believed that the occurrence of muscular dystrophy was a fluke. There was no reason why it occurred, and they informed my parents that to their understanding, the odds of their having another child with the birth defect were unlikely. This led them to decide to have another child. Like my brother, I also was born with the same form of muscular dystrophy. This really perplexed the doctors not only because my parents had another baby with the disease but also because I wasn't as severely impacted by its limitations.

However, following the birth of a second child with the neuromuscular condition, the doctors again insisted that someone on one side of the family had to have had the condition. They even wondered whether a family member had a baby with the same or similar condition but never took the baby home. This was common at that time, as children with birth defects were generally institutionalized because it was an embarrassment to families to have children with impairments. It was also believed that parents couldn't provide the needed specialized care. If this were the case, the doctors believed that whoever in the family may have had a child with muscular dystrophy wouldn't want to admit to it, being ashamed or embarrassed, because of the belief that everyone wants the perfect baby.

Following the doctor's recommendation, my parents again went back to their parents to examine both sides of the family. It was emphasized that it was important to know whether there was any family history of muscular dystrophy so the doctors could more efficiently treat me and my brother. Again, as with the previous search, the second attempt to identify anyone in the family who may have had the same or similar condition also proved unsuccessful. No one in the family reported having any family members with any physical disabilities. Because of the absence of any disclosure, it was suggested that my parents not have any more children because it couldn't be guaranteed that they wouldn't have another child with the physical impairments. With each of our births, it was also recommended that they not bring us home, as the doctors attempted to tell my parents that we would never grow up to be anything, to have independent lives, and would demand a lot of care. Such communication was especially true after I was born. The doctors tried to explain that my parents already had their hands full with taking care of a child with a severe physical impairment. Trying to take care of two would be too much and too overwhelming. In both cases, my parents opted not to listen to the doctors, so they took me home with them; about 2 years later, they had their third child. Again, a boy was born with the same physical impairments, but with less impairment than I had.

Following the birth of my parents' third child, the physicians were perplexed as to how parents who had no history of muscular dystrophy on either side of the family could have three children with the condition. The only thing they were left to believe was that my mother as a child had been misdiagnosed as having polio. They believed that it could have been an easy mistake because at the time many children were getting sick with polio, and the symptoms my mother recalled experiencing as a child were similar to the impairments experienced with polio. This perception existed for several years until my younger brother was 15 years old. Around that time, my mother and he concurrently had a muscle biopsy, a process in which they had a small piece of muscle removed from their thigh to be analyzed. This analysis revealed that each had the same condition, and then these results were compared to the biopsy results my older brother and I had as young children. Thus, as had long been expected, my mother did in fact have muscular dystrophy.

But our lives continued, and my parents successfully raised three children with muscular dystrophy. Each of us completed high school and went on to college. My older brother obtained a job as an advocate for individuals with various impairments after leaving Boston University, I was a senior at Northeastern University, and my younger brother entered the first year at the University of Massachusetts at Amherst after earning an AA degree from Newbury Junior College. However, after my brothers and I had begun to move forward with our lives, my mom found that her mother started to have slight problems with memory, which in the early days was minimal but then slowly progressed. This would eventually lead her to bring her mother to be seen by a doctor because she was concerned that there may be something more serious than normal aging. She was told that her mother did in fact have major health problems and that she was in the early stages of Alzheimer disease.

As the disease would progress, my mom would be faced with one of the most difficult decisions that no child ever looks forward to making regarding one's parent. She would realize that despite existing support systems, her mother was no longer safe living on her own, and my mom would have to make the decision that she was unable to care for her mother's needs and would have to put her in a nursing home. She knew that her mother wouldn't want that, as she'd always made it clear that she wanted to remain and die in her own home with her dignity. However, my mom knew that a nursing home was the only real option available, fearing that not acting so would result in her mother doing something that would result in serious injury or, worse yet, put a neighbor at risk in the elderly housing complex where she was living.

During this process of placing her mother in a nursing home, my mother needed to obtain a variety of information about her mother for the nursing home, which included a determination of eligibility for Medicaid, which is the insurance company that covers the nursing home expenses. One item needed was my grandmother's birth certificate, leading my mother to call the city hall in the town of Kennebunkport, Maine. That is the town where my grandmother had always reported being born and raised. However, this was unsuccessful because when speaking with the town's city hall administrator, my mother was told that there was no record of anyone with the name my mother had provided. A bit confused, my mother followed the recommendation of the city hall employee, which was to check neighboring towns in the event my grandmother had been mistaken. Though my mother found it difficult to believe that her mother wouldn't know the town where she'd been born, she wondered whether she had been born in a different city and just raised in Kennebunkport. My mother spent days calling numerous city halls in those cities and towns surrounding Kennebunkport. All of these calls were unsuccessful, as none of the cities or towns had any record of anyone being born there with her mother's name.

After days of numerous phone calls, feeling frustrated, my mother contacted her mother's sister to ask for assistance and inquired where her mother was born. To my mother's shock, she found out that her mother was adopted as a child. This frustrated my mother. She could only think of why her mother never mentioned this, especially, during the early years in which she and my father were checking both of their family's backgrounds to see whether there was any history of muscular dystrophy on either side of the family. In further conversation with her aunt, my mother indeed discovered that her mother was aware that she did in fact have muscular dystrophy. But for reasons my own mother will never understand, her mother was apparently embarrassed by this diagnosis and her mother told the doctors treating my mother as a child to tell her it was polio, not muscular dystrophy.

After this revelation, my mother was extremely confused, understandably frustrated, and angry that her mother kept this information from her. Her mother was a registered nurse and should have known that muscular dystrophy is a genetic disorder and not the result of something she or my mother had done wrong that resulted in this impairment. Even more aggravating for my mother was how her mother could remain silent about this information when she, my father, and the doctors were working with both sides of the family to explore whether there was any history of the impairment. My mother found herself not knowing how she should feel or how to approach this topic with her mother. Her mother probably wouldn't have a clear understanding of her reasoning behind the decision or understand the frustration my mother was dealing with. Alzheimer disease had robbed her mother of an ability to comprehend anything beyond simple childlike questions and reasoning. She had to figure out herself how to deal with the anger and frustration she had toward her mother, which she knew would be difficult. My mom was unable to resolve questions regarding her mother's decision-making, as well as how to set aside these feelings. She knew she had to do this, because she could see her mother quickly withering away day by day as the Alzheimer disease progressed and knew that things were only going to get worse. Therefore, for her mother to be properly cared for at that time and in the later years of her life, and knowing the effects Alzheimer diseases would continue to have, she had to put these feelings aside if she were to make sure that her mother's needs were met.

Though my mother didn't—and probably never would—totally understand or forgive her mother for what she did at that time, my mother was able to put these feelings aside and put her mother into a nursing home where she was properly cared for during the final few years of her life. I don't know how my mother was able to do this, as I knew how she felt, though I do know it took a great deal of strength. She would have drawn on the same strength and courage it took to raise three children with physical impairments during a time when most parents would have had their children placed in an institution, which was recommended when my brother and I were born.

During my lifetime, I've gone through numerous changes due to the progression of my impairment. I started as an individual who was able to walk, then to one who walked and used a manual wheelchair when having to go for any distances or when my legs were sore and weak due to fatigue, and then to one who used a manual chair at all times because I was no longer able to walk, though I was able to perform all activities of daily living. Currently, I require the use of an electric wheelchair for mobility and rely on a personal care attendant to assist me with all activities of daily living.

Though I have dealt with and will continue to deal with rough times that are associated with a progressive form of a physical impairment, I truly can't complain about my life. I have completed both bachelor's and master's degrees from two major universities in Boston and have always had a great job. In most instances, such accomplishments are not true for individuals with major impairments. When people first meet me, whether they are personal care attendants, colleagues, students, or clients, they tend to be surprised at my positive outlook on life. I think they believe they probably would be angry if they were in my situation. But perhaps they would not be angry, since I believe that most people with various limitations learn to make the most out of life. Of course, there will always be some people who will never be able to accept their life, choosing instead to be bitter and angry about their situation and wishing they were dead. Some of these people will indeed die, whether through willing themselves to die or from self-induced or assisted suicide.

Concerning my positive outlook on life, I attribute most of this attitude to my parents. They wouldn't allow me or my two brothers to sit back and feel sorry for ourselves or use our disability as an excuse for not doing something. My mother particularly served as a personal inspiration for us. Though she also has muscular dystrophy, she taught us through example how to live and make the most out of life. She believes that having a disability doesn't entitle one to look for pity from others or to feel sorry for oneself.

My mother even advocated early in my life, fighting with the local school board, that my brothers and I be integrated and mainstreamed into regular classes with our nondisabled peers, years before the Massachusetts public law, Chapter 766, was enacted guaranteeing equal public education for children with disabilities.

Feeling sorry for ourselves was not an option. While in high school, it was instilled in us that we were expected to go to college and to get ahead in life and to get a good job. Continued education was a necessity. Though I received Social Security benefits as an individual with a disability, my parents made it clear it was only while in school that I would collect benefits and would not do so for life. Having a job was an important value for my parents, and they insisted that my brothers and I were to have jobs every summer, with a majority of the money to be set aside to pay for college. This value is one that stuck with me. Since earning a bachelor's degree, I've always had a job, even when, because of a dramatic change in my impairment, I had to take time off from work. Each time I knew I would return to work. Not working was never an option in my mind, though the doctors would have preferred that I only collect disability benefits. I believe that having a job is important because it allows people to understand that individuals with disabilities are capable of working and can be productive members of society who shouldn't feel sorry for themselves because of their limitations.

Another belief I value that allows me to have a positive outlook on life is that there is always someone worse off than myself. When I was 11 years old and had recently undergone surgery for scoliosis, I was sent to a residential school for children with disabilities for 4 years. This school was wired via television cameras to the classrooms, which allowed me to participate in the school curriculum while recuperating from the surgery. Because the local junior high school where I was born and raised was inaccessible to individuals with physical impairments, I attended this "hospital school." While attending the school, I went home on weekends and holidays. I realized that half of the students lived there lbecause their family wanted nothing to do with them, choosing to make them wards of the state and to be forgotten about. But as a young boy I hated to be away from my family, and during this time I gained an appreciation of how fortunate I was. I realized that my parents cared for and loved me and only sent me to this "hospital school" because it was the only viable option for my junior high education.

Many at this school had no one and would be there until they were 21. Then they would leave the school and at that time not know what would happen to them. I also feel fortunate because I was born with my disability and it's the only life I've known. Compared to those who acquire an impairment due to a traumatic event or an illness, I've always said that if I had to have a disability, I'm glad I was born with it. Yes, there have been changes in my condition resulting in a loss of independence. But I grew up knowing that I was going to experience exacerbations with this neuromuscular impairment. The only thing I had to live with was not knowing when the condition would get worse and to what extent the change would be. If an individual acquires his or her impairment later in life, with one's life turned upside down with no warning that the life he or she was used to is suddenly taken away, for that person the adjustment is extremely difficult if he or she does make any adjustment at all.

In addition, I've always been thankful that my impairment affects my body and not my mind. I do not consider myself better than someone else with a different condition. But I'd rather have it the way that I am even though I depend a great deal on assistance from others. Importantly, despite my physical limitations, I'm able to understand my needs and direct others on how to assist me with my needs, and with my intact cognitive functions I have earned two college degrees and maintain a great job. These are just my personal beliefs, and I do not ever intend to insult those who have severe, cognitive impairments, such as traumatic brain injuries or Alzheimer disease.

My final belief that has allowed me to maintain a positive attitude is the conviction that God doesn't put more on one's plate than one is able to manage. Though I am not a very religious individual, I do not want to convey the impression that I've never been angry about my situation or bitter and depressed, wishing that I was dead. There have been numerous times when I wonder why I don't understand what it's all about and why it happened to me; I can't wait to ask God what it was all about. However, in time I always come around to the beliefs that have allowed me to adjust and make the most out of my life and realize how lucky I am.

I have always been asked, "If there was a cure for muscular dystrophy would I take it?" People are usually amazed when I state that I would decline. Why I decline a hypothetical cure is because this is the only life I know and I feel, because of the reasons discussed, that I am truly blessed for my life. I believe that having this impairment allows me, despite my limitations, to serve as an example that one is still able to have a happy and productive life.

LIFE LESSONS TAUGHT TO ME BY MY DISABILITY

ALFRED H. DEGRAFF

At the age of 18 years, I dove off a pier on Martha's Vineyard and experienced a cervical spinal cord injury. I became, and remain, a quadriplegic dependent on motorized wheelchair mobility, daily physical help from personal assistants (PAs), and enough prescription medications to make several pharmaceutical companies financially dependent on me.

That was almost 40 years ago. I'm convinced from experience that my severe physical disability becomes more valuable to me and to society with each passing year. Although it initially takes a burst of courage and coping skills to acknowledge and "accept" a fresh disability in its infancy, the real test of skills is one's adequacy to support and maintain his or her disability lifestyle over the long haul, decade after decade. Does the person have the staying power to survive daily health crises, hundreds of whining and immature PAs, and, for many, a chronic depression that makes addictions and suicide seem so attractive?

For some people, I'm convinced that the disability lifestyle is no longer viewed as a meaningless tragedy, but instead as a meaningful gift teaching life lessons. People with disabilities encounter an endless stream of opportunities for unique experiences, learning, and growth.

My disability has gifted me with wisdom about humanity that I wouldn't have been able to realize, or realize in such detail and depth, had I been able-bodied. This wisdom has given the disability a sense of worth. What follows is my "top 10" list of life lessons—my personal statement of what my disability has meant to me by way of personal experiences, learning, and growth. To many of my able-bodied peers without insightful experiences, these are nice clichés—the text of refrigerator magnets. Instead, for many of us with disabilities, these are lessons acquired from repeated experiences or crises. While coping with an active crisis, these lessons reveal themselves in response to our often-desperate plea to make sense of the situation: "Please show me what I'm to learn from this experience."

I have learned that I have the choice of living this disability lifetime as a victor or a victim. Although I attempt to live optimistically as a victor, I have found that no matter how deeply I might occasionally slip into the victim role, a return route is always made available to me.

Living with a lifelong disability isn't easy. I have found that much of my success or failure has been dependent on how I view life. There is a big difference between whether I choose to be a victim or a victor. And I truly do always have a choice.

As a victim at various times, I have chosen to go through life in a semi-hopeless frame of mind: "Why me? I'll never get ahead, because I'm stuck in this wheelchair." Those who take up full-time residence as a victim erroneously believe they find comfort in wallowing in the anger, grief, sorrow, depression, and despair.

As a victor, I'm presented with the same rough times as the victim; however, I work hard at staying in control of my disability and the quality of my life. As a victim, the nucleus of my daily life is my disability, and my lifestyle becomes a consequence of what my disability permits. As a victor, my soul or spirit is my nucleus, and the disability, like other personal characteristics, is one of many electrons orbiting around my soul or spirit.

I have learned the importance of taking the time to formally grieve a loss, instead of unemotionally trivializing or dismissing it with denial.

Life with a disability is one with many losses. We have lots of opportunities and need to practice grieving. We repeatedly have the choice of grieving now or grieving later—of paying now or paying later. There are many factors, outside the scope of this essay, that give us no choice but to grieve later or grieve over a long duration in bite-size pieces.

When we delay, we are sometimes sentenced to carry the weight of the loss's baggage. Grief baggage can manifest itself in many forms, including sorrow, frustration, anger, and depression.

When possible, I try to grieve my losses soon, to defuse grieving of its depressing power, and to move on. The relative absence of unaddressed grief is one of the elements that can reward us with that desirable state we call inner peace.

I have learned that life does not randomly expose me to coincidences, accidents, or seemingly meaningless tragedies. Instead, I am routinely meant to encounter learning and growth opportunities that are sent to me in a variety of disguises.

The Rolling Stones have sung, "You can't always get what you want, but if you try, sometimes you get what you need." The Dalai Lama was articulate in countering with, "Remember that not getting what you want is sometimes a wonderful stroke of luck." More recent, there has been yet another outlook that states, "Be careful of what you ask for, you might receive it."

My personal experience has shown me that if I am open to recognizing and learning from life's lessons and flowing with life's rhythms instead of fighting or fleeing from them, then a whole world of benefits can open up to me.

I have learned that if I were given the opportunity either to shed my disability and return to the experiences, knowledge, and values that I had at the time of my disabling injury or to keep my current disability with the wisdom it has taught me, I would usually choose to retain my disability.

What about those unique experiences—some joyful and some painful—that I would not have encountered without my paralysis? I usually take full advantage of them. Regardless of whether they were good or bad memories, I have usually succeeded in learning and growing because of them.

I have had firsthand experience in needing, receiving, and then returning human compassion. My disability has also given me first-person insights into prejudice, bigotry, discrimination, injustice, poverty, caring, love, support, integrity, and many other human qualities and inequalities.

I'm not saying I enjoy having my disability; however, it has enabled me to learn much more about humanity and life than I could have learned in an able-bodied lifetime. It's now been almost 40 years of these specialized experiences, learning, and growth. Were I actually presented with the chance of walking away from my wheelchair—but also the need to leave behind the insights I've acquired—I really doubt I'd accept walking back to the starting line of wisdom.

I have learned that it is never appropriate for me to try to shift my responsibilities, which are rightfully mine and for which I am capable of managing, to others and then to blame them when my needs aren't accommodated.

I have learned that I should never blame any provider for not doing what I should be doing for myself. In addition, I am always ultimately responsible for an aide failing to do a task or doing it incompletely. Most of the assistance an aide gives me is the face-to-face kind. I am right there and have a continual responsibility to do QC, or quality control. If an aide has helped me get dressed and I arrive at my downtown office to find that I am wearing shoes but no socks, is my morning aide to blame? I don't think so.

Sure, I am annoyed that the aide totally spaced out on where my socks were this morning after remembering them for the previous 7 months. However, I have decided that my responsibility to watch my help providers is more realistic than to attempt to hold anyone responsible for performing my help routine flawlessly with no mistakes. Indeed, I never hold a PA responsible for memorizing every detail of my routine. In the books I've written about PA management, I refer to working with an aide as analogous to dancing. I expect each PA in each work shift to occasionally forget a detail—a dance step. As the PA and I dance through the routine's tasks and I sense he or she has forgotten the next "step," it's my responsibility to subtly remind the PA of the next step so we can keep on dancing.

I have learned that I am the only valid source for my own joy, sorrow, and inner peace. My own inner peace most often occurs when my actions are in harmony and authentic with my perception of spiritual intentions.

Not only am I solely responsible for my own happiness, for answers to my own life questions, and for coordinating the help required to maintain my health but no one else will care as much as I if I fail to reach my goals or permit my health to decline.

A rock star who became addicted to drugs and then went through recovery acknowledges that others can't be held responsible for his happiness or the consequences of not achieving happiness. This rock star believed that "we are who we choose to be" . . . "you've got to save yourself . . ." and "nobody knows what you want . . . and nobody will be as sorry if you don't get it."

I have learned that there is a difference between physical pain and emotional suffering. Physical pain is objective and physiological; emotional suffering is subjective and psychological. While I sometimes cannot control the physical pain, I usually do have the choice and ability to control the much more powerful suffering that is created in my mind.

There are psychological ways of alleviating many kinds of emotional suffering. What the mind has the power to create, it also has the power to take away. From many personal experiences, I have learned the difference between the different feelings of physical pain and emotional suffering. I can assure myself of my ability to control suffering, and this has saved my life several times.

I have learned about the powerful advantages and life-sustaining utility there are in making maximum use of mental discipline. I've participated in many workshops and seminars that taught me skills of self-hypnosis, healing mental imagery, and progressive relaxation. I had been routinely using these skills to consciously lower stress and relax, mindfully reduce constrictive asthma, and even attempt to imagine genital orgasms that I could no longer feel. My increasing skills at mind control had resulted in perhaps a 90% success rate for these varied objectives, while enabling me to occasionally reduce my need for prescription medications.

I have learned to live for today—in the present—because yesterday is gone and tomorrow might never happen. Today's events will never happen again, nor should they. Perhaps the predominant daily challenge I have in living with my disability is in creating and maintaining a set of activities and goals that make life sufficiently interesting and important to merit my getting out of bed each morning.

When I first acquired my disability, I spent a lot of time living in the past. I would look at what I could no longer physically do and think back to the good old days when I was able-bodied and could do those things. This is, of course, a setup for depression—concentrating on and aspiring to do what we cannot. If someone with diabetes lies in bed all day and thinks about hot fudge sundaes, he will get depressed. Crosby, Stills, and Nash, in the song "Judy Blue Eyes," sing, "Don't let the past remind us of what we are not now."

People with disabilities should be cautious about reminiscing constantly about missing their able-bodied past or fantasizing about the shape of the future after their ship comes in (for example, after they win the lottery) and how much better than their current lifestyle the future will be. Sometimes, when I repeatedly procrastinate about becoming involved in interesting events, I think of Stephen Levine. In his book *A Year to Live* (1997), he cites one quite effective way to identify one's current life purpose: Vividly imagine that you are going to die exactly 1 year from today. Ask yourself what priorities you consequently have during this final year of your life!

I have learned the difference between accepting my own disability and society accepting it. For my own acceptance, I should formally acknowledge it, accept my limitations, and then concentrate instead on living within my abilities. If I concentrate on limitations and loss, I will become depressed. For the social acceptance of my disability, I should mostly ignore it. If I speak mostly about my disability instead of my true personal self and interests, it is unfortunately my disability that people will most remember.

During my undergraduate years, I lived purposely in a campus residence hall to facilitate my socialization. Disability-related discussions would crop up occasionally, but for a tiny minority of time. I didn't deny I had a disability or forbid my dorm mates "to talk about it"; instead, we had more important and interesting topics. One evening, a couple of friends popped into my room and asked if I wanted to join them in casing out a new bar within walking distance from our living area. Out of curiosity, I asked whether the entrance or interior had unavoidable steps. In response, they looked at each other and became very apologetic, "Oh, Al, we're so sorry, we forgot that was a concern." I grinned ear to ear and assured them they weren't guilty of anything. Indeed, they primarily invited me and my personal interests and not the wheelchair. I felt quite honored that those were my friends' priorities!

So in conclusion to this essay, while I stay in continual communication with the physical and psychological aspects of my disability, it is essential that I concurrently transcend—rise above—this disability and its limitations. It is important that I be able to look beyond the limitations of the disability in order to see the benefits that it offers.

As my abilities decrease with progressing years and disability, it has become increasingly important for me to use my daily time, energy, and stamina as efficiently as possible. My daily aerobic workouts, my requirement for "smart food" quality nutrition, and other health measures are more important to me than to my able-bodied peers.

It has been said that freedom in life is not necessarily doing what one wishes, whenever one wishes to do so. Instead, true freedom is the ability to face, cope with, and successfully get through each of life's unpredictable crises. I believe that my disability and limitations have ironically taught me many lessons about freedom—wisdom that I would not have realized as an able-bodied person.

REFERENCES

Arata, T. (1990). The dance [Recorded by G. Brooks]. On *If tomorrow never comes* [CD]. Capitol Nashville.

Dion, K., Berscheid, E., & Walster, E. (1972). What is beautiful is good. *Journal of Personality and Social Psychology, 24*, 285–290. https://doi.org/10.1037/h0033731

Dutta, A., & Kundu, M. (2007). Psychosocial adjustment to disability: A multi-ethnic approach. In P. Leung, C. Flowers, W. Talley, & P. Sanderson (Eds.), *Multicultural issues in rehabilitation and allied health* (pp. 1–21). Aspen Professional Services.

Gray, F. (1969). *Scoremanship: The sensational new approach to success with women.* Bantam.

Levine, S. (1997). *A year to live: How to live this year as if it were your last.* Bell Tower.

Power, P. W., & Dell Orto, A. E. (1980). *Role of the family in the rehabilitation of the physically disabled.* University Park Press.

Power, P. W., & Dell Orto, A. E. (2004). *Families living with chronic illness and disability* (pp. 271–277). Springer Publishing Company.

Power, P. W., Dell Orto, A. E., & Blechar-Gibbons, M. (1988). *Family interventions throughout chronic illness and disability.* Springer Publishing Company.

Wallace, M. (1978). *Black macho and the myth of the superwoman.* Dial Press.

Williams, M. (1975). *The velveteen rabbit.* Avon.

Woods-Giscombé, C. (2010). Superwomen schema: African American women's views on stress, strength, and health. *Qualitative Health Resources, 20*(5), 668–683. https://doi.org/10.1177%2F1049732310361892

Wright, B. (1983). *Physical disability: A psychosocial approach* (2nd ed.). Harper & Row.

INDEX

ableist microaggressions
  bystander interventions
    ascribed stereotypic trait broadening, 208
    asking for clarification, 209
    disarm microaggressions, 211–212
    external support/validation, 212
    metacommunication explicit, 209
    naming, 208
    perpetrator, 209–211
    perspicacity, 207–208
    undermining metacommunication, 208
  counselors
    collaborative approach, 205
    cultural humility, 205–206
    cultural orientation, 205
    defensiveness, 206
    experimental study, 204
    group multicultural orientation, 206
    incompetence, 204
    metacommunication, 206
    recommendations, 206–207
    seven-step action plan, 206
  domains
    denial of disability-related experience, 201
    denial of identity, 201
    denial of privacy, 201
    de-sexualization, 203
    expectation of helplessness, 201–202
    infantilization, 202–203
    patronization, 202
    secondary gain, 202
    second-class citizenship, 203
    spread effect, 202
  gender minority, 204
  intersectional identities, 203
  LGBTQ participants, 204
  racism, 200
  sexual minority community, 204
ableism
  behavioral discrimination, 73–74
  insider–outsider distinction, 71–72
  intentional or unintentional, 74–76
  internalized, 77
  navigation
    advocacy activities, 80–81
    attitudes, 81
    disability culture and identity promotion, 78

  diversity education and workshop opportunities, 78
  identity-first language, 80
  person-first language, 79–80
  as outsider privilege, 76–77
  racism, 200
  stigmatization, 71
abortion laws, 94
abuse and relationship violence
  disproportionate risk, 352
  emotional abuse, 352
  financial abuse, 352
  intersectional identities, 352–353
  intimate partner violence (see intimate partner violence)
  physical abuse, 352
  sexual abuse, 352
ACA. See Affordable Care Act
acceptance and commitment therapy (ACT), 113
acceptance of disability, 60
Acceptance of Disability Scale (ADS) and Revised ADS (ADS-R), 117–118, 223
activities of daily living (ADLs), 452
activity theory of aging, 384
ACT program. See Assertive Community Treatment program
AD. See autonomic dysreflexia
ADA. See Americans with Disabilities Act
ADAA. See Americans with Disabilities Amendments Act
ADAPT. See American Disabled for Attendant Programs Today
adaptational approach, parenting reaction, 240
adapted motivational interviewing (AMI), 478–479
addiction, 313
ADEA. See Age in Employment Act of 1967
adjustment
  chronic illness and disability (CID) adaptation, 113
  definition, 124
adjustment theories
  acquired disability, 142–144
  chaos and complexity theory (CCT), 140–141
  coping vs. succumbing framework, 127
  disability centrality model (DCM), 133–135
  ecological models
    disability nature, 135–136
    environmental influences, 137–138
    personal characteristics, 136–137

adjustment theories (*cont.*)
  good-fortune comparison, 142
  recurrent/integrated model, 138–139
  reevaluation changes, 127
  somatopsychology, 132–133
  stage models
    assumptions, 128
    defense mobilization, 128–130
    final adjustment/reintegration, 131–132
    initial impact, 128
    initial realization, 130
    retaliation, 131
  transactional model of coping, 139–140
  value change system, 141–142
advocacy, 466–468
  activities, ableism, 80–81
  organizations, 99–100
aesthetic aversion, 23
Affordable Care Act (ACA), 96, 329
African American family, 248–249
Age in Employment Act of 1967 (ADEA), 391
aging population
  activity theory, 384
  assessment, 385–388
  career assessment, 386
  continuity theory, 384
  counseling
    case managers, 389
    casework, 389
    education and training implications, 393–394
    e-health, 390
    life review therapy (LRT), 390
    life span developmental research, 389
    mental health inequalities, 389
    practice implications, 393
    problem-solving approach, 390
    research implications, 394
    solution-focused approaches, 391
    whole person wellness paradigm, 389
  developmental models, 383
  disengagement theory, 384
  functional assessments, 386
  life experiences, 388
  mental health assessment, 386–387
  proactive employer response
    Age in Employment Act of 1967 (ADEA), 391
    benefit plans, 392
    human resource policies and practices, 392
    human resources (HR) practices, 392
    intergenerational conflict and concerns, 392–393
    job application process, 391
    managers, 392
  serious mental illness (SMI), 385
  socioecological models, 383–384
  subjective assessment, 386
  substance use, 385
  theoretical and clinical implications, 384–385
  vocational assessment, 386
  workplaces and workers, 382

Alcohol, Smoking and Substance Involvement Screening
    Test (ASSIST), 387
Alcohol Use Disorders Identification Test (AUDIT), 387
allyship, 80, 98–99
American Association of Retired Persons (AARP), 291
American Disabled for Attendant Programs Today
    (ADAPT), 88, 99
American Federation of the Physically Handicapped
    (AFPH), 87
American Rehabilitation Counseling Association
    (ARCA), 106
Americans with Disabilities Act (ADA), 26, 32, 50–51,
    75, 200, 318, 356, 418
  and accessibility, 89–90
  enforcement entity and purview, 90
Americans with Disabilities Amendments Act
    (ADAA), 59
Americans with Disabilities for Attendant Programs
    Today (ADAPT), 467
AMI. *See* adapted motivational interviewing
amyotrophic lateral sclerosis (ALS), Teplow's perspective,
    513–517
anger, chronic illness and disability adaptation, 112–113
anticipatory grief response, 286
antipsychotic medication, 44
anxiety, 128
  chronic illness and disability (CID) adaptation, 112
  provoking situations, 22
appraisal-focused approaches, 115
Arab families, 251–252
Architectural Barriers Act, 89
Asexualization Act, 40
Asian American families, 249–250
Assertive Community Treatment (ACT) program, 47
asset values, 142
ASSIST. *See* Alcohol, Smoking and Substance
    Involvement Screening Test
assistive technology
  BMAT, 427–430
  definition, 417–418
  device, 419
  education, 420
  employment, 420–421
  ethical orientation, 422–423
  HAAT model, 425–426
  high-tech, 422
  history and legislative influence, 418–419
  leisure and community involvement, 421
  low-tech, 421
  mid-tech, 421–422
  MPT model, 426–427
  needs and usage rates, 419–420
  SETT model, 424–425
  universal design, 430–431
Assistive Technology Provider (ATP), 423
asylums, 39
asylum seeker. *See also* immigrants
  definition, 368
  etiology, 369

medical and mental health screenings, 373–374
social–emotional development, 370
attitude survey and disability
affective component, 18
ambivalence, 28–29
behavioral component, 18
cognitive component, 18
competence, 20
definition, 18
empirical studies, 19
fundamental negative bias, 19
inherent problems, 18
negative attitudes, 21–26
physical attractiveness, 19–20
poorly validated measures, 17
positive attitudes, 26–27
socially desirable, 17
social skills, 20
stereotypical attitudes, 20–21
AUDIT. *See* Alcohol Use Disorders Identification Test
Autism Spectrum Conditions-Enhancing Nurture and
Development (ASCEND), 294
autonomic dysreflexia (AD), 184
aversive racism, 198

balanced family, 241
bargaining, adjustment theories, 128–129
behavioral discrimination, ableism, 73–74
behavioral microaggressions, 198
bifurcation points, 140
Biopsychosocial Model of Assistive Technology Team
Collaboration (BMAT)
device abandonment, 428–429
interdisciplinary collaboration, 429
medical and psychosocial aspects, 428
multidisciplinary collaboration, 429
process example, 430
terminology needs, 428
transdisciplinary collaboration, 429–430
bladder and bowel accidents, 184
blaming the victim concept, 21, 23
blindness, Macarena Pena's experience, 497–500
BMAT. *See* Biopsychosocial Model of Assistive
Technology Team Collaboration
body dissatisfaction, 475
body image
chronic illness and disability (CID) adaptation, 109
cognitive reframing interventions, 479
eating disorders, 477–478
self-compassion intervention (SCI), 479–480
body positive movement, 460
body surveillance, 475
Buddhist religion, 437

cannabinoids, 312
caregiver burden, 237
caregiver stress, grieving process, 283–284

Catholicism, 437
CCT. *See* chaos and complexity theory
Centers for Independent Living (CILs), 468
CFS. *See* Clinical Frailty Scale
chaos and complexity theory (CCT)
butterfly effect, 140
complex systems, 140
dynamic systems, 140
fixed-point attractors, 140
limited cycle/periodic attractors, 140
non-linearity, 140
self-organization, 141
self-similarity, 141
strange attractors, 140
characterological self-blame, 131
Character Strengths, 406
childhood, negative attitudes, 22
Children's attitudes toward disability, 30
child with a disability (CWD)
demographic factors, 442–443
family perspective, 441–442
interactionist approach, 442
psychodynamic approach, 441
psychosocial approach, 441
chloral hydrate, 40
chlorpromazine, 44
chronic illness and disability (CID)
assessment
ADS and ADS-R, 117–118
PAIS, 117
PAIS-SR, 117
POMS, 118
RIDI, 118
body image, 109
coping strategies
appraisal, 114
categories, 114–115
definition, 114
models, 115–117
tripartite taxonomic structure, 114–115
counselors, 106–107
family caregiver (*see* family caregivers)
grief response, 281–282
loss and grief, 108–109
psychological maladjustment, 125
psychological responses
acceptance and adjustment, 113
anger/hostility, 112–113
denial, 112
depression, 112
negative and positive affectivity, 111
posttraumatic growth, 113–114
shock and anxiety, 112
psychosocial adaptation, 106
psychosocial reaction-specific interventions, 119
quality of life (*see* quality of life)
self-concept, 109–110
self-management, 120
stigmatization, 110

chronic illness and disability (CID) (*cont.*)
    stress, 107–108
    theory-driven interventions, 119
    trauma and crisis, 108
    uncertainty and unpredictability, 111
chronic sorrow, 237
CID. *See* chronic illness and disability
cisgender, 171
Civil Rights Act, 88, 461
civil rights, U.S., 90–91
    autonomy and decision-making, 92–93
    community living, 93
    financial wellness, 91–92
    parenting and disability, 93–94
    political access and voting, 94–95
Clinical Frailty Scale (CFS), 12
Clubhouse approach, 405
cognitive appraisal mechanisms, 111
cognitive behavioral therapy
    intimate partner violence (IPV), 163
    social media, 479
cognitive disabilities, sexuality, 181
cognitive schema, 138
cognitive trauma therapy for battered women
        (CTT-BW), 163
collaboration, trauma-informed care, 162
communication, disability culture, 78
Community Mental Health Centers Act of 1963, 46
competent person, 20
complex grief
    chronic illnesses and disabilities, 281–282
    "continuing bonds" therapy, 279–280
    culturally specific issues, 279
    functional psychological consequence, 279
    risk factors, 279
    therapeutic relationship, 279
complicated grief, 277
compound caregiver, 293
congenital disabilities, 124
conservation of resources (COR) theory, 116–117
conservatorships, 92–93
contact hypothesis, 81
containment of disability effect, value change, 141–142
continuity theory of aging, 384
control, 150
coping strategies
    chronic illness and disability (CID)
        appraisal, 114
        categories, 114–115
        conservation of resources (COR) theory, 116–117
        crisis and coping model, 115–116
        models, 115–117
        stress-appraisal-coping, 115
    definition, 114
    tripartite model, 115
COR theory. *See* conservation of resources theory
counseling intervention
    aging population (*see* aging population)
    identity development (*see* identity development)

intimate partner violence (IPV), 161–162
COVID-19, 483, 485
    intellectual disability, 52
    online videoconferencing platforms, 53
    spinal cord injuries (SCIs), 52
    telehealth adoption, 52, 53
    therapeutic relationship risk, 52–53
Crime Victims with Disabilities Awareness Act, 193
criminal justice system involvement, substance use
        disorders, 325–326
Crisis Intervention Team (CIT) programs, 48
cultural humility, 205–206
CWD. *See* child with a disability

DCM. *See* disability centrality model
DCS. *See* Disability Centrality Scale
deaf, Cassandra Cantu's experience, 493–494
Deferred Action for Childhood Arrivals (DACA)
        program, 369
Degraff's experience of physical disability, 529–532
Delighted–Terrible Scale, 134
denial
    adjustment, 129–130
    chronic illness and disability (CID) adaptation, 112
Department of Housing and Urban Development
        (HUD), 90
depressants, 312
depression
    chronic illness and disability (CID) adaptation, 112
    intimate partner violence, 156
Devins's illness intrusiveness model, 134, 226–227
DIDS. *See* Disability Identity Development Scale
disability activism, 88
disability advocacy organizations, 467
disability centrality model (DCM)
    centrality, 227–228
    considerations, 229–230
    Devins's illness intrusiveness model, 134
    domain importance, 228
    domain salience, 228
    empirical support, 134
    life domains, 135
    multiple sclerosis, 134, 228
    objective and subjective measures, 133–134
    psychosocial well-being, 227
    self-report instrument, 228
    subjective QOL, 227
    testable hypotheses, 229
    theoretical underpinnings, 133
    value change, 229
Disability Centrality Scale (DCS), 134, 223–224
disability culture
    ableism, 78–79
    functions, 57
    sociopolitical stances, 58
    values, 57
disability group identity, 110
disability identity, 487. *See also* identity development

ableism, 78–79
    internal and external experience, 56–57
    models
        acceptance, 60
        Darling and Heckert model, 60
        diversity model, 59
        four-status model, 60–61
        medical model, 58
        passive awareness, 60
        political disability identity, 60
        social model, 59
        superman/woman complex, 60
    in rehabilitation psychology, 56
    and scholarship, 56–57
    self-concept, 56
    self development, 56
Disability Identity Development Scale (DIDS), 63
Disability Identity Scale, 62–63
disability language, 64
disability-related counseling competencies, 106
disability rights movement, 87–88
Disability simulation exercises, 32
disabled parents, civil rights, 93–94
disarm microaggressions, 211–212
disengagement theory of aging, 384
dissociatives, 312
distorted body image
    cognitive reframing interventions, 479
    eating disorders, 477–478
    self-compassion intervention (SCI), 479–480
diversity model of disability, 59
domestic violence. See also intimate partner violence
    physical and mental health disorders, 158–159
    physical health problems, 155–156
    resilience of women survivors, 161
    vulnerabilities and mental health, 156–158
Down syndrome (DS), 94, 175
Drug-Free Workplace Act of 1998, 326–327
drug overdose deaths, 316–317
drug use disorder (DUD), health impact, 316
durable medical equipment (DME), 428

eating disorders, 477–478
    cognitive reframing interventions, 479
    motivational interviewing (MI), 478
education
    assistive technology, 420
    experiential sensitivity exercises, 31
    media portrayals, 32
    parenting experience
        family engagement, 267, 269
        Partnership Capacity Matrix, 266
        vision statement, 268, 269
    simulation activities, 31
educational disadvantage, 75
Education for All Handicapped Children Act, 13, 419
electroconvulsive therapy (ECT), 43
emergency preparedness, Henderlong's experience, 494–497

emotional abuse, 352
emotional prejudice, 77
emotional reactions, families and disability, 237
emotion-focused coping strategy, 129
emotion-focused strategies, 114
empathogens, 313
empathy, 77
Employee Assistance Program (EAP), 334
employment
    assistive technology, 420–421
    immigrants, 370
    oppression and disenfranchisement, 457–458
    substance use disorders
        disclosure and workplace accommodations,
            334–335
        workplace policies, 333–334
        workplace stigma, 332–333
empowerment, trauma-informed care, 162
environmental inequities, 458–460
environmental microaggressions, 198
epigenetic principle, 383
Equal Employment Opportunity Commission
    (EEOC), 332
erectile dysfunction (ED), 185
Erikson theory of psychosocial development, 126, 383
ethnic minority and disability, 24
eudaimonia, 219
eugenics movement, 9, 40
existential angst, 23
exosystem, 384
exploitation, 150

Facebook depression and fatigue, 475
Fair Food Network Double Up Food Bucks (DUFB), 410
Fair Housing Act of 196, 93
Fairweather Community Lodge Programs, 47
families and disability
    access to coping resources, 238
    adjustment models, 239–240
    belief systems, 238
    childhood illness
        anger, 242
        child's age, 242
        denial, 242
        grandparents, 243–244
        grief, 242
        intellectual disabilities, 243
        mother's and father's reactions, 243
        outside placement decisions, 244
    coping strategies, 240–241
    cultural differences, 247–255
    emotional reactions, 237
    family history, 239
    healthy family, 236
    marital discord, 238
    parenting reaction perspectives, 240
    parents with disability, 245–246
    partner with disability

families and disability (*cont.*)
    divorce rate, 245
    multiple sclerosis (MS), 244
    social isolation, 244
    spinal cord injury (SCI), 244–245
  protective factors, 238
  relationships and communication styles, 239
  risk factors, 238
  sibling with disability, 246–247
  stress reactions, 237–238
  traditional family model, 236
  in United States, 236
Family Caregiver Alliance, 291, 304
family caregivers
  chronic illness and disability
    aging adults, 295
    caregiving tasks, 292
    clinical implications, 304–305
    compound caregiver, 293
    and culture, 303–304
    family psychoeducation (FPE), 299–300
    family–school partnership (FSP), 300–301
    family support practices, 293
    gender differences, 293
    health and psychological impact, 295–296
    parent management training (PMT), 298–299
    peer support, 302–303
    poor family adjustment risk factors, 293–294
    positive caregiving outcomes, 296–297
    posttraumatic growth (PTG), 298
    psychosocial impacts, 296
    research implications, 305–306
    resilience, 297
    respite support, 301–302
    self-compassion, 297–298
    spouse's transition, 292–293
    young adults and adults, 294
    young children, 294
  definition, 291
  demographic characteristics, 292
  diversity, 292–293
family-centered decision-making (FCDM), 304
family functioning, 241
family psychoeducation, chronic illness and disability,
    299–300
family readiness groups (FRGs), 341
family resilience model, 239
family–school partnership, chronic illness and disability,
    300–301
FCDM. *See* family-centered decision-making
fear of contamination, 23
fear of missing out (FOMO), 475
Federal Communications Commission (FCC), 90
feminist therapy, intimate partner violence, 164
fertility issues, 185–186
fibromyalgia syndrome, positive psychology
    interventions, 407
financial abuse, 352
financial wellness, U.S. civil rights, 91–92

fixed-point attractors, 140
food insecurity, 409
forced sterilization laws, 94
fortification, disability culture, 78
Freud's psychosexual theory of development, 383
functional/interactional perspective, disability, 436
functionalist approach, parenting reaction, 240
functional support, adjustment, 137

gay oppression, 461–462
gender identity, 171
genderqueer, 171
Geriatric Anxiety Scale, 387
Geriatric Depression Scale, 387
Gibson Disability Identity Development Scale, 63
grief, dying, and death
  caregiver stress, 283–284
  chronic illness and disability (CID), 281–282
  complex, 279–280
  complicated grief, 277
  critical incidents, 277
  cultural and spiritual sensitivity, 277
  cultural expression, 276
  definition, 276–277
  end-of-life decisions, 287–288
  level of care transition
    anticipatory grief response, 286
    case management, 286
    end-of-life decision-making tasks, 285–286
    guilt experience, 285
    psychosocial stressors and traumas, 285
  measurement, 277
  military culture, 276
  model of linear progression, 277
  older adults, 282–283
  persistent complex bereavement disorder, 277–278
  prolonged grief disorder (PGD), 278–279
  psychological and emotional reaction, 276
  therapeutic interactions, 276
  trauma, 280–281
guardianships, 92–93

HAAT model. *See* Human Activity Assistive Technology
    model
hallucinogenics, 312
handicap, definition, 27
handicapism, 435
healthcare, U.S.
  accessibility, 98
  affordability, 96–97
  inequality, 96
  quality care, 97
  violations and devaluations, 95
healthy family, 236
Hearing Handicap Inventory for the Elderly–Screening
    Version, 388
hedonia, 219

Help America Vote Act, 95, 410
highlight reel, 475
high-tech assistive technologies, 422
Hinduism, 437
hopes and home, Chris's perspective, 503–507
Housing First (HF) program, 330
Human Activity Assistive Technology (HAAT) model, 425–426
Human Performance model (HP), 425
hydrotherapeutic techniques, mental illness, 41

ICD. *See* internet communication disorder (ICD)
ICDIDH. *See* International Code of Impairment, Disease, and Handicap
IDEA. *See* Individuals with Disabilities Education Act
identity development
  congenital and acquired disability adaptation
    meaning-making process, 62
    self-concept, 61–62
  counseling
    ableism, 64
    client-centered approach, 64
    disability community, 65–66
    Disability-Identity Circle activity, 66
    microaggressions, 64–65
    narrative approaches, 66
  identity measures
    Disability Identity Development Scale (DIDS), 63
    Gibson Disability Identity Development Scale, 63
    Personal Identity Scale, 63
    qualitative methods, 62
    quantitative measurement, 62–63
    Questionnaire on Disability Identity and Opportunity, 63
identity-first language, 80
identity, sexuality, 170
identity synthesis, 56
iDisorders, 475, 477
IDS. *See* Issues in Disability Scale
illegal aliens, 367
illness intrusiveness, 111, 226–227
illness uncertainty, 111
immigrants
  adjustment issue, 370
  complex trauma, 371
  culturally sensitive approaches, 376–377
  definition, 367–368
  employment, 370
  government-driven disaster response, 372–373
  humanitarian crisis and efforts, 371, 372
  medical and mental health screenings, 373–374
  mental and physical assessment, 375–376
  military's contribution, 373
  multicultural counseling approaches, 375
  postmigration, 374
  prevalence and incidence, 368
  Strategic Foresight Initiative action plan, 372–373
  triage, 375

working alliance, 377–378
Immigration and Nationality Act (INA), 367
immigration processing system, 369
Immigration Restriction League (IRL), 6
impairment, definition, 27
INA. *See* Immigration and Nationality Act
indigenous American families
  cultural trauma, 253
  extended family system, 254
  health disparities, 254
  health issues, 253
  life expectancy, 253
  rituals and ceremonies, 254
  social construct of disability, 253–254
  traditional parenting roles, 254
  tribes, 253
Individuals with Disabilities Education Act (IDEA), 13, 59, 258, 418–419
inequality, 451
ingroup favoritism
  minimal group paradigm, 73
  outgroup homogeneity effect, 74
  social script, 73
institutionalization
  adjustment, 138
  sexual abuse, 191
intellectual and developmental disability (IDD)
  research, 260
intellectual disability, 98
intentional ableism, 74–75
interactionist approach, parenting reaction, 240
internalized ableism, 77
internalized anger, 131
internalized oppression
  ableism, 463
  factors contributing, 463–464
  health and well-being, 463
  negative stereotypes, 463
  social groups, 462
International Code of Impairment, Disease, and Handicap (ICDIDH), 430–431
internet communication disorder (ICD), 473, 476
intimacy, sexuality, 170
intimate partner violence (IPV), 352
  abuse, 148
  anxiety and PTSD, 157, 158
  cognitive behavioral therapy, 163
  counseling intervention, 161–162
  cultural competency, 164–165
  culturally competent principles, 359
  depression, 156
  disability-related accommodations, 358
  ecological context
    bidirectional effects, 357
    gender identity, 357
    geographical location, 356–357
    historical influences, 355
    housing insecurity, 356
    socioeconomic status, 355–356

intimate partner violence (IPV) (*cont.*)
  feminist therapy, 164
  help-seeking barriers
    COVID-19 pandemic, 154–155
    deaf community, 153
    immigrant women, 154
    inability to admit, 151–152
    IPV program accessibility barriers, 152
    LGBTQ women, 153
    rural communities, 153–154
  LGBTQ+ individuals, 354
  LGBTQ populations, 149–150
  low self-esteem and self-worth, 156–157
  mental health interventions, 148
  person-centered therapy, 163–164
  physical and mental health disorders, 158–159
  physical health problems, 155–156
  physical violence, 354
  psychological aggression, 354
  psychosocial disparities, 159–160
  resilience of women survivors, 161
  safety procedures, 358
  self-harm, 158
  sexual violence, 354
  stalking, 354
  transgender individuals, 353
  trauma-informed care, 162–163
  United States, 148
intimidation, 150
Inventory of Complicated Grief (ICG), 277
IPV. *See* intimate partner violence
isolation, 150
Issues in Disability Scale (IDS), 28

Ladder of Adjustment scale, 134, 135
Latinx families, 250–251
Law Enforcement and Mental Health Project Act of
    2000, 48
lawful permanent resident (LPR), 367
Leadership Education in Neurodevelopmental and Other
    Related Disabilities (LEND), 265–266
League of the Physically Handicapped (LPH), 8
learning disability, sexuality, 180–181
lesbian, gay, bisexual, transgender, queer/questioning
    (LGBTQ) populations, 353
  abuse, 354
  intimate partner violence (IPV), 149–150, 153, 160
  microaggressions, 204
  substance use disorder, 325
leucotomy, 43–44
leukotome, 43
Lewinian "life space", 72
Lewin's somatopsychology theory, 132–133
Livneh's conceptual framework
  antecedents, 224
  components, 224
  continuous approach, 225
  dichotomous view, 225

  ecological models, 225
  process component, 224–225
  QOL outcomes, 225–226
loss and grief, chronic illness and disability adaptation,
    108–109. *See also* grief, dying, and death
low-tech assistive technologies, 421

macroaggressions, 200
macro interventions, well-being
  community-based services, 409
  economic resource gaps, 409–410
  political engagement, 410–411
  unemployment and underemployment, 410
marital discord, 238
Matching Person and Technology (MPT) model,
    426–427
Medicaid, 96–97
medical model of disability, 58
medical perspective, disability, 435
Memory Care Home Solutions (MCHS) program, 301
mental health disorders
  PTSD, 320
  social media, 473, 475–477
  substance use disorders, 320
  women, 156–158
Mental Health Study Act, 46
Mental Health Treatment Tool Kit, 347
mental illness classification, 45–46
mental illness treatment
  client-centered therapy, 44
  convulsive therapies, 43
  and criminal justice system, 48
  current issues, 50–51
  deinstitutionalization, 46–47
  drug treatments, 40
  electroconvulsive therapy (ECT), 43
  fever therapy, 43
  hydrotherapy, 41
  Middle Ages, 37–38
  moral treatments, 40
  19th-century America, 39–40
  psychoanalysis, 44
  psychosurgery, 43–44
  psychotropic medication, 44
  sexual and physical abuse, 48–49
  shock therapies, 43
  sterilization, reproduction control, 40–41
  stigmatized beliefs about, 49–50
  talk therapy, 44
  World War II (WWII) veterans, 45
mental retardation (MR), 246
mesosystem, 383–384
metaverse, 475
metrazol injections, 43
microaggressions, 64–65. *See also* ableist
    microaggressions
  aversive racism, 198
  behavioral, 198

environmental, 198
   vs. macroaggressions, 200
   marginalized groups, 198
   micro-assault, 198–199
   micro-invalidation, 199
   oppression, 198
   psychological dilemmas, 199–200
   unintentional ableism, 74
   verbal, 198
micro-invalidation, 199
microsystem, 383
mid-tech assistive technology, 421–422
Migration Policy Institute (MPI), 368
military culture
   deployments
      emotional stages, 341–342
      family readiness groups (FRGs), 341
   organizational structure, 340
   service members, 340
      children, 343–344
      intimate relationships, 342
      mental health, 340–341
      mothers, 342
      negative consequences, 342
      positive aspects, 342
      romantic partners, 344
      spouse, 342–343
      support sources and benefits, 340
   subcultures, 340
   veterans (see veterans)
military sexual trauma (MST), 346
mindfulness-based health wellness program, 408
minimal group paradigm, ingroup favoritism, 73
model of linear progression, 277
Moos's crisis and coping model, 115–116
motivational interviewing (MI), 478
mourning and depression theory, 130–131
mourning concept, 130
Multidimensional Acceptance of Loss Scale (MALS), 223
multiple sclerosis (MS), 244
   Jessica Henry's experience, 501–503
   positive psychology interventions, 407
   Tosca Appel's experience, 510–513
muscular dystrophy, Winske's experience, 524–529

naïve realism, 72
National Alliance for Caregiving (NAC), 291
National Alliance of Mental Illness (NAMI) Basics, 302
National Association of Recovery Residences (NARR), 330–331
National Coalition of Anti-Violence Programs (NCAVP), 353
National Council on Independent Living (NCIL), 99–100
National Health and Nutrition Examination Survey database, 484
National Institute on Drug Abuse (NIDA), 328, 385
National Resource Directory (NRD), 347
Native American women

abuse and neglect, 353
   intimate partner violence. See intimate partner violence (IPV)
negative attitudes
   aesthetic aversion, 23
   anxiety-provoking situations, 22
   attributional origins, 21
   blaming the victim concept, 21
   childhood influences, 22
   disability as punishment for sin, 21–22
   disability-related factors, 24
   existential angst, 23
   minority status, 24
   prejudice-inviting behavior, 24
   psychodynamic factors, 23
   sociocultural conditioning, 22
negative medical experiences, 98
neurotransmitters, 313
nonlinear behavior, 140
novelty shock crisis, 237

Occupational Health and Safety (OSHA) rules, 423
older adults. See also aging population
   grief and loss, 282–283
opioids, 312, 317
oppression and disenfranchisement
   education, 456–457
   employment, 457–458
   environmental Inequities, 458–460
   healthcare and health costs, 458
   internalized, 462–464
   psychosocial cost, 461–462
   racial and ethnic disparities, food insufficiency, 455–456
   social and economic cost, 455–456
   supplemental security income (SSI), 455
outgroup homogeneity effect, ingroup favoritism, 74
overprotection, 93

PACID. See psychosocial adaptation to chronic illness and disability
PAIS-SR. See Psychological Adjustment to Illness Scale-Self Report
parental leadership
   family engagement, 269
   LEND programs, 265–266
parenting and disability
   child welfare system, 186
   intellectual impairment, 187
   legislative changes, 188
   parental rights termination, 186–187
   skills training, 187
   societal concerns, 187
parenting experience, disabled children
   culturally responsive interventions, 260
   developmental disability, 258
   disability stigma, 258

parenting experience, disabled children (*cont.*)
    Down syndrome in children, 257
        education, 266–269
        family history, 259, 263, 265–267, 269
        federal policy, 271
        inequities, 259
        intellectual and developmental disability (IDD)
            research, 260
        local policy, 271
        parental adaptation research, 260
        religion and spirituality, 261–262
        resiliency approach, 260
        state policy, 271
    education
        family engagement, 267, 269
        Partnership Capacity Matrix, 266
        vision statement, 268, 269
    family-centered approach, 258, 262
    healthcare and health services, 264–266
    parental leadership, 262–263
    policy and legislation, 257–258
    policymaking, 270
    Taiwanese mothers, autistic children, 260
parent management training (PMT), chronic illness and
        disability, 298–299
partial hospitalization programs (PHPs), 328
Partnership Capacity Matrix, 266
Patient Health Questionnaire (PHQ-9), 387
Patient-Reported Outcomes Measurement Information
        System (PROMIS), 218
Paul Egan's experience with disability, 517–519
PCBD. *See* persistent complex bereavement disorder
peer support, chronic illness and disability, 302–303
People First advocacy group, 88
people with disabilities in United States, treatment
        history
    Clinical Frailty Scale (CFS), 12
    current attitudes, 14
    early immigration legislation
        antidisability legislation, 6
        1907 Immigration Act, 7
        Immigration Restriction League (IRL), 6
        physical impairments, 8
    equality movements
        Education for All Handicapped Children Act, 13
        Rehabilitation Act, 13
        Smith–Fess Act, 12
        Vocational Rehabilitation Act Amendments, 13
    eugenics movement, 9, 13, 14
    new eugenics movement, 11–12
    SOFA scores, 12
    sterilization program, 9–10
    survival-of-the-fittest concept, 15
    triage protocols, 11
    Ugly Laws, 10–11
Permanent Supportive Housing (PSH), 330
PERMA Theory of Well-Being, 406
persistent complex bereavement disorder (PCBD),
        276–278

Personal Identity Scale, 63
person-centered therapy, intimate partner violence
        (IPV), 163–164
person-first language, 79–80, 86
PGD. *See* prolonged grief disorder
physical abuse, 352
physical attractiveness, 19–20
physical disabilities
    domestic violence, 155–156
    sexuality, 179–180
physically attractive people, 19–20
physical/mental impairment, disability, 435
physical therapy, mental illness, 40
physical violence, 354
political disability identity, 60
position disability activism, 60
positive attitudes, 26–27
positive disability group identity, 110
positive psychology and wellness interventions
    empirical support, 407–408
    mindfulness-based health wellness program, 408
    positive psychology, 406
    rehabilitation counseling, 406
    theories, 406–407
post-Americans with Disabilities Act, 88–89
posttraumatic growth (PTG)
    chronic illness and disability (CID), 113–114
    family caregiver, 298
posttraumatic stress disorder (PTSD)
    chronic pain conditions, 320
    cognitive behavioral therapy, 163
    cognitive model, 346
    intimate partner violence (IPV), 157
    mental health disorder, 320
    military-connected individuals, 345
    veterans, 346
poverty and disability. *See also* oppression and
        disenfranchisement
    in America, 454–455
    nuance of, 455
prefrontal lobotomy, 43–44
prejudice, chronic illness and disability adaptation, 110
prejudice-inviting behavior, 24
privilege, 150
problem-focused approaches, 114
problem-focused coping strategy, 129
Profile of Mood States (POMS), 118
Program for the Education and Enrichment of
        Relationship Skills (PEERS), 299
prolonged grief disorder (PGD), 276, 278–279
PROMIS. *See* Patient-Reported Outcomes Measurement
        Information System
prostitution, 181
Protestantism, 437
psychiatric disabilities, treatment history
    American colonies, 39
    COVID-19 pandemic, 51–53
    mental illness, 37–41
    mental illness treament. *See* mental illness treament

public's perception, 41–42
social security beneficiaries, 49
psychodynamic approach, parenting reaction, 240
Psychological Adjustment to Illness Scale-Self Report
    (PAIS-SR), 117, 223
psychological aggression, 354
psychological centrality, 227
psychological well-being, 220
psychosocial adaptation to chronic illness and disability
    (PACID). See also chronic illness and
    disability
    Devins's Illness Intrusiveness Model, 226–227
    Disability Centrality Model (DCM), 227–230
    Livneh's conceptual framework, 224–226
Psychosocial Adjustment to Illness Scale (PAIS), 117
psychosocial approach, parenting reaction, 240
psychosurgery, 43–44

QDIO. See Questionnaire on Disability Identity and
    Opportunity
quality of life (QOL), 111
    chronic illness and disability (CID) adaptation, 111
    CID adaptation
        Devins's Illness Intrusiveness Model, 226–227
        Disability Centrality Model (DCM), 227–230
        Livneh's conceptual framework, 224–226
    construct, 216
    definition, 219
    elements, 219
    eudaimonia, 219
    hedonia, 219
    history and development, 216–218
    Neuro-QoL measurement system, 218
    patient-reported outcome measures (PROMs),
        217–218
    patient-reported outcomes (PROs), 218
    psychological well-being, 220
    in rehabilitation counseling
        ADS and ADS-R, 223
        clinical perspective, 221
        DCS, 223–224
        Multidimensional Acceptance of Loss Scale, 223
        outcome indicators, 221
        program evaluation perspective, 221
        psychosocial adaptation/adjustment measures,
            221, 222
        RAND 36-Item Health Survey, 224
        RIDI and PAIS-SR, 223
    subjective well-being, 219–220
    WHOQOL-100 development, 218
Quality of Life in Neurological Disorders (Neuro-QoL), 218
Questionnaire on Disability Identity and Opportunity
    (QDIO), 63

RAND 36-Item Health Survey, 224
RAND Medical Outcomes Study 36-Item Short-Form
    Health Survey, 118

Reaction to Impairment and Disability Inventory (RIDI),
    118, 223
Recognize, Assist, Include, Support and Engage (RAISE)
    Family Caregiver Act, 304
recruitment, disability culture, 78
refugees. See also immigrants
    definition, 367–368
    medical and mental health screenings, 373–374
    mental and physical assessment, 375
    natural disasters, 483–484
    working alliance, 376–378
Rehabilitation Act, 418
Rehabilitation Act of 1973, 88
Rehabilitation Engineering Society of North America
    (RESNA), 423
relationship status, disability identity, 60
religion and disability
    adjustment/adaptations, 438
    contextual factors and trends, 439–440
    family perspectives, 440–443
    medical model, 438
    social model, 438
    and spirituality
        COVID-19 pandemic, 446
        definition, 443–444
        dimensions, 445
        ecograms, 447
        hope and religious coping, 446
        individual perspectives, 444–445
        mental disabilities, 446
        rehabilitation counselors and approaches, 446–447
    in United States
        Buddhist religion, 437
        Catholicism, 437
        cultural concept, 436
        First Amendment, 436
        Hinduism, 437
        Jewish immigration, 437
        Protestantism, 437
reproductive aspects, sexuality, 170
resiliency model of family, 239
resilient families, 241
Resources for Enhancing Alzheimer's Caregiver Health
    (REACH) II program, 302
retaliation, adjustment, 131
rheumatoid arthritis
    Neumann's experience, 519–524
    positive psychology interventions, 407

SAI. See Spiritual Assessment Inventory
schizophrenia, 182
SCI. See spinal cord injury
SCM. See stereotype content model
secular proactive measures, 438
self-blame behavior, adjustment, 131
self-compassion, family caregiver, 297–298
self-concept, chronic illness and disability adaptation,
    109–110

self-defense strategies, 193–194
self-esteem, and body image, 174–175
self-harm, intimate partner violence, 158
self-stigma, 324
sensory impairments, 191, 246
sensuality, sexuality, 170
Sequential Organ Failure Assessment (SOFA), 12
serious mental illness (SMI), 181–182
Serviceman's Readjustment Act of 1944, 344
SETT model. *See* Student, Environment, Task, and Tool
    model
severity, disability, 136
sexual abuse, 352
    frequency, 190–191
    legislation and trends, 193–194
    women with disabilities, 192
        assistance barriers, 193
        disability services, 192
        physical and emotional isolation, 192
        stereotypical assumptions and stereotypes, 192
        violence-induced disability, 192
sexuality
    body image
        and gender identity, 172–173
        and self-esteem, 174–175
    components, 170
    definition, 170–171
    people with disabilities
        chronic health conditions, 182–183
        cognitive disabilities, 181
        disability type, 176–177
        fertility issues, 185–186
        gender-based values and social roles, 173
        learning disability, 180–181
        parenting, 186–188
        and partnering desires, 175–176
        physical disabilities, 179–180
        preimplantation and prenatal screening, 190
        psychiatric Illness, 181–182
        relationship types, 177–179
        reproductive choice, 186
        reproductive health and sterilization, 186
        severity impact, 177
        sex education, 188–189
        sex therapy, 189
        sexual functioning, 184–185
        sexual orientation, 183–184
        sexual surrogacy, 189
    persons without disabilities, 176
    stigmatization, 171–172
sexualization, sexuality, 170
sexual orientation, 170, 183–184
sexual violence, 354
shared decision-making (SDM), family caregiver, 304
shock
    adjustment, 128
    chronic illness and disability (CID) adaptation, 112
Smith–Fess Act, 12
social comparison theory, 474, 475

social consciousness toward disability
    education, 30–32
    individuals' contact with disable persons, 30
social construct model of disability, 27
Social currency, 473
social group identity, 56
social identity theory, ingroup favoritism, 73
social inaccessibility, 94
social injustice and poverty
    African countries
        children with disabilities, 453–454
        Christian fatalism, 453
        cultural and religious beliefs, 453, 454
        Ethiopia and Sierra, 454
        juju, West Africa, 453
        Nepal, 454
        Nigeria, 453
    disenfranchised and vulnerable group, 452
    root causes, 452
social justice
    and advocacy, 466–468
    American Counseling Association, 464
    counselors, 465–466
social media
    behavioral change intervention, 478–479
    body positive movement, 460
    cognitive reframing interventions, 479
    empowerment, 460–461
    human relationships, 472
    mental health, 475–477
    neoliberal inclusionism, 461
    self-compassion intervention (SCI), 479–480
    self-representations, 460
    social constructs, 473–474
    social networking sites, 472
    theoretical frameworks, 474–475
    time spent on, 472–473
    women and body image
        body surveillance, 477
        eating disorders, 477–478
        westernized ideal feminine body image, 477
    yoga practices, 460
social model of disability, 58, 59
social networking site addiction, 473, 476
social perspective, disability, 436
Social Security Act, 9, 96
Social Security Administration (SSA) programs, 49
Social Security Disability Insurance (SSDI), 91
social skills, attitude measurements, 20
social support, adjustment, 137
social worker attitudes, mental illness
    burden perceptions, 26
    demographic variables, 25–26
    environmental barriers, 26
    media portrayals of disability, 24–25
sociocultural conditioning, attitudes, 22
socioecological models of aging, 383–384
socio-motivational process, ingroup favoritism, 73
spinal cord injury (SCI), 184–185, 244–245

Spiritual Assessment Inventory (SAI), 447
spirituality and religion
    COVID-19 pandemic, 446
    definition, 443–444
    dimensions, 445
    ecograms, 447
    hope and religious coping, 446
    individual perspectives, 444–445
    mental disabilities, 446
    rehabilitation counselors and approaches, 446–447
spouses, military, 342–343
SSI. *See* supplemental security income
stability, disability, 136
stereotype content model (SCM), 77
stereotypical attitudes, 20–21
sterilization program, 9–10
stigmatization
    ableism, 71
    chronic illness and disability (CID) adaptation, 110
    substance use disorders
        self-stigma, 324
        structural discrimination, 323–324
stimulants, 312
Strategic Foresight Initiative (SFI) action plan, 372–373
stress
    chronic illness and disability adaptation, 107–108
    families and disability, 237–238
    women, 155
stress-appraisal-coping model, 115
Student, Environment, Task, and Tool (SETT) model, 424–425
subjective well-being, 219–220
subordination of physique, value change, 141
Substance Abuse and Mental Health Services Administration (SAMHSA), 333, 476
substance use disorder (SUD)
    and addiction, 313
    aging population, 385
    Americans with Disabilities Act (ADA)
        Drug-Free Workplace Act, 326–327
        employment, legal guidelines, 327
        legal and illegal substances, 326
    chronic pain conditions, 320
    criminal justice system involvement, 325–326
    diagnosis, 315–316
    as disease, 314
    drug overdose deaths, 316–317
    employment and recovery framework, 317
        disclosure and workplace accommodations, 334–335
        workplace policies, 333–334
        workplace stigma, 332–333
    evidence-based practices, 329
    harm reduction programs, 321–322
    health impact, 316
    impact on families, 320–321
    and marginalized identities, 324–325
    medication-assisted treatment (MAT), 329
    mental health disorder, 320

opioid crisis, 317
    psychotherapies, 329–330
    recovery, 328–329
    recovery housing programs, 330–331
    social determinants of health
        community level factors, 319
        employment status, 318
        individual level factors, 318
        interpersonal level, 319
        social relationship and home status factors, 319
        societal level factors, 319
    social media, 476
    stigma, 322–324
    stimulant overdoses, 318
    substance categories, 312–313
    symptoms, 314–315
    traumatic brain injury (TBI), 320
    treatment settings and modalities, 327–328
    veterans, 346
SUD. *See* substance use disorder
supplemental security income (SSI), 91, 455
Support for Patients and Communities (SUPPORT) Act, 331

TASH organization, 100
Team Red, White & Blue (RWB) service organization, 347
Tech Act, 418
trait ascription bias, ingroup favoritism, 74
transactional model of coping, 139–140
transgender, 171, 183, 353
transorbital lobotomy, 43
transsexuals, 183
transvestites, 183
trauma
    chronic illness and disability (CID) adaptation, 108
    and grief, 280–281
trauma-informed care, intimate partner violence (IPV), 162–163
trauma-informed messages (TIM), 163
traumatic brain injury (TBI)
    sexuality, 181
    veteran, 346, 348
Treatment and Education of Autistic and related Communications handicapped Children (TEACHH) program, 299
trustworthiness, trauma-informed care, 162

Ugly Laws, 10–11
uncertainty emotions, 129
underemployment, 410
unemployment, 410
unification, disability culture, 78
unintentional ableism, 74–75
United Home Care Services (UHCS), 302
United Nations Convention on the Rights of Persons with Disabilities (UNCRPD), 93

United States laws and policies
    advocacy and policy change, 98–99
    Americans With Disabilities Act, 89–90
    civil rights, 90–95
    healthcare
        accessibility, 98
        affordability, 96–97
        inequality, 96
        quality care, 97
        violations and devaluations, 95
    historical context, 86–87
        disability rights movement, 87–88
        post-Americans with Disabilities Act, 88–89
universal design (UD), 430–431
U.S. Citizenship and Immigration Services (USCI), 367
U.S. Department of Housing and Urban Development
    (HUD), 330
U.S. Department of Justice (DOJ), 90, 93
U.S Department of Transportation (DOT), 90
U.S. Equal Opportunity Commission (EEOC), 90

vaguebooking, 475
value change system, 141–142
valued social roles, 405
verbal microaggressions, 198
veterans
    common life issues, 345
    honorable discharges, 344
    mental health and physical health
        formal programs, 347
        moral injury, 346
        post-9/11–era veterans, 346
        PTSD, 346
        reunification programs, 347
        sexual assaults, 346
        substance use disorders, 346
        Team Red, White & Blue (RWB) service
            organization, 347
        traumatic brain injury, 346, 348
        veteran treatment courts, 348
    vocational rehabilitation, 348–349
Veterans Health Administration Vocational
    Rehabilitation (VHA VR), 348–349

Violence Against Women Act (VAWA), 160, 193
visibility, disability, 136
Vocational and Educational Services for Individuals with
    Disabilities (VESID), 173
Vocational Rehabilitation Act Amendments, 13
vocational rehabilitation, veterans, 348–349
voting and political site access, 94–95
Voting Rights Act of 1965, 95
vulnerability, 150

well-being and quality of life
    counseling practice, 411–414
    definition, 401–402
    individual functioning
        autonomy and personal choice, 405
        physical and mental health, 405–406
        social connectedness and supports, 404–405
        valued social roles, 405
    internal and external contributors, 403
    micro and macro-level interventions, 412–414
    positive psychology interventions (PPT)
        empirical support, 407–408
        mindfulness-based health wellness program, 408
        positive psychology, 406
        rehabilitation counseling, 406
        theories, 406–407
    social determinants of health
        environments, 408
        macro interventions, 409–411
        resources, 408
wellness education group intervention, 408
wheelchair-using exercise, 31
whole person wellness paradigm, 389
women with disabilities (WDs)
    ableism, 149
    abusive tactics, 149
    intersectionality, 150–151
    intimate partner violence (*see also* intimate partner
        violence)
    sexuality, 172
    vulnerability, 148
Workforce Innovation and Opportunity Act of 2014
    (WIOA), 270